2 MINUTE MEDICINE'S
THE CLASSICS IN MEDICINE™

Summaries of Clinically Relevant and Recent Landmark Studies, 2e (The Classics Series)

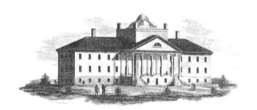

SECOND EDITION

ANDREW CHEUNG, MD
Managing Editor, 2 Minute Medicine Publishing Group
University Health Network, Toronto
University of Toronto School of Medicine

DEEPTI S KARHADE, DMD, MS
Managing Editor, 2 Minute Medicine Publishing Group
Harvard School Dental of Medicine

MARC D. SUCCI, MD
Editor-in-Chief, 2 Minute Medicine Publishing Group
Mass General Brigham
Harvard Medical School

2 Minute Medicine™
Physician Press™
2 Minute Medicine, Inc.
PO Box 140373
Boston, MA 02114
USA

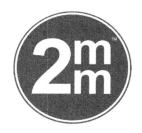

ISBN-13: 978-0-9963042-3-8

Copyright © 2023 by 2 Minute Medicine, Inc. All rights reserved. Except as permitted under the United States Copyright Act of 1976, no part of this publication may be reproduced in any form or by any means, including photocopying, or used by any information storage and retrieval system without prior written permission from 2 Minute Medicine, Inc. This book and the individual contributions contained in it are protected under copyright by the Publisher.

NOTICES/TERMS OF USE

This book is protected by copyright. No works may be reproduced in any form or by any means, including photocopying, or used by any information storage and retrieval system without written permission from 2 Minute Medicine, Inc. Your right to use the work may be terminated if you fail to comply with these terms. You may use this work for non-commercial and personal use only, any other use is strictly prohibited. You may not decompile, disassemble, reverse engineer, reproduce, modify, create derivative works based upon, transmit, distribute, disseminate, sell, publish or sublicense the work or any part of it without written permission from 2 Minute Medicine, Inc. This work contains information derived from peer-reviewed medical journals, which is constantly changing. While every effort has been made to provide accurate up-to-date information, some information may become out-of-date. This text may not reflect these changes. No article or chapter should be construed as medical advice and is not intended as such by the contributors, authors, editors, or by 2 Minute Medicine, Inc. This work is provided as-is. 2 Minute Medicine, Inc makes no guarantees or warranties as to the accuracy or completeness of the contents of this book, including information accessed through hyperlinks or otherwise and expressly disclaims any warranty. With respect to any drug or pharmaceutical products identified, readers are advised to check the most current information provided (i) on procedures featured or (ii) by the manufacturer of each product to be administered, to verify the recommended dose or formula, the method and duration of administration, and contraindications. It is the responsibility of practitioners, relying on their own experience and knowledge of their patients, to make diagnoses, to determine dosages and the best treatment for each individual patient, and to take all appropriate safety precautions. To the fullest extent of the law, 2 Minute Medicine, Inc shall not be liable to you or anyone else for any inaccuracy, error or omission, regardless of cause, in the work or for any damages resulting therefrom. Under no circumstances shall 2 Minute Medicine, Inc be liable for any indirect, incidental, special, punitive, consequential or similar damages that result from the use of or inability to use the work, even if any of them has been advised of the possibility of such damages. This limitation of liability shall apply to any claim or cause whatsoever whether such claim or cause arises in contract, tort or otherwise.

Library of Congress Cataloging-in-Publication Data
Names: Succi, Marc D., editor | Cheung, Andrew, editor | Karhade, Deepti, S. editor
Title: The Classics in Medicine / [edited by] Marc D. Succi, Andrew Cheung, Deepti Karhade
Other titles: The classics in medicine (Succi)
Description: Summaries of Clinically Relevant and Recent Landmark Studies, 2e (the Classics Series) | Boston, MA: 2 Minute Medicine, [2023] | Includes bibliographical references and index.
Identifiers: LCCN (applied for) | ISBN 978-0-9963042-3-8
Subjects: LCSH: Medicine. | Cardiology. | Clinical trials.
Classification: LCC RC46 | NLM WB115 | DDC 616

Project Manager: Marc Succi, Andrew Cheung, Deepti S. Karhade
Content Strategist: Marc Succi, Andrew Cheung, Deepti S. Karhade
Cover Art: The Anatomy Lesson of Dr. Nicolaes Tulp; 1632, Rembrandt Harmenszoon van Rijn.

2 Minute Medicine™
Physician Press™
2 Minute Medicine, Inc.
PO Box 140373
Boston, MA 02114
USA

Explore other books in 2 Minute Medicine's *The Classics Series*™

2 Minute Medicine's The Classics in Radiology: Summaries of Clinically Relevant & Recent Landmark Studies, 1e (The Classics Series)
Marc D. Succi, Ravi Gottumukkala, MD

Available at Amazon, iTunes, Barnes & Noble, and bookstores worldwide

"In general, we look for a new law by the following process. First, we guess it. Then we compute the consequences of the guess to see what would be implied if this law that we guessed is right. Then we compare the result of the computation to nature, with experiment or experience, compare it directly with observation, to see if it works. If it disagrees with experiment, it's wrong.

In that simple statement is the key to science.

It doesn't make any difference how beautiful your guess is. It doesn't make any difference how smart you are, who made the guess, or what his name is.

If it disagrees with experiment it's wrong. That's all there is to it."

-Richard P. Feynman, PhD

Winner of the Nobel Prize in Physics (1965)

This page left intentionally blank.

DEDICATION

This book is dedicated to the late Dr. Mario Succi, 2 Minute Medicine's very first customer of the 1st edition of this book.

-Marc Succi, MD

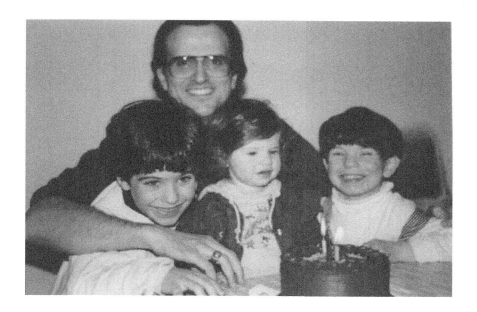

This page left intentionally blank.

PREFACE

The authors would like to express a sincere appreciation for the academic culture at Harvard Medical School, Massachusetts General Hospital and Mass General Brigham. It is only through voluntary collaboration and academic camaraderie that ventures such as this book are possible. We have received support from countless individuals across departments.

To my husband, Aditya, and my parents, Anil and Nandini, thank you for your unwavering and infinite love and support. To my mentors and the patients that I have had the privilege of caring for as a doctor, thank you for all that you have taught me.
- DSK

To my father, who was the very first customer to buy the 1st edition of this book and has always been my greatest supporter, confidant, and mentor.
- MDS

This is the second edition in the popular 2 Minute Medicine's The Classics in Medicine series, adding over 150 new study summaries of key landmark trials, including a special COVID-19 section. 2 Minute Medicine™ presents a comprehensive and updated authoritative, curated, and physician-written collection of summaries of the key landmark trials in medicine – over 300 study summaries in total. Every physician, health professional, and trainee should have a working knowledge of these trials to both understand and make daily evidence-based clinical decisions. With contributions from renowned medical faculty and practicing physicians at top institutions, 2 Minute Medicine's The Classics in Medicine: Summaries of Clinically Relevant and Recent Landmark Studies, 2e (the Classics Series) is an indispensable tool for the practicing physician or trainee. The textbook edition is organized into Classics by Specialty and includes trials from the following fields: General Medicine and Chronic Disease, Cardiology, Critical and Emergent Care, Endocrinology, Gastroenterology, Hematology and Oncology, Imaging, Infectious Disease, Nephrology, Neurology, Pediatrics, Psychiatry, Pulmonology, Surgery, and COVID-19.

-Marc Succi, Andrew Cheung, Deepti Karhade

This page left intentionally blank.

Effectively Using this Book

A note on the specialties included:

Medicine is a fluid study of the human condition. While modern medicine is segmented into various subspecialties, the reality is that illness does not respect these artificial boundaries. Thus, many of these trials could fit appropriately under the heading of several specialties in this book. In an effort to prioritize readability, the editors organized each trial under only one specialty. Furthermore, some specialties (e.g., endocrinology) do not carry their own heading. Instead, they are interspersed throughout the other specialties within this book.

A note on language:

In general, most of the trials included in this text were designed by investigators to discern causal links. These trials have generally stood the test of reproducibility over time, earning them inclusion into this collection. Thus, in many instances this text uses definitive causal terminology (e.g., "reduced", "lowered", etc.) as opposed to associative terminology (e.g., "is linked with a lower risk") to denote strong, time-tested data. While causal links by definition include an association, the inverse is not necessarily true.

A note on study abbreviations:

While one would benefit greatly from reading this book front-to-back, the summaries stand-alone. They are designed so that the reader may look up a study and read one particular summary, and thus we continually redefine abbreviations anew for each individual summary. The choice of abbreviations defined differ by study as they are tailored to individual summaries to maximize readability.

A note on references:

The e-book edition encourages efficient reading and seamless study. As such, every summarized study has a "clickable" hyperlink near the mid-page which, when "tapped" with the reader's finger, will open up the e-reader/tablet/phone internet browser and link directly to the original text by the publishing journal. This allows the reader to access the original paper instantly (journal subscription and internet access not included). The paperback edition includes full written references.

CONTRIBUTORS

This text is made possible by the authors and journals that published the original trials as well as the work of numerous contributors at various medical schools and hospitals.

Andrew Cheung, MD | University of Toronto

Deepti S. Karhade, DMD, MS | The Harvard School of Dental Medicine

Marc D. Succi, MD | Massachusetts General Hospital

Contributing Authors

Lewis R. First, MS, MD | Vermont Children's Hospital

Benjamin Laguna, MD | University of California San Francisco

Aaron Maxwell, MD | Brown Alpert Medical School

Aimee Li, MD | University of Ottawa

Milana Bogorodskaya, MD | Case Western Reserve University

Evan Chen, BSc | Stanford School of Medicine

Adrienne Cheung, BHSc | University of British Columbia School of Medicine

Lauren Ko, BSc | Harvard Medical School

Shaidah Deghan, MSc | University of Toronto School of Medicine

Michael Milligan, BSc | Harvard Medical School

Dylan Wolman, MD | Stanford University

Leah H. Carr, MD | Seattle Children's Hospital

Leah Bressler, MD, MPH | Northwestern Memorial Hospital

Dayton McMillan, BSc | Harvard Medical School

David Wang, BSc | University of Toronto School of Medicine

Aliya Ramjaun, BHSc, MSc | University of Toronto School of Medicine

Jimmy Roebker, BSc, MBA | University of Cincinnati School of Medicine

Masis Isikbay, BSc | Harvard Medical School

David Arsanious, MD | University of Vermont College of Medicine

Xu Gao, BSc | University of Cincinnati School of Medicine

Kiera Liblik, BSc | Queen's School of Medicine

Thomas Su, BS | The University of Texas at Austin

Michael Pratte, BS | University of Ottawa Faculty of Medicine

Matthew Lin, MD | University of Vermont College of Medicine

Sze Wah Samuel Chan, MD | McMaster University

Harsh Shah, BS, MPH, MS | Mayo Clinic Alix School of Medicine

Rebecca Seliga, BSc | University of Ottawa Faculty of Medicine

Avneesh Bhangu, BMSc | Queen's School of Medicine

Shayna Bejaimal, MD | University of Toronto Faculty of Medicine

Jack Lennon, Ma | Adler University

Cyrus Ayubcha, BA, MSc | Harvard Medical School

Teddy Z. Guo, BMSc | McMaster University

Jessie Willis, BSc | University of Ottawa Faculty of Medicine

Neel Mistry, BSc | University of Ottawa Faculty of Medicine

This page left intentionally blank.

CONTENTS

DEDICATION vii
PREFACE ix
EFFECTIVELY USING THIS BOOK xi
CONTRIBUTORS xiii
CONTENTS xvii

I. General Chronic Disease 35

The HMPS I: Adverse events in patients and negligence 36

The HMPS II: Characterizing adverse events in hospitalized patients 38

The DASH trial: Diet change significantly reduces blood pressure 40

The HOT trial: Diastolic blood pressure targets in hypertension 42

The UKPDS: Reducing diabetes-related morbidity and mortality 44

Symptom-triggered benzodiazepine treatment for alcohol withdrawal 47

The CATIE trial: High rates of medication discontinuation in schizophrenic patients 49

The STAR*D trials I: Medication augmentation for depression 51

The STAR*D trials II: Switching antidepressants in depression management 53

The ENHANCE trial: Simvastatin and ezetimibe in familial hypercholesterolemia 55

The JUPITER: Rosuvastatin reduces the risk of major cardiovascular events in healthy patients 57

The RAVE trial: Rituximab induces remission in ANCA-associated vasculitis 59

II. Cardiology 61

The BHAT: Propranolol after acute myocardial infarction 62

The LRC-CPPT 1: Cholestyramine and coronary heart disease 64

The V-HeFT I: Hydralazine and isosorbide dinitrate reduce mortality in heart failure 66

The CONSENSUS: Enalapril reduces mortality in severe heart failure 68

The CAST: Anti-arrhythmic agents increase risk of death in patients after myocardial infarction 70

The V-HeFT II: Enalapril reduces mortality in heart failure when compared to hydralazine and isosorbide 72

The SOLVD trial: Enalapril reduces mortality in heart failure with reduced ejection fraction 74

The SAVE trial: Captopril reduces mortality after acute myocardial infarction 76

The CARE trial: Pravastatin reduces risk of coronary events 78

The DIG trial: Digoxin reduces hospitalization in patients with systolic heart failure 80

The MERIT-HF trial: Metoprolol reduces mortality in patients with symptomatic heart failure 82

The RALES trial: Spironolactone reduces mortality in heart failure patients . 84

The ATLAS trial: Angiotensin converting enzyme inhibitor dosing in chronic heart failure 86

The HOPE trial: Ramipril reduces cardiovascular events in high-risk patients with normal ejection fractions 88

The MIRACL trial: Atorvastatin reduces recurrent ischemia after acute coronary syndrome 90

The CHADS2 score: Stroke risk in atrial fibrillation 92

The REMATCH trial: Left ventricular assist devices reduce mortality in heart failure 95

The Val-HeFT trial: Valsartan reduces morbidity in chronic heart failure 97

The MADIT-II: Prophylactic defibrillators reduce mortality in left ventricular dysfunction 99

The COPERNICUS trial: Carvedilol reduces mortality in severe chronic heart failure 101

The ALLHAT: Thiazide diuretics as first-line antihypertensive therapy 103

The AFFIRM trial: Rate-control vs. rhythm-control in atrial fibrillation 105

The EPHESUS: Eplerenone reduces mortality in heart failure after myocardial infarction 107

The CHARM-Added trial: Adding candesartan to ACE inhibitor reduces mortality in heart failure 109

The CHARM-Preserved trial: Candesartan reduces hospitalization in heart failure with preserved ejection fraction 111

The CHARM-Alternative trial: Candesartan reduces mortality in heart failure 113

The VALIANT trial: Valsartan vs. captopril in patients with acute myocardial infarction and heart failure 115

The PROVE IT trial: High-dose atorvastatin reduces mortality after acute coronary syndrome 117

The CLARITY trial: Clopidogrel reduces arterial reocclusion after myocardial infarction 119

The TNT trial: Intensive statin therapy in coronary heart disease 121

The SCD-HeFT: ICD vs. amiodarone for congestive heart failure 123

The COMMIT: Metoprolol and clopidogrel in patients with acute myocardial infarction 125

The COURAGE trial: Percutaneous coronary intervention does not improve mortality in stable coronary artery disease 127

The TRITON-TIMI 38 trial: Prasugrel reduces recurrent infarction after acute coronary syndrome 129

The ONTARGET: Telmisartan non-inferior to ramipril in improving cardiovascular outcomes in high-risk populations 131

The ACCOMPLISH trial: Benazepril plus amlodipine reduces cardiovascular events 133

The SYNTAX trial: Coronary bypass superior to percutaneous coronary intervention for triple-vessel or left main artery disease 135

The ROMICAT 1 trial: Coronary computed tomographic angiography highly sensitive for acute coronary syndrome in patients with acute chest pain 137

The ACTIVE trial: Dual antiplatelet therapy in atrial fibrillation 139

The RE-LY trial: Dabigatran non-inferior to warfarin for stroke prevention in atrial fibrillation 141

The PLATO trial: Ticagrelor vs. clopidogrel for acute coronary syndrome . 143

The MADIT-CRT trial: Cardiac resynchronization therapy in heart failure . 145

The RACE-II trial: Lenient vs. strict rate-control in atrial fibrillation 147

The SHIFT: Ivabradine in congestive heart failure 149

The HAS-BLED score: Bleeding risk in atrial fibrillation 151

The EMPHASIS-HF trial: Eplerenone reduces mortality in mild systolic heart failure 155

The RIVAL trial: Radial vs. femoral artery access for percutaneous coronary intervention 157

The PRECOMBAT trial: Percutaneous coronary intervention vs. coronary bypass in left main coronary artery stenosis 159

The ARISTOTLE trial: Apixaban superior to warfarin for stroke prophylaxis in atrial fibrillation 161

Medical management superior to stenting for stroke related to intracranial arterial stenosis 163

The ROCKET AF: Rivaroxaban non-inferior to warfarin for stroke prophylaxis in atrial fibrillation 165

The ROMICAT 2 trial: Coronary computed tomographic angiography shortens hospital stay for acute chest pain 167

The FREEDOM trial: Coronary bypass graft vs. PCI in diabetic patients ... 169

The WOEST trial: Double vs. triple therapy in patients requiring PCI and anticoagulation 171

The RE-ALIGN trial: Dabigatran vs. warfarin for mechanical heart valves. 173

The ICAP trial: Colchicine in acute pericarditis 175

The PARADIGM-HF trial: Combo angiotensin-neprilysin inhibitor superior to enalapril in heart failure 177

The DAPT trial: Extended dual antiplatelet therapy after drug eluting stents 179

The BRIDGE trial: Periprocedural bridging in patients with atrial fibrillation 181

Liraglutide associated with lower incidence of death from CV causes in type 2 diabetics 183

The FOURIER trial: PCSK9 inhibitor significantly reduces the risk of cardiovascular events 185

xx

The POET trial: oral antibiotics in stable endocarditis patients noninferior to intravenous treatment 187

The PARTNER 3 Trial: Transcatheter aortic-valve replacement versus surgery 189

The DAPA-HF trial: Dapagliflozin in patients with heart failure 191

The VICTORIA trial: Vericiguat in high-risk heart failure 193

Early rhythm control therapy for atrial fibrillation 195

Rivaroxaban noninferior to warfarin in patients with atrial fibrillation and bioprosthetic mitral valves 196

The EARLY-AF Trial: Catheter cryoballoon ablation for atrial fibrillation .. 198

The EMPEROR-Preserved trial: Empagliflozin in heart failure 200

III. Critical, Emergent and Pulmonary Care 203

Initial trial of conservative management for splenic injury 204

Magnesium sulfate in torsade de pointes 206

CT insensitive to mediastinal lymph node metastasis in bronchogenic carcinoma 208

The DIGAMI trial: Insulin-glucose infusion in diabetics with acute myocardial infarction 210

Ottawa ankle rules reduce the rate of referral for ankle radiography 212

The NINDS trial: Tissue plasminogen activator in acute ischemic stroke improves functional outcomes 215

The Rockall score: Risk assessment after acute upper gastrointestinal hemorrhage 217

The TRICC trial: Restrictive transfusion in intensive care does not increase mortality 218

The ARMA trial: Lower tidal volume ventilation in acute respiratory distress syndrome 220

The CAPRICORN trial: Carvedilol reduces mortality after acute myocardial infarction 222

The Canadian CT Head Rule 224

The CURE trial: Clopidogrel reduces mortality after acute coronary syndrome 226

The Rivers trial: Early goal-directed therapy reduces mortality in severe sepsis and septic shock 228

Mild hypothermia improves neurological outcome after cardiac arrest 230

Voriconazole superior to amphotericin B for invasive aspergillosis 232

Canadian C-Spine Rules superior to NEXUS Low-Risk Criteria for detecting cervical-spine injuries 234

The SAFE trial: Normal saline vs. albumin for fluid resuscitation 238

The ICTUS trial: Early invasive vs selectively invasive management for acute coronary syndrome 240

Fleischner Society Guidelines, 2005 Statement: Limited CT follow-up recommended for small, solitary, pulmonary nodules 242

Delayed antimicrobial therapy linked with higher mortality in septic shock. 246

The TORCH trial: Combination of salmeterol and fluticasone in COPD 248

The CORTICUS trial: Hydrocortisone does not reduce mortality in septic shock 250

The ACCORD trial: Intensive glucose control associated with increased mortality 252

The UPLIFT trial: Tiotropium improves quality of life in chronic obstructive pulmonary disease 254

The NICE-SUGAR trial: Intensive glycemic control harmful in the intensive care unit 256

Clinical rules accurately predict children at low risk of clinically-important traumatic brain injury 258

The SOAP-II trial: First-line vasopressor for shock management 261

The CRASH-2 trial: Tranexamic acid reduces mortality in trauma patients.. 263

The ACURASYS trial: Neuromuscular blockade in early acute respiratory distress syndrome 265

The LACTATE trial: Early lactate-guided therapy in intensive care patients 267

Fleischner Society Guidelines, 2013 Update: Frequent CT follow-up recommended for subsolid pulmonary nodules 269

The PROSEVA trial: Proning in severe ARDS 271

INPULSIS: Nintedanib for Idiopathic Pulmonary Fibrosis 273

The SEPSISPAM trial: Mean arterial pressure targets in septic shock 275

The TRISS trial: Transfusion thresholds in septic shock 276

RE-VERSE AD trial: Idarucizumab for the Reversal of Anticoagulation by Dabigatran 278

ANNEXA-A and ANNEXA-R Trials: Andaxanet Alfa for Reversal of Apixaban and Rivaroxaban 280

SALT-ED: Normal Saline versus Balanced Crystalloids in Noncriticaly Ill Adults 282

TRAPS: Rivaroxaban vs. Warfarin for Secondary Prevention in Antiphospholipid Syndrome 284

IV. Gastroenterology 287

The Child-Pugh score: Prognosis in chronic liver disease and cirrhosis 288

The Harvey-Bradshaw Index is a practical alternative to the Crohn's Disease Activity Index in measuring disease severity 290

CT evaluation in pancreatitis strongly correlates with patient outcomes 295

Endoscopic biliary drainage in acute cholangitis 297

Prednisolone vs. placebo in severe alcoholic hepatitis 299

Transjugular intrahepatic portosystemic shunt effective in preventing recurrent variceal hemorrhage 301

Omeprazole vs placebo for bleeding peptic ulcer 303

Magnetic resonance based preoperative evaluation for perianal fistulas superior to traditional clinical method and improve surgical outcomes 305

Intravenous omeprazole after endoscopy reduces rebleeding in patients with peptic ulcers 308

Decrease in symptom severity linked to infliximab Crohn's treatment 310

The MELD score: Predicting survival in end-stage liver disease 312

Ceftriaxone vs. norfloxacin for prophylaxis in patients with cirrhosis and gastrointestinal bleeding 314

Omeprazole before endoscopy in patients with gastrointestinal bleeding 316

Early transjugular intrahepatic portosystemic shunt in cirrhosis and variceal bleeding 318

The COGENT: Omeprazole with antiplatelet therapy in upper gastrointestinal bleeding 320

Weekly semaglutide effective for decreasing body weight in obesity 322

V. Hematology/Oncology 325

The Milan Criteria: Liver transplantation is effective for treating cirrhotic patients with unrespectable hepatocellular carcinomas 326

Vena caval filters in pulmonary embolism prophylaxis 329

Arterial chemoembolization improves survival in non-resectable hepatocellular carcinoma 331

No survival difference between lumpectomy and mastectomy for breast cancer 333

OPTN and UNOS update policy regarding hepatocellular carcinoma 335

The CLOT trial: Dalteparin vs warfarin for venous thromboembolism in malignancy 337

Finasteride significantly reduces the incidence of prostate cancer 339

Radiofrequency thermal ablation superior to percutaneous ethanol injection in hepatocellular carcinoma 341

Dexamethasone effective as an initial therapy for immune thrombocytopenic purpura 343

The Wells DVT criteria: A clinical prediction model for deep vein thrombosis 345

Hepatocellular carcinoma screening reduces mortality in high risk patients . 348

Intraperitoneal chemotherapy improves advanced ovarian cancer survival .. 350

The RAPTURE trial: Radiofrequency ablation effective and safe in lung cancer 352

The RECIST 1.1 trial: Measuring tumor burden to assess response to therapy 354

The PLCO trial 1: PSA and digital rectal examination in prostate cancer screening 359

Stereotactic body radiotherapy as a state of the art treatment option in inoperable non-small cell lung cancer 361

Immune-related response criteria captures tumor response to therapy 363

The RE-COVER trial: Dabigatran non-inferior to warfarin in treating acute venous thromboembolism 366

The EINSTEIN-DVT trial: Rivaroxaban in acute deep vein thrombosis 368

The NLST trial: CT screening reduces lung cancer mortality 370

The EINSTEIN-PE trial: Rivaroxaban to treat pulmonary embolism 372

The PLCO trial 2: Flexible sigmoidoscopy in colon cancer screening 374

The ATLAS trial: Duration of adjuvant tamoxifen in estrogen receptor-positive breast cancer 376

The AMPLIFY trial: Apixaban for treatment of venous thromboembolism 378

The SOME trial: Screening for occult malignancy in unprovoked venous thromboembolism 380

VI. Imaging 383

Bosniak classification system differentiates benign renal cysts from cystic carcinoma 384

Ultrasound sensitive for appendicitis, improves outcomes 387

Compression ultrasound identifies proximal deep venous thrombosis with high sensitivity and specificity 389

Fewer adverse drug reactions occur with nonionic than ionic contrast media 391

Visualization of noncystic masses on transvaginal ultrasound sensitive and specific for ectopic pregnancy 394

MRI reveals lumbar intervertebral disk herniations are common in asymptomatic individuals 397

Breast ultrasound sensitive for cancer, carries a low false positive rate 399

Magnetic resonance cholangiopancreatography diagnoses bile duct obstruction with high sensitivity and specificity 401

Chemical shift and gadolinium-enhanced MRI identifies adrenal adenomas with high specificity and acceptable sensitivity 403

Hepatic arterial phase imaging more sensitive than portal venous phase in the detection of hepatic lesions and arterioportal shunting 406

CT-guided percutaneous lung biopsies more effective for larger pulmonary nodules 409

Percutaneous ethanol injection safe and effective in hepatocellular carcinoma 411

Rapid CT contrast washout differentiates adrenal adenomas from nonadenomas 413

Endovaginal ultrasound highly sensitive screen for endometrial cancer 421

Breast MRI most sensitive screening modality in high-risk patients 424

MRI enhances diagnostic certainty of ovarian cancer following indeterminate ultrasound 427

MRI effective for the assessment of acute appendicitis in pregnancy 429

The PIOPED II trial: CT sensitive and specific for pulmonary embolism ... 431

Breast density increases the risk of cancer and hinders mammographic detection 433

Detection of advanced colorectal neoplasia by CT colonography comparable to optical colonoscopy 436

MRI offers an alternative to endoscopic assessment of disease activity and severity in ileocolonic Crohn's disease 439

LI-RADS outlines standards for liver imaging studies assessing HCC 444

Ovarian cancer screening does not reduce mortality 449

CT scans increase the risk of malignancy in children and young adults 451

Increased use of pediatric CT poses significant oncogenic risk 453

LUNG-RADS criteria increases positive predictive value for lung cancer detection in high-risk patients 455

Combination mammography and breast tomosynthesis improves breast cancer screening 459

Coronary CT angiography not superior to functional testing in cardiac risk management 462

PI-RADS version 2: Standardized acquisition, interpretation, and reporting of prostate MRI 465

The SOME trial: Screening for occult malignancy in unprovoked venous thromboembolism 469

Fleischner Society Guidelines, 2017 Update: Consolidated follow-up recommendations for incidental solid and subsolid pulmonary nodules 471

VII. Infectious Disease 477

Albumin in cirrhotic patients with spontaneous bacterial peritonitis 480

Adjuvant dexamethasone improves outcomes in adult bacterial meningitis . 482

The CURB-65 score: Risk stratifying patients with community-acquired pneumonia 484

Quadrivalent HPV vaccine in young women 486

Tenofovir-emtricitabine more effective and safer than zidovudine-lamivudine in HIV treatment 488

Vancomycin superior to metronidazole for severe C. difficile diarrhea 490

Early initiation of antiretroviral therapy significantly improves HIV survival 492

Fidaxomicin vs. vancomycin in C. difficile infection 494

Early antiretroviral therapy reduces HIV-1 transmission in couples 496

Fecal transplantation in recurrent C. difficile infection 498

The iPrEx trial: Preexposure prophylaxis reduces HIV transmission in men and transgender women who have sex with men 500

The VALENCE Trial: Sofosbuvir–ribavirin for hepatitis C 502

STOP-IT Trial: Short-course antimicrobial therapy in the treatment of intraabdominal infection 504

On-demand preexposure prophylaxis decreases HIV infection in high-risk men 506

Bezlotoxumab associated with lower recurrence of C. difficile infection: The MODIFY I and II trials 508

VIII. Nephrology 511

The MDRD trial: Protein intake and blood pressure control in renal insufficiency 512

Non-contrast CT sensitive and specific for kidney stones 514

The IDNT: Irbesartan protects from renal deterioration in diabetic nephropathy 516

The RENAAL trial: Losartan in diabetic nephropathy 518

Percutaneous radiofrequency ablation effective in small, exophytic renal cell carcinoma 520

The CHOIR trial: Targeting lower hemoglobin levels in patients with anemia and chronic kidney disease 522

The ADVANCE trial: Intensive glycemic control reduces the risk of nephropathy in diabetes 524

The Symplicity HTN-2 trial: Renal denervation effective for treatment-resistant hypertension 526

Gadolinium-containing contrast associated with nephrogenic fibrosing dermopathy and systemic fibrosis 528

The DOSE trial: Loop diuretic strategies in acute decompensated heart failure 530

The CREDENCE trial: The effect of canagliflozin on renal function 532

IX. Neurology 535

The NASCET: Carotid endarterectomy in symptomatic stenosis 536

The SPAF trial: Warfarin and aspirin reduce the risk of stroke in atrial fibrillation 538

Interferon beta-1b reduces exacerbations in relapsing-remitting multiple sclerosis 540

The WARSS: Warfarin vs. aspirin in preventing recurrent ischemic stroke.. 542

Aspirin vs. warfarin in atherosclerotic intracranial stenosis 544

The CARESS trial: Dual antiplatelet therapy superior to monotherapy in symptomatic carotid stenosis 546

Donepezil and vitamin E in Alzheimer's disease 548

The ESPRIT trial: Aspirin with dipyridamole after cerebral ischemia 550

The SPARCL trial: Atorvastatin reduces the risk of stroke in patients with recent stroke or transient ischemic attack 552

The ABCD2 score: Risk of stroke after transient ischemic attack 554

CT not sufficient to rule out early subarachnoid hemorrhage 557

Thrombolysis harmful in acute ischemic strokes with large area of parenchymal hypoattenuation 559

Diffusion-weighted MRI highly sensitive for acute stroke 562

The ISAT trial: endovascular coiling superior to neurosurgical clipping in selected patients with aneurysmal subarachnoid hemorrhage 564

The ECASS III trial: Administering alteplase up to 4.5 hours after onset of acute ischemic stroke improves neurological outcomes 566

MR CLEAN: Intraarterial Treatment for Acute Ischemic Stroke 568

Intraarterial therapy and t-PA increase reperfusion and functional independence after acute ischemic stroke 570

Thrombectomy between 6 and 24 hours after acute stroke reduces disability: The DAWN trial 577

POINT trial: Clopidogrel and Aspirin for Acute Ischemic Stroke 579

OVIVA trial: Oral versus Intravenous Antibiotics for Bone and Joint Infection 581

X. Obstetrics and Gynecology 583

Antenatal steroids promote fetal lung maturity 584

A standard for fetal growth in pregnancy 586

HELLP syndrome is variant of preeclampsia 588

Low maternal serum α-fetoprotein associated with fetal aneuploidy 590

Atypia predicts progression to endometrial cancer 592

Nurses' Health Study: Postmenopausal estrogen associated with cardiovascular risk 594

Human papillomavirus infection is associated with adenocarcinoma of the cervix 596

Folic acid for prevention of neural tube defects 598

Preterm infants benefit from delayed cord clamping 600

Anal sphincter disruption common with forceps-assisted vaginal delivery ... 602

The ACTG 076 Trial: Zidovudine for reduction of maternal-infant HIV transmission 604

Cervical length indicates risk of preterm delivery 606

Adverse pregnancy outcomes linked to thrombophilias 608

Uterine artery embolization effective for uterine fibroids 610

Doppler velocimetry predicts fetal anemia 612

The Term Breech Trial: Cesarean delivery improves perinatal outcome 614

The TARGET trial: Anastrazole superior to tamoxifen for breast cancer 616

The ORACLE trial: Antibiotics improve preterm outcomes 618

The MAGPIE trial: Magnesium lowers eclampsia risk 620

The WHI trial: Risks outweigh benefits of combination hormone replacement therapy 622

Progesterone injections for recurrent preterm birth 624

The TOLAC study: Risks of labor after Cesarean delivery 626

Head cooling improves outcome in neonatal encephalopathy 628

Intraperitoneal chemotherapy improves advanced ovarian cancer survival .. 630

The HAPO trial: Hyperglycemia and adverse pregnancy outcomes 632

Magnesium for the prevention of cerebral palsy... 634

XI. Ophthalmology 637

The ONTT: Intravenous steroids lead to faster visual recovery in optic neuritis 638

The EVS: Vitrectomy results in better visual outcomes for light-perception patients 640

The CNTG trial: Intra-ocular pressure reduction slows progression of normal-tension glaucoma 642

The AREDS1: Zinc and antioxidant supplementation reduce progression of age-related macular degeneration in high-risk patients 644

The OHTS trial: Topical ocular hypotensive medication reduces risk of open-angle glaucoma 646

The EMGT: Reducing intraocular pressure slows progression of glaucoma 648

The AREDS2: No benefit from additional carotenoid and omega-3-fatty acid supplementation to original AREDS formulation 650

XII. Pediatrics 653

Childhood febrile seizure characteristics associated with epilepsy diagnosis 654

Initial guidelines for prolonged fever in children 656

Artificial surfactant improves respiratory distress syndrome in infants 658

IVIg with aspirin reduces coronary aneurysms in Kawasaki disease 660

Prone sleeping position and heavy bedding associated with sudden infant death syndrome 662

Lead exposure in childhood associated with worse cognitive performance .. 664

PROS network study examines pubertal onset by race/ethnic groups 666

Transcutaneous bilirubinometry linked to decreased serum testing and cost in infants 668

The ACE trial: Adverse childhood exposures associated with poor health in adulthood 670

Sleep-disordered breathing associated with poor academics and surgical improvement 672

The Bogalusa Heart Study: Childhood weight status and cardiovascular risk factors 674

Kocher Criteria differentiates pediatric septic arthritis and transient synovitis of the hip 676

Antibiotic Group B Streptococcus prophylaxis linked with reduced neonatal infection 679

Parental input in oncology-related palliation and pain relief for children 681

Laboratory values and treatment associated with DKA-related cerebral edema in children 683

Earlier diagnosis and improved cystic fibrosis nutritional status with newborn screening 685

MMR vaccine not associated with autism 687

Clinical prediction rule stratifies pediatric bacterial meningitis risk 689

RSV positivity associated with less serious bacterial infection risk in infants 691

Computerized order system linked with increased pediatric mortality 693

Antibiotic prophylaxis and UTI prevention in children 695

PECARN Prediction rules for children at a low risk of clinically-important traumatic brain injury 697

XIII. Surgery 699

The Lee index: Risk of perioperative cardiac events 700

The NETT: Lung-volume-reduction surgery in emphysema 702

The CARP trial: Preoperative revascularization prior to elective vascular surgery 704

The POISE trial: Perioperative use of beta-blockers 706

The POISE 2 trial: Aspirin increases risk of major bleeding after noncardiac surgery 708

The INVEST trial: Limited added utility of vertebroplasty versus sham surgery 710

The PANTER trial: Open necrosectomy vs. step-up approach for necrotizing pancreatitis 713

The EVAR I trial: Endovascular vs. open abdominal aortic aneurysm repair 715

The EVAR II trial: Endovascular approach when unfit for open aortic aneurysm repair... 717

The CREST: Stenting versus endarterectomy for carotid stenosis 719

The PIVOT: Radical prostatectomy versus observation 721

XIV. COVID-19 723

COVID-19 pneumonia patients in Wuhan, China 724

COVID-19 epidemiologic characteristics in Wuhan, China 726

Characteristics of COVID-19 pneumonia patients 727

Novel coronavirus identified from patients with pneumonia in Wuhan, China 728

Sequencing of COVID-19: Comparison to SARS and bat coronavirus 730

COVID-19 patient characteristics across Mainland China 732

5-day versus 10-day course of remdesivir in patients with severe COVID-19 734

The ACTT-1: Remdesivir for the treatment of COVID-19 736

BNT162b2 mRNA vaccine for COVID-19 prevention 738

The EMPACTA trial: Tocilizumab reduced COVID-19 disease-related adverse health outcomes 740

The COVE Trial: mRNA-1273 vaccine for preventing COVID-19 742

The RECOVERY trial: Dexamethasone decreased mortality in hospitalized COVID-19 patients 744

Interleukin-6 receptor antagonist treatment improves outcomes in patients with COVID-19 infection.. 746

Nationwide vaccination campaign with BNT162b2 (Pfizer–BioNTech) mRNA vaccine reports high immunogenicity across all age groups................ 748

Mixed vaccination with ChAdOx1-S followed by BNT162b2 induces a robust humoral immune response 750

Inactivated whole-virion SARS-CoV-2 vaccine reduces rates of symptomatic COVID-19 infections... 752

Heparin in noncritically ill COVID-19 patients 754

Third dose of BNT162b2 COVID-19 vaccine effective at decreasing risk of hospitalization... 756

INDEX	759
BIBLIOGRAPHY	767
STATISTICS ABBREVIATIONS	799
NOTES	800

This page left intentionally blank.

I. General Chronic Disease

"The thing that doesn't fit is the thing that's the most interesting, the part that doesn't go according to what you expected."

- Richard P. Feynman, PhD

The HMPS I: Adverse events in patients and negligence

1. This study determined that adverse events occurred in 3.7% of hospitalizations.

2. About 28% of adverse events occurring in the hospital were attributed to negligence.

Original Date of Publication: February 1991

Study Rundown: The Harvard Medical Practical Study (HMPS) I identified a significant burden from iatrogenic injury, recognizing that a substantial proportion of adverse events in the hospital lead to permanent disability or death. Of note was the significant number of adverse events resulting from substandard care, which may be reduced by quality assurance measures. Increasing age was identified as an important risk factor for the occurrence of adverse events, likely reflecting more complicated illness and poorer health. Limitations of the study included the difficulty of evaluating negligence and degree of disability from hospital records; however, the validity and reliability of the review process were tested and found to be reasonably high with 89% sensitivity in screening for adverse events and 89% agreement on the presence of an adverse event. Other strengths of the study were the large sample size and the use of a random sample which allowed extrapolation to population estimates. In summary, the HMPS I was one of the earliest and largest efforts to quantify the incidence of adverse events and their impacts. It also determined that many adverse events were preventable, and these findings justified greater investment in quality improvement initiatives.

In-Depth [retrospective case review]: The HMPS I results are based on the review of 30 121 records from a random sample of 2 671 863 non-psychiatric patients in New York in 1984. Records were first screened by nurses and medical record analysts. Those identified as positive for the occurrence of an adverse event were independently reviewed by 2 physicians. Physicians identified 1278 adverse events, of which 306 were due to negligence. From this, the statewide incidence rate of adverse events was estimated to be 3.7%, while approximately 27.6% of these events were the result of negligence. The majority of adverse events led to disability that resolved in less than 6 months; however, 2.6% led to permanent total disability and 13.6% resulted in death. Rates of adverse events were positively correlated with increasing age ($p < 0.0001$) and negligence was more frequently implicated with increasing severity of adverse events, causing 22% of events leading to temporary disability and 51% of events resulting in death ($p < 0.0001$). The percentage of adverse events due to negligence did not vary between clinical specialties.

Brennan TA, Leape LL, Laird NM, Hebert L, Localio AR, Lawthers AG, et al. Incidence of Adverse Events and Negligence in Hospitalized Patients. New England Journal of Medicine. 1991 Feb 7;324(6):370–6.

The HMPS II: Characterizing adverse events in hospitalized patients

1. Drug-related complications were the most common type of adverse event in hospitalized patients.

2. Adverse events due to negligence in hospitalized patients were more likely to cause serious disability or death than adverse events not attributed to negligence.

Original Date of Publication: February 1991

Study Rundown: Many adverse events in hospitalized patients are not preventable due to current limitations in medical knowledge or capabilities. Advances in scientific knowledge and medical technology may reduce the frequency of these events over time. However, many errors in management can be prevented with the development and implementation of clinical practice guidelines and quality assurance programs. The HMPS produced reliable estimates of rates of adverse events in hospital as well as the proportion of those events attributable to management error and negligence. The study also identified high-risk groups and areas where rates of negligence were highest, both of which can be targeted with quality assurance programs. The study supports the use of systems analysis and disciplinary action in instances of negligence to minimize the significant consequences of adverse events in hospitalized patients. In summary, by further characterizing the adverse events identified in HMPS I, the findings from the HMPS II study have been fundamental in guiding the development of quality improvement initiatives by identifying priorities for the field of patient safety.

In-Depth [retrospective case review]: Published in NEJM in 1991, the results of the HMPS II further analyzed the adverse events described in HMPS I by classifying the type of adverse event, where the event occurred (inside or outside hospital), those most likely to result in serious disability, the type of management error responsible, and those most likely to be due to negligence. As described in the HMPS I summary, this investigation included a random sample of 30 195 hospital records from the state of New York in 1984. Records were reviewed independently for the occurrence of adverse events. Drug-related complications were the most common single type of adverse event. The proportion of adverse events attributed to negligence varied between categories, with 17% of operative adverse events, 75% of diagnostic mishaps, and 77% of therapeutic mishaps attributed to negligent care. Adverse events due to negligence in hospitalized patients were more likely to cause serious disability or death than adverse events not attributed to negligence.

Leape LL, Brennan TA, Laird N, Lawthers AG, Localio AR, Barnes BA, et al. The Nature of Adverse Events in Hospitalized Patients. New England Journal of Medicine. 1991 Feb 7;324(6):377–84.

The DASH trial: Diet change significantly reduces blood pressure

1. A "combination" diet rich in fruits and vegetables and low in saturated and total fat significantly reduced blood pressure in comparison to the typical American diet.

2. Blood pressure reductions were observed in the setting of stable weight, unchanged sodium intake, and consumption of no more than 2 alcoholic drinks per day.

Original Date of Publication: April 1997

Study Rundown: At the time of the Dietary Approaches to Stop Hypertension (DASH) trial, national guidelines recommended reduced salt intake, weight control, and reduced alcohol consumption as nutritional means of controlling high blood pressure. Observational studies suggested that increased vegetable consumption could reduce blood pressure as well, but follow-up trials assessing the effect of individual nutrients on blood pressure were inconclusive. The DASH trial sought to assess the effect of dietary patterns, rather than individual nutrients, on blood pressure control. Results showed that, in comparison to a typical American diet low in fruits and vegetables, a diet rich in fruits and vegetables (the "fruit-and-vegetable" diet) significantly reduced systolic and diastolic blood pressure, while a "combination" diet rich in fruits and vegetables and low in saturated and total fat showed a greater reduction in blood pressure. Blood pressure reductions were greater in hypertensive participants than non-hypertensive participants. Notably, the reduction in blood pressure in hypertensive participants was similar in magnitude to reductions achieved through mono-drug therapy.

A strength of this trial was the large proportion of minorities enrolled - > 60% of participants were from minority groups for all 3 experimental diets. This was done to reflect the disproportionate burden of hypertension in minority populations. Moreover, diets in the study were designed so that the salt content was kept at 3 g/day. Participants were also allowed to consume 1-2 alcoholic beverages per day, and weight-loss was not a required goal. These findings suggest that the blood pressure reduction achieved the DASH diets are meant to complement, rather than supplant, current recommendations to reduce salt and alcohol consumption. Limitations of the trial include the lack of long-term assessment of the DASH diet's efficacy, as the trial consisted only of an 11-week feeding period. Notably, patients' ease of adherence to the diet was also not evaluated. In summary, the DASH trial showed that dietary modification involving increased vegetable and fruit consumption and decreased fat consumption offers an additional approach to lowering blood pressure.

In-Depth [randomized controlled trial]: The DASH trial was a randomized, multi-centered trial that enrolled 459 participants. Eligible participants were at least 22 years of age, did not take any antihypertensive medication, and had an average systolic blood pressure (BP) greater than 160 mmHg and a diastolic BP of 80-95 mmHg. Exclusion criteria included poorly controlled diabetes, hyperlipidemia, a cardiovascular event in the previous 6 months, BMI> 35, renal insufficiency, alcoholic beverage intake > 14 drinks/week, and unwillingness to stop taking medications or dietary supplements. Approximately 150 participants were randomized to each of the following diets: 1) the control diet (i.e., low in vegetables and fruit with a fat content similar to the typical American diet), 2) the "vegetable-and-fruit" diet (i.e., higher in vegetables and fruit), and 3) the "combination" diet (i.e., higher in vegetables and fruit and lower in fats). For each group, participants' BPs were screened at baseline first, then all participants were given the control diet for 3 weeks. Afterward, participants in the "vegetable-and-fruit" diet and the "combination" diet were switched to their respective diet, and all diets were continued for an additional 8 weeks. Diets were designed to include commonly available foods in different forms (fresh, frozen, etc.), and all foods were prepared similarly and using the same brand-name items at each study center.

Results showed a reduction in systolic BP of 2.8 mmHg ($p < 0.001$) and diastolic by 1.1 mmHg ($p = 0.07$) in the "vegetable and fruit" diet compared to the control diet. The "combination" diet reduced systolic BP by 5.5 mmHg ($p < 0.001$) and diastolic BP by 3.0 mmHg ($p < 0.001$). For participants with hypertension, the "combination" diet reduced systolic BP by 11.4 mmHg ($p < 0.001$) and diastolic BP by 5.5 mmHg ($p < 0.001$). For participants without hypertension, the "combination" diet reduced systolic BP by 3.5 mmHg ($p < 0.001$) and diastolic BP by 2.1 mmHg ($p = 0.003$).

Appel LJ, Moore TJ, Obarzanek E, Vollmer WM, Svetkey LP, Sacks FM, et al. A Clinical Trial of the Effects of Dietary Patterns on Blood Pressure. New England Journal of Medicine. 1997 Apr 17;336(16):1117–24.

The HOT trial: Diastolic blood pressure targets in hypertension

1. In hypertensive patients, there were no significant differences between different diastolic blood pressure (dBP) targets (≤90 mmHg, ≤85 mmHg, ≤80 mmHg) with regards to the risk of major cardiovascular events.

2. In patients with diabetes, treating to a target ≤80 mmHg led to significantly fewer major cardiovascular events and cardiovascular death compared to those treated to a target ≤90 mmHg.

3. Antihypertensive therapies were generally well tolerated, with common complaints including dizziness, leg edema, and coughing.

Original Date of Publication: June 1998

Study Rundown: While previous evidence had shown that treating hypertension reduced cardiovascular morbidity and mortality, it was thought that those with treated hypertension had higher risk of developing cardiovascular complications compared to normotensive individuals. The purpose of the Hypertension Optimal Treatment (HOT) trial was to determine whether different dBP targets led to different rates of major cardiovascular events (myocardial infarction, stroke, cardiovascular death). Moreover, the study explored whether adding low-dose acetylsalicylic acid (ASA) to antihypertensive therapy would further also major cardiovascular outcomes.

In summary, the HOT trial demonstrated that there were no significant differences between the different dBP targets (≤90 mmHg, ≤85 mmHg, ≤80 mmHg) in terms of risk of major cardiovascular events. In patients with diabetes mellitus, it was shown that targeting a dBP of ≤80 mmHg led to significant reductions in the risk of major cardiovascular events and cardiovascular mortality, when compared with a target of ≤90 mmHg. In these patients with treated hypertension, concurrent low-dose ASA also led to significantly lower rates of major cardiovascular events and myocardial infarction compared to those taking placebo. Antihypertensive therapy was generally well tolerated, with some patients complaining of dizziness, headache, leg edema, and coughing. Treatment with ASA led to significantly higher rates of nonfatal major bleeding compared to placebo.

In-Depth [randomized controlled trial]: This multicenter, randomized controlled trial involved 18 790 patients from 26 different countries. Patients were eligible for the trial if they were between 50-80 years of age and had hypertension with diastolic blood pressure between 100-115 mmHg. Included patients were randomly assigned to one of the 3 dBP target groups (≤90 mmHg, ≤85 mmHg, or ≤80 mmHg) and to treatment with either ASA 75 mg daily or placebo.

All patients were started on the long-acting calcium channel blocker felodipine at a dose of 5 mg daily, and additional therapy was provided to reach the randomized target blood pressure. Angiotensin-converting-enzyme (ACE) inhibitor or beta-blocker was added at step 2. Steps 3 and 4 involved dosage titrations (i.e., increasing felodipine to 10 mg daily and doubling the dose of the ACE inhibitor/beta-blocker, respectively). Step 5 involved the addition of a diuretic. The primary outcome was major cardiovascular events, defined as all myocardial infarctions and strokes (fatal and nonfatal), and all other cardiovascular deaths. Deaths occurring within 28 days of an event were labeled as fatal.

Patients were followed for an average of 3.8 years. The mean dBP achieved in the ≤90 mmHg, ≤85 mmHg, and ≤80 mmHg groups were 85.2 mmHg, 83.2 mmHg, and 81.1 mmHg, respectively. There were no differences between the three groups with regards to major cardiovascular events ($p = 0.50$). Moreover, there were no differences between the groups in the risk of all stroke ($p = 0.74$), all myocardial infarction ($p = 0.05$), cardiovascular mortality ($p = 0.49$), or total mortality ($p = 0.32$). In diabetic patients, patients in the ≤80 mmHg group experienced significantly lower rates of major cardiovascular events (RR 2.06, 95%CI 1.24 to 3.44, $p = 0.005$), and specifically cardiovascular mortality (RR 3.0, 95%CI 1.28 to 7.08, $p = 0.016$), when compared to patients in the ≤90 mmHg group. Patients taking ASA had significantly fewer major cardiovascular events (RR 0.85, 95%CI 0.73 to 0.99, $p = 0.03$) and myocardial infarctions (HR 0.64, 95%CI 0.49 to 0.85, $p = 0.002$) compared to those receiving placebo.

Generally, antihypertensive therapies were well-tolerated, with common side effects being dizziness, headache, lower extremity edema, flushing, and coughing. ASA was linked with significantly higher risk of nonfatal major bleeding as compared with placebo (RR 1.8, $p < 0.001$).

Hansson L, Zanchetti A, Carruthers SG, Dahlöf B, Elmfeldt D, Julius S, et al. Effects of intensive blood-pressure lowering and low-dose aspirin in patients with hypertension: Principal results of the Hypertension Optimal Treatment (HOT) randomised trial. The Lancet. 1998;351(9118):1755-1762.

The UKPDS: Reducing diabetes-related morbidity and mortality

1. For patients with type 2 diabetes mellitus (T2DM), pharmacologic blood glucose control with sulfonylureas or insulin significantly reduced the risk of microvascular complications, but not macrovascular complications.

2. Metformin therapy significantly reduced diabetes-related and all-cause mortality.

3. Strict control of blood pressure in T2DM reduced the risk of both microvascular and macrovascular complications, along with diabetes-related mortality.

Original Date of Publication: September 1998

Study Rundown: The United Kingdom Prospective Diabetes Study (UKPDS) produced a number of publications exploring the effectiveness of different interventions in reducing diabetes-related morbidity and mortality. In this report, we highlight 3 of the most influential papers yielded from this initiative: 1) UKPDS 33, which explored the use of sulfonylureas and insulin, 2) UKPDS 34, which examined the effects of metformin, and 3) UKPDS 38, looking at the effects of tight blood pressure control in patients with T2DM.

UKPDS 33 and 34 demonstrated that intensive blood glucose control with sulfonylureas, insulin, and/or metformin significantly reduced the incidence of microvascular complications of T2DM when compared to lifestyle modifications alone (i.e., diet and weight control). In these studies, microvascular complications were defined as retinopathy, vitreous hemorrhage, neuropathy, and renal failure. Pharmacologic therapy using any of these agents was associated with significant reductions in hemoglobin A1c (HbA1c) levels. There were no significant differences between pharmacologic therapy and lifestyle modifications alone in terms of the development of macrovascular complications (i.e., coronary artery disease, peripheral arterial disease, cerebrovascular disease). Metformin, however, was shown to significantly reduce diabetes-related and all-cause mortality. With regards to blood pressure control, UKPDS 38 demonstrated that treatment with angiotensin converting enzyme (ACE) inhibitors or beta blockers to lower blood pressure below 150/85 mmHg was associated with significantly reduced microvascular complications, macrovascular complications, and diabetes-related deaths when compared to control subjects with less tight blood pressure control (i.e., < 180/105 mmHg).

In summary, the use of pharmacologic agents (i.e., sulfonylureas, insulin, metformin) in patients with T2DM significantly reduced their risk for developing microvascular complications. Because metformin significantly reduced diabetes-related mortality, all-cause mortality and had low-risk of hypoglycemia, it is often considered the first-line pharmacotherapy in managing T2DM in present-day clinical practice. Moreover, tight blood pressure control was shown to reduce the incidence of microvascular and macrovascular complications, as well as diabetes-related mortality. The long duration, effective randomization, and large study population of the UKPDS are factors that have made these findings highly influential.

In-Depth [randomized controlled studies]: In UKPDS 33 and 34, patients with newly diagnosed T2DM aged 25-65 were recruited from 23 participating centers and followed over 10 years. Both papers were randomized trials that allocated patients to different treatment groups or conventional management, which involved only lifestyle modifications. UKPDS 33 demonstrated that median HbA1c levels were significantly lower in the treatment group (i.e., patients receiving sulfonylureas or insulin) at 7.0% compared to 7.9% for the control group ($p < 0.0001$). Moreover, the risk of microvascular complications was significantly reduced in the treatment group (RR 0.75; 95%CI 0.60-0.93). Patients in the treatment group, however, did experience significantly higher rates of hypoglycemic episodes than the control group ($p < 0.0001$). Similarly, treating patients with T2DM with metformin was found to be beneficial in UKPDS 34. When compared to conventional therapy (i.e., lifestyle changes alone), treatment with metformin was found to reduce diabetes-related death (RR 0.58; 95%CI 0.37-0.91) and all-cause mortality (RR 0.64; 95%CI 0.45-0.91). Moreover, metformin therapy was linked with fewer hypoglycemic episodes than treatment with sulfonylureas and insulin.

In UKPDS 38, which assessed the effects of blood pressure control, patients with newly diagnosed T2DM were again recruited from 23 participating hospitals and were followed over 10 years. Blood pressure was measured at clinic visits every 3-4 months. Patients were randomized to either tight blood pressure control (i.e., < 150/85 mmHg) or less tight control (i.e., < 180/105 mmHg). Patients were treated with ACE inhibitors or beta-blockers to achieve target blood pressures. It was found that patients in the tight control group experienced a 32% reduction in the risk of diabetes-related morality compared to the less tight group ($p = 0.019$). Diabetes-related mortality was defined as deaths resulting from myocardial infarction, sudden death, stroke, peripheral vascular disease, renal disease, hyperglycemia, or hypoglycemia. In addition, the risk of macrovascular complications was demonstrated to be 34% lower in the tight control group (p = 0.019).

UK Prospective Diabetes Study (UKPDS) Group. *Intensive blood-glucose control with sulphonylureas or insulin compared with conventional treatment and risk of complications in patients with type 2 diabetes (UKPDS 33). The Lancet. 1998 Sep 12;352(9131):837–53.*

UK Prospective Diabetes Study (UKPDS) Group. *Effect of intensive blood-glucose control with metformin on complications in overweight patients with type 2 diabetes (UKPDS 34). Lancet. 1998 Sep 12;352(9131):854–65.*

UK Prospective Diabetes Study (UKPDS) Group. *Tight blood pressure control and risk of macrovascular and microvascular complications in type 2 diabetes: UKPDS 38. UK Prospective Diabetes Study Group. BMJ. 1998 Sep 12;317(7160):703–13.*

Symptom-triggered benzodiazepine treatment for alcohol withdrawal

1. For patients withdrawing from alcohol, symptom-triggered pharmacologic therapy decreased detoxification time without compromising the safety or comfort of the patient.

2. Symptom-triggered individualized benzodiazepine administration significantly reduced the intensity and duration of oxazepam use during withdrawal treatment.

Original Date of Publication: May 2002

Study Rundown: Fixed doses of benzodiazepines are considered the first-line pharmacologic approach when treating patients with alcohol withdrawal. In this landmark study, withdrawing patients were randomized into 2 groups: 1) patients who underwent individualized treatment with oxazepam in response to withdrawal symptoms or 2) patients were treated with a fixed amount of oxazepam with additional doses given only as needed. It was determined that the symptom-triggered patient group not only used 6 times less oxazepam but also experienced a shorter treatment duration than did the fixed-schedule group of patients. The difference in oxazepam use was not tied to any changes in safety, withdrawal intensity, or comfort level of the patients. In summary, this study supports the use of symptom-triggered benzodiazepine administration in patients suffering alcohol withdrawal.

In-Depth [randomized controlled trial]: In this double-blinded randomized controlled trial, an uninvolved pharmacist randomized all 117 eligible patients admitted to the alcohol treatment inpatient program, a clinic associated with the Lausanne University hospital, into clusters of 10 participants to either the symptom-triggered or fixed schedule group. Fixed-schedule subjects received a 30 mg dose of oxazepam every 6 hours, and subsequently, 8 doses of 15 mg. Shortly after administration, patients would be administered additional drugs depending on their Clinical Institute Withdrawal Assessment for Alcohol Scale (CIWA-Ar) score. Symptom-triggered subjects received a placebo every 6 hours and were administered oxazepam only if their CIWA-Ar score reached certain pre-determined thresholds. In comparing the 2 groups, only 39% in the symptom-triggered group were treated with oxazepam, which stood in great contrast to the 100% treated in the fixed schedule group (p < .001). The mean total oxazepam dose administered to the symptom-triggered and fixed-schedule groups were 37.5

mg and 231.4 mg (p < .001) respectively. The mean duration of treatment in the symptom triggered group was 20.0 hours, which was significantly lower than the mean duration time of 62.7 hours in the fixed schedule group (p < .001). Despite these differences, there were no distinctions in comfort level noted between individuals in the 2 groups, as measured by comparing the CIWA-Ar scores of each patient.

Daeppen J, Gache P, Landry U, et al. Symptom-triggered vs fixed-schedule doses of benzodiazepine for alcohol withdrawal: A randomized treatment trial. Arch Intern Med. 2002 May 27;162(10):1117–21.

The CATIE trial: High rates of medication discontinuation in schizophrenic patients

1. Approximately 74% of schizophrenic patients discontinued their medications before 18 months, with the median being 6 months.

2. Olanzapine was found to have a significantly longer time to discontinuation than quetiapine or risperidone.

3. Olanzapine was associated with significantly more weight gain and increases in glycosylated hemoglobin, cholesterol, and triglycerides when compared to the other antipsychotics.

Original Date of Publication: September 2005

Study Rundown: Antipsychotic drugs form the foundation of schizophrenia management. Typical antipsychotic drugs were first developed and are highly effective in managing psychotic symptoms, though they are now linked with a high-risk of extrapyramidal side effects. Atypical antipsychotics were subsequently developed and promised lower risk of such side effects, though limited evidence existed to support these claims. This double-blind, randomized controlled study sought to compare the relative effectiveness of atypical and typical antipsychotics, in addition to evaluating claims that atypical antipsychotics have a better side effect profile. The Clinical Antipsychotic Trials of Intervention Effectiveness (CATIE) trial demonstrated that schizophrenic patients discontinued their antipsychotics at very high rates, thereby limiting the effectiveness of drug therapy. Olanzapine was found to be significantly more effective than other atypical antipsychotics (i.e., quetiapine and risperidone) in terms of time to discontinuation. However, olanzapine was associated with significantly more weight gain and increases in glycosylated hemoglobin, cholesterol, and triglyceride levels. This study was funded by the National Institute of Mental Health. Pharmaceutical companies contributed drug supplies for the study and advice regarding dosing; they were not otherwise involved in the design of the study, or the analyses and interpretation of its results.

In-Depth [randomized controlled trial]: A total of 1493 patients were recruited from 57 different centers across the United States, and were randomly assigned to receive olanzapine (7.5-30 mg daily), quetiapine (200-800 mg daily), risperidone

(1.5-6 mg daily), ziprasidone (40-160 mg daily), or perphenazine (8-32 mg daily); all medications were administered as identical-appearing capsules. Patients were included in the study if they were between 18 and 65 years of age, if they were diagnosed with schizophrenia, and if they were able to take antipsychotics. The primary outcome was the discontinuation of treatment for any reason. It was thought that this measure would represent the efficacy, safety, and tolerability of different treatment options. Secondary outcomes included reasons for discontinuation and scores on the Positive and Negative Syndrome Scale (PANSS) and the Clinical Global Impression (CGI) scale. Approximately 74% of patients discontinued their assigned treatment before the 18 month mark, with the median time to discontinuation being about 6 months. The time to discontinuation was significantly longer in the olanzapine group, when compared to the quetiapine (HR 0.63), risperidone (HR 0.75), ziprasidone (HR 0.76), and perphenazine group (HR 0.78). After adjusting for multiple comparisons, however, significant differences only remained between olanzapine and quetiapine/risperidone. The study also demonstrated that PANSS and CGI scores significantly improved over time. Notably, olanzapine was significantly associated with greater weight gain, as well as greater increases in glycosylated hemoglobin, total cholesterol, and triglycerides when compared to the other study drugs.

Lieberman JA, Stroup TS, McEvoy JP, Swartz MS, Rosenheck RA, Perkins DO, et al. Effectiveness of Antipsychotic Drugs in Patients with Chronic Schizophrenia. New England Journal of Medicine. 2005 Sep 22;353(12):1209–23.

The STAR*D trials I: Medication augmentation for depression

1. In patients who have not experienced remission of depression despite vigorous treatment with a selective serotonin-reuptake inhibitor (SSRI), augmentation of treatment by adding bupropion or buspirone achieved remission in approximately 30% of patients.

2. There were no significant differences between drug groups in terms of remission rates.

Original Date of Publication: March 2006

*The Sequenced Treatment Alternatives to Relieve Depression (STAR*D) trials explored the management of patients who had refractory depression despite treatment with a SSRI. Two papers were published based on data from the STAR*D trials in NEJM in 2006, which involved outpatients with nonpsychotic major depression who had not experienced remission with citalopram alone. In both papers, the primary outcome measure was remission with a score of < 7 on the Hamilton Rating Scale for Depression (HRSD-17), while secondary outcome measurement of remission and response was done using the Quick Inventory of Depressive Symptomatology (QIDS-SR-16). Patients in this study were given the option to 1) augment their therapy by adding other agents or 2) switch to another therapy.*

Study Rundown: The use of medications to augment SSRI therapy is common practice in the treatment of depression, though no previous randomized controlled trials had explored this issue. This paper demonstrated that in patients with refractory depression despite vigorous SSRI treatment, augmenting therapy by adding bupropion or buspirone to existing SSRI therapy can help achieve remission in approximately 30% of patients. While there were no significant differences between the bupropion and buspirone groups in terms of remission rates, patients in the bupropion group were adherent to treatment for significantly longer periods of time, and experienced higher reductions in QIDS-SR-16 scores.

In-Depth [randomized controlled trial]: A total of 565 patients were recruited and randomized to either receive 1) sustained-release bupropion or 2) buspirone, in addition to citalopram, an SSRI. There were no significant differences in remission rates between the two groups based on HSRD-17 scores (29.7% for bupropion group, 30.1% for buspirone group). Similarly, remission and response rates based on QIDS-SR-16 scores were not significantly different between the groups. Patients in the bupropion group were adherent to treatment for significantly longer than those in the buspirone group (10.2 weeks vs. 9.2 weeks, p = 0.01). Moreover, patients in the bupropion group experienced significantly higher reductions in QIDS-SR-16 scores at the end of the study when compared to the buspirone group.

Trivedi MH, Fava M, Wisniewski SR, Thase ME, Quitkin F, Warden D, et al. Medication Augmentation after the Failure of SSRIs for Depression. New England Journal of Medicine. 2006 Mar 23;354(12):1243–52.

The STAR*D trials II: Switching antidepressants in depression management

1. In cases where citalopram failed or could not be tolerated, approximately 1 in 4 patients experienced remission of their depression symptoms by switching to sustained-release bupropion, sertraline, or extended-release venlafaxine.

Original Date of Publication: March 2006

Study Rundown: Apart from augmentation, switching to a different antidepressant represents another option for managing patients who do not experience depression remission despite treatment with an SSRI. This trial examined patients suffering from refractory depression after a trial of citalopram. It demonstrated that switching to another medication resulted in approximately 1 in 4 patients experiencing remission of their symptoms with sustained-release bupropion, sertraline, or extended-release venlafaxine. A strength of the STAR*D studies is the few criteria for inclusion and exclusion, which suggests that these findings may be generalizable to an outpatient population. Limitations included the lack of a placebo control group and the fact that treatment delivery was unblinded. Interestingly, the rates of remission with switching medications were lower than the remission rates observed with augmenting therapy. Part of this may be attributed to the differences in patient pools seen in the 2 studies (i.e., the "medication switch" study having a larger proportion of patients who could not tolerate citalopram) and the inadequate doses/treatment durations. Nevertheless, this study demonstrated clinically meaningful remission rates when switching to other antidepressants.

In-Depth [randomized controlled trial]: A total of 727 outpatients with non-psychotic depression were enrolled. All patients had been previously treated with citalopram and had not experienced remission or could not tolerate citalopram. Patients were randomized to switch from citalopram to 1) sustained-release bupropion (a norepinephrine-dopamine reuptake inhibitor, NDRI), 2) sertraline (another SSRI), or 3) extended-release venlafaxine (a serotonin-norepinephrine reuptake inhibitor, SNRI). Remission rates were not significantly different between the 3 treatment groups, as measured by HSRD-17 scores (21.3% in the bupropion group, 17.6% in the sertraline group, 28.4% in the venlafaxine group). Moreover, the 3 groups were not significantly different with regards to response/remission rates, or time to response/remission, as measured by QIDS-SR-16 scores, nor were they significantly different in terms of their rates of side effects or serious adverse events.

Rush AJ, Trivedi MH, Wisniewski SR, Stewart JW, Nierenberg AA, Thase ME, et al. Bupropion-SR, Sertraline, or Venlafaxine-XR after Failure of SSRIs for Depression. New England Journal of Medicine. 2006 Mar 23;354(12):1231–42.

The ENHANCE trial: Simvastatin and ezetimibe in familial hypercholesterolemia

1. In patients with familial hypercholesterolemia, simvastatin and ezetimibe combination therapy did not result in significant differences in carotid artery thickness when compared to treatment with simvastatin alone.

2. Treatment with simvastatin and ezetimibe resulted in significantly greater reductions in low-density lipoprotein (LDL) cholesterol, triglyceride, and C-reactive protein levels as compared to treatment with simvastatin alone.

3. There were no significant differences between the 2 groups in the rates of adverse events or drug discontinuation.

Original Date of Publication: April 2008

Study Rundown: Ezetimibe is a cholesterol-absorption inhibitor that lowers plasma cholesterol by decreasing the amount of cholesterol absorption in the small intestine. This drug is often used in combination with statins, and this combination has been shown to further reduce levels of LDL when compared to statins alone. However, no prior large-scale randomized clinical trial had been conducted to assess the effect of adding ezetimibe to statins on atherosclerosis progression. In the Ezetimibe and Simvastatin in Hypercholesterolemia Enhances Atherosclerosis Regression (ENHANCE) trial, 720 patients with familial hypercholesterolemia were randomized to receive simvastatin with placebo or simvastatin with ezetimibe. After 24 months of therapy, there was no significant difference between the groups in mean change in intima-media thickness of the carotid arteries. Nevertheless, patients that took combination therapy rather than simvastatin alone experienced greater reductions in LDL cholesterol, triglyceride, and C-reactive protein levels.

In-Depth [randomized controlled trial]: This double-blinded randomized control trial was originally published in the NEJM in 2008. It was conducted at 18 centers in the United States, Canada, South Africa, Spain, Denmark, Norway, Sweden, and the Netherlands. Patients were eligible for the study if they were between 30-75 years of age and had been diagnosed with familial hypercholesterolemia by genotyping or World Health Organization diagnostic criteria. Exclusion criteria included having high-grade stenosis/occlusion of the carotid artery, a history of carotid endarterectomy/stenting, homozygous familial hypercholesterolemia, New York Heart Association class III or IV congestive heart failure, and cardiac arrhythmia. All patients underwent a screening phase, a single-blind 6-week placebo run-in period, and a double-blind study period lasting 24 months. The primary outcome was the mean change in intima-media thickness of the carotid arteries, as measured by ultrasonography of the carotid arteries.

A total of 720 patients with familial hypercholesterolemia were randomized into 2 treatment groups: 1) simvastatin 80 mg daily with placebo or 2) simvastatin 80 mg daily and ezetimibe 10 mg daily. In the simvastatin-only group, the mean change in thickness was 0.0058 ± 0.0037 mm, while it was 0.0111 ± 0.0038 mm in the simvastatin-ezetimibe group, an insignificant difference ($p = 0.29$). Patients in the simvastatin-ezetimibe group experienced a 16.5% greater reduction in LDL levels compared with the simvastatin-only group ($p < 0.01$). Patients in the combination group also experienced significantly greater reductions in triglyceride and C-reactive protein levels, when compared with simvastatin alone ($p < 0.01$). There were no significant differences between the two groups in the rates of adverse events and medication discontinuation.

Kastelein JJP, Akdim F, Stroes ESG, Zwinderman AH, Bots ML, Stalenhoef AFH, et al. Simvastatin with or without Ezetimibe in Familial Hypercholesterolemia. New England Journal of Medicine. 2008 Apr 3;358(14):1431–43.

The JUPITER: Rosuvastatin reduces the risk of major cardiovascular events in healthy patients

1. In patients with average low density lipoprotein (LDL) cholesterol levels and elevated C-reactive protein, rosuvastatin reduced the risk of a first major cardiovascular event compared to placebo.

2. Rosuvastatin therapy also significantly reduced the risk of all-cause mortality compared to placebo.

3. The study was terminated early and did not meet the prespecified number of primary endpoints needed to be sufficiently powered.

Original Date of Publication: November 2008

Study Rundown: Similar to present day, at the time of this study statins were commonly used medications in the treating patients with vascular disease and known hyperlipidemia. Clinical observations, however, revealed that myocardial infarctions and strokes were occurring in patients with normal levels of LDL, and in whom statin therapy would not be warranted based on consensus guidelines. Similarly, C-reactive protein, a marker of inflammation, was known to be a predictor of vascular events. The Justification for the Use of Statins in Prevention: an Intervention Trial Evaluating Rosuvastatin (JUPITER) sought to determine whether statin therapy could help prevent major cardiovascular events in patients with LDL levels below treatment thresholds, but who also had elevated CRP levels. Investigators successfully demonstrated that prescribing rosuvastatin to patients with LDL levels below treatment thresholds, but with elevated C-reactive protein levels, significantly reduced the rate of first major cardiovascular events as compared to placebo. Of note, the rates of adverse events were similar in the 2 groups. It must be noted that this trial was terminated early with a median follow-up less than 2 years. As a result, the trial did not have the prespecified 520 confirmed primary endpoints needed to be sufficiently powered.

In-Depth [randomized controlled trial]: A total of 17 802 patients were enrolled and randomized as part of the JUPITER. In order to be eligible, patients needed to meet age requirements ($\geq$ 50 years of age for men, $\geq$ 60 years of age for women), have no history of cardiovascular disease, have an LDL cholesterol < 130 mg/dL, and have a high-sensitivity C-reactive protein level $\geq$ 2.0 mg/L.

Exclusion criteria included previous or current use lipid-lowering therapy, current use of post-menopausal hormone-replacement therapy, evidence of hepatic dysfunction, elevated creatine kinase level, creatinine > 2.0 mg/dL (176.8 μmol/L), diabetes, and uncontrolled hypertension. Moreover, patients with inflammatory conditions (e.g., severe arthritis, lupus, inflammatory bowel disease) were excluded. Eligible patients were randomized to treatment with either rosuvastatin 20 mg daily or placebo. Follow-up occurred up to 60 months after randomization. The primary outcome was the occurrence of a first major cardiovascular event (i.e., nonfatal myocardial infarction, nonfatal stroke, hospitalization for unstable angina, arterial revascularization procedure, or death from cardiovascular cause).

Patients were followed for a median of 1.9 years. The rate of the primary endpoint was significantly lower in the rosuvastatin group as compared with the placebo group (HR 0.56; 95%CI 0.46-0.69). This was driven by significant reductions in all components of the primary endpoint, except for hospitalization for unstable angina (HR 0.59; 95%CI 0.32-1.10). Notably, patients treated with rosuvastatin experienced a significant reduction in all-cause mortality when compared to those treated with placebo (HR 0.80; 95%CI 0.67-0.97). The rates of adverse events reported were similar for both groups (p = 0.60). The rates of myopathy (p = 0.82), newly diagnosed cancer (p = 0.51), gastrointestinal disorder (p = 0.43), and elevations in hepatic transaminases (p = 0.34) were similar between both groups.

Ridker PM, Danielson E, Fonseca FAH, Genest J, Gotto AM, Kastelein JJP, et al. Rosuvastatin to Prevent Vascular Events in Men and Women with Elevated C-Reactive Protein. New England Journal of Medicine. 2008 Nov 20;359(21):2195–207.

The RAVE trial: Rituximab induces remission in ANCA-associated vasculitis

1. Rituximab was non-inferior to cyclophosphamide in inducing remission of severe ANCA-associated vasculitis.

2. There were no significant differences between both groups in the rates of total, serious, or non-disease-related adverse events.

Original Date of Publication: July 2010

Study Rundown: The combination of cyclophosphamide and a glucocorticoid has long been the standard of treatment for ANCA-associated vasculitides. The Rituximab in ANCA-Associated Vasculitis (RAVE) trial demonstrated that rituximab was non-inferior to cyclophosphamide in inducing remission in severe ANCA-associated vasculitis when used alongside glucocorticoids. Moreover, there were no significant differences between the 2 groups in the rates of total, severe, or non-disease-related adverse events. The authors noted that their trial only included patients with severe ANCA-associated vasculitis, thereby limiting its generalizability. Others have also criticized this trial for its short follow-up and point to the paucity of data regarding long-term efficacy and safety. Rituximab subsequently received approval from the Food and Drug Administration for use in treating certain ANCA-associated vasculitides. One group has also recommended the use of rituximab while cautioning the lack of data about long-term effects.

In-Depth [randomized controlled trial]: The RAVE trial was a randomized, double-blind, double-dummy, non-inferiority trial examining the efficacy of rituximab in inducing remission of severe ANCA-associated vasculitis. Patients were eligible if they had Wegner's granulomatosis or microscopic polyangiitis, positive serum assays for proteinase 3-ANCA or myeloperoxidase-ANCA and a Birmingham Vasculitis Activity Score for Wegener's Granulomatosis (BVAS/WG) of 3 or more. Both patients with new diagnoses and relapsing disease were eligible for the trial. Eligible participants were randomized to receive either rituximab (375 mg/m^2 IV weekly for 4 weeks) or cyclophosphamide (2 mg/kg, with adjustments for renal insufficiency) with a subsequent switch to azathioprine if remission was achieved between 3-6 months. Both groups were also treated with glucocorticoids (i.e., 1-3 pulses of methylprednisolone, with subsequent prednisone tapered according to symptomology). The primary endpoint was a BVAS/WG score of 0 and successful completion of prednisone taper at 6 months.

A total of 197 patients with ANCA-associated vasculitis were enrolled in the trial. Approximately 64% of patients in the rituximab group and 53% of the patients in the cyclophosphamide group reached the primary endpoint, and this treatment difference met the criterion for non-inferiority (p < 0.001). The difference between the 2 groups was not statistically significant. There were no significant differences between the groups in the rates of total, severe, or non-disease-related adverse events.

Stone JH, Merkel PA, Spiera R, Seo P, Langford CA, Hoffman GS, et al. Rituximab versus Cyclophosphamide for ANCA-Associated Vasculitis. New England Journal of Medicine. 2010 Jul 15;363(3):221–32.

II. Cardiology

> "A fact is a simple statement that everyone believes. It is innocent, unless found guilty. A hypothesis is a novel suggestion that no one wants to believe. It is guilty, until found effective."
>
> - Edward Teller, PhD

The BHAT: Propranolol after acute myocardial infarction

1. This large, randomized trial was the first to demonstrate that propranolol significantly reduced mortality after acute myocardial infarction when compared with placebo.

Original Date of Publication: March 1982

Study Rundown: The Beta-Blocker Heart Attack Trial (BHAT) was established in 1977 to study whether daily administration of propranolol after a myocardial infarction would lead to a reduction in total mortality. Prior to this study, beta-blockers were well known to reduce myocardial oxygen demand and suppress arrhythmias. They were also widely used in the setting of coronary artery disease, although numerous studies exploring this question were inconclusive due to small sample sizes and study design issues.

In summary, patients with recent hospitalization for myocardial infarction experienced significantly lower all-cause mortality when taking propranolol rather than placebo. Moreover, propranolol therapy led to significantly lower rates of cardiovascular mortality and sudden death. Patients taking propranolol experienced significantly higher rates of bronchospasm and diarrhea, but fewer instances of palpitations when compared to placebo. The BHAT was the first large, randomized trial to demonstrate a significant reduction in mortality when treating patients with recent myocardial infarction with a beta-blocker, and beta-blockade remains a staple in the management of acute myocardial infarction.

In-Depth [randomized controlled trial]: The BHAT was a double-blinded, placebo-controlled, randomized trial conducted at 31 institutions in the United States and Canada. Patients were eligible for the study if they were between 30-69 years of age and hospitalized for acute myocardial infarction. Exclusion criteria included contraindications to propranolol (e.g., marked bradycardia), a history of severe heart failure or asthma, other life-threatening illness, a need for cardiac surgery, or a previous need for beta-blocker therapy. A total of 3837 were enrolled and randomized to treatment with propranolol 40 mg every eight hours or placebo. The propranolol dose was subsequently titrated up to 60 mg or 80 mg every eight hours.

The majority of patients enrolled in this study were white males, comprising over 80% of the study population. Compared with patients who received placebo, those in the propranolol group experienced significantly lower all-cause mortality (7.2% vs. 9.8%, p < 0.005). Patients taking propranolol also experienced significantly lower cardiovascular mortality (6.6% vs. 8.9%, p < 0.01), arteriosclerotic heart disease mortality (6.2% vs. 8.5%, p < 0.01), and sudden death (3.3% vs. 4.6%, p < 0.05) compared to those treated with placebo.

There were significantly more instances of bronchospasm (31.3% vs. 27.0%, p < 0.005) and diarrhea (5.5% vs. 3.6%, p < 0.01) in the propranolol group, though palpitations were more common in the placebo group (10.8% vs. 15.1%, p < 0.001).

Beta-Blocker Heart Attack Trial Research Group. A randomized trial of propranolol in patients with acute myocardial infarction. JAMA. 1982;247(12):1707-1714.

The LRC-CPPT 1: Cholestyramine and coronary heart disease

1. This trial was one of the first large, randomized studies to demonstrate that reducing lipid levels with cholestyramine could significantly lower death from CHD and nonfatal myocardial infarction, when compared to placebo.

Original Date of Publication: January 1984

Study Rundown: CHD remains a significant cause of death and disability around the world. In the 1970s, some observational data showed a direct relationship between serum lipid levels, particularly low-density lipoprotein cholesterol (LDL-C), and risk of CHD. It was suspected that LDL-C was heavily involved in the pathophysiology of atherosclerosis and thereby responsible for CHD. It was also understood at the time that serum lipid levels could be altered by changing diet and taking medications, though a causal relationship between cholesterol levels and CHD had yet been firmly established.

The Lipid Research Clinics Coronary Primary Prevention Trial (LRC-CPPT) was a large randomized trial started in the mid-1970s to address this relationship. Patients were largely high-school educated white men with elevated cholesterol levels. They were randomized to treatment with either cholestyramine or placebo, in addition to cholesterol-lowering diet and nutritional counseling. Treatment with cholestyramine led to significantly larger reductions in total cholesterol and LDL-C levels when compared to placebo therapy. Patients taking cholestyramine also experienced significantly lower rates of death from CHD and nonfatal myocardial infarction. Despite the study's homogeneous population and limited generalizability, this was one of the first large-scale randomized trials to demonstrate a consistent reduction in CHD after lipid lowering therapy.

In-Depth [randomized controlled trial]: This double-blind, placebo-controlled, randomized trial was conducted at 12 sites in the United States. Men between 35 and 59 years of age, with a plasma cholesterol level ≥6.9 mmol/L (265 mg/dL) and LDL-C level ≥ 4.9 mmol/L (190 mg/dL) were recruited for the study. Exclusion criteria included triglyceride levels averaging > 3.387 mmol/L (300 mg/dL), type III hyperlipoproteinemia, clinical manifestations of CHD (e.g., myocardial infarction, angina pectoris, ECG abnormalities, heart failure), diabetes mellitus, hypothyroidism, nephrotic syndrome, obesity, and hypertension. A total of 3806 participants were randomized to treatment with either cholestyramine 24 g daily or an equivalent amount of placebo and followed for an average of 7.4 years. All patients were offered a cholesterol-lowering diet along with nutritional counseling. The primary endpoint was a composite of death from CHD and nonfatal myocardial infarction. Other endpoints were all-cause mortality, atherothrombotic brain infarction, and arterial peripheral vascular disease.

Compared to placebo, treatment with cholestyramine significantly reduced total cholesterol (8.5%, $p < 0.001$) and LDL-C (12.6%, $p < 0.001$). At 7 years, the primary endpoint occurred significantly less frequently in the cholestyramine group as compared with the placebo group (8.1% vs. 9.8%; risk reduction 19%, 90%CI 3 to 32%, $p < 0.05$). There were significantly fewer CHD deaths (1.6% vs. 2.0%; risk reduction 24%) and nonfatal myocardial infarctions (6.8% vs. 8.3%; risk reduction 19%) in patients taking cholestyramine. There were no significant differences between the 2 groups in the incidence of brain infarction or peripheral vascular disease, and no difference in all-cause mortality. Gastrointestinal side effects were common during the trial. In the first year, the rate of such side effects were significantly higher in the cholestyramine group (68% vs. 43%). These rates were quite similar by year 7 (29% vs. 26%).

Lipid Research Clinics Program. The lipid research clinics coronary primary prevention trial results: Reduction in incidence of coronary heart disease. JAMA. 1984;251(3):351-364.

The V-HeFT I: Hydralazine and isosorbide dinitrate reduce mortality in heart failure

1. In patients with congestive heart failure, the combination of hydralazine and isosorbide dinitrate significantly reduced mortality compared to placebo.

2. This was one of the first large randomized trials to demonstrate a significant mortality benefit in the treatment of congestive heart failure.

Original Date of Publication: June 1986

Study Rundown: Prior to the 1980s, few options were available in heart failure treatment, with digitalis and diuretics being the only medications used to relieve symptoms. Subsequent efforts to treat heart failure focused on altering hemodynamics, and it was hypothesized that reducing preload and afterload using isosorbide dinitrate and hydralazine, respectively, could improve outcomes. The Vasodilator-Heart Failure Trial I (V-HeFT I) sought to explore the effects of using a combination of hydralazine and isosorbide dinitrate in managing heart failure. In summary, this trial demonstrated that treating patients with congestive heart failure with hydralazine-isosorbide dinitrate significantly reduced mortality compared to placebo for the initial 3-year period. This study was one of the first to demonstrate a significant reduction in mortality with heart failure treatment.

In-Depth [randomized controlled trial]: A total of 642 patients were randomized to treatment with placebo, prazosin 2.5 mg 4 times per day, or hydralazine 37.5 mg-isosorbide dinitrate 20 mg 4 times per day. Patients with chronic congestive heart failure were recruited from 11 Veterans Administration hospitals in the United States. Patients were eligible for the trial if they were male, between 18-75 years of age, and had congestive heart failure, as determined by evidence of cardiac dilatation (i.e., increased cardiothoracic size on chest x-ray, left ventricular dilatation on echocardiogram) or left ventricular impairment and reduced exercise tolerance. Patients were excluded if they had reduced exercise tolerance due to chest pain, rather than fatigue/breathlessness, myocardial infarction in the recent 3 months, or substantial disease to limit 5-year survival. Over the initial 2-year period, Cox regression demonstrated a significant 34% reduction in mortality (95%CI 4-54%) in the hydralazine-isosorbide dinitrate group compared with the placebo group. By 3 years, the hydralazine-isosorbide dinitrate group experienced a 36% reduction in mortality (95%CI 11-54%). Beyond 3 years, the data was insufficient to draw any conclusions.

Cohn JN, Archibald DG, Ziesche S, Franciosa JA, Harston WE, Tristani FE, et al. Effect of Vasodilator Therapy on Mortality in Chronic Congestive Heart Failure. New England Journal of Medicine. 1986 Jun 12;314(24):1547–52.

The CONSENSUS: Enalapril reduces mortality in severe heart failure

1. In patients with severe heart failure, treatment with enalapril significantly reduced the risk of mortality at 6 months and 1 year when compared with placebo.

2. The reduction in mortality was attributed to significantly lower risk of mortality resulting from progression of heart failure.

3. Patients on enalapril were significantly more likely to suffer from hypotension compared to those receiving placebo.

Original Date of Publication: June 1987

Study Rundown: In 1987, few therapies for heart failure were supported by well-conducted, randomized trials. Most patients were treated with digoxin and diuretics for symptomatic relief. The V-HeFT I, originally published in 1986, was one of the first studies to demonstrate mortality benefit in the treatment of heart failure, as patients receiving the combination of hydralazine and isosorbide dinitrate had significantly lower mortality than patients on placebos. It was suspected that hydralazine and isosorbide improved outcomes by optimizing cardiac hemodynamics in reducing both preload and afterload. At the time of the Cooperative North Scandinavian Enalapril Survival Study (CONSENSUS), some evidence suggested that angiotensin-converting-enzyme (ACE) inhibitors had beneficial effects on cardiac hemodynamics and heart failure symptoms. As a result, the CONSENSUS was conducted to determine the effects of enalapril on mortality in severe heart failure. In summary, patients being treated with enalapril experienced significantly lower mortality at both 6 month and 1-year follow-up when compared to those on placebo. This effect was driven by a significant reduction in mortality due to heart failure progression. Of note, the trial was terminated early by the Ethical Review Committee on the basis of ethical considerations given the large reduction in mortality observed in the enalapril group.

In-Depth [randomized controlled trial]: The CONSENSUS was a randomized trial conducted at 35 centers in North Scandinavia (6 centers in Finland, 12 in Norway, 17 in Sweden). Patients were eligible for the trial if they had severe congestive heart failure defined as New York Heart Association (NYHA) class IV symptoms, with radiographically determined enlarged heart size (i.e., > 600 mL/m² body surface area in men, > 550 mL/m² in women). All patients were on treatment with digoxin and diuretics. Exclusion criteria included acute pulmonary edema, hemodynamically significant aortic or mitral valve stenosis, myocardial infarction within the previous 2 months, unstable angina, planned cardiac surgery, right heart failure secondary to pulmonary disease, and serum creatinine concentration > 300 μmol/L. Patients were randomized to treatment with enalapril (i.e., starting at 5 mg twice daily, titrated up to 20 mg twice daily) or placebo. The primary endpoints were 6 month mortality and cause of death.

The study was terminated early by the Ethical Review Committee after a total of 253 patients had undergone randomization. Patients in the enalapril group experienced significantly lower 6 month mortality compared to patients receiving placebo (26% vs. 44%, RRR 40%, $p < 0.002$). Mortality at 1 year was also significantly lower in patients being treated with enalapril (36% vs. 52%, RRR 31%, $p < 0.001$). There were no significant differences between the 2 groups in the rates of sudden cardiac death ($p > 0.25$), though patients being treated with enalapril were significantly less likely to die from heart failure progression compared to those on placebo (22 vs. 44, $p < 0.001$). Similar numbers of patients from both groups withdrew from the study (14% in the placebo group, 17% in the enalapril group), though more patients withdrew from the enalapril group due to hypotension compared to those on placebo (7 on enalapril, 0 on placebo).

The CONSENSUS Trial Study Group. Effects of enalapril on mortality in severe congestive heart failure: Results of the Cooperative North Scandinavian Enalapril Survival Study (CONSENSUS). The New England Journal of Medicine. 1987;316(23):1429-1435.

The CAST: Anti-arrhythmic agents increase risk of death in patients after myocardial infarction

1. The use of class IC anti-arrhythmic agents flecainide and encainide in patients following myocardial infarction with left ventricular dysfunction increased the risk of death due to arrhythmia and shock.

Original Date of Publication: March 1991

Study Rundown: Ventricular arrhythmia is a major cause of cardiac death following myocardial infarction. Thus, the Cardiac Arrhythmia Suppression Trial (CAST) sought to determine whether suppression of ventricular ectopy with class IC anti-arrhythmic drugs in patients with a recent myocardial infarction would improve outcomes, including mortality. Unfortunately, the results demonstrated an increased risk of death from arrhythmia and any cause in those patients receiving these drugs following myocardial infarction. This increased incidence of arrhythmia-associated death was not matched correspondingly with an increased incidence of non-lethal events involving arrhythmia. This study was one of the first to encourage practicing caution in the use of anti-arrhythmic drugs in patients with cardiovascular disease, including following acute myocardial infarction. In summary, this study highlighted that the use of class IC antiarrhythmic agents flecainide and encainide for suppression of ventricular ectopy should be avoided in patients post-myocardial infarction, as they carry excess risk of mortality.

In-Depth [randomized controlled trial]: This trial enrolled 1498 patients. Patients with a recent myocardial infarction, ventricular dysfunction, and asymptomatic or mildly symptomatic ventricular arrhythmia were eligible for this study. The study employed an initial open-label titration period to identify patients who responded to at least 1 drug with 80-90% suppression of ventricular arrhythmia. The patients were then randomized to receive either study drug or placebo. The primary end-point was death or cardiac arrest with resuscitation, either of which occurring secondary to arrhythmia. The trial was originally planned to last 3 years, but was discontinued a year early due to results suggesting excess death in the treatment arm. Findings demonstrated that death from arrhythmia was significantly increased in the treatment group receiving flecainide or encainide as compared to those receiving placebo (relative rate (RR) 2.64; 95%CI 1.60-4.36). Mortality from any cause was also significantly more likely in the treatment arms (RR 2.38; 95%CI 1.59-3.57).

Echt DS, Liebson PR, Mitchell LB, Peters RW, Obias-Manno D, Barker AH, et al. Mortality and Morbidity in Patients Receiving Encainide, Flecainide, or Placebo. New England Journal of Medicine. 1991 Mar 21;324(12):781–8.

The V-HeFT II: Enalapril reduces mortality in heart failure when compared to hydralazine and isosorbide

1. In patients with heart failure, patients treated with enalapril experienced significantly lower mortality at 2-years when compared to patients on hydralazine and isosorbide dinitrate.

2. Patients treated with enalapril experienced significantly higher serum creatinine levels and higher potassium levels than patients on the combination of hydralazine and isosorbide dinitrate.

Original Date of Publication: August 1991

Study Rundown: Heart failure is a common condition where the heart cannot pump adequately to meet the body's metabolic demands. It has been estimated that almost 6 million people in the United States suffer from heart failure, and the prevalence continues to rise steadily. Over the past few decades, numerous advances have been made in the treatment of heart failure. The Veterans Administration Cooperative Vasodilator-Heart Failure Trial I (V-HeFT I), completed in 1985, was one of the first randomized trials to demonstrate a mortality benefit with heart failure therapy. It showed that treating heart failure patients with hydralazine and isosorbide dinitrate significantly reduced their mortality when compared with placebo. Subsequently, the CONSENSUS trial demonstrated that enalapril significantly reduced mortality in patients with severe heart failure. This landmark study, th V-HeFT II, sought to directly compare enalapril with the combination of hydralazine and isosorbide dinitrate in patients with heart failure who were also being treated with digoxin and diuretics. In summary, patients being treated with enalapril experienced significantly lower mortality at 2-years when compared with those on hydralazine and isosorbide dinitrate. Over the entire follow-up period, however, there was no significant difference between the 2 groups in terms of all-cause mortality. Despite the mortality benefit, patients being treated with enalapril were significantly more likely to experience rises in serum creatinine levels and had higher potassium levels than patients on the combination.

In-Depth [randomized controlled trial]: This randomized trial was conducted at 13 participating Veterans Affairs medical centers. Patients were eligible for the study if they were between 18 and 75 years old and had evidence of cardiac dysfunction (i.e., cardiothoracic ratio ≥0.55 on chest radiography, left ventricle internal diameter > 2.7 cm/m² of body-surface area at diastole on echocardiography, or ejection fraction < 0.45 on radionuclide imaging) with reduced exercise tolerance. Patients were excluded if they had myocardial infarction or cardiac surgery in the 3 months prior to randomization, angina pectoris limiting exercise or requiring long-term medical therapy, serious obstructive valvular disease, obstructive lung disease, or other diseases to limit life expectancy. Eligible patients were randomized to treatment with enalapril (i.e., starting at 5 mg daily, titrated up to 20 mg daily) or the combination of hydralazine (i.e., starting at 37.5 mg daily, titrated up to 300 mg daily) and isosorbide (i.e., starting at 40 mg daily, titrated up to 160 mg daily). The primary endpoint was 2-year mortality.

A total of 804 patients were enrolled and randomized as part of the trial. Average follow-up time for the trial was 2.5 years (range 0.5-5.7 years). At 2 years, mortality was significantly lower in the enalapril group as compared to those taking hydralazine and isosorbide (p = 0.016). There were no significant differences between the enalapril and hydralazine/isosorbide groups in all-cause mortality for the duration of the study period (32.8% vs. 38.2%, p = 0.08). Further analysis of the mortality data demonstrated significantly lower risk of sudden death without warning (p = 0.015) and with warning (p = 0.032). There were no significant differences between the 2 groups in the rates of hospitalization for heart failure. Patients in the enalapril group experienced significantly higher rates of serum creatinine rise after 1 year (p = 0.02) and significantly higher potassium levels (p < 0.01) than patients treated with hydralazine and isosorbide.

Cohn JN, Johnson G, Ziesche S, Cobb F, Francis G, Tristani F, et al. A comparison of enalapril with hydralazine-isosorbide dinitrate in the treatment of chronic congestive heart failure. The New England Journal of Medicine. 1991;325(5):303-310.

The SOLVD trial: Enalapril reduces mortality in heart failure with reduced ejection fraction

1. Enalapril significantly reduced the risk of all-cause mortality in patients with congestive heart failure (CHF) and reduced left ventricular ejection fraction (LVEF) compared to placebo.

2. Patients being treated with enalapril had a significantly higher risk of developing elevated serum potassium levels and serum creatinine levels.

Original Date of Publication: August 1991

Study Rundown: At the time of the Studies of Left Ventricular Dysfunction (SOLVD) trial, some evidence existed to support that angiotensin converting enzyme (ACE) inhibitors improved hemodynamic stability and reduced mortality in CHF patients. One such study was the CONSENSUS trial, which was published several years before the SOLVD trial. The CONSENSUS trial, however, only included patients with New York Heart Association (NYHA) Class IV CHF. Given the results of prior studies, researchers in the SOLVD trial hypothesized that treatment with an ACE inhibitor would be beneficial to all patients with CHF with reduced ejection fraction, regardless of their NYHA classification. The SOLVD trial demonstrated that treatment with enalapril significantly reduced mortality and frequency of hospitalizations for heart failure in patients with CHF when compared with placebo. Prior to enrollment in the trial, there was a run-in period where participants received enalapril for several days followed by approximately 2 weeks of placebo. This was used as a tool to identify patients who would not tolerate the experimental drug and to assess compliance. This method, however, potentially underestimated the risks of treatment by screening out patients that may have poorly tolerated the drug. It also weakened the external validity of the trial by narrowing the study population of the trial. Nevertheless, this study demonstrated that ACE inhibitor treatment was significant beneficial for patients with all NYHA classes of CHF with reduced ejection fraction.

In-Depth [randomized controlled trial]: This study, conducted at 83 different hospitals in 3 different countries, randomized 2569 patients with LVEF ≤35% to receive either enalapril or placebo. Patients were excluded if they were already taking an ACE inhibitor as part of their CHF management, if they were > 80 years of age, or if they were hemodynamically unstable or had severe co-morbidities, such as unstable angina, recent MI, severe pulmonary disease, or severe chronic kidney disease. A run-in period prior to enrollment in the trial included 2-7 days of enalapril 2.5 mg twice daily to assess for adverse reactions and noncompliance, followed by a 14-17 day placebo phase. Doses of enalapril for the treatment group varied from 2.5-10 mg twice daily and were based on the patient's tolerance of the drug by the participating physician. If a patient's heart failure worsened over the course of the study, the patient was switched over to open-label treatment.

Patients were followed for an average of 41 months. The study outcomes included all-cause mortality, specific causes of mortality, hospitalizations for heart failure, and all hospitalizations. The mortality rate in the treatment group was significantly lower than that of the placebo group (35.2% vs. 39.7%; $p < 0.0036$). The patients in the enalapril group also had a significant decrease in deaths due to progressive heart failure or arrhythmia (16.3% vs. 19.5%; $p < 0.0045$). Post-hoc sub-group analyses showed that enalapril was beneficial in all 4 NYHA classes of CHF. The enalapril group had higher incidence of elevated serum potassium levels (6.4% vs. 2.5%, $p < 0.01$) and creatinine levels (10.7% vs. 7.7%, $p < 0.01$) than the placebo group.

The SOLVD Investigators. Effect of enalapril on survival in patients with reduced left ventricular ejection fractions and congestive heart failure. New England Journal of Medicine. 1991 Aug 1;325(5):293–302.

The SAVE trial: Captopril reduces mortality after acute myocardial infarction

1. Treating patients with captopril after acute myocardial infarction (MI) with asymptomatic left ventricular (LV) dysfunction reduced mortality from cardiovascular causes (i.e., atherosclerotic heart disease, progressive heart failure).

2. The captopril group experienced lower rates of hospitalization due to heart failure and recurrent MI.

Original Date of Publication: September 1992

Study Rundown: The Survival and Ventricular Enlargement (SAVE) trial was a randomized controlled trial that sought to explore the effects of captopril on mortality and morbidity in patients suffering from acute MI and asymptomatic LV dysfunction. In previous animal studies, angiotensin converting enzyme (ACE) inhibitors like captopril were shown to delay ventricular remodeling, and help preserve function after MI. The SAVE trial was the first to demonstrate that treating patients with acute MI and asymptomatic LV dysfunction with an ACE inhibitor reduced morbidity and mortality. These benefits were thought to result from ACE inhibitors slowing the remodeling process that takes place after patients suffer MIs. The findings have since been replicated in other trials (e.g., TRACE trial), systematic reviews, and meta-analyses. In patients suffering from an acute MI and asymptomatic LV dysfunction, early initiation of and continued treatment with captopril can significantly reduce cardiovascular mortality, hospitalization due to heart failure, and recurrent MIs.

In-Depth [randomized controlled trial]: The trial was conducted at 45 centers across North America. A total of 2231 patients took part in the study and were randomized to receive either captopril or placebo. Patients were followed for a minimum of 2 years, though mean follow-up was 42 months. Inclusion criteria were age between 21-80 years, being between 3-16 days away from a recent MI, and LV ejection fraction ≤40% as determined by radionuclide ventriculography. Exclusion criteria included not being randomized within 16 days after an MI, a relative contraindication to ACE inhibitors or need for symptomatic heart failure or hypertension management, serum creatinine > 221 μmol/L (or 2.5 mg/dL), and unstable post-infarction course. The endpoints included all-cause mortality, death from cardiovascular causes, heart failure hospitalization, and rate of recurrent MI.

Patients randomized to receive captopril experienced a significantly reduced all-cause mortality (RRR 19%, 95%CI 3-32%, p = 0.019) and mortality from cardiovascular causes (RRR 21%, 95%CI 5-35%, p = 0.014) compared to the placebo group. Specifically, captopril was associated with significant reductions in mortality from atherosclerotic heart disease and progressive heart failure (RRR 36%, 95%CI 4-58%, p = 0.032). Moreover, the captopril group demonstrated a significant decrease in hospitalization because of heart failure (RRR 22%, 95%CI 4-37%, p = 0.019) and recurrent MIs (RRR 25%, 95%CI 5-40%, p = 0.015) compared to placebo.

Pfeffer MA, Braunwald E, Moyé LA, Basta L, Brown EJ, Cuddy TE, et al. Effect of Captopril on Mortality and Morbidity in Patients with Left Ventricular Dysfunction after Myocardial Infarction. New England Journal of Medicine. 1992 Sep 3;327(10):669–77.

The CARE trial: Pravastatin reduces risk of coronary events

1. Statin therapy reduced the risk of coronary events in patients with known coronary artery disease and low-density lipoprotein levels (LDL) > 125 mg/dL.

2. The reduction in coronary events with statin therapy was found to be greater in women and patients with higher pretreatment LDL levels.

Original Date of Publication: October 1996

Study Rundown: Serum cholesterol levels have long been considered important risk factors for the development of coronary artery disease, and previous studies have demonstrated that lowering cholesterol levels in patients with high cholesterol significantly reduces the risk of coronary events. The Cholesterol and Recurrent Events (CARE) trial examined the effect of lowering LDL levels on the incidence of coronary events in patients with known coronary artery disease and average cholesterol levels. The study demonstrated that treating such patients with pravastatin to lower LDL levels significantly reduced the risk of the composite endpoint of fatal coronary artery disease or nonfatal myocardial infarction when compared to placebo. This difference was driven by a reduction in the rate of nonfatal myocardial infarctions, as there was no significant difference in mortality from coronary artery disease. Notably, women and patients with higher pretreatment LDL levels experienced significantly greater risk reductions than men and patients with lower pretreatment LDL levels, respectively. In summary, this trial supports the use of statin therapy to lower cholesterol levels patients with known coronary artery disease and LDL levels > 125 mg/dL.

In-Depth [randomized controlled trial]: A total of 4159 patients from 80 centers across Canada and the United States were randomized. Patients were eligible if they had an acute myocardial infarction 3-20 months prior to randomization, were between 21-75 years of age, had total cholesterol levels of < 240 mg/dL, had LDL cholesterol levels between 115-174 mg/dL, had fasting triglyceride levels < 350 mg/dL, had fasting glucose levels < 220 mg/dL (12.2 mmol/L), had left ventricular ejection fractions of ≥25%, and did not have symptomatic congestive heart failure. Patients were randomized to receive pravastatin 40 mg daily or placebo and followed for a median of 5.0 years. The primary endpoint was a composite of fatal coronary artery disease or nonfatal myocardial infarction.

Patients treated with pravastatin experienced significantly lower rates of the primary endpoint as compared with patients taking placebo (RR 24%; 95%CI 9-36%). This difference was driven by a significant reduction in nonfatal myocardial infarctions (RR 23%; 95%CI 4-39%), as there was no significant difference in death from coronary artery disease. The risk of revascularization (i.e., coronary artery bypass graft, percutaneous transluminal coronary angioplasty) was significantly lower in patients taking pravastatin (RR 27%; 95%CI 15-37%). Women experienced significantly larger reductions in the risk of coronary events compared to men (p = 0.05 for interaction between sex and outcomes). Of note, results differed according to pretreatment LDL levels. Patients with LDL > 150 mg/dL experienced a larger risk reduction compared to those with LDL between 125-150 mg/dL at baseline (35% vs. 26%, p = 0.03 for interaction between pretreatment LDL and risk reduction).

Sacks FM, Pfeffer MA, Moye LA, Rouleau JL, Rutherford JD, Cole TG, et al. The Effect of Pravastatin on Coronary Events after Myocardial Infarction in Patients with Average Cholesterol Levels. New England Journal of Medicine. 1996 Oct 3;335(14):1001–9.

The DIG trial: Digoxin reduces hospitalization in patients with systolic heart failure

1. **Digoxin significantly reduced hospitalizations in patients with systolic heart failure.**

2. **Digoxin was most beneficial in patients with low ejection fractions (EFs) and poor functional status (NYHA III-IV).**

Original Date of Publication: February 1997

Study Rundown: Digoxin, a cardiac glycoside derived from the extracts of the foxglove plant *Digitalis purpurea*, has a long history of use in the treatment of heart disease. It acts primarily as a positive inotrope by inhibiting the sarcolemmal Na-K ATPase pump and consequently increasing myocardial intracellular calcium concentrations. Prior to the Digitalis Investigation Group (DIG) trial, digoxin was commonly prescribed for patients with heart failure with the intention of improving contractility and thus cardiac output. There was no substantial evidence, however, suggesting that the use of digoxin improved long-term outcomes in patients with heart failure. This landmark randomized controlled trial enrolled 6800 patients and sought to examine the long-term effects of digoxin on mortality and hospitalization in patients suffering from systolic heart failure.

The DIG trial provided evidence that digoxin significantly reduced the number of hospitalizations in patients with heart failure. This effect was greatest for those with low ejections fractions and poor functional status. Although the study did not show any mortality benefit, digoxin was not linked to increased mortality, as had been demonstrated with other positive inotropes. This study indicated that to reduce hospitalizations, the addition of digoxin should be considered for patients with systolic heart failure (EF < 0.45) who continue to have poor functional status (NYHA III-IV) and are already optimized on a beta-blocker and angiotensin converting enzyme inhibitor.

In-Depth [randomized controlled trial]: This trial was conducted at 302 clinical centers in the United States and Canada. Patients were eligible for the trial if they had heart failure with left ventricular EF $\leq$ 0.45 and were in normal sinus rhythm. Included patients were randomized to either receive digoxin or placebo. The primary outcome studied was death from any cardiovascular cause.

Secondary outcomes included hospitalization or death from worsening of heart failure. A total of 6800 patients were randomized as part of the trial. There was no significant difference in mortality from any cause between the digoxin and placebo groups (RR 0.99; 95%CI 0.91-1.07; p = 0.80). Patients in the digoxin group, however, were significantly less likely to be hospitalized for worsening of heart failure (RR 0.72; 95%CI 0.66-0.79; p < 0.001). Subgroup analysis showed that the benefit of digoxin on a combined outcome of mortality and hospitalization for heart failure was greatest in patients with low ejection fractions (EF < 0.25) and functional status (NYHA III-IV).

The Digitalis Investigation Group. The Effect of Digoxin on Mortality and Morbidity in Patients with Heart Failure. New England Journal of Medicine. 1997 Feb 20;336(8):525–33.

The MERIT-HF trial: Metoprolol reduces mortality in patients with symptomatic heart failure

1. In patients with symptomatic heart failure and reduced ejection fraction, the addition of metoprolol to standard therapy reduced all-cause mortality by 34% compared to placebo.

2. Similar findings were reported in the CIBIS-II trial.

Original Date of Publication: June 1999

Study Rundown: This trial investigated effect of adding metoprolol to standard therapy in the treatment of patients with decreased ejection fraction and symptomatic heart failure. Adding metoprolol controlled/extended release to standard optimum therapy (i.e., a diuretic and angiotensin converting enzyme (ACE) inhibitor reduced all-cause mortality by 34% in patients with symptomatic heart failure compared to placebo. Another study published around the same time, the Cardiac Insufficiency Bisoprolol Study II (CIBIS-II), reported similar findings. Of note, the study was funded by grants from a pharmaceutical company. In summary, adding metoprolol controlled release/extended release to optimum standard therapy in symptomatic heart failure (NYHA class II-IV) reduces all-cause mortality.

In-Depth [randomized controlled trial]: A total of 3991 patients were enrolled in the study and randomized to receive either metoprolol controlled release/extended release (12.5 mg for NYHA class III-IV, 25 mg for NYHA class II) once daily or placebo. The study was conducted at 313 sites in 13 European countries and the United States. Patients were included if they had symptomatic heart failure (i.e., New York Heart Association functional class II-IV) for at least 3 months, a left ventricular ejection fraction less than 0.40 in the 3 months before enrollment, a stable clinical condition in the 2 week run-in phase for the study, and were taking optimum standard therapy (i.e., combination of diuretics and ACE inhibitor).The trial was stopped early on the recommendation of the independent safety committee, as the predefined criterion for ending the study had been met. There was a significant reduction in all-cause mortality in the metoprolol group compared to the placebo group, with a relative risk of 0.66 (95%CI 0.53-0.81). Specifically, there were significantly fewer cardiovascular deaths, sudden deaths, and deaths from aggravated heart failure in the metoprolol group.

MERIT-HF Study Group. Effect of metoprolol CR/XL in chronic heart failure: Metoprolol CR/XL Randomised Intervention Trial in-Congestive Heart Failure (MERIT-HF). The Lancet. 1999 Jun 12;353(9169):2001–7.

The RALES trial: Spironolactone reduces mortality in heart failure patients

1. Adding 25 mg of spironolactone to standard therapy reduced all-cause mortality in heart failure patients with an ejection fraction < 35%.

Original Date of Publication: September 1999

Study Rundown: Progression of heart failure is thought to be related to physiological neuroendocrine compensation of the body to decreased effective circulating volume - the activation of the sympathetic and renin-angiotensin-aldosterone system, which lead to myocardial remodeling and subsequent progressive reduction in cardiac output. The Randomized Aldactone Evaluation Study (RALES) trial looked at the latter system, particularly the role of aldosterone blockade in treating heart failure. At the time of this study's completion, there was controversy amongst physicians in using aldosterone-inhibitors, like spironolactone, for the treatment of heart failure as it was assumed that angiotensin converting enzyme (ACE) inhibitors, which were well established as standard of care for the condition, already offered effective aldosterone blockade by inhibiting its production. Furthermore, many clinicians exhibited caution in using spironolactone, as it was thought that adding this medication to standard therapy would increase the risk of serious hyperkalemia. Increasing evidence, however, suggested that ACE inhibitors did not effectively suppress the production of aldosterone in the long-term. Thus, the RALES trail was launched in order to investigate the role of aldosterone-receptor antagonism in the treatment of advanced heart failure. Specifically, the trial sought to determine whether spironolactone would reduce mortality in patients with advanced heart failure, who were already on standard medical therapy.

This landmark study supported the use of spironolactone, in addition to standard medical therapy, to reduce mortality and hospitalizations in patients with heart failure. Based upon the study's findings, aldosterone antagonism with spironolactone should be considered for patients with a left ventricular ejection fraction (LVEF) < 35% and New York Heart Association (NYHA) Class III-IV symptoms, despite optimization of standard therapy. A subsequent study conducted in 2004 demonstrated an abrupt increase in the prescription of spironolactone after the publication of the RALES trial, and showed a rapid rise in morbidity and mortality associated with hyperkalemia. Thus, calls were made for closer monitoring of patients being prescribed spironolactone.

In-Depth [randomized controlled trial]: The study involved 1663 patients from 195 centers in 15 countries. Inclusion criteria were functional NYHA class III-IV, LVEF < 35%, and current treatment with standard therapy (i.e., ACE inhibitor and loop diuretic). Most patients were also on digoxin. Patients were randomly assigned to either the treatment arm (i.e., standard therapy and spironolactone 25-50 mg daily) or the placebo arm (i.e., standard therapy and placebo). The trial was scheduled to run for 3 years, but was discontinued early at 24 months due to the clear benefit of spironolactone. Patients treated with spironolactone experienced significantly lower mortality than those treated with placebo (RR 0.70; 95%CI 0.60-0.82; p < 0.001), which was driven by significantly lower rates of death due to progressive heart failure and sudden cardiac death. The spironolactone group also had significantly lower rates of hospitalization for worsening heart failure (RR 0.65; 95%CI 0.54-0.77; p < 0.001). The rates of gynecomastia and breast pain were significantly higher in the spironolactone group (p < 0.001), while there was no difference between the groups in the risk of serious hyperkalemia.

Pitt B, Zannad F, Remme WJ, Cody R, Castaigne A, Perez A, et al. The Effect of Spironolactone on Morbidity and Mortality in Patients with Severe Heart Failure. New England Journal of Medicine. 1999 Sep 2;341(10):709–17.

The ATLAS trial: Angiotensin converting enzyme inhibitor dosing in chronic heart failure

1. When compared to a lower dose, high-dose angiotensin converting enzyme (ACE) inhibitors were associated with a significantly reduced risk of hospitalization or death in patients with chronic heart failure.

Original Date of Publication: December 1999

Study Rundown: At the time, physicians often prescribed ACE inhibitors to patients with chronic heart failure in lower doses than proven effective by large-scale studies. Nonetheless, convincing research on the comparative benefits of high dose and low dose ACE inhibitors was severely lacking. The Assessment of Treatment with Lisinopril and Survival (ATLAS) trial randomized 3164 patients to receive low- or high-dose of the ACE inhibitor lisinopril for 29-58 months. This study demonstrated that compared with those in the low-dose group, patients in the high-dose treatment group experienced a significantly lower risk of death or hospitalization for any reason. The high-dose group also had significantly fewer hospitalizations for heart failure. These findings suggested that patients with heart failure due to left ventricular systolic dysfunction should not be maintained on low doses of ACE inhibitor unless they are intolerant of higher doses. Rather, tolerant patients should be placed on a higher doses of ACE inhibitors due to increased effectiveness.

In-Depth [randomized controlled trial]: The ATLAS study randomly assigned 3164 patients with New York Heart Association (NYHA) class II to IV heart failure and an ejection fraction of $\leq 30\%$ to treatment with either a high-dose (32.5-35 mg daily) or low-dose (2.5-5.0 mg daily) of lisinopril, an ACE inhibitor. The trial was conducted in 287 hospitals across 19 countries. The duration of follow-up ranged from 39 to 58 months.

The trial found that patients randomized to receive high-dose lisinopril experienced a 12% lower risk of hospitalization or death for any reason (p = 0.002) and 24% fewer hospitalizations for heart failure (p = 0.002) as compared to patients in the low-dose group. Patients in the high-dose group did experience dizziness and renal insufficiency more frequently. However, these side effects did not lead to lower compliance with medication in the high-dose group.

Packer M, Poole-Wilson PA, Armstrong PW, Cleland JGF, Horowitz JD, Massie BM, et al. Comparative Effects of Low and High Doses of the Angiotensin-Converting Enzyme Inhibitor, Lisinopril, on Morbidity and Mortality in Chronic Heart Failure. Circulation. 1999 Dec 7;100(23):2312–8.

The HOPE trial: Ramipril reduces cardiovascular events in high-risk patients with normal ejection fractions

1. **Ramipril significantly reduced the risk of cardiovascular events including myocardial infarction, stroke and death in high risk-patients without left ventricular dysfunction.**

Original Date of Publication: January 2000

Study Rundown: Prior to the publication of the Heart Outcomes Prevention Evaluation (HOPE) trial, the benefit of angiotensin converting enzyme (ACE) inhibitors had been well established in improving long-term outcomes for patients with heart failure associated with reduced left ventricular ejection fraction. There was also evidence of the value of these medications in controlling blood pressure, particularly in diabetic patients with microalbuminuria. At the time, however, there was limited evidence as to whether ACE inhibitors provided any cardiovascular protection in the absence of left ventricular dysfunction. That is, there was uncertainty as to whether the blockade of the renin-angiotensin system offered any inherent benefit in improving cardiac outcomes in high-risk populations, independent of its effect on blood pressure or preventing the progression of systolic heart failure. This landmark study evaluated the effect of ramipril on major cardiovascular events in high-risk patients over 55 years old with normal ejection fractions.

This trial was the first to provide evidence for the potential benefit of ACE inhibitors for vascular protection in preventing adverse cardiac outcomes among a broad range of high-risk patients with normal ejection fractions. Patients assigned to receive ramipril had significantly less cardiovascular-related complications. After its publication, there was some criticism that the blood pressure lowering effect of ramipril may have accounted for the improved cardiac outcomes, as opposed to the medication itself. However, most patients did not have baseline hypertension in this study and the difference in blood pressure between the 2 groups was minor. Even in the absence of reduced ejection fraction or high blood pressure, the addition of ramipril for high-risk patients at least 55 years of age may be considered for protection against adverse cardiovascular outcomes and death.

In-Depth [randomized controlled study]: This large, double-blind, randomized control study included 9541 patients from 281 centers internationally. Inclusion criteria were age ≥55 years, a history of coronary artery disease, stroke, peripheral vascular disease, or diabetes, and one additional cardiovascular risk factor (e.g., hypertension, dyslipidemia, cigarette smoking, documented microalbuminuria). Patients with known low ejection fraction (EF < 40%), history of heart failure, or who were already on an ACE inhibitor were excluded from this study. Patients were randomized to either receive 1) placebo or 2) ramipril titrated up to 10 mg daily. Primary outcome was a composite of myocardial infarction, stroke, or death from cardiovascular causes.

The trial lasted a total of 5 years. The rate of the primary outcome was significantly lower in patients being treated with ramipril as compared with placebo (RR 0.78; 95%CI 0.70-0.86). This finding held true among a broad range of patients in this study. Subgroup analysis showed that the benefit of ramipril was consistent despite sex, age, cardiac risk factors, presence of diabetes, evidence of cardiovascular disease, baseline blood pressure, or evidence of microalbuminuria. The most common adverse effect of ramipril was cough.

Yusuf S, Sleight P, Pogue J, Bosch J, Davies R, Dagenais G. Effects of an angiotensin-converting-enzyme inhibitor, ramipril, on cardiovascular events in high-risk patients. The Heart Outcomes Prevention Evaluation Study Investigators. New England Journal of Medicine. 2000 Jan 20;342(3):145–53.

The MIRACL trial: Atorvastatin reduces recurrent ischemia after acute coronary syndrome

1. In patients with a recent acute coronary syndrome (ACS), atorvastatin 80 mg daily reduced the risk of recurrent ischemia.

2. This study did not demonstrate a significant reduction in death, cardiac arrest, or nonfatal acute myocardial infarction with statin therapy, as compared to placebo.

Original Date of Publication: April 2001

Study Rundown: Previous studies had demonstrated that reducing cholesterol levels with statins was linked to a reduction in the risk of mortality and cardiac events. The Myocardial Ischemia Reduction with Aggressive Cholesterol Lowering (MIRACL) trial demonstrated that providing atorvastatin 80 mg daily 24-96 hours after the onset of an ACS reduced the risk of recurrent ischemia as compared to placebo. In summary, treating patients with ACS with atorvastatin was associated with a significant reduction in the risk of recurrent symptomatic myocardial ischemia requiring rehospitalization in the 16 weeks following an ACS. Given that this was a large, international, multicenter trial, the findings are generalizable to patients with ACS in different settings, with different ethnicities and risk profiles. Based on these findings, statins are commonly prescribed for patients who have suffered acute coronary syndromes, in hopes of reducing the risk of recurrent ischemia.

In-Depth [randomized controlled trial]: The MIRACL trial enrolled 3086 patients from 122 centers in Europe, North America, South Africa, and Australasia. Patients were eligible if they were ≥18 years of age and had chest pain > 15 minutes duration in the 24 hours prior to presentation. Exclusion criteria included serum cholesterol levels > 270 mg/dL (7 mmol/L), plans for coronary revascularization at the time of screening, evidence of Q-wave myocardial infarction (MI) in the past 4 weeks, and coronary artery bypass surgery in the past 3 months. Patients were randomized to receive atorvastatin 80 mg daily or placebo for 16 weeks after an ACS. The primary endpoint was a composite of death, cardiac arrest, nonfatal acute MI, or recurrent symptomatic myocardial ischemia requiring emergency rehospitalization.

At 16 weeks, patients receiving atorvastatin had significantly lower rates of the composite endpoint compared to those taking placebo (RR 0.84; 95%CI 0.70-1.00, p = 0.048), with an absolute risk reduction of 2.6% (NNT = 38). Notably, there was no significant difference between the groups in the risk of death, nonfatal acute MI, or cardiac arrest. The difference in the primary endpoint was due to a reduction in the risk of recurrent symptomatic myocardial ischemia (RR 0.74; 95%CI 0.57-0.95). The risk of abnormal liver transaminase levels was significantly higher in the atorvastatin group (2.5% vs. 0.6%, p < 0.001).

Schwartz GG, Olsson AG, Ezekowitz MD, et al. Effects of atorvastatin on early recurrent ischemic events in acute coronary syndromes: The miracl study: a randomized controlled trial. JAMA. 2001 Apr 4;285(13):1711–8.

The CHADS2 score: Stroke risk in atrial fibrillation

1. The CHADS2 index was an accurate predictor of stroke in patients with non-rheumatic atrial fibrillation.

2. Presently, CHADS2 scores are used to aid decisions regarding the need for anti-thrombotic therapy.

Original Date of Publication: June 2001

Study Rundown: The CHADS2 index combined risk factors identified in the Atrial Fibrillation Investigators (AFI) and the Stroke Prevention and Atrial Fibrillation (SPAF) investigations to create a new clinical prediction model for stroke in patients with atrial fibrillation. This study validated the 3 tools and found that CHADS2 predicts stroke with greater accuracy than both the AFI and SPAF schemes. CHADS2 scores may be used to guide decisions regarding the need for anti-thrombotic therapy (i.e., aspirin for low-risk patients, warfarin for high-risk patients), particularly in identifying low-risk patients who may benefit from aspirin therapy. Strengths of the study include wide representation of regions within the United States and generalizability of results to frail, elderly patients. The CHADS2 index includes a limited set of risk factors for stroke and may neglect other important risk factors.

In-Depth [randomized controlled trial]: This study evaluated the predictive accuracy of the AFI and SPAF stroke classification schemes, as well as the CHADS2 index, a new stroke-risk prediction model created by combining the AFI and SPAF schemes. CHADS2 is an acronym for the risk factors considered and their score value. One point is assigned for any of the following risk factors: recent congestive heart failure, hypertension, age ≥ 75 years, and diabetes mellitus. Two points were added if there is a history of stroke or transient ischemic attack.

Risk factor	Points
Congestive heart failure	1
Hypertension	1
Age ≥75 years	1
Diabetes mellitus	1
Stroke or transient ischemic attack	2

Table I. Risk factors and score values

The study included 1733 patients between ages 65 to 95 years with non-rheumatic atrial fibrillation. Stroke rate increased by a factor of 1.5 for each 1-point increment in CHADS2 score ($p < 0.001$) and the CHADS2 index was found to predict stroke with greater accuracy than both the AFI and SPAF schemes with a c statistic of 0.82.

CHADS2 score	Stroke rate per 100 patient-years
0	1.9
1	2.8
2	4.0
3	5.9
4	8.5
5	12.5
6	18.2

Table II. CHADS2-score and stroke rate per 100 patient years

Gage BF, Waterman AD, Shannon W, Boechler M, Rich MW, Radford MJ. Validation of clinical classification schemes for predicting stroke: Results from the national registry of atrial fibrillation. JAMA. 2001 Jun 13;285(22):2864–70.

The REMATCH trial: Left ventricular assist devices reduce mortality in heart failure

1. In patients with end-stage heart failure on optimal medical therapy, treatment with a left ventricular assist device (LVAD) significantly reduced the risk of all-cause mortality when compared with medical therapy alone.

2. The difference in mortality was observed at 1 year, while no significant differences were observed at the 2-year mark.

Original Date of Publication: November 2001

Study Rundown: In patients with severe heart failure, cardiac transplantation has been shown to provide considerable benefit, though the supply of donor hearts is incredibly limited and has been approximated at about 3000 per year. As a result, much research has focused on mechanical means of improving myocardial function, and several such LVADs have been developed through the National Institutes of Health artificial-heart program. Several devices have been previously approved by the Food and Drug Administration as bridging therapy to transplantation, though none have been studied as long-term alternatives to transplantation. The Randomized Evaluation of Mechanical Assistance for the Treatment of Congestive Heart Failure (REMATCH) trial explored whether a specific type of LVAD, when used in the long-term, would reduce mortality in patients with end-stage heart failure who are not eligible for cardiac transplantation when compared with optimal medical therapy. In summary, this study found that treating end-stage heart failure patients with this LVAD significantly reduced the risk of mortality 1-year after randomization, though this difference was no longer seen at the 2-year mark.

In-Depth [randomized controlled trial]: This trial was conducted at 20 cardiac transplantation centers across the United States. A total of 129 patients were randomized to treatment with either LVAD or optimal medical therapy. Adults with chronic end-stage heart failure were eligible for the trial. End-stage heart failure was defined as New York Heart Association (NYHA) class IV symptoms for at least 90 days, left ventricular ejection fraction (LVEF) < 25%, peak oxygen consumption < 12 mL/kg/min or continued need for intravenous inotropes for symptomatic hypotension, or worsening renal function/pulmonary congestion. The inclusion criteria were subsequently broadened, though only 5 patients were included under these broader criteria. The primary endpoint was all-cause mortality.

The study was terminated when the predetermined threshold of 92 deaths was reached. The risk of mortality was significantly lower in the group that received LVAD when compared to those on medical therapy (RR 0.52; 95%CI 0.34-0.78). The Kaplan-Meier estimates of survival demonstrated significantly reduced mortality in the LVAD group at the 1-year mark (p = 0.002), though this difference was not significant at the 2-year mark (p = 0.09). Patients in the LVAD group were significantly more likely to experience a serious adverse event compared to those on medical therapy (RR 2.35; 95%CI 1.86-2.95), including nonneurologic bleeding, neurologic dysfunction, supraventricular arrhythmia, and peripheral embolic events.

Rose EA, Gelijns AC, Moskowitz AJ, Heitjan DF, Stevenson LW, Dembitsky W, et al. Long-term use of a left ventricular assist device for end-stage heart failure. The New England Journal of Medicine. 2001;345(20):1435-1443.

The Val-HeFT trial: Valsartan reduces morbidity in chronic heart failure

1. Valsartan, an angiotensin-receptor blocker (ARB), reduced morbidity, but not mortality, in heart failure patients when added to background therapy.

2. As an exception, valsartan was associated with increased morbidity and mortality in patients already receiving both an angiotensin converting enzyme (ACE) inhibitor and beta-blocker.

Original Date of Publication: December 2001

Study Rundown: Angiotensin II contributes to cardiac remodeling that leads to decreased left ventricular function and progressive heart failure. At the time of the study in 2001, ACE inhibitors and beta-blockers were the standard therapies for heart failure. This study demonstrated that treatment with the ARB valsartan in addition to previously prescribed therapy could further decrease patient morbidity. Patient mortality, however, was not significantly different when compared to placebo, and valsartan was linked to increased morbidity and mortality in the subgroup of patients already receiving both an ACE inhibitor and beta-blocker. The study's results do not generalize to patients already receiving ARBs, who were excluded from this study. Additionally, approximately 90% of the study's participants were white. In the study's black population, consisting of African American and South African patients, the effect of valsartan was not statistically significant. Finally, valsartan was associated with only a moderate increase in ejection fraction when compared with other prior trials involving ACE inhibitors and beta-blockers. In summary, the Val-HeFT trial demonstrated an important role for ARBs in the management of heart failure.

In-Depth [randomized controlled trial]: This randomized, double-blinded, placebo-controlled, trial involved 302 centers in 16 countries. A total of 5010 patients with documented left ventricular dilatation and at least 2 weeks of treatment with ACE inhibitors, diuretics, digoxin, or beta-blockers were stratified according to previously prescribed beta-blocker treatment and randomized to receive valsartan or placebo. Two primary endpoints were measured: 1) mortality alone and 2) the combined endpoint of mortality and morbidity (defined as cardiac arrest with resuscitation, hospitalization for heart failure, etc.). The combined endpoint of mortality and morbidity was significantly lower with valsartan (RR 0.87; 97.5%CI 0.77-0.97) than placebo, which was attributed to a decreased number of hospitalizations for heart failure (p < 0.001). There was no significant difference in mortality alone (RR 1.02; 98%CI 0.88-1.18).

Cohn JN, Tognoni G. A Randomized Trial of the Angiotensin-Receptor Blocker Valsartan in Chronic Heart Failure. New England Journal of Medicine. 2001 Dec 6;345(23):1667–75.

The MADIT-II: Prophylactic defibrillators reduce mortality in left ventricular dysfunction

1. There was a 31% reduction in the risk of death associated with implantation of a defibrillator in patients with a previous myocardial infarction and left ventricular dysfunction, when compared to conventional therapy.

2. Rates of hospitalization for heart failure were not significantly elevated in the defibrillator group.

Original Date of Publication: March 2002

Study Rundown: The Multicenter Automatic Defibrillator Implantation Trial II Investigators (MADIT-II) examined the potential survival benefit of an implantable defibrillator in patients with a previous myocardial infarction and left ventricular dysfunction (without requiring patients to undergo electrophysiological testing for inducible arrhythmias). The results indicated that an implantable defibrillator may significantly improve outcomes along with appropriate drug therapy. Of note, a slightly higher rate of hospitalization with heart failure was observed in the defibrillator group, though this did not reach statistical significance. Further investigations, including electrophysiologic testing, as inclusion criteria may help to determine the specific groups for whom implantation of a defibrillator would be most beneficial with minimal risk. In summary, the findings of this trial determined that implantation of a defibrillator should be considered in patients with myocardial infarction and reduced ejection fraction as a prophylactic measure for sudden cardiac death.

In-Depth [randomized controlled trial]: The trial assessed the survival benefit of prophylactic defibrillator implantation in patients with a previous myocardial infarction and an ejection fraction of ≤0.30. A total of 1232 patients were assigned to receive an implantable defibrillator or to conventional medical therapy in a 3:2 ratio. After an average follow-up of 20 months, the trial found a significant 31% reduction in risk of death in the defibrillator group compared to the conventional therapy group (HR 0.69; 95%CI 0.51-0.93, $p = 0.016$). Subgroup analyses did not reveal any differences in this effect based on a number of factors, including age, gender, ejection fraction, and QRS interval. Serious complications associated with defibrillator therapy were uncommon. A slightly higher, though nonsignificant, rate of hospitalization with heart failure in the defibrillator group compared to conventional therapy.

Moss AJ, Zareba W, Hall WJ, Klein H, Wilber DJ, Cannom DS, et al. Prophylactic Implantation of a Defibrillator in Patients with Myocardial Infarction and Reduced Ejection Fraction. New England Journal of Medicine. 2002 Mar 21;346(12):877–83.

The COPERNICUS trial: Carvedilol reduces mortality in severe chronic heart failure

1. Adding carvedilol to the management of patients with severe heart failure was associated with a significant, 35% relative risk reduction in mortality.

2. In this patient population, carvedilol was also associated with significantly reduced risks of hospitalization and serious adverse effects, as well as improvement in symptoms.

Original Date of Publication: October 2002

Study Rundown: The landmark Carvedilol Prospective Randomized Cumulative Survival (COPERNICUS) trial provided further support to the already established and growing body of evidence supporting the use of beta-blockers in the treatment of heart failure. Prior to COPERNICUS, the randomized controlled trials MOCHA and PRECISE had demonstrated that carvedilol was associated with reductions in mortality and hospitalizations for patients with mild-moderate heart failure. The COPERNICUS trial investigated the benefit of carvedilol in patients with severe heart failure, defined as New York Heart Association (NYHA) class III-IV and a left ventricular ejection fraction (LVEF) < 25%. Results from this randomized, placebo-controlled trial showed that carvedilol therapy was associated with a 35% relative risk reduction in mortality. For this reason, the study was terminated 1 year early. Carvedilol was also associated with a similar reduction in the combined risk of death or hospitalization for cardiovascular reasons/heart failure. Patients receiving carvedilol were also significantly more likely to report improvement in symptoms. Furthermore, carvedilol was associated with significantly reduced risk of serious adverse events, including heart failure, sudden death, cardiogenic shock and ventricular tachycardia.

In-Depth [randomized controlled trial]: The COPERNICUS enrolled 2289 patients. Patients were eligible for the study if they reported symptoms of dyspnea or fatigue at minimal exertion and had a LVEF< 25%. These patients were optimized medically on a diuretic and an angiotensin converting enzyme (ACE) inhibitor or angiotensin receptor II blocker (ARB) upon entry to the study. Digitalis, spironolactone, amiodarone and vasodilators were permitted but not required for eligibility. Study patients were randomized to receive either 1) carvedilol titrated to a target dose of 25mg twice per day or 2) placebo. The primary endpoint studied was all-cause mortality. Secondary endpoints were combined risk of death or hospitalization, either due to cardiovascular reason or heart failure, as well as improvement or worsening of symptoms by global patient assessment. Serious adverse events were also studied.

While the study was terminated a year early, patients were followed for a mean of 10.4 months. Results showed that risk of mortality was significantly reduced for those patients receiving carvedilol (12.8% vs. 19.7%, $p = 0.00013$). Carvedilol therapy was also associated with significantly reduced rates of hospitalization for heart failure (17.1% vs. 23.7%, $p = 0.0001$) or for any reason (32.2% vs. 38.1%, $p = 0.003$). These effects were consistent in the subgroup analysis, which included sex, age, location, left ventricular function, as well etiology of heart failure (i.e., ischemic vs. non-ischemic). In the global patient assessment, significantly more patients reported moderate to marked improvement in symptoms and were less likely to show moderate to marked worsening. Significantly fewer patients in the carvedilol group experienced serious adverse events, such as worsening of heart failure ($p < 0.0001$), sudden death ($p = 0.016$), cardiogenic shock ($p = 0.003$) and ventricular tachycardia ($p = 0.019$), as compared to the placebo group.

Packer M, Fowler MB, Roecker EB, Coats AJS, Katus HA, Krum H, et al. Effect of Carvedilol on the Morbidity of Patients With Severe Chronic Heart Failure Results of the Carvedilol Prospective Randomized Cumulative Survival (COPERNICUS) Study. Circulation. 2002 Oct 22;106(17):2194–9.

The ALLHAT: Thiazide diuretics as first-line antihypertensive therapy

1. There were no significant differences in the rates of fatal coronary artery disease or nonfatal myocardial infarction when comparing thiazide diuretics with angiotensin converting enzyme (ACE) inhibitors or calcium channel blockers (CCBs) for hypertension management.

Original Date of Publication: December 2002

Study Rundown: Hypertension is considered a major risk factor for cardiovascular disease and blood pressure control is an international priority. Some studies have estimated that 26.4% of the global population suffered from hypertension in 2000, and this number is expected to increase to 29.2% in 2025, affecting an estimated 1.56 billion people. While antihypertensive medication therapy has been shown to reduce the risk of adverse outcomes in hypertensive patients, there are many antihypertensive agents available and questions remained regarding the best choice for initial therapy. The earliest studies demonstrated benefits associated with using thiazides and beta-blockers (BB), though many new agents were subsequently introduced into practice, including ACE inhibitors and CCBs. The Antihypertensive and Lipid-Lowering Treatment to Prevent Heart Attack Trial (ALLHAT) focused specifically on high-risk patients - it sought to determine whether there were significant differences in rates of cardiovascular events when using different first-line antihypertensive agents, such as ACE inhibitors (i.e., lisinopril), CCBs (i.e., amlodipine), alpha-blockers (i.e., doxazosin), and thiazides (i.e., chlorthalidone). The alpha-blocker arm was terminated early, as chlorthalidone was found to be superior to doxazosin. In summary, there were no significant differences in the rates of fatal coronary artery disease (CHD) or nonfatal myocardial infarction when comparing chlorthalidone with amlodipine or lisinopril for hypertension management. Because thiazide diuretics are often cheaper than other options, it was recommended that they be considered first-line therapy for hypertension based on the findings of this study.

In-Depth [randomized controlled trial]: The study involved 33 357 participants and had a mean follow-up of 4.9 years. Patients were eligible for the study if they were ≥55 years of age and had stage 1 or 2 hypertension with ≥1 additional risk factor (i.e., previous myocardial infarction, stroke, left ventricular hypertrophy, type 2 diabetes, current cigarette smoking, low high-density lipoprotein). Exclusion criteria were a history of heart failure and/or left ventricular ejection fraction < 35%. The primary outcome was fatal CHD or nonfatal myocardial infarction, while the secondary outcomes were all-cause mortality, fatal/nonfatal stroke, combined CHD, and combined cardiovascular disease.

Chlorthalidone was found to be superior to doxazosin, and the alpha-blocker arm was terminated early. In the comparison between amlodipine and chlorthalidone, there were no significant differences in the primary (RR 0.98; 95%CI 0.90-1.07) or secondary outcomes. Amlodipine, however, was associated with a significantly higher risk of heart failure, particularly hospitalized/fatal heart failure ($p < 0.001$). The comparison between lisinopril and chlorthalidone again demonstrated no significant differences in the primary (RR 0.99; 95%CI 0.91-1.08) or secondary outcomes; but, lisinopril use was associated with significantly elevated risk of stroke, combined cardiovascular disease, heart failure, hospitalized/treated angina, and coronary revascularization. Moreover, participants in the lisinopril group had significantly higher follow-up systolic blood pressure.

The ALLHAT Officers and Coordinators for the ALLHAT Collaborative Research Group. Major outcomes in high-risk hypertensive patients randomized to angiotensin-converting enzyme inhibitor or calcium channel blocker vs diuretic: The antihypertensive and lipid-lowering treatment to prevent heart attack trial (allhat). JAMA. 2002 Dec 18;288(23):2981–97.

The AFFIRM trial: Rate-control vs. rhythm-control in atrial fibrillation

1. Compared to rhythm-control, rate-control resulted in a lower incidence of adverse events and no significant difference in mortality in patients with atrial fibrillation.

Original Date of Publication: December 2002

Study Rundown: The Atrial Fibrillation Follow-up Investigation of Rhythm Management (AFFIRM) trial compared two common strategies for managing atrial fibrillation: rhythm-control and rate-control. Patients were anticoagulated in both approaches to address the increased risk of thromboembolic disease in atrial fibrillation. Prior to this study, both rhythm-control and rate-control were considered acceptable strategies, though rhythm-control was often the initial therapy. Rhythm-control involves the use of cardioversion and antiarrhythmic medications to maintain normal sinus rhythm, and this was thought to have benefits of lowering the stroke risk and allowing anticoagulation therapy to be discontinued. At the time of this study's publication, proponents of the rate-control method argued that rate-control medications were far less toxic than antiarrhythmics, and that there were likely no differences between the methods in terms of patient-important outcomes.

To address this conflict, the AFFIRM trial was designed to assess the differences in long-term outcomes associated with these 2 treatment approaches. Patients in the rhythm-control group could be treated with specific antiarrhythmic agents or cardioversion, as decided by their treating physician. Rate-controlled patients were managed using beta blockers (BBs), calcium channel blockers (CCBs), digoxin, or a combination of these medications. In summary, there was no significant difference between the groups in mortality or the rate of the composite secondary endpoint of death, disabling stroke, disabling anoxic encephalopathy, major bleeding, and cardiac arrest. The risk of torsade de pointes, cardiac arrest, and hospitalization, however, were significantly higher in the rhythm-control group.

In-Depth [randomized controlled trial]: A total of 4060 patients were enrolled in the trial and followed for a mean of 3.5 years. They were randomized to the rhythm-control strategy (i.e., treatment with antiarrhythmic medications) or the rate-control strategy (i.e., controlling heart rate with BBs, CCBs and digoxin). Patients were included if they were ≥65 years of age, they had atrial fibrillation that was likely to be recurrent, long-term treatment of their atrial fibrillation was warranted, and they were eligible for anticoagulation therapy. The primary endpoint was mortality. The secondary endpoint was a composite of death, disabling stroke, disabling anoxic encephalopathy, major bleeding, and cardiac arrest. There was no significant difference in mortality between the groups (HR 1.15; 95%CI 0.99-1.34). The rate of the secondary endpoint was also not significantly different between the two groups. There was a significantly higher incidence of torsade de pointes, cardiac arrest (i.e., pulseless electrical activity, bradycardia, or other rhythm), and hospitalization after baseline in the rhythm-control group compared to the rate-control group. It was also demonstrated that individuals in the rhythm-control group experienced significantly higher incidence of adverse drug events, including pulmonary events, gastrointestinal events, bradycardia, and prolongation of the QT interval ($p < 0.001$). There was no significant difference between the groups in the incidence of stroke.

Wyse DG, Waldo AL, DiMarco JP, Domanski MJ, Rosenberg Y, Schron EB, et al. A comparison of rate control and rhythm control in patients with atrial fibrillation. New England Journal of Medicine. 2002 Dec 5;347(23):1825–33.

The EPHESUS: Eplerenone reduces mortality in heart failure after myocardial infarction

1. Eplerenone reduced all-cause mortality in patients with heart failure and left ventricular dysfunction (LVEF ≤40%) after myocardial infarction (MI) compared with placebo.

2. Eplerenone treatment in this setting significantly reduced mortality from cardiovascular causes and hospitalizations for cardiovascular issues.

Original Date of Publication: April 2003

Study Rundown: At the time of the Eplerenone Post-Acute Myocardial Infarction Heart Failure Efficacy and Survival Study (EPHESUS), aldosterone blockade was linked to a reduced mortality in severe systolic heart failure (as demonstrated in the RALES trial) and prevented ventricular remodeling in patients after an acute MI. It was hypothesized that starting a mineralocorticoid antagonist after an acute MI would be beneficial, and the EPHESUS was designed to test this proposition. In summary, the trial demonstrated that treatment with eplerenone 3-14 days after an acute MI significantly reduced mortality and the rate of hospitalization for heart failure. It has been noted that EPHESUS started randomization several months after data from the RALES trial was published, and one criticism that has been leveled at the EPHESUS was regarding their choice of mineralocorticoid antagonist. While the rates of gynecomastia have been lower with eplerenone as compared with spironolactone, the costs of treatment with eplerenone are considerably higher. Moreover, the RALES trial had demonstrated a much larger relative risk reduction in all-cause mortality with spironolactone, thus, some have suggested that EPHESUS should have been conducted with spironolactone instead.

In-Depth [randomized controlled trial]: This multicenter, randomized controlled study was conducted at 674 centers in 37 countries. 6642 patients were recruited and randomized to treatment with either eplerenone or placebo in addition to optimal management 3-14 days after suffering an acute MI. Other inclusion criteria were LVEF ≤40% and clinical findings of heart failure (i.e., pulmonary rales, pulmonary congestion on x-ray, third heart sound). Patients with diabetes did not need clinical evidence of heart failure in order to be included because of their increased risk of cardiovascular events. Patients were excluded if they were using potassium-sparing diuretics, had a serum creatinine > 220 μmol/L, or had a serum potassium > 5.0 mmol/L. There were two primary endpoints: 1) time to death from any cause and 2) time to death from cardiovascular causes or first hospitalization for a cardiovascular event.

The incidence of both primary endpoints - death from any cause (RR 0.85; 95%CI 0.75-0.96) and death from/hospitalization for cardiovascular causes (RR 0.87; 95%CI 0.79-0.95) - were significantly lower in the eplerenone group as compared to the placebo group. Patients in the eplerenone group also had a significantly lower rate of sudden cardiac death (RR 0.79; 95%CI 0.64-0.97) and significantly fewer hospitalizations for heart failure (RR 0.85; 95%CI 0.74-0.99). There were significantly more episodes of serious hyperkalemia noted in the eplerenone group compared to the placebo group (5.5% vs. 3.9%, p = 0.002). Patients receiving eplerenone also had significantly more gastrointestinal issues (19.9% vs. 17.7%, p = 0.02).

Pitt B, Remme W, Zannad F, Neaton J, Martinez F, Roniker B, et al. Eplerenone, a Selective Aldosterone Blocker, in Patients with Left Ventricular Dysfunction after Myocardial Infarction. New England Journal of Medicine. 2003 Apr 3;348(14):1309–21.

The CHARM-Added trial: Adding candesartan to ACE inhibitor reduces mortality in heart failure

1. Angiotensin-converting-enzyme (ACE) inhibitors have been shown to significantly reduce mortality in patients with heart failure, and it was hypothesized that adding an angiotensin-receptor blocker (ARB) would provide further clinical benefit.

2. The addition of candesartan to ACE inhibitor treatment led to significant reductions in cardiovascular mortality and hospitalization for heart failure when compared to placebo.

3. Patients taking candesartan experienced significantly higher rates of serum creatinine elevation and hyperkalemia.

Original Date of Publication: September 2003

Study Rundown: Angiotensin II is the end product of the renin-angiotensin system, and it has been shown to be involved in the process of cardiac remodeling. ACE inhibitors, which impede the conversion of angiotensin I to angiotensin II, have been shown to reduce mortality in patients with congestive heart failure. It had also been shown, however, that angiotensin II production continues despite patients taking target doses of ACE inhibitors. Thus, it was hypothesized that adding ARBs would provide better inhibition of angiotensin II and potentially improve outcomes in patients with congestive heart failure. The Candesartan in Heart failure: Assessment of Reduction in Mortality and morbidity (CHARM)-Added trial was conducted to determine the effects of adding candesartan to the treatment of patients with congestive heart failure who were already on an ACE inhibitor. Adding candesartan significantly reduced the risk of both cardiovascular death and hospitalization for heart failure when compared with placebo. Patients in the candesartan group experienced significantly higher rates of increased serum creatinine and hyperkalemia.

Previously, the Val-HeFT had found that adding valsartan to conventional therapy (i.e., 93% of patients were taking ACE inhibitors) led to no significant reduction in cardiovascular mortality, but did reduce the risk of hospitalization for heart failure. Authors of the CHARM-Added trial suggested that these differences could potentially be explained by the use of different ARBs and differences in dosing between the 2 studies. Current recommendations suggest considering a combination of ACE inhibitor and ARB only if aldosterone antagonists are not tolerated, though this combination may be harmful.

In-Depth [randomized controlled trial]: The CHARM-Added trial involved 2548 patients with a median follow-up of 41 months. Patients were eligible for the trial if they were ≥18 years of age, had left-ventricular ejection fraction (LVEF) ≤40%, had New York Heart Association (NYHA) class II-IV symptoms, and were already treated with an ACE inhibitor for 30 days or longer. Patients were randomized to receive either candesartan (i.e., started at 4 or 8 mg daily, titrated up to 32 mg daily) or placebo. The primary outcome was cardiovascular death or admission to hospital for the management of worsening heart failure.

Patients in the candesartan group experienced significantly lower rates of the primary outcome when compared to those in the placebo group (aHR 0.85; 95%CI 0.75-0.96). Patients on candesartan experienced significantly lower risk of cardiovascular death (aHR 0.83; 95%CI 0.71-0.97) and hospitalization for heart failure (aHR 0.83; 95%CI 0.71-0.97) compared to patients taking placebos. The candesartan group had significantly higher numbers of patients with increased serum creatinine levels ($p = 0.0001$), hyperkalemia ($p < 0.0001$), or any adverse event or laboratory abnormality ($p = 0.0003$).

McMurray JJ, Ostergren J, Swedberg K, Granger CB, Held P, Michelson EL, et al. Effects of candesartan in patients with chronic heart failure and reduced left-ventricular systolic function taking angiotensin-converting-enzyme inhibitors: The CHARM-Added trial. The Lancet. 2003;362(9386):767-771.

The CHARM-Preserved trial: Candesartan reduces hospitalization in heart failure with preserved ejection fraction

1. In patients with heart failure and preserved ejection fraction, candesartan was not associated with a significant reduction in the rate of cardiovascular death, but was linked to a significant reduction in the rate of hospitalization for heart failure as compared with placebo.

Original Date of Publication: September 2003

Study Rundown: A large body of evidence exists supporting various interventions to improve outcomes in heart failure with reduced left-ventricular ejection fraction (LVEF). The SOLVD and ATLAS trials demonstrated that treatment with angiotensin converting enzyme (ACE) inhibitors was linked to a significant reduction in mortality among heart failure patients with reduced LVEF. The Val-HEFT and CHARM-Alternative trials demonstrated the benefits of angiotensin-receptor blocker (ARB) therapy, while the MERIT-HF and COPERNICUS trials supported the use of beta-blockers. The RALES, EMPHASIS-HF, and EPHESUS trials provide evidence for aldosterone blockade in these patients and the MADIT-II trial found that prophylactic implantable defibrillators also reduced mortality.

At the time of the Candesartan in Heart failure: Assessment of Reduction in Mortality and morbidity (CHARM)-Preserved trial, many guidelines for heart failure management did not specifically address treating patients with preserved ejections fractions. Given that there was some evidence to support the use of ACE inhibitors in treating heart failure with preserved ejection fraction, the aim of the CHARM-Preserved trial was to explore whether angiotensin blockade using an ARB would have similar benefits. In summary, there were no significant differences between the candesartan and placebo groups in terms of the rate of cardiovascular death and hospitalization for heart failure. There was a small but significant reduction in hospitalizations for heart failure, while there was a significantly higher rate of adverse events in the candesartan group.

In-Depth [randomized controlled trial]: This trial included 3025 patients from 618 centers in 26 countries. Patients were eligible for the study if they were 18 years of age or older, had New York Heart Association (NYHA) functional class II-IV symptoms for at least 4 weeks, had a history of hospital admission for a cardiac reason, and had LVEF > 40%. Eligible patients were randomized to receive either candesartan or placebo. The primary outcome was cardiovascular death or unplanned admission to hospital for the management of worsening heart failure. Secondary outcomes included several combinations of cardiovascular death, admission to hospital for heart failure, non-fatal myocardial infarction, non-fatal stroke, coronary revascularization, all-cause mortality, and new development of diabetes.

There was no significant difference between the candesartan and placebo groups in terms of the rate of the primary outcome (adjusted HR 0.86; 95%CI 0.74-1.00, p = 0.051). Specifically, there was no significant difference between the groups in terms of the rate of cardiovascular death (adjusted HR 0.95; 95%CI 0.76-1.18, p = 0.635). The rate of hospital admission for heart failure was significantly reduced in the candesartan group as compared with the placebo group (adjusted HR 0.84; 95%CI 0.70-1.00, p = 0.047). The rates of study-drug discontinuation due to adverse events or laboratory abnormalities were significantly higher in the candesartan group (17.8% vs. 13.5%, p = 0.001), with the most common causes being rising creatinine (4.8% vs. 2.4%, p = 0.0005), hypotension (2.4% vs. 1.1%, p = 0.009), and hyperkalemia (1.5% vs. 0.6%, p = 0.029), all of which were elevated in the candesartan group.

Yusuf S, Pfeffer MA, Swedberg K, Granger CB, Held P, McMurray JJV, et al. Effects of candesartan in patients with chronic heart failure and preserved left-ventricular ejection fraction: the CHARM-Preserved Trial. Lancet. 2003 Sep 6;362(9386):777–81.

The CHARM-Alternative trial: Candesartan reduces mortality in heart failure

1. Candesartan therapy significantly reduced cardiovascular death and hospital admission for chronic heart failure in patients with heart failure, reduced ventricular function, and angiotensin receptor blocker (ACE) inhibitor intolerance.

2. Candesartan was well-tolerated in patients with previous intolerance to ACE inhibitors.

Original Date of Publication: September 2003

Study Rundown: ACE inhibitors have been shown to effectively reduce morbidity and mortality in patients with symptomatic heart failure, but intolerance to ACE inhibitors occurs frequently. Angiotensin-receptor blockers (ARB) are an alternative agent that may be used to inhibit the renin-angiotensin-aldosterone system but evidence of its effectiveness in reducing long-term clinical events was limited at the time this study was conducted. The Candesartan in Heart failure: Assessment of Reduction in Mortality and morbidity (CHARM)-Alternative trial was one arm of the CHARM-Overall program assessing the effectiveness of candesartan compared to placebo in patients with symptomatic heart failure and reduced left-ventricular systolic function, who could not tolerate ACE inhibitors. Results of the study showed a significant reduction in cardiovascular death and hospital admission due to heart failure in the candesartan group. In summary, an ARB should be considered in patients with symptomatic chronic heart failure, reduced ventricular function, and an intolerance to ACE inhibitors.

In-Depth [randomized controlled trial]: This study randomized 2028 patients to receive an ARB (i.e., candesartan) or placebo and investigated the long-term clinical outcomes. The CHARM-Alternative trial included patients with symptomatic chronic heart failure and left-ventricular ejection fraction of 40% or less who had a previously documented intolerance to ACE inhibitors. The primary outcome of cardiovascular death or hospital admission for CHF occurred in 33% of patients in the candesartan group and 40% of patients in the placebo group (HR 0.77; 95%CI 0.67-0.89; p = 0.0004). This reduction in the primary outcome in the candesartan group was significant and was maintained when non-fatal myocardial infarction, non-fatal stroke and coronary revascularization were included in the composite outcome. Study drug discontinuation was similar between the treatment and placebo groups suggesting that candesartan was well-tolerated in this population of patients in spite of previously documented intolerance to ACE inhibitors.

Granger CB, McMurray JJV, Yusuf S, Held P, Michelson EL, Olofsson B, et al. Effects of candesartan in patients with chronic heart failure and reduced left-ventricular systolic function intolerant to angiotensin-converting-enzyme inhibitors: the CHARM-Alternative trial. Lancet. 2003 Sep 6;362(9386):772–6.

The VALIANT trial: Valsartan vs. captopril in patients with acute myocardial infarction and heart failure

1. In patients with acute myocardial infarction and heart failure/evidence of left ventricular dysfunction, patients treated with valsartan and captopril experienced similar all-cause mortality.

2. Valsartan and captopril were found to be non-inferior with regards to death from cardiovascular causes, recurrent myocardial infarction, and hospitalization for heart failure in this patient population.

3. The combination of valsartan and captopril increased the rate of adverse events without improving survival when compared to treatment with captopril alone.

Original Date of Publication: November 2003

Study Rundown: A number of large randomized, controlled trials have previously demonstrated that angiotensin-converting-enzyme (ACE) inhibitors reduced the risk of death and major nonfatal cardiovascular events after myocardial infarction. Angiotensin-receptor blockers (ARBs) represent another way of inhibiting the renin-angiotensin system, and may potentially be more effective than ACE inhibitors in blocking the effects of angiotensin. Moreover, it has been hypothesized that concurrent treatment with an ACE inhibitor and an ARB may be a more effective treatment strategy to reduce the risk of cardiovascular events after a myocardial infarction.

The Valsartan in Acute Myocardial Infarction (VALIANT) trial sought to determine whether valsartan, an ARB, alone or in combination with captopril, an ACE inhibitor, would lead to better outcomes than treatment with an ACE inhibitor alone. This trial found that using valsartan in patients with acute myocardial infarction and heart failure/left ventricular dysfunction resulted in similar all-cause mortality when compared to captopril. Valsartan was found to be non-inferior to captopril for death from cardiovascular causes, recurrent infarction, and hospitalization for heart failure. When comparing combination therapy with captopril alone, there were no significant differences for any of the outcomes. Thus, valsartan is another option for renin-angiotensin blockade in patients with acute myocardial infarction and at high-risk of cardiovascular events.

In-Depth [randomized controlled trial]: A total of 14 703 patients from 24 countries were randomized in a 1:1:1 ratio to treatment with valsartan only, captopril only, or a combination of the 2. All patients 18 years of age or older, with acute myocardial infarction (0.5-10 days prior to randomization) complicated by clinical or radiographic heart failure, left ventricular dysfunction (ejection fraction ≤35% on echocardiogram, ≤40% on radionuclide ventriculography), or both were eligible for the trial. Patients were excluded if they had systolic blood pressure < 100 mmHg, serum creatinine < 2.5 mg/dL (or 221 µmol/L), intolerance or contraindication to ACE inhibitor or ARB, clinically significant valvular disease, or another disease known to limit life expectancy. The primary outcome was all-cause mortality, while the secondary outcome was a composite of death from cardiovascular causes, recurrent myocardial infarction, or hospitalization for heart failure.

The median follow-up was 24.7 months. There was no significant difference between the valsartan and captopril groups in all-cause mortality (HR 1.00; 97.5%CI 0.90-1.11; p = 0.98). All-cause mortality was also found to be similar when comparing combination therapy with captopril alone (HR 0.98; 97.5%CI 0.89-1.09; p = 0.73). The 3 groups were also similar in terms of the rate of the secondary endpoint, with no significant differences between valsartan and captopril (HR 0.95; 97.5%CI 0.88-1.03; p = 0.20) or between combination therapy and captopril (HR 0.97; 97.5%CI 0.89-1.05).

The discontinuation rates were significantly higher in the combination group, as compared with captopril alone (19.0% vs. 16.8%, p = 0.007). Dose reduction for hypotension was significantly more common in the combination and valsartan groups when compared with the captopril group (18.2%, 15.1%, and 11.9%, respectively; p < 0.05). There were also significantly higher rates of permanent discontinuation of therapy due to adverse events in the combination group when compared to captopril alone (9.0% vs. 7.7%; p < 0.05).

Pfeffer MA, McMurray JJ, Velazquez EJ, Rouleau JL, Køber L, Maggioni AP, et al. Valsartan, captopril, or both in myocardial infarction complicated by heart failure, left ventricular dysfunction, or both. The New England Journal of Medicine. 2003;349(20):1893-1906.

The PROVE IT trial: High-dose atorvastatin reduces mortality after acute coronary syndrome

1. High-dose atorvastatin was associated with a 16% reduction in death or major cardiovascular events compared to standard pravastatin therapy following an acute coronary syndrome (ACS).

2. The protective effect of intensive lipid-lowering was evident in the first 30 days of therapy and was consistent across pre-specified subgroups.

Original Date of Publication: April 2004

Study Rundown: The REVERSAL trial first suggested that intensive lipid-lowering therapy may be superior to standard therapy; however, this trial was not designed to assess clinical outcomes. The Pravastatin or Atorvastatin Evaluation and Infection Therapy (PROVE IT) trial pursued this implication by comparing the standard pravastatin dose to high-dose atorvastatin and measured a composite end point of death from all-causes and major cardiovascular events. The magnitude of the improvement with intensive lipid-lowering over standard therapy was comparable to the benefit seen when comparing statins to placebo. The effect was apparent early on after therapy initiation and was consistent over the mean 2-year follow up period. It is uncertain to what extent the difference in statins may have contributed to the difference in outcomes. Future studies may explore the effect of varying doses of a single statin. The results of the PROVE IT trial challenged guidelines at the time by suggesting that target low-density lipoprotein (LDL) levels should be lower in patients following an ACS. In summary, intensive lipid-lowering with high-dose atorvastatin may further reduce the risk of mortality or major cardiovascular events compared to a standard dose of pravastatin in patients with recent ACS.

In-Depth [randomized controlled trial]: The PROVE IT trial randomly assigned 4162 patients who had been hospitalized within the previous 10 days for an ACS to receive a standard regimen of 40 mg pravastatin daily or an intensive regimen of 80 mg atorvastatin daily. The primary outcome measured was the time to death from any cause, myocardial infarction, unstable angina requiring hospitalization, revascularization or stroke. During follow-up, the LDL cholesterol levels reached were significantly lower in the atorvastatin group, with values of 2.46 mmol/L in the pravastatin group and 1.60 mmol/L in the atorvastatin group (p < 0.001). There was a 16% reduction in the hazard ratio for the primary outcome in the atorvastatin group compared to the pravastatin group (95%CI 5-26%; p = 0.005). No significant difference was detected in the rate of discontinuation because of adverse events or patient preference; however, a significantly greater proportion of patients in the atorvastatin group had elevated alanine aminotransferase levels.

Cannon CP, Braunwald E, McCabe CH, Rader DJ, Rouleau JL, Belder R, et al. Intensive versus Moderate Lipid Lowering with Statins after Acute Coronary Syndromes. New England Journal of Medicine. 2004 Apr 8;350(15):1495–504.

The CLARITY trial: Clopidogrel reduces arterial reocclusion after myocardial infarction

1. The early addition of clopidogrel to standard therapy reduced the incidence of infarct-related arterial reocclusion within 30 days following myocardial infarction (MI).

2. The addition of early clopidogrel was associated with improved outcomes of coronary angiography and a decreased need for early/emergent angiography during the event.

3. There were no differences in major bleeding, minor bleeding, or intracranial hemorrhage incidence between the clopidogrel group and the control group.

Original Date of Publication: March 2005

Study Rundown: It is well known that platelet activation and aggregation have a significant role in the initiation and propagation of coronary artery thrombosis. As a result, antiplatelet agents are part of the standard management of acute coronary syndromes. Aspirin, which inactivates the cyclooxygenase enzyme, inhibits platelet aggregation and has been shown to help reduce the rate of reocclusion after MI. Clopidogrel is another antiplatelet agent that acts by blocking ADP receptors on platelets.

The Clopidogrel as Adjunctive Reperfusion Therapy (CLARITY-TIMI 28) trial sought to determine whether early treatment with clopidogrel in addition to standard aspirin and fibrinolytic therapy would produce better outcomes than standard therapy alone in the treatment of ST-elevation MI (STEMI). The study showed that early treatment with clopidogrel resulted in a significant improvement in outcomes. The early clopidogrel group had a significantly lower incidence of persistent arterial occlusion or reocclusion, as well as improved outcomes on all angiography measures. There was also a significant decrease in the need for early or emergent angiography in the clopidogrel group and a significant decrease in the incidence of recurrent MI within 30 days of the first event. No significant difference in 30-day mortality from cardiovascular events was shown, however this study was not powered to assess the impact of intervention on mortality. In summary, this study showed that early treatment with clopidogrel in addition to standard management of STEMI significantly improved patient outcomes in regards to coronary arterial patency. This study has had meaningful impact on STEMI management and has impacted ACCF and AHA guidelines.

In-Depth [randomized controlled trial]: This large, multicenter, double-blinded, randomized, placebo-controlled trial involved enrollment of 3491 patients with an acute STEMI at 319 sites to receive early clopidogrel or placebo along with standard therapy, including aspirin and fibrinolytic agents. Patients between the age of 18-75 years who presented with ST elevation and an episode of chest pain that lasted > 20 minutes within 12 hours of randomization were eligible. Patients who had received clopidogrel in the past 7 days, had a history of coronary artery bypass grafting, presented with cardiogenic shock, or who were scheduled to receive coronary angiography within 48 hours regardless of clinical indication were excluded. Eligible patients received a 300 mg loading dose of clopidogrel followed by 75 mg daily maintenance dose, which was continued to the day of angiography. If a patient did not undergo angiography, it was continued until day 8 or discharge from hospital, whichever was sooner. Patients were followed up to 30 days after randomization. The primary outcome was evidence of infarct-related arterial occlusion on angiography or death/recurrent MI before angiography, day 8 of hospitalization, or hospital discharge. The study demonstrated that early treatment with clopidogrel resulted in a 6.7% absolute reduction of the primary end point (21.7% vs. 15%; 95%CI 24-47%, $p < 0.001$). There was no significant difference in the rate of death from any cardiovascular cause between the groups. The study also demonstrated no significant difference in incidence of major or minor bleeding or intracranial hemorrhage between the 2 groups ($p = 0.64$, $p = 0.17$, and $p = 0.38$, respectively).

Sabatine MS, Cannon CP, Gibson CM, López-Sendón JL, Montalescot G, Theroux P, et al. Addition of Clopidogrel to Aspirin and Fibrinolytic Therapy for Myocardial Infarction with ST-Segment Elevation. New England Journal of Medicine. 2005 Mar 24;352(12):1179–89.

The TNT trial: Intensive statin therapy in coronary heart disease

1. In patients with stable coronary heart disease (CHD), high-dose atorvastatin significantly reduced the risk of major cardiovascular events when compared to low-dose.

2. Patients in the high-dose group experienced significantly higher rates of adverse events, though the rate of statin-related myalgias were similar in the 2 groups.

Original Date of Publication: April 2005

Study Rundown: Numerous studies exist to support the effectiveness of statins in secondary prevention of major cardiovascular events. At the time this study was conducted, guidelines recommended an LDL target of 2.6 mmol/L (100 mg/dL) in patients with stable coronary heart disease (CHD). Several smaller studies, however, suggested more aggressive LDL targets could provide clinical benefit. The Treating to New Targets (TNT) trial was conducted to gauge the safety and effectiveness of lowering LDL targets among patients with stable CHD.

In summary, this prospective, randomized controlled trial found that a higher dose of atorvastatin (80 mg daily compared to 10 mg daily) was associated with greater reductions in LDL. Patients in the high-dose group experienced a significant reduction in the rate of major cardiovascular events (death from CHD, nonfatal myocardial infarction, fatal/nonfatal stroke, resuscitation after cardiac arrest). There was no difference between the groups in all-cause mortality. The rate of adverse events was significantly higher in the high-dose group, though the rate of statin-related myalgias were similar in the 2 groups. This trial provided evidence to support higher doses of statin therapy in patients with stable CHD.

In-Depth [randomized controlled trial]: This prospective, double-blind, randomized trial was conducted at 256 institutions in 14 countries. Patients were eligible for the trial if they had a history of clinically evident CHD (previous myocardial infarction, previous or current angina, history of coronary revascularization) and were between 35 and 75 years of age. During the 8-week run-in, all patients received 10 mg of atorvastatin daily in an open-label fashion. At the end of this period, patients with LDL < 3.4 mmol/L (130 mg/dL) underwent randomization. In total, 10 001 patients were randomized to either 10 mg daily (low-dose) or 80 mg daily (high-dose) of atorvastatin daily, and were followed for a median of 4.9 years. The primary outcome was the occurrence of a major cardiovascular event (death from CHD, nonfatal myocardial infarction, fatal/nonfatal stroke, resuscitation after cardiac arrest).

At randomization, the 2 cohorts had similar serum LDL levels. By 12 weeks after randomization, LDL levels were significantly higher in the low-dose group (101 mg/dL or 2.6 mmol/L vs. 77 mg/dL or 2.0 mmol/L) and this difference was maintained throughout the follow-up period. The rate of the primary outcome was significantly lower in the high-dose group, as compared with the low-dose group (8.7% vs. 10.9%; HR 0.78, 95%CI 0.69-0.89, p < 0.001). This was driven by significantly lower rates of nonfatal myocardial infarction (HR 0.78, 95%CI 0.66-0.93, p = 0.004) and fatal/nonfatal stroke (HR 0.75, 95%CI 0.59-0.96, p = 0.02). There was no difference between the groups in terms of all-cause mortality (p = 0.92). More adverse events were observed in the high-dose group (8.1% vs 5.8%, p < 0.001). There were similar rates of statin-related myalgias in both groups (p = 0.72), though the high-dose group had significantly more patients with persistently elevated aminotransferase levels (p < 0.001).

LaRosa JC, Grundy SM, Waters DD, Shear C, Barter P, Fruchart JC, et al. Intensive lipid lowering with atorvastatin in patients with stable coronary disease. The New England Journal of Medicine. 2005;352(14):1425-1435.

The SCD-HeFT: ICD vs. amiodarone for congestive heart failure

1. In patients with congestive heart failure (CHF) and reduced ejection fraction, mortality was significantly lower in patients who received an implantable cardioverter-defibrillator (ICD) compared those who did not receive one.

2. In these patients, amiodarone did not confer a favorable survival benefit as compared to placebo.

Original Date of Publication: January 2005

Study Rundown: Patients with CHF are at higher risk of sudden cardiac death, often secondary to cardiac arrhythmias, despite being treated with conventional medical therapy. Amiodarone and ICDs were identified as 2 potential approaches to prevent death in this patient population. Amiodarone had been previously studied in patients with CHF, though the findings were inconclusive. Similarly, some evidence supported the effectiveness of ICDs in this setting, though the trials were small. Moreover, most previous studies had explored the use of amiodarone and ICDs in patients who had recently suffered myocardial infarctions or ventricular arrhythmia, and were not generalizable to patients with CHF who did not experience these events.

The Sudden Cardiac Death in Heart Failure Trial (SCD-HeFT) was designed to evaluate amiodarone and ICDs in the treatment of patients with mild-to-moderate CHF. In patients with New York Heart Association (NYHA) class II or III symptoms and left ventricular ejection fraction (LVEF) ≤35%, ICD treatment led to a significant reduction in mortality when compared with placebo. There were no significant differences in mortality when comparing the amiodarone and placebo groups. Although this study suffered from high rates of study drug discontinuation, it provides strong evidence in support of ICDs in patients with stable CHF and reduced LVEF.

In-Depth [randomized controlled trial]: A total of 2521 patients were randomized for this study. All patients ≥18 years of age, with NYHA class II or III symptoms, and with LVEF ≤35% were eligible for the trial. Patients were randomized equally to treatment with placebo, amiodarone (weight-adjusted maintenance dosing after initial loading), or Medtronic single-chamber ICD programmed to shock-only mode. The primary endpoint was death from any cause.

The median follow-up was 45.5 months for all surviving patients. The median dose of amiodarone used was 300 mg daily. A total of 29% of the placebo group, 28% of the amiodarone group, and 22% of the ICD group died during the course of this study. There were no significant differences in mortality between the amiodarone and placebo groups (28% vs. 29%; HR 1.06 97.5%CI 0.86 to 1.30, p = 0.53). Patients treated with ICD experienced significantly lower mortality when compared with those taking placebo (22% vs. 29%; HR 0.77, 97.5%CI 0.62 to 0.96, p = 0.007). Drug discontinuation rates were high, with 22% of the placebo group and 32% of the amiodarone group discontinuing their drug therapies. Patients in the amiodarone group experienced significantly higher rates of tremor (4%, p = 0.02) and hypothyroidism (6%, p < 0.001). Approximately 5% of patients receiving ICDs experienced a significant complication at the time of implantation (surgical correction, hospitalization, new/unanticipated drug therapy), while 9% of patients experienced such complications later.

Bardy GH, Lee KL, Mark DB, Poole JE, Packer DL, Boineau R, et al. Amiodarone or an implantable cardioverter-defibrillator for congestive heart failure. The New England Journal of Medicine. 2005;352(3):225-237.

The COMMIT: Metoprolol and clopidogrel in patients with acute myocardial infarction

1. Adding early metoprolol did not further decrease the risk of death after myocardial infarction (MI) compared to conventional fibrinolytic therapy alone.

2. Use of early metoprolol decreased the risk of reinfarction and ventricular fibrillation, but increased the risk of cardiogenic shock.

3. Adding clopidogrel to aspirin decreased the combined risk of death, reinfarction, or stroke post-MI, without significantly increasing the risk of major bleeding.

Original Date of Publication: November 2005

Study Rundown: The Clopidogrel and Metoprolol in Myocardial Infarction Trial (COMMIT) featured a 2x2 factorial design, in which patients with acute myocardial infarction were treated with 1) metoprolol or placebo and 2) aspirin plus clopidogrel or aspirin plus placebo. The study assessed the effect of adding early metoprolol (intravenous then oral) to conventional fibrinolytic therapy in patients with a recent MI. This aim was motivated by the fact that previous studies had only evaluated early beta-blockade before fibrinolytic therapy had become routine. Moreover, it was thought that beta-blockers would decrease the risk of cardiac rupture associated with fibrinolytic therapy alone. COMMIT showed that the addition of metoprolol did not result in significantly fewer deaths compared to fibrinolytic therapy alone. Use of metoprolol did decrease the rate of reinfarction and ventricular fibrillation, but this was counterbalanced by an increase in cardiogenic shock, particular in patients with moderate heart failure (i.e., Killip class II or III).

The study assessed also the effect of adding clopidogrel to aspirin in the treatment of patients with a recent MI. Aspirin, which acts by blocking the thromboxane pathway of platelet aggregation, had been previously shown to reduce mortality post-MI, and it was thought that clopidogrel, which inhibits platelet aggregation via an adenosine 5'-diphosphate-mediated pathway, might reduce mortality even further. Findings from COMMIT showed that the addition of clopidogrel resulted in a significant post-MI reduction in death, reinfarction, and stroke in patients, without a significant risk of bleeding regardless of the patient's age. A limitation of the study was the possibility that instances of rapid reduction in blood pressure might have correctly indicated to physicians that metoprolol was administered rather than placebo. In summary, the COMMIT trial suggested that beta-blocker therapy may be more appropriately started only after a patient has been stabilized hemodynamically post-MI, with the aim of preventing reinfarction and fibrillation. In contrast, adding clopidogrel to aspirin should be considered for all patients with a suspected acute MI, especially given clopidogrel's modest cost and minimal required monitoring.

In-Depth [randomized controlled trial]: The COMMIT was a large, randomized, placebo-controlled trial with a 2x2 factorial design (metoprolol vs. placebo and clopidogrel plus aspirin vs. aspirin alone) involving 45 852 patients. On-site audits were performed at hospitals, and study drug packs were systematically checked to ensure that correct contents were packaged. Patients who presented with ST elevation, ST depression, or left-bundle branch block within 24 hours of a suspected acute MI were eligible. Patients at risk of adverse effects from beta blockade (e.g., low heart rate, hypotension, cardiogenic shock) or from antiplatelet therapy (e.g., bleeding, allergic reaction) were excluded. Eligible patients received metoprolol or placebo doses for intravenous infusion, followed by a 4-week supply of 1) oral metoprolol or placebo and 2) clopidogrel plus aspirin or placebo plus aspirin. The co-primary outcomes for the assessment of both clopidogrel and metoprolol were 1) the composite of death, reinfarction, cardiac arrest (metoprolol only), and stroke (clopidogrel only), and 2) death from any cause. There was no difference in death from any cause with the use of metoprolol (OR 0.99; 95%CI 0.92-1.05). Metoprolol use was associated with a significantly decreased risk of reinfarction (OR 0.82; 95%CI 0.72-0.92) and ventricular fibrillation (OR 0.83; 95%CI 0.75-0.93), but increased risk of cardiogenic shock (OR 1.30; 95%CI 1.19-1.41). Clopidogrel use resulted in a reduction in death, reinfarction, or stroke (OR 0.91; 95%CI 0.86-0.97), without a significantly increased risk of major bleeding regardless of age.

Chen ZM, Pan HC, Chen YP, Peto R, Collins R, Jiang LX, et al. Early intravenous then oral metoprolol in 45,852 patients with acute myocardial infarction: randomised placebo-controlled trial. Lancet. 2005 Nov 5;366(9497):1622–32.

Chen ZM, Jiang LX, Chen YP, Xie JX, Pan HC, Peto R, et al. Addition of clopidogrel to aspirin in 45,852 patients with acute myocardial infarction: randomised placebo-controlled trial. Lancet. 2005 Nov 5;366(9497):1607–21.

The COURAGE trial: Percutaneous coronary intervention does not improve mortality in stable coronary artery disease

1. The addition of percutaneous cutaneous intervention (PCI) to optimal medical therapy for patients with stable coronary artery disease did not improve mortality or cardiovascular outcomes.

Original Date of Publication: April 2007

Study Rundown: The Clinical Outcomes Utilizing Revascularization and Aggressive Drug Evaluation (COURAGE) trial was the first to provide evidence that in patients with stable coronary artery disease, the addition of PCI to optimal medical therapy does not provide any mortality benefit or improve cardiovascular outcomes. A subsequent report from the COURAGE investigators demonstrated that patients who received PCI were free of angina and had improvements in various quality of life parameters at 3 months after the intervention, though this difference was not sustained at 36 months. Optimization of medical therapy alone without PCI is sufficient for initial treatment of patients with stable coronary artery disease. The addition of PCI to optimal medical therapy likely does not improve mortality or cardiovascular outcomes as evidenced by the COURAGE trial.

In-Depth [randomized controlled trial]: A total of 2287 patients with stable coronary artery disease, objective evidence of myocardial ischemia, and significant disease in at least 1 major coronary artery were enrolled in this study. Patients were randomized to 2 groups: 1) optimal medical therapy alone or 2) optimal medical therapy with PCI. All patients were optimized medically on an angiotensin converting enzyme (ACE) inhibitor or angiotensin receptor blocker (ARB), antiplatelet therapy (acetylsalicylic acid or clopidogrel), as well as a combination of beta-blockers, calcium channel blockers and nitrates. All patients also received aggressive lipid optimizing therapy. The primary outcome studied was a composite of death from any cause and non-fatal myocardial infarction. The median follow-up period was 4.6 years. In patients undergoing PCI, 89% achieved clinical success. There was no significant difference in the primary outcome between the groups (HR 1.05; 95%CI 0.87-1.27; p = 0.62). Furthermore, rates of hospitalization for acute coronary syndrome were not significantly different between the groups (HR 1.07; 95%CI 0.84-1.37; p = 0.56). The need for subsequent revascularization procedures (PCI or coronary artery bypass graft) was, however, significantly higher in the medical therapy group as compared to the PCI group (32.6% vs. 21.1%, p < 0.001).

Boden WE, O'Rourke RA, Teo KK, Hartigan PM, Maron DJ, Kostuk WJ, et al. Optimal Medical Therapy with or without PCI for Stable Coronary Disease. New England Journal of Medicine. 2007 Apr 12;356(15):1503–16.

The TRITON-TIMI 38 trial: Prasugrel reduces recurrent infarction after acute coronary syndrome

1. Prasugrel was significantly more effective than clopidogrel in reducing the incidence of recurrent myocardial infarction (MI) in patients presenting with acute coronary syndrome (ACS), though there was no difference in mortality between the groups tested.

2. Patients treated with prasugrel had a significantly higher incidence of fatal major bleeding compared to clopidogrel.

Original Date of Publication: November 2007

Study Rundown: Current ACS management guidelines call for treatment with dual antiplatelet therapy, usually consisting of aspirin and clopidogrel, a thienopyridine. However, it is known that there is much interpatient variability in the metabolism of clopidogrel, which may lead to variable efficacy of the drug in different patients. Prasugrel, a newer thienopyridine, was known to be more rapid and less variable in its platelet-binding activity. This trial sought to determine whether treatment with prasugrel and aspirin produced better outcomes than the standard treatment with clopidogrel and aspirin in the management of patients with ACS. The study demonstrated that prasugrel was significantly more effective than clopidogrel at reducing the incidence of recurrent myocardial infarctions.

Notably, the study did not show a significant mortality benefit with using prasugrel. Moreover, researchers found that prasugrel use was linked to significantly higher incidence of major bleeding, both related to instrumentation and also spontaneous bleeding. While analysis of net clinical benefit still showed preference for prasugrel, stratification of groups revealed that prasugrel showed no clinical net benefit for patients who had a prior history of a cerebral vascular accident or transient ischemic attack, are above 75 years of age, or are below 60 kg for weight. In summary, this study showed that prasugrel was more effective than clopidogrel in preventing recurrent myocardial infarctions and subsequent deaths, but also increased the risk of major bleeding. Overall, the net clinical benefit of prasugrel provides evidence for its use in ACS management, but it must be used with caution. Patients should be counseled of the increased risk of bleeding with this drug over clopidogrel.

In-Depth [randomized controlled trial]: This trial was a large, multicenter, double-blinded, randomized controlled trial that enrolled 13 608 patients with acute coronary syndrome at 707 sites to receive either prasugrel or clopidogrel along with aspirin as part of the dual antiplatelet regimen for ACS management. Patients who presented with symptoms lasting greater than 10 minutes within 72 hours of enrollment, had a TIMI score greater than 3, had > 1 mm ST segment change, or had an increased blood level of biomarker of cardiac necrosis were eligible. Patients who had received any thienopyridine in the past 5 days, had an increased risk of bleeding, or another contraindication to antiplatelet therapy were excluded. Eligible patients received a loading dose of a single antiplatelet agent and were continued on daily maintenance dosing along with a low-dose aspirin (75 to 162 mg daily). Patients were followed for 6-15 months, with study visits performed at hospital discharge, 30 days, 90 days, and every 3 months after that. The primary outcome was a composite of the rate of death related to cardiovascular events, non-fatal myocardial infarction, or non-fatal stroke in the follow-up period.

The study demonstrated that treatment with prasugrel was associated with significantly reduced incidence of the primary outcome when compared to clopidogrel (HR 0.81; 95%CI 0.73-0.90). A significant reduction in the primary endpoint was seen in the prasugrel group at 3 days and the trend persisted throughout the follow-up period. The difference between the groups was attributed to a significant decrease in the rate of recurrent myocardial infarctions (HR 0.76; 95%CI 0.67-0.85) in the prasugrel group compared to the clopidogrel group. There was no significant difference between the groups in terms of mortality, though prasugrel use was linked with significantly lower rates of urgent target-vessel revascularization (HR 0.66; 95%CI 0.54-0.81) and stent thrombosis (HR 0.48; 95%CI 0.36-0.64). The prasugrel group had a significantly higher incidence of fatal major bleeding compared to clopidogrel group (0.4% vs. 0.1%, p = 0.002).

Wiviott SD, Braunwald E, McCabe CH, Montalescot G, Ruzyllo W, Gottlieb S, et al. Prasugrel versus Clopidogrel in Patients with Acute Coronary Syndromes. New England Journal of Medicine. 2007 Nov 15;357(20):2001–15.

The ONTARGET: Telmisartan non-inferior to ramipril in improving cardiovascular outcomes in high-risk populations

1. The angiotensin receptor blocker (ARB) telmisartan was non-inferior to the angiotensin converting enzyme (ACE) inhibitor ramipril in improving cardiovascular outcomes in high-risk populations.

2. Telmisartan was associated with significantly less angioedema and cough compared to ramipril.

3. The combination of telmisartan and ramipril in high-risk populations did not offer additional benefit compared to ramipril alone, and was associated with increased risk of complications.

Original Date of Publication: April 2008

Study Rundown: ARBs reduce the activation of the renin-angiotensin-aldosterone system by blocking the angiotensin-II (ANG-II) receptor. At the time of their introduction, there was uncertainty as to whether ARBs were a viable alternative to ACE inhibitors. It was thought that ARBs would be associated with fewer adverse effects, as ARBs, unlike ACE inhibitors, do not reduce bradykinin degradation (which is associated with cough and angioedema). One of the indications for ACE inhibitors is to prevent cardiac events in high-risk patients without systolic heart failure, as shown in the Heart Outcomes Prevention Evaluation (HOPE) trial. The purpose of the Ongoing Telmisartan Alone and in Combination with Ramipril Global Endpoint Trial (ONTARGET) was to determine whether the ARB, telmisartan, was a non-inferior alternative to ramipril in improving cardiac outcomes (a composite of death from cardiovascular causes, myocardial infarction, stroke, or hospitalization for heart failure) in a similar patient population. The study also investigated whether combination therapy with both telmisartan and ramipril offered additional benefit to ramipril alone.

This study demonstrated that telmisartan was a non-inferior alternative to ramipril in reducing cardiac outcomes in high-risk patients, and was associated with a significantly lower risk of cough and angioedema. Combination therapy with both drugs, however, did not appear to provide additional benefit as compared to ramipril alone and was associated with increased adverse effects including renal failure. For improving cardiac outcomes, an ARB can be considered as an alternative for high-risk patients who are not able to tolerate ACE inhibitor therapy. Combination therapy with an ARB and an ACE inhibitor should be avoided.

In-Depth [randomized controlled trial]: This trial enrolled 25 620 patients from 40 countries. Patients were eligible for inclusion if they were considered high-risk for adverse cardiac outcomes, that is if they had coronary, peripheral, or cerebrovascular disease, or diabetes mellitus with end-organ damage. Patients underwent double-blind randomization to 1 of 3 groups receiving 1) 80 mg telmisartan daily, 2) 5 mg ramipril, or 3) a combination of both drugs. The primary outcome was a composite of death from cardiovascular causes, myocardial infarction, stroke, or hospitalization for heart failure. The main secondary outcome was a composite of death from cardiovascular causes, myocardial infarction, or stroke, which was the primary outcome in the HOPE trial.

With regards to the primary outcome, telmisartan was found to be non-inferior to ramipril ($p = 0.004$) and also non-superior (RR 1.01; 95%CI 0.94-1.09). The rate of the main secondary outcome was also similar between the groups (RR 0.99; 95%CI 0.91-1.07; $p = 0.001$ for non-inferiority). Patients receiving telmisartan were significantly less likely to develop cough and angioedema than those receiving ramipril (RR 0.26; $p < 0.001$). The combination of the drugs, however, was non-superior to ramipril alone (RR 0.99; 95%CI 0.92-1.07). Patients receiving both drugs were more likely to develop hypotensive symptoms (RR 2.75; $p < 0.001$), syncope (RR 1.95; $p = 0.03$), diarrhea (RR 3.28; $p < 0.001$) and renal impairment (RR 1.58; $p < 0.001$) than those receiving ramipril alone.

The ONTARGET Investigators. Telmisartan, Ramipril, or Both in Patients at High Risk for Vascular Events. New England Journal of Medicine. 2008 Apr 10;358(15):1547–59.

The ACCOMPLISH trial: Benazepril plus amlodipine reduces cardiovascular events

1. Benazepril plus amlodipine offered the same effect at reducing blood pressure in hypertensive patients as benazepril plus hydrochlorothiazide (HCTZ).

2. Benazepril plus amlodipine was more effective than benazepril plus HCTZ at reducing cardiovascular events in hypertensive patients at risk for such events.

Original Date of Publication: December 2008

Study Rundown: The Avoiding Cardiovascular events through Combination therapy in Patients Living with Systolic Hypertension (ACCOMPLISH) trial sought to compare a thiazide with a calcium channel blocker (CCB) as a combination therapy with an angiotensin converting enzyme (ACE) inhibitor in reducing cardiovascular events in patients with hypertension. Patients with hypertension and cardiovascular risk factors were randomized to treatment with benazepril plus amlodipine or benazepril plus HCTZ. In summary, patients in the benazepril-amlodipine group experienced significantly lower rates of the primary outcome compared to those in the benazepril-HCTZ group. This was due to a significant reduction in the rates of fatal/nonfatal myocardial infarction, while there was no significant difference in the rate of death from cardiovascular causes. This study demonstrated that adding a CCB to an ACE inhibitor reduces the risk of myocardial infarction when compared to adding a thiazide diuretic for blood pressure control in hypertensive patients. It is important to note that a pharmaceutical company was significantly involved in the execution of the study, from coordination to data analysis. Moreover, the study was stopped early by the executive committee, as preliminary results met premature termination conditions.

In-Depth [randomized controlled trial]: A total of 11 506 patients from 548 centers in the United States, Sweden, Norway, Denmark, and Finland were randomized to receive either 1) benazepril plus amlodipine or 2) benazepril plus HCTZ. Patients were started on therapy with either benazepril 20 mg and amlodipine 5 mg daily or benazepril 20 mg and HCTZ 12.5 mg daily. Patients were eligible if they had hypertension, a history of coronary events/myocardial infarction/revascularization/stroke, impaired renal function, peripheral artery disease, left ventricular hypertrophy, or diabetes mellitus. Medication doses were adjusted in the first 3 months to maintain a blood pressure ≤140/90, or ≤130/80 in patients with diabetes and kidney disease. Patients were followed every 6 months, and dose adjustments were performed during these visits. The primary endpoint was a composite of cardiovascular events or death from cardiovascular causes. Of note, the study was funded by a pharmaceutical company, which was also involved in overseeing coordination, data gathering, and data analysis.

Mean blood pressures were 131.6/73.3 mmHg in the benazepril-amlodipine group and 132.5/74.4 mmHg in the benazepril-hydrochlorothiazide group. The mean difference in blood pressure was 0.9 mm Hg systolic and 1.1 mm Hg diastolic ($p < 0.001$). The trial was terminated early by the executive committee. Patients in the benazepril-amlodipine group experienced a significantly lower rate of the primary endpoint as compared with patients in the benazepril-HCTZ group (HR 0.80; 95%CI 0.72-0.90), with an absolute risk reduction of 2.2%. This difference was attributed to significantly lower rates of fatal and nonfatal myocardial infarction in the benazepril-amlodipine group (HR 0.78; 95%CI 0.62-0.99), while there was no significant difference between the 2 groups in death from cardiovascular causes.

Jamerson K, Weber MA, Bakris GL, Dahlöf B, Pitt B, Shi V, et al. Benazepril plus Amlodipine or Hydrochlorothiazide for Hypertension in High-Risk Patients. New England Journal of Medicine. 2008 Dec 4;359(23):2417–28.

The SYNTAX trial: Coronary bypass superior to percutaneous coronary intervention for triple-vessel or left main artery disease

1. In severe coronary artery disease, coronary artery bypass graft (CABG) was superior to percutaneous coronary intervention (PCI) in reducing the need for repeat vascularization.

2. This study suggested CABG should remain the standard of care for severe coronary artery disease, despite being associated with a higher risk of stroke.

Original Date of Publication: March 2009

Study Rundown: The Synergy between Percutaneous Coronary Intervention with Taxus and Cardiac Surgery (SYNTAX) trial was the first large, multicenter, randomized controlled trial comparing CABG to PCI in severe coronary artery disease. This non-inferiority trial demonstrated that CABG was superior to PCI in preventing a composite measure of death, and this was driven by a decrease in the need for repeat revascularization. CABG, however, was associated with a significantly higher rate of stroke compared to PCI. Strengths of this study included the fact that it was conducted at 85 centers across North America and Europe and that it assessed all-comers with severe coronary artery disease. Criticisms of the study included the limited follow-up of 12 months and that most study participants were male. Thus, in patients with severe coronary artery disease, the SYNTAX trial suggests that CABG remain the standard of care, given reduced rate of the primary endpoint at the 12 month mark.

In-Depth [randomized controlled trial]: The SYNTAX trial, published in 2009 in NEJM, sought to determine the optimal mode of revascularization, CABG or PCI for patients with severe coronary artery disease; that is, previously untreated triple-vessel or left main artery disease. In this non-inferiority trial, the primary endpoint was a composite of death from any cause, stroke, myocardial infarction, or repeat revascularization in the 12 month period after randomization. A total of 3075 patients were included in the trial. Of these patients, 1800 were randomized to either CABG or PCI. For the other 1275, there was only 1 suitable treatment option, and they were enrolled in registries for either CABG or PCI. The majority of patients studied were male (78%). There were no significant differences between the groups in terms of preprocedural rates of major adverse cardiac or cerebrovascular events. At 12 months, there was a significantly lower rate of the primary endpoint in the CABG group compared to PCI (12.4% vs. 17.8%, p = 0.002), which was driven by a significant reduction in the need for repeat revascularization (5.9% vs. 13.5%, p < 0.001). Notably, when compared to PCI, there was a significantly higher rate of stroke in the CABG group.

Serruys PW, Morice M-C, Kappetein AP, Colombo A, Holmes DR, Mack MJ, et al. Percutaneous Coronary Intervention versus Coronary-Artery Bypass Grafting for Severe Coronary Artery Disease. New England Journal of Medicine. 2009 Mar 5;360(10):961–72.

The ROMICAT 1 trial: Coronary computed tomographic angiography highly sensitive for acute coronary syndrome in patients with acute chest pain

1. In patients presenting with chest pain and a low to intermediate risk of acute coronary syndrome (ACS), computed tomographic coronary angiography (CTCA) demonstrated high sensitivity and negative predictive value for acute coronary syndrome.

Original Date of Publication: May 2009

Study Rundown: Chest pain is one of the most common patient complaints and accounts for over 100 million emergency department visits every year in the U.S. alone. Most patients presenting with chest pain have not suffered an ACS, though many are admitted to hospital for further monitoring and testing. CTCA is a rapid test that can identify significant stenoses in the coronary arteries, though its utility in chest pain evaluation was unclear having only been assessed in several small studies.

The Rule Out Myocardial Infarction using Computer Assisted Tomography 1 (ROMICAT 1) trial was a blinded prospective cohort study that sought to determine whether CTCA was useful in assessing patients with acute chest pain and low to intermediate risk of ACS. The absence of coronary artery disease on CTCA demonstrated sensitivity of 100% and negative predictive value (NPV) of 100% for ACS. Thus, CTCA may be of high utility in evaluating patients with chest pain in the emergency department and facilitate more rapid discharge of patients with low to intermediate likelihood of ACS. Additional radiation exposure remains one of the limitations inherent in this technology, though decreasingly so with modern techniques including prospective electrocardiogram (ECG) triggering.

In-Depth [prospective cohort]: This study examined 368 patients who were > 18 years of age, presented to the emergency department with chest pain lasting > 5 minutes in the previous 24 hours, had initially normal troponin levels and ECG, were suspected to have ischemic chest pain, were admitted to the hospital to rule out myocardial infarction (MI), and were able to perform a breath hold of 10-15 seconds. Exclusion criteria included initial elevation in troponin or CK-MB levels, new diagnostic ECG changes (ST-segment elevation or depression ≥1 mm or T wave inversions > 4 mm in 2 contiguous leads), hemodynamic or clinical instability, known allergy to iodinated contrast, and history of established coronary artery disease (previous stent implantation or coronary bypass grafting).

CT imaging was performed using a 64-slice scanner (Sensation 64, Siemens Medical Solutions) with iodinated contrast. Patients with heart rate > 60 beats/min received intravenous metoprolol 5-20 mg, unless their systolic blood pressure was < 100 mmHg. Axial images were reconstructed using a retrospectively ECG-gated algorithm. The presence of significant coronary artery stenosis was defined as any luminal obstruction > 50% in any coronary segment.

By CTCA, 183 patients (50%) were found to have no coronary disease. In this cohort, identifying no plaque demonstrated a sensitivity and NPV of 100% (95%CI 89-100%) and 100% (95%CI 98-100%), respectively, for ACS. Finding any plaque yielded a specificity of 54% (95%CI 49-60%) for ACS with positive predictive value (PPV) of 17%. The absence of significant coronary stenosis demonstrated a sensitivity of 77% (95%CI 59-90%) and NPV of 98%, while the presence of coronary stenosis demonstrated specificity of 87% (95%CI 83-90%) and PPV of 35%. Additionally, both plaque and stenosis, as assessed on CTA, predicted ACS independent of cardiovascular risk factors or TIMI risk score (AUC 0.88, 0.82 versus 0.63, respectively; all $p < 0.05$).

Hoffmann U, Bamberg F, Chae CU, Nichols JH, Rogers IS, Seneviratne SK, et al. Coronary Computed Tomography Angiography for Early Triage of Patients With Acute Chest Pain The ROMICAT (Rule Out Myocardial Infarction using Computer Assisted Tomography) Trial. J Am Coll Cardiol. 2009 May 5;53(18):1642–50.

The ACTIVE trial: Dual antiplatelet therapy in atrial fibrillation

1. In patients with atrial fibrillation who require anticoagulation but cannot tolerate warfarin, dual anti-platelet therapy may be a potential alternative for stroke prophylaxis.

2. Clopidogrel, in addition to daily aspirin, was associated with a significantly reduced incidence of stroke, but increased incidence of major bleeding in patients with atrial fibrillation when compared to treatment with aspirin alone.

Original Date of Publication: May 2009

Study Rundown: Atrial fibrillation is a common arrhythmia characterized by uncoordinated contractions of the atria, thereby resulting in blood stasis and increased risk of thromboembolic disease. The CHADS2 score is a commonly used score to estimate a patient's annualized risk of stroke by assessing age and comorbidities. Stroke prophylaxis with antiplatelets or anticoagulants is generally recommended with a CHADS2 score of 1 or more. While vitamin K antagonists, like warfarin, remain the most commonly used anticoagulants for stroke prophylaxis in atrial fibrillation, they are not suitable for many patients due to drug interactions, elevated risk of intracranial bleeds, and monitoring requirements, amongst other reasons. Originally published in 2009, the purpose of the Atrial Fibrillation Clopidogrel Trial with Irbesartan for Prevention of Vascular Events (ACTIVE) trial was to explore whether adding clopidogrel to aspirin for stroke prophylaxis would be more effective than aspirin alone, in patients who were considered unsuitable for warfarin. In summary, the trial found that the addition of clopidogrel significantly reduced the risk of stroke, but also significantly increased the risk of major bleeding.

In-Depth [randomized controlled trial]: The study involved 7554 participants from 580 centers in 33 countries. Patients were eligible for the trial if they had atrial fibrillation at enrolment or ≥2 episodes of intermittent atrial fibrillation in the past 6 months, and at least 1 risk factor for stroke (e.g., ≥75 years, hypertension, previous stroke, left ventricular ejection fraction < 45%). Patients were excluded if they required a vitamin K antagonist or clopidogrel, or if they had risk factors for hemorrhage (e.g., peptic ulcer disease in past 6 months, previous intracerebral hemorrhage, significant thrombocytopenia, alcohol abuse). Participants were randomly assigned to receive either clopidogrel 75 mg daily or a matching placebo. All participants were also prescribed 75-100 mg of aspirin daily. Follow-up occurred over a median of 3.6 years. The primary outcome was a composite measure comprised of strokes, myocardial infarctions, non-central nervous system systemic embolism, or death from vascular causes. Patients in the clopidogrel group experienced significantly lower risk of the primary outcome compared to patients taking aspirin alone (RR 0.89; 95%CI 0.81-0.98). This difference was driven by a significant reduction in the risk of stroke (RR 0.72; 95%CI 0.62-0.83). Compared to those receiving aspirin alone, the rates of major bleeding were significantly higher in the group receiving clopidogrel (RR 1.57; 95%CI 1.29-1.92), occurring most commonly in the gastrointestinal tract.

ACTIVE Investigators, Connolly SJ, Pogue J, Hart RG, Hohnloser SH, Pfeffer M, et al. Effect of clopidogrel added to aspirin in patients with atrial fibrillation. New England Journal of Medicine. 2009 May 14;360(20):2066–78.

The RE-LY trial: Dabigatran non-inferior to warfarin for stroke prevention in atrial fibrillation

1. High-dose dabigatran was superior to warfarin in the prevention of strokes in patients with atrial fibrillation, while low-dose dabigatran was non-inferior to warfarin in preventing strokes in this population.

2. There was lower risk of major hemorrhage with low-dose dabigatran compared to warfarin, while there was similar rate of major hemorrhage with high-dose dabigatran as compared to warfarin.

Original Date of Publication: September 2009

Study Rundown: Anticoagulation with warfarin, a vitamin K antagonist, has long been the standard of care for preventing thromboembolic strokes in high-risk patients with atrial fibrillation. Warfarin, however, is limited by the need for frequent monitoring due to its narrow therapeutic window, as well as its variable pharmacokinetics and drug interactions. Furthermore, its use is associated with a significant risk of major bleeding. Dabigatran, a direct thrombin inhibitor, is a newer oral anticoagulant introduced within the last decade as a possible alternative to warfarin. There is evidence for its use in venous thromboembolism (VTE) prophylaxis after total knee or hip arthroplasty, as well as in the treatment of acute VTE. At the time of this study, no evidence, existed for the use of dabigatran in the context of atrial fibrillation in the prevention of stroke. The Randomized Evaluation of Long-Term Anticoagulation Therapy (RE-LY) trial compared low- (110 mg PO BID) and high-dose (150 mg PO BID) dabigatran with dose-adjusted warfarin in preventing stroke in at risk patients with atrial fibrillation.

Dabigatran was found to be non-inferior to warfarin in the prevention of stroke in at-risk patients with atrial fibrillation, and was associated with an overall lower risk of major bleeding and intracranial hemorrhage. For those at-risk patients requiring anticoagulation for the prevention of stroke in the context of atrial fibrillation, dabigatran could be considered as an alternative to warfarin in those patients with a creatinine clearance > 30 mL/min, as dabigatran is renally cleared. A major criticism of the RE-LY trial was the high risk of bias created by the unblinded administration of warfarin. Moreover, it has been noted that the incidence of intracranial hemorrhage with warfarin observed in this study was much higher than previously reported rates and reasons for this are unclear.

In-Depth [randomized controlled trial]: This large, randomized, double-blinded, controlled trial included 18 113 patients from 951 clinical centers in 44 countries. Patients were randomized to 3 groups: 1) dose-adjusted warfarin titrated to INR of 2.0-3.0, 2) low-dose dabigatran (110 mg PO twice per day), or 3) high-dose dabigatran (150 mg PO twice per day). Patients were eligible for the trial if they had atrial fibrillation documented on electrocardiogram and at least 1 high-risk feature (e.g., previous stroke or transient ischemic attack, a left ventricular ejection fraction < 40%, New York Heart Association (NYHA) class II or higher symptoms, age > 75 years or between 65-74 years with diabetes mellitus/hypertension/coronary artery disease). Notably, dabigatran administration was blinded, while warfarin administration was unblinded. The primary outcome studied was stroke or systemic embolism. The primary safety outcome was major hemorrhage.

The trial lasted a total of 2 years. The rate of stroke or systemic embolism was significantly lower in patients that received high-dose dabigatran as compared to warfarin (RR 0.66; 95%CI 0.53-0.82), and there was no significant difference in major bleeding between these 2 groups (p = 0.31). Furthermore, low-dose dabigatran was non-inferior to warfarin in preventing strokes (RR 0.91; 95%CI 0.74-1.11), but it was associated with a significant reduction in risk of major bleeding (RR 0.80; 95%CI 0.69-0.93). Intracranial hemorrhage was significantly less common in both dabigatran groups compared to warfarin (p < 0.001). Rate of major gastrointestinal bleeding was significantly higher for patients receiving high-dose dabigatran as compared to the warfarin group (p < 0.001). There was no significant difference in mortality between all groups.

Connolly SJ, Ezekowitz MD, Yusuf S, Eikelboom J, Oldgren J, Parekh A, et al. Dabigatran versus Warfarin in Patients with Atrial Fibrillation. New England Journal of Medicine. 2009 Sep 17;361(12):1139–51.

The PLATO trial: Ticagrelor vs. clopidogrel for acute coronary syndrome

1. Treatment with ticagrelor significantly reduced mortality among patients with acute coronary syndrome (ACS) when compared to clopidogrel.

2. Ticagrelor treatment did not significantly increase the incidence of major bleeding.

Original Date of Publication: September 2009

Study Rundown: Clopidogrel is a commonly used medication in the management of ACS. A previous study comparing prasugrel, another oral antiplatelet agent, with clopidogrel demonstrated a significant reduction in the risk of coronary thrombotic events, but no improvement in mortality. The Platelet Inhibition and Patient Outcomes (PLATO) trial compared the use of ticagrelor, a newer and more potent oral platelet inhibitor, with clopidogrel in treating patients with ACS. In summary, patients treated with ticagrelor experienced significantly lower rates of death from vascular causes, myocardial infarction, or stroke at 12 months when compared to patients on clopidogrel. This was driven by both significant reductions in the rate of death from vascular causes and myocardial infarction. Moreover, there was no significant difference between the 2 groups in the rate of major bleeding.

In-Depth [randomized controlled trial]: This study was a multicenter trial, which randomized patients to treatment with clopidogrel or ticagrelor in addition to aspirin after ACS. Patients were eligible for the study if they were hospitalized for ACS with or without ST-segment elevation, with symptom onset in the previous 24 hours. Patients were excluded if they had contraindications to clopidogrel, they received fibrinolytic therapy in the 24 hours prior to randomization, they needed oral anticoagulation, they had an increased risk of bradycardia, or they were being treated with a strong cytochrome P-450 3A inhibitor or inducer. The primary endpoint was a composite of death from vascular causes, myocardial infarction, or stroke. Major life-threatening bleeding was defined as fatal bleeding, intracranial bleeding, intrapericardial bleeding with cardiac tamponade, shock/hypotension as a result of bleeding, hemoglobin decrease ≥ 5.0 g/dL, or need for transfusion of ≥ 4 units of packed red blood cells.

A total of 18 624 patients were recruited from 862 centers in 43 countries. At 12 months, the primary endpoint occurred significantly less in the ticagrelor group as compared with the clopidogrel group (HR 0.84; 95%CI 0.77-0.92). This difference was driven by significant reductions in rates of myocardial infarction (HR 0.84; 95%CI 0.75-0.95) and death from vascular causes (HR 0.79; 95%CI 0.69-0.91) in the ticagrelor group. The rates of major bleeding were not significantly different between the 2 groups (HR 1.04; 95%CI 0.95-1.13). Notably, the rate of fatal intracranial bleeding was significantly higher in the ticagrelor group compared to the clopidogrel group ($p = 0.02$).

Wallentin L, Becker RC, Budaj A, Cannon CP, Emanuelsson H, Held C, et al. Ticagrelor versus Clopidogrel in Patients with Acute Coronary Syndromes. New England Journal of Medicine. 2009 Sep 10;361(11):1045–57.

The MADIT-CRT trial: Cardiac resynchronization therapy in heart failure

1. In patients with heart failure, reduced left ventricular ejection fraction, and prolonged QRS> 130 ms, treatment with cardiac resynchronization therapy (CRT), in addition to implantable cardioverter-defibrillator (ICD), significantly reduced the risk of heart failure events when compared with patients only receiving ICD.

2. The rates of device-related complications were similar between the 2 groups both in short- and long-term follow-up.

Original Date of Publication: October 2009

Study Rundown: In patients with severe heart failure and reduced left ventricular ejection fraction, treatment with an ICD has been shown to reduce mortality. On the other hand, prolonged defibrillator therapy has been shown to increase the likelihood of suffering from heart failure events. CRT involving biventricular pacing has been shown to reduce the risk of heart failure exacerbation in specific patients with severe heart failure. The purpose of the Multicenter Automatic Defibrillator Implantation Trial with Cardiac Resynchronization Therapy (MADIT-CRT) trial was to determine whether CRT in combination with an ICD would reduce the risk of death or nonfatal heart failure events in patients with left ventricular ejection fraction (LVEF) < 30%, QRS > 130 ms, and New York Heart Association (NYHA) class I or II symptoms. In summary, patients treated with ICD-CRT were significantly less likely to experience nonfatal heart failure events when compared to those treated with ICD alone. There was no significant difference between the groups in all-cause mortality. Notably, this study was stopped prematurely because prespecified efficacy thresholds were achieved.

In-Depth [randomized controlled trial]: This study was conducted at 110 centres from across Canada, the United States, and Europe. A total of 1820 patients were randomized to receive either ICD only or ICD-CRT. Patients were eligible for the study if they were 21 years or older, with NYHA class I or II symptoms, sinus rhythm, LVEF < 30%, and QRS duration > 130 ms. All eligible patients also had an indication for ICD. Exclusion criteria included an existing indication for CRT, NYHA class III or IV symptoms, previous coronary artery bypass grafting, or myocardial infarction in the 3 months prior to randomization.

The primary endpoint was all-cause mortality or nonfatal heart failure events, and analysis was performed using intention-to-treat principle.

The trial was stopped prematurely after prespecified efficacy threshold was achieved. The primary endpoint was significantly less likely to occur in the ICD-CRT group as compared with the ICD group (HR 0.66; 95%CI 0.52-0.84). This difference was driven by a significant reduction in nonfatal heart failure events (HR 0.59; 95%CI 0.47-0.74), while there was no difference between the groups in all-cause mortality (HR 1.00; 95%CI 0.69-1.44). These findings were true for both patients with ischemic and non-ischemic cardiomyopathy. One death occurred in the ICD-CRT group after device implantation due to pulmonary embolism. In the first 30 days after device implantation, the rates of pneumothorax, infection, and pocket hematoma were similar between the 2 groups. Rates of device-related adverse events were also similar in longer term follow-up.

Moss AJ, Hall WJ, Cannom DS, Klein H, Brown MW, Daubert JP, et al. Cardiac-resynchronization therapy for the prevention of heart-failure events. The New England Journal of Medicine. 2009;361(14):1329-1338.

The RACE-II trial: Lenient vs. strict rate-control in atrial fibrillation

1. Lenient rate-control was found to be non-inferior to strict rate-control in managing patients with atrial fibrillation.

2. Compared to strict rate-control, lenient rate-control was achieved with lower doses of medication and fewer medications.

Original Date of Publication: April 2010

Study Rundown: Atrial fibrillation is the most prevalent sustained cardiac arrhythmia. It is a condition characterized by tachycardia and irregular heart rate, which often results due to disorganized electrical signaling in the atria. The condition is associated with an increased risk of stroke, and anticoagulation is an important management consideration. Previously, rate-control and rhythm-control were both considered acceptable options for management. The AFFIRM and RACE trials demonstrated, however, that rate-control was not inferior and was also associated with fewer adverse events compared to rhythm-control. As a result, rate-control is now often the first-line approach for treating atrial fibrillation, along with appropriate anticoagulation. While certain guidelines suggested stricter rate-control would reduce symptoms, reduce the incidence of heart failure, and improve survival, these recommendations were not evidence-based. The risk of certain adverse events was higher in patients undergoing stricter rate-control, including bradycardia and syncope. The RACE-II trial was a randomized, controlled trial designed to explore whether lenient rate-control (i.e., target resting heart rate < 110 bpm) was inferior to strict rate-control (i.e., target resting heart rate < 80 bpm, < 110 bpm during exercise) in reducing the incidence of cardiovascular events in patients with atrial fibrillation. In summary, there was no significant difference between the strategies in the risk of death from cardiovascular causes, hospitalization for heart failure, stroke, systemic embolism, major bleeding, and arrhythmic events.

In-Depth [randomized controlled trial]: The study was conducted at 33 centers in the Netherlands and involved 614 patients. Patients were eligible if they had atrial fibrillation for up to 12 months, were ≤80 years of age, had a mean resting heart rate > 80 bpm, and were using oral anticoagulation therapy. Included patients were randomized to the lenient control strategy (i.e., target resting heart rate < 110 bpm) or the strict control strategy (i.e., target resting heart rate < 80 bpm, < 110 bpm during exercise). The primary outcome was a composite of death from cardiovascular causes, hospitalization for heart failure, stroke, systemic embolism, major bleeding, and arrhythmic events (e.g., syncope, sustained ventricular tachycardia, and cardiac arrest). Secondary outcomes included components of the primary outcome, along with all-cause mortality, symptoms, and functional status. At the end of the follow-up period, the resting heart rates were 85±14 and 76±14 in the lenient- and strict-control groups, respectively ($p < 0.001$). It was found that lenient control was noninferior to strict control in preventing the primary outcome (HR 0.84; 90%CI 0.58-1.21). Moreover, there was no significant difference in all-cause mortality (HR 0.91; 90%CI 0.52-1.59). There were no significant differences between the groups in symptoms associated with atrial fibrillation such as dyspnea, fatigue, and palpitations. Additionally, there was no significant difference between the groups in terms of heart failure functional status.

Van Gelder IC, Groenveld HF, Crijns HJGM, Tuininga YS, Tijssen JGP, Alings AM, et al. Lenient versus Strict Rate Control in Patients with Atrial Fibrillation. New England Journal of Medicine. 2010 Apr 15;362(15):1363–73.

The SHIFT: Ivabradine in congestive heart failure

1. In patients with congestive heart failure (CHF) and baseline heart rate > 70 beats per minute (bpm), ivabradine significantly reduced the risk of heart failure hospitalization and death from heart failure compared to placebo.

2. Compared to those on placebo, patients taking ivabradine experienced significantly higher rates of atrial fibrillation, asymptomatic and symptomatic bradycardia.

Original Date of Publication: August 2010

Study Rundown: CHF is a common condition across much of the developed world and is a significant source of morbidity and mortality. Current therapies for CHF, including angiotensin-converting-enzyme (ACE) inhibitors and beta-blockers, work in part by reducing cardiac workload and harmful remodeling. However, even with maximally tolerated doses of beta-blockers, many patients still present with elevated heart rates, a factor linked to increased rates of hospitalization and cardiovascular death. Ivabradine, a novel inhibitor of the "funny current" (I_f) channels, was found to selectively reduce heart rate in preclinical studies. The Systolic Heart failure with the I_f inhibitor ivabradine Trial (SHIFT) sought to investigate the effect of ivabradine on patients with CHF.

This multinational, randomized controlled trial compared adding ivabradine or placebo to standard therapy in patients with CHF and a baseline heart rate > 70 bpm. In summary, patients receiving ivabradine achieved significant reductions in their average resting heart rate and experienced lower rates of cardiovascular death and hospitalization for CHF than those taking placebo. This study is limited in its generalizability, as patients with arrhythmias and severe CHF were excluded. Nevertheless, the results do suggest that heart rate plays a significant role in the progression of heart failure, and that the introduction of ivabradine may improve outcomes.

In-Depth [randomized controlled trial]: This multinational, double-blind, randomized controlled trial was conducted in 677 institutions in 37 countries. A total of 6558 adults with stable symptomatic heart failure, a prior hospitalization for CHF, an ejection fraction < 35%, and a resting heart rate > 70 bpm were enrolled in the study. These participants were all maintained on standard medical therapy and randomly assigned to receive placebo or a twice-daily dose of ivabradine titrated to achieve a heart rate between 50 and 60 bpm. Exclusion criteria included recent myocardial infarction in the preceding 2 months, ventricular or atrioventricular pacing for > 40% of the day, atrial fibrillation or flutter, and symptomatic hypotension. Patients were followed for a median of 22.9 months. The primary outcome was a composite endpoint of cardiovascular death or hospitalization for worsening CHF.

Compared to the placebo group, heart rates in patients taking ivabradine were reduced by 10.9 bpm (95%CI 10.4-11.4 bpm). Patients in the ivabradine group experienced significantly lower rates of the primary outcome compared to those on placebo (HR 0.82, 95%CI 0.75-0.90, p < 0.0001). The effect was driven mainly by reduced rates of hospitalization (HR 0.74; 95%CI 0.66-0.83, p < 0.0001) and lower mortality from heart failure (HR 0.74, 95%CI 0.58-0.94, p = 0.014, respectively). In total, there were fewer adverse events reported in the ivabradine group than in the placebo group, although ivabradine was associated with increased rates of atrial fibrillation (p = 0.012), asymptomatic bradycardia (p < 0.0001), symptomatic bradycardia (p < 0.0001), and visual disturbances (p < 0.0001).

Swedberg K, Komajda M, Böhm M, Borer JS, Ford I, Dubost-Brama A, et al. Ivabradine and outcomes in chronic heart failure (SHIFT): A randomised placebo-controlled study. The Lancet. 2010;376(9744):875-885.

The HAS-BLED score: Bleeding risk in atrial fibrillation

1. The HAS-BLED score is an easy-to-remember and easy-to-apply tool that has good predictive accuracy for the risk of major bleeding in patients with atrial fibrillation.

2. Since its publication, the HAS-BLED score has been validated in a large cohort study of 7329 patients.

Original Date of Publication: November 2010

Study Rundown: In atrial fibrillation impaired atrial contraction leads to blood stasis within the atria, thereby increasing the risk of thrombus formation and cardioembolic stroke. The CHADS2 score was developed to identify patients with atrial fibrillation who are at higher risk of stroke and who should therefore be treated with oral anticoagulation. Treatment with oral anticoagulants, however, increases one's risk of bleeding. The HAS-BLED score was developed in response to the need for tools to estimate the risk of major bleeding in patients with atrial fibrillation. Originally published in 2010, the score consists of 7 factors: hypertension, abnormal renal/liver function, stroke, bleeding history or predisposition, labile international normalized ratio (INR), elderly (>65 years), and drugs/alcohol use concomitantly. This study demonstrated that the HAS-BLED score had good predictive accuracy for major bleeding in the overall cohort of patients, but performed much better in patients on antiplatelet agents or no antithrombotic therapy. When compared to the HEMOR2RHAGES scheme, the HAS-BLED score consists of fewer factors and only requires clinical assessment or routine bloodwork. The HAS-BLED score has since been validated in a larger cohort study published in the Journal of the American College of Cardiology.

In-Depth [retrospective cohort]: This study utilized a cohort of patients that were identified from the prospectively developed Euro Heart Survey on Atrial Fibrillation database. Patients in the database were followed for 1 year to determine survival and incidence of major adverse events, including major bleeding (i.e., hemoglobin drop > 2 g/L or requiring transfusion). The HAS-BLED score was constructed by identifying bleeding risk factors from a derivation cohort and adding consistent risk factors for major bleeding found in recent systematic reviews. The final score included hypertension (systolic > 160 mmHg), abnormal renal (dialysis, renal transplantation, or creatinine ≥200 umol/L) or liver function (chronic liver disease, or biochemical evidence), stroke, bleeding history or predisposition, labile INR (therapeutic time in range < 60%), elderly (>65 years), drugs/alcohol use concomitantly.

Of the 5272 patients in the Euro Heart Survey on Atrial Fibrillation, 3456 did not have mitral valve stenosis or valvular surgery and were included in this study. The HAS-BLED score was compared with the HEMOR2RHAGES scheme, a previously developed tool for estimating the risk of bleeding. C statistics were calculated to determine the predictive accuracy of each model using various sets of patients. The HAS-BLED score had C statistics of 0.72 (95%CI 0.65-0.79) for the overall cohort, 0.69 (95%CI 0.59-0.80) for patients on oral anticoagulants, 0.91 for patients on antiplatelet agents (95%CI 0.83-1.00), and 0.85 for patients on no antithrombotic therapy (95%CI 0.00-1.00). The HEMOR2RHAGES scheme had C statistics of 0.66 (95%CI 0.57-0.74) for the overall cohort, 0.64 (95%CI 0.53-0.75) for patients on oral anticoagulants, 0.83 for patients on antiplatelet agents (95%CI 0.68-0.98), and 0.81 for patients on no antithrombotic therapy (95%CI 0.00-1.00). *The HAS-BLED score is detailed below:*

Clinical characteristic	Points awarded
Hypertension	1
Abnormal renal and liver function (1 each)	1 or 2
Stroke	1
Bleeding history or predisposition	1
Labile INR	1
Elderly (>65 years)	1
Drugs or alcohol (1 each)	1 or 2

Table I. Clinical characteristics and points awarded

HAS-BLED score	Number of patients	Bleeds per 100 patient-years
0	798	1.13
1	1,286	1.02
2	744	1.88
3	187	3.74
4	46	8.70
5	8	12.50
6	2	0.0
7	0	-
8	0	-
9	0	-

Table II. HAS-BLED score, number of patients and bleeds per 100 patient-years

Pisters R, Lane DA, Nieuwlaat R, de Vos CB, Crijns HJGM, Lip GYH. A novel user-friendly score (has-bled) to assess 1-year risk of major bleeding in patients with atrial fibrillation: The euro heart survey. Chest. 2010 Nov 1;138(5):1093–100.

The EMPHASIS-HF trial: Eplerenone reduces mortality in mild systolic heart failure

1. Eplerenone significantly reduced mortality in patients suffering from heart failure with reduced systolic function (left ventricular ejection fraction [LVEF] ≤30%, or 30-35% if QRS> 130 ms) and mild symptoms (New York Heart Association [NYHA] class II) when compared with placebo.

2. The incidence of hyperkalemia was significantly higher in the eplerenone group.

Original Date of Publication: January 2011

Study Rundown: Mineralocorticoid antagonists significantly improved survival in patients with severe systolic heart failure (i.e., LVEF< 35% and NYHA class III/IV symptoms) in the RALES trial and in patients with heart failure after myocardial infarction in the EPHESUS trial. The purpose of the EMPHASIS-HF trial was to explore the effects of adding eplerenone, a type of mineralocorticoid antagonist, to evidence-based therapy in patients with systolic heart failure and only mild symptoms (i.e., LVEF< 35% and NYHA class II symptoms). Results showed that eplerenone significantly reduced the risk of death from cardiovascular causes and hospitalization for heart failure. While there was a significantly higher risk of hyperkalemia in the eplerenone group, there were no significant differences between the groups in the rate of drug withdrawal for hyperkalemia. This study, along with the RALES and EPHESUS trials, demonstrated that mineralocorticoid antagonism in patients with symptomatic systolic heart failure was linked with improved mortality and reduced hospitalization. One criticism of the trial was that the study population only differed from the RALES population based on their subjective NYHA classification. Thus, critics argued that it was difficult to determine whether there was really a true enough difference between the study populations. While the NYHA classification is subjective, it is a strong prognostic tools for heart failure patients, and the rates of mortality observed in the EMPHASIS-HF trials were much lower than those seen in the RALES trial, suggesting there was a difference in the severity of disease.

In-Depth [randomized controlled trial]: This trial involved 2737 patients recruited at 278 centers in 29 countries. Patients were considered eligible for the trial if they were ≥55 years of age, had NYHA class II symptoms, LVEF≤30% (or

30-35% if QRS> 130 ms), and were being treated with angiotensin-converting enzyme inhibitor/angiotensin receptor blocker and a beta-blocker at recommended or maximal tolerated doses, unless contraindicated. Patients were excluded if they were having acute myocardial infarction, NYHA class III/IV symptoms, serum potassium > 5.0 mmol/L, glomerular filtration rate < 30 mL/min/1.73m^2, a need for potassium-sparing diuretic, or any other clinically significant coexisting condition. The primary outcome was a composite of death from cardiovascular causes or a first hospitalization for heart failure. Secondary outcomes included hospitalization for heart failure or death from any cause, death from any cause, and death from cardiovascular causes, among others.

A total of 1364 patients were randomized to the eplerenone group, while 1373 were randomized to the placebo group. At 3 years after randomization, the eplerenone group experienced a significantly lower rate of the primary outcome (HR 0.63; 95%CI 0.54-0.74) when compared to placebo. Notably, the eplerenone group experienced significantly lower rates of both death from cardiovascular causes (HR 0.76; 95%CI 0.61-0.94) as well as hospitalization for heart failure (HR 0.58; 95%CI 0.47-0.70). Moreover, patients treated with eplerenone also experienced significantly lower rates of death from any cause (HR 0.76; 95%CI 0.62-0.93) and hospitalization for any reason (HR 0.77; 95%CI 0.67-0.88). While rates of hyperkalemia were significantly higher in the eplerenone group (8.0% vs 3.7%, $p < 0.001$), there were no significant differences in the rates of study drug withdrawal for hyperkalemia between the 2 groups.

Zannad F, McMurray JJV, Krum H, van Veldhuisen DJ, Swedberg K, Shi H, et al. Eplerenone in Patients with Systolic Heart Failure and Mild Symptoms. New England Journal of Medicine. 2011 Jan 6;364(1):11–21.

The RIVAL trial: Radial vs. femoral artery access for percutaneous coronary intervention

1. The composite outcome of death, myocardial infarction (MI), stroke, and non-coronary artery bypass graft-related major bleeding did not differ between radial and femoral access for percutaneous coronary intervention (PCI).

2. Radial artery access was associated with a significantly lower rate of vascular complications when compared to femoral access.

Original Date of Publication: April 2011

Study Rundown: For patients with acute coronary syndromes (ACS), vascular access for PCI via the femoral artery is associated with a substantial risk of bleeding, particularly at the access site. Vascular access via the radial artery may reduce bleeding risks since the site is more superficial and compressible. Observational studies suggested that radial access may also be associated with a lower risk of death and MI. The Radial Vs Femoral (RIVAL) trial was the first large, randomized, controlled trial that compared radial access for PCI to femoral access. Results revealed that radial and femoral access did not differ in the rate of the composite primary outcome, which consisted of death, MI, stroke, and non-coronary artery bypass graft (CABG)-related major bleeding. Vascular access site complications, however, were significantly reduced with radial access compared to femoral. In particular, radial access was associated with a decreased risk of developing large hematomas and pseudoaneurysms requiring closure. Finally, there was a significant interaction between the primary outcome and the volume of radial PCIs performed by the medical center. One potential limitation of the study was the overall low rate of major bleeding, which may have prevented the detection of a significant difference in non-CABG-related bleeding due to radial versus femoral access. This may have been due to the study's use of experienced, high-volume interventional cardiologists whose technical skills may be superior to those of other cardiologists. In summary, the RIVAL trial demonstrated that radial and femoral artery access for PCI are equally effective in managing ACS. Radial access, while potentially more difficult to establish, may be preferable due to the significantly lower risk of vascular complications, as compared with femoral access.

In-Depth [randomized controlled trial]: The RIVAL trial was a randomized, parallel group, multicenter trial. A total of 7021 patients were enrolled in the trial and underwent randomization. Patients were eligible if they had a diagnosis of ACS and were planning to undergo PCI. Patients were excluded if they presented in cardiogenic shock, had peripheral vascular disease, or a history of previous CABG surgery. Recruited cardiologists were required to have expertise in both radial and femoral artery access, including at least 50 radial procedures. In the end, 3507 participants were randomized to radial access and 3514 participants were randomized to femoral access. The primary outcome was a composite of death, MI, stroke, and non-CABG-related major bleeding at 30 days. There was no difference in the occurrence of the primary outcome between the radial and femoral groups (HR 0.92; 95%CI 0.72-1.17). There was an observed interaction between the primary outcome and a medical center's volume of radial access (HR 0.49, 95%CI 0.28-0.87). Radial access was associated with significantly fewer vascular complications, including development of large hematoma (HR 0.40; 95%CI 0.28-0.57) and pseudoaneurysm needing closure (HR 0.30; 95%CI 0.13-0.71).

Jolly SS, Yusuf S, Cairns J, Niemelä K, Xavier D, Widimsky P, et al. Radial versus femoral access for coronary angiography and intervention in patients with acute coronary syndromes (RIVAL): a randomised, parallel group, multicentre trial. Lancet. 2011 Apr 23;377(9775):1409–20.

The PRECOMBAT trial: Percutaneous coronary intervention vs. coronary bypass in left main coronary artery stenosis

1. In patients with left main coronary artery stenosis, angioplasty with sirolimus-eluting stents was noninferior to coronary artery bypass grafting (CABG) in preventing subsequent cardiac and cerebrovascular events.

2. Percutaneous coronary intervention (PCI) patients experienced a significantly higher incidence of ischemia-driven target vessel revascularization compared to coronary artery bypass graft patients

3. Because of low event rates, the study was underpowered.

Original Date of Publication: May 2011

Study Rundown: The Premier of Randomized Comparison of Bypass Surgery versus Angioplasty Using Sirolimus-Eluting Stent in Patients with Left Main Coronary Artery Disease (PRECOMBAT) trial compared PCI to CABG in patients with left main coronary artery stenosis. Prior to this study, some evidence suggested that PCI may be an acceptable alternative to CABG in certain patients with left main disease, though outcomes had never been assessed in a large, randomized trial. In the PRECOMBAT trial, patients with left main coronary artery stenosis were treated with PCI with a sirolimus-eluting stent or CABG and were followed for 2 years after randomization. PCI with sirolimus-eluting stents was found to be non-inferior to CABG for left main coronary artery stenosis at 12 months with respect to the primary outcome. At 2 years, the rates of major coronary events, cerebrovascular events, and all-cause mortality were similar in patients being treated with PCI or CABG. Of note, patients treated with PCI experienced significantly higher rates of ischemia-driven target vessel revascularization when compared with CABG patients at the 2-year mark. In summary, this study shows that PCI was noninferior to CABG in treating left main coronary artery stenosis with regards to the primary composite endpoint (i.e., major adverse cardiac or cerebrovascular events). As a result of low event rates, however, the study was underpowered and the study authors have noted that these findings should not be clinically directive.

In-Depth [randomized controlled trial]: This trial was conducted at 13 centers across South Korea. Patients were eligible for the study if they were ≥18 years of age and had received a diagnosis of stable angina, unstable angina, silent ischemia, or non-ST-elevation myocardial infarction (NSTEMI), with more than 50% stenosis of the left main coronary artery. Eligible patients also needed to be candidates for CABG or PCI as determined heir treating physicians and surgeons. The primary endpoint was a composite of death from any cause, myocardial infarction, stroke, and ischemia-driven target vessel revascularization in the 12 months following randomization.

A total of 600 patients were enrolled and randomized as part of the trial. At 12 months, 8.7% of patients in the PCI group and 6.7% of patients in the CABG group experienced primary endpoints (absolute risk difference 2.0%; 95%CI -1.6 to 5.6%; p = 0.01 for non-inferiority). At 24 months, there were no significant differences between the 2 groups with regards to the primary endpoint (HR 1.50; 95%CI 0.90-2.52). Ischemia-driven target vessel revascularization (i.e., repeat revascularization with stenosis of 50% and ischemic signs/symptoms or 70% without ischemic signs/symptoms) was significantly higher in the PCI group at 24 months (HR 2.18; 95%CI 1.10-4.32).

Park S-J, Kim Y-H, Park D-W, Yun S-C, Ahn J-M, Song HG, et al. Randomized Trial of Stents versus Bypass Surgery for Left Main Coronary Artery Disease. New England Journal of Medicine. 2011 May 5;364(18):1718–27.

The ARISTOTLE trial: Apixaban superior to warfarin for stroke prophylaxis in atrial fibrillation

1. Apixaban was superior to warfarin in preventing stroke in patients with atrial fibrillation.

2. Apixaban therapy had a decreased risk of intracranial hemorrhage compared to warfarin.

3. There was no difference in gastrointestinal (GI) bleeding risk between apixaban and warfarin.

Original Date of Publication: September 2011

Study Rundown: Warfarin is a vitamin K antagonist that has long been the mainstay of anticoagulation therapy for prevention of thromboembolic stroke in patients with atrial fibrillation. Recently, apixaban, a direct Xa inhibitor, was introduced to the market. It has a much wider therapeutic range, does not require monitoring, and 25% of it is cleared by the kidneys. The Apixaban for Reduction in Stroke and Other Thromboembolic Events in Atrial Fibrillation (ARISTOTLE) was a landmark trial that sought to address whether apixaban was superior to warfarin in reducing the risk of thromboembolic stroke in patients with atrial fibrillation. The trial demonstrated that apixaban was superior in preventing thromboembolic strokes in patients with atrial fibrillation when compared to warfarin. In addition, there was a significant reduction in the risk of bleeding in patients treated with apixaban compared to warfarin. While the high cost of apixaban limits its widespread use, for patients in whom warfarin is contraindicated, apixaban offers an effective, safe anticoagulation alternative to warfarin.

In-Depth [randomized controlled trial]: This study was a multicenter, blind, randomized controlled trial that assigned 18 206 patients with atrial fibrillation to either standard warfarin therapy or apixaban therapy for thromboembolism prophylaxis. All patients had a documented history of atrial fibrillation or atrial flutter at least twice in the past 12 months and all had at least 1 additional risk factor for stroke. The primary outcome in the study was rate of thromboembolic stroke or a systemic embolism. The secondary outcome was death from all causes.

Patients were followed for 1.8 years and all adverse effects of therapy were documented.

The apixaban group experienced a significant reduction in thromboembolic stroke compared to the warfarin group (HR 0.79, 95%CI 0.66-0.95) but no difference in the rate of systemic embolism (HR 0.89, 95%CI 0.44-1.75). There was also a significant reduction in all-cause mortality in the apixaban group compared to the warfarin group (HR 0.89; 95%CI 0.80-0.998). Apixaban treatment also significantly reduced the risk of major bleeding as compared to warfarin (HR 0.69, 95%CI 0.6-0.8). On further examination, the apixaban group had a significantly lower rate of intracranial bleeds but no difference in the rate of GI bleeding in comparison to warfarin. When the primary outcome results were examined in subgroups, apixaban proved to be better than warfarin in all subgroups except for the younger population (i.e., patients less than 65 years of age), who fared better with warfarin therapy.

Granger CB, Alexander JH, McMurray JJV, Lopes RD, Hylek EM, Hanna M, et al. Apixaban versus Warfarin in Patients with Atrial Fibrillation. New England Journal of Medicine. 2011 Sep 15;365(11):981–92.

Medical management superior to stenting for stroke related to intracranial arterial stenosis

1. The risk of early stroke after angioplasty and stenting of intracranial atherosclerotic lesions was higher than expected, while the risk of stroke with aggressive medical therapy alone was lower than expected.

2. The probability of ischemic stroke, symptomatic brain hemorrhage, and non-stroke related death after stenting plus medical management was significantly greater than medical management alone.

Original Date of Publication: September 2011

Study Rundown: Atherosclerotic intracranial arterial stenosis is an important cause of ischemic stroke and a major predictor of recurrent stroke following an initial event. Combination antiplatelet therapy and risk factor management have long been regarded as mainstays in the treatment and prevention of recurrent stroke. However, with the approval of the first self-expanding nitinol stent by the Food and Drug Administration (FDA) in 2005 for use in patients with atherosclerotic intracranial arterial stenosis, percutaneous transluminal angioplasty and stenting (PTAS) in addition to antithrombotic therapy emerged as a potential alternative approach towards the treatment of high-risk patients.

In the randomized controlled trial conducted by Chimowitz and colleagues, the safety and efficacy of PTAS and medical therapy was compared to medical therapy alone in high-risk patients with intracranial arterial stenosis. The results of this trial showed that aggressive medical management alone was superior to PTAS plus medical management, demonstrating a lower risk of recurrent ischemic stroke.

In-Depth [randomized controlled trial]: This study was conducted in 50 sites across the United States. To be considered eligible for participation in the study, patients must have experienced a transient ischemic attack (TIA) or nondisabling stroke within 30 days of enrollment, attributed to intracranial arterial stenosis of 70-99% of a major intracranial artery. Arterial stenosis was verified angiographically. Patients with tandem extracranial or intracranial stenosis, an occlusion located proximally or distally to the target intracranial lesion, or bilateral intracranial vertebral artery stenosis were excluded. Following screening and consent, patients were randomized to receive PTAS and medical management or medical management alone. Medical therapy consisted of 325 mg of aspirin and 75 mg of clopidogrel, both administered daily for 90 days after enrollment, as well as management of primary (elevated systolic blood pressure and low-density lipoprotein (LDL) cholesterol levels) and secondary risk factors (diabetes, elevated non-high-density lipoprotein (non-HDL) cholesterol levels, smoking, excess weight and sedentarism) through a lifestyle modification program. Primary endpoints of the study included ischemic stroke, symptomatic brain hemorrhage, and non-stroke related death within 30 days after enrollment, as well as ischemic stroke in the territory of the qualifying lesion beyond 30 days of enrollment.

A total of 451 patients were randomized to receive either PTAS and medical therapy (n = 224; mean age 61.0 years, SD 10.7; 56.7% male) or medical therapy alone (n = 227; mean age 59.5 years, SD 11.8 years; 63.9% male). There were no significant differences between the groups with respect to baseline patient characteristics. In the PTAS group, the probability of experiencing any primary end point within 30 days after enrollment was considerably higher at 14.7% compared to 5.8% in the medical management group (p = 0.002). In addition, while no patients in the medical management group experienced symptomatic brain hemorrhage during the 30-day follow-up period, 10 of the 33 strokes (30.3%) in the PTAS group resulted in this outcome (p = 0.04). Over 1 year of follow-up, the probability of experiencing a primary endpoint was also significantly greater in the PTAS group (20.2%) compared to the medical management group (12.2%) (p = 0.009).

Chimowitz MI, Lynn MJ, Derdeyn CP, Turan TN, Fiorella D, Lane BF, et al. Stenting versus aggressive medical therapy for intracranial arterial stenosis. The New England Journal of Medicine. 2011 Sep;365(11):993-1003.

The ROCKET AF: Rivaroxaban non-inferior to warfarin for stroke prophylaxis in atrial fibrillation

1. Rivaroxaban was non-inferior to warfarin in preventing strokes and systemic embolism.

2. Compared to warfarin, rivaroxaban reduced the rates of critical, fatal, and intracranial bleeding.

Original Date of Publication: September 2011

Study Rundown: Warfarin is the standard for anticoagulation in patients with atrial fibrillation to prevent thromboembolic events. However, accompanying warfarin therapy are challenging pharmacokinetics, extensive food and drug interactions, and need for international normalized ratio (INR) monitoring. In recent years, investigators have studied new oral anticoagulants for use in atrial fibrillation. A main advantage of these agents is that they do not require frequent INR monitoring. Dabigatran, a direct thrombin inhibitor, was shown to be a possible alternative to warfarin in the RELY trial. Rivaroxaban is another new oral anticoagulant. It acts to prevent thrombus formation by being a direct factor Xa inhibitor. The Rivaroxaban Once Daily Oral Direct Factor Xa Inhibition Compared with Vitamin K Antagonism for Prevention of Stroke and Embolism Trial in Atrial Fibrillation (ROCKET AF) was published in 2011. The trial demonstrated that rivaroxaban was non-inferior to warfarin in preventing stroke and systemic embolism. The use of rivaroxaban was also associated with significantly lower rates of critical bleeding, fatal bleeding, and intracranial hemorrhage when compared to warfarin. Thus, in patients with non-valvular atrial fibrillation who are at elevated risk of stroke or systemic embolism, rivaroxaban may be considered as an alternative to warfarin in those patients with a creatinine clearance > 30mL/min.

In-Depth [randomized controlled trial]: This large, randomized, controlled trial included 14 264 patients from 1178 clinical centers in 45 countries. Patients were included if they had nonvalvular atrial fibrillation, demonstrated on electrocardiography, and were at moderate-to-high risk for stroke (i.e., CHADS2 score ≥2). Patients were randomized to 2 groups: 1) rivaroxaban 20 mg daily, or 15 mg daily if creatinine clearance was 30-49 mL/min, or 2) warfarin with dose titrated to INR of 2.0-3.0. The primary outcome studied was a composite of stroke (i.e., both ischemic and hemorrhagic) and systemic embolism. The primary safety outcome was a composite of major and non-major bleeding events that were clinically relevant. In the intention-to-treat population, there was no significant difference in the incidence of the primary endpoint between the rivaroxaban and warfarin groups, thereby demonstrating non-inferiority (HR 0.88; 95%CI 0.74-1.03). With regard to the primary safety endpoint, there was no significant difference between the 2 groups in terms of the incidence of major and non-major bleeding events that were clinically relevant (HR 1.03; 95%CI 0.96-1.11). A further analysis of major bleeding events, however, demonstrated that the rivaroxaban group experienced significantly lower rates of critical bleeding (HR 0.69; 95%CI 0.53-0.91), fatal bleeding (HR 0.50; 95%CI 0.31-0.79), and intracranial hemorrhage (HR 0.67; 95%CI 0.47-0.93) compared to the warfarin group.

Patel MR, Mahaffey KW, Garg J, Pan G, Singer DE, Hacke W, et al. Rivaroxaban versus Warfarin in Nonvalvular Atrial Fibrillation. New England Journal of Medicine. 2011 Sep 8;365(10):883–91.

The ROMICAT 2 trial: Coronary computed tomographic angiography shortens hospital stay for acute chest pain

1. In patients presenting to the emergency department with acute chest pain, evaluation with coronary computed tomographic angiography (CTCA) led to significantly shorter hospital stays compared to standard care.

2. There were no undetected acute coronary syndromes (ACSs) in either group and no significant difference between the groups in the rate of major adverse cardiovascular events (MACE) at 28 days.

Original Date of Publication: July 2012

Study Rundown: The Rule Out Myocardial Infarction/Ischemia Using Computer Assisted Tomography 1 (ROMICAT 1) trial was a prospective cohort study that demonstrated the high sensitivity and negative predictive value of CTCA in patients with low to intermediate risk of ACS. The ROMICAT 2 trial was a randomized controlled trial that compared a strategy incorporating CTCA with standard care in assessing patients presenting to the emergency department with chest pain. Patients in the CTCA group experienced significantly shorter hospital stays and higher rates of direct discharge from the emergency department compared to those receiving standard care. Moreover, there were no cases of undetected ACS in either group, and no significant difference in the rate of major adverse cardiovascular events (MACE) at 28 days after the index visit.

In-Depth [randomized controlled trial]: The study involved 1000 patients recruited from 9 centers across the U.S. who were randomized in a 1:1 ratio to evaluation involving CTCA or to standard evaluation. Patients were eligible for the trial if they were 40-74 years of age, had chest pain or an angina equivalent lasting > 5 minutes in the 24 hours prior to presenting, and warranted further risk stratification to rule out acute coronary syndrome (ACS) according to the assessing physician. Exclusion criteria included history of known coronary artery disease, new diagnostic ischemic changes on the initial electrocardiogram (ECG), initial elevated troponin, creatinine > 132.6 μmol/L (>1.5 mg/dL), iodine contrast allergy, and body mass index > 40.

At least 64-slice CT technology was required, and both retrospectively ECG-gated and prospectively ECG-triggered CTCAs were allowed. The primary endpoint was length of hospital stay. Secondary endpoints included time to diagnosis, rate of direct discharge from the emergency department, and resource utilization. The secondary safety endpoints were undetected ACS and MACE (death, myocardial infarction, unstable angina, or urgent coronary revascularization) within 28 days, and periprocedural complications (stroke, bleeding, anaphylaxis, renal failure).

The mean length of hospitalization was 7.6 hours shorter for patients in the CTA group compared to those undergoing standard evaluation ($p < 0.001$). Patients undergoing CTCA also experienced significantly shorter time to diagnosis ($p < 0.001$), and had significantly higher rates of direct discharge from the emergency department (47% versus 12%, $p < 0.001$). There were no undetected ACSs and no significant differences between the groups in the rate of MACE at 28 days ($p = 0.18$) or periprocedural complications ($p = 0.50$).

Patients in the CTA group had significantly higher rates of diagnostic testing ($p < 0.001$) and functional testing ($p < 0.001$) than those in the standard group. Moreover, there was a trend towards higher rates of coronary angiography ($p = 0.06$) and revascularization ($p = 0.16$) in those who underwent CTA, though the costs of care were not significantly different between the two groups for the index visit and follow-up period ($p = 0.65$).

Hoffmann U, Truong QA, Schoenfeld DA, Chou ET, Woodard PK, Nagurney JT, et al. Coronary CT Angiography versus Standard Evaluation in Acute Chest Pain. The New England Journal of Medicine. 2012 Jul 26;367(4):299–308.

The FREEDOM trial: Coronary bypass graft vs. PCI in diabetic patients

1. In patients with diabetes and multivessel disease, coronary artery bypass grafting (CABG) was shown to be superior to percutaneous coronary intervention (PCI) with drug-eluting stents in reducing the risk of all-cause mortality and nonfatal myocardial infarction.

2. Patients treated with PCI experienced a smaller risk of nonfatal stroke, but also had significantly higher rates of revascularization within a year of their procedure compared to those treated with CABG.

Original Date of Publication: December 2012

Study Rundown: Patients with multivessel coronary artery disease regularly undergo revascularization, and a large portion of these patients have diabetes. Prior studies have demonstrated that diabetic patients have greater survival when they receive CABG rather than balloon angioplasty, and as a result, guidelines at the time favored CABG for revascularization. There have been significant advances in PCI over the past few decades, particularly with the advent of drug-eluting stents. As a result, it remains unclear whether CABG or PCI was more suitable for multivessel disease in the context of diabetes.

The Future Revascularization Evaluation in Patients with Diabetes Mellitus: Optimal Management of Multivessel Disease (FREEDOM) trial sought to address this question. Patients with diabetes and multivessel disease were randomized to undergo PCI with drug-eluting stents or CABG in addition to standard medical therapy, and subsequently followed for minimum of 2 years. In summary, CABG was found to be superior to PCI in reducing all-cause mortality and nonfatal myocardial infarctions in this patient population. Compared to PCI, CABG was linked with a small but significant increase in the risk of nonfatal stroke. Nevertheless, this trial supports the use of CABG over PCI in diabetic patients with multivessel disease.

In-Depth [randomized controlled trial]: This randomized controlled trial was conducted at 140 centers around the world. To be included, patients had to have diabetes and angiographically confirmed multivessel disease with stenosis > 70% in 2 or more major coronary arteries in at least 2 major coronary-artery territories.

Patients with left main coronary stenosis were excluded. A total of 1900 patients met these criteria and underwent randomization to either PCI with drug-eluting stents or CABG, where arterial revascularization was encouraged. All patients were treated to optimize their medical risk factors (e.g., low-density lipoprotein levels, blood pressure, glycated hemoglobin), and the primary outcome was a composite of all-cause mortality, nonfatal myocardial infarction, and nonfatal stroke.

The rate of the primary outcome was significantly higher in patients receiving PCI than in those receiving CABG at 5 years (26.6% vs. 18.7%, absolute difference 7.9%, 95%CI 3.3 to 12.5%, $p = 0.005$). This was driven by lower rates of all-cause mortality (absolute difference 5.4%, 95%CI 1.5 to 9.2%, $p = 0.049$) and nonfatal myocardial infarction ($p < 0.001$). Patients treated with PCI experienced significantly fewer strokes than those treated with CABG ($p = 0.03$). Significantly higher rates of repeat revascularization within 1 year were observed in the PCI compared to CABG group (12.6% vs. 4.8%, $p < 0.001$).

Farkouh ME, Domanski M, Sleeper LA, Siami FS, Dangas G, Mack M, et al. Strategies for multivessel revascularization in patients with diabetes. The New England Journal of Medicine. 2012;367(25):2375-2384.

The WOEST trial: Double vs. triple therapy in patients requiring PCI and anticoagulation

1. In patients requiring percutaneous coronary intervention (PCI) and long-term oral anticoagulation, treating with clopidogrel alone (i.e., double therapy) significantly reduced the risk of bleeding when compared to a combination of aspirin and clopidogrel (i.e., triple therapy).

2. There were no differences between the 2 groups in the risk of myocardial infarction, stroke, target vessel revascularization, or stent thrombosis.

Original Date of Publication: March 2013

Study Rundown: Many patients, like those with atrial fibrillation or mechanical heart valves, require long-term oral anticoagulation. A significant proportion of these patients also suffer from ischemic coronary artery disease requiring PCI, and subsequently, require dual antiplatelet therapy in addition to anticoagulation. Combining these therapies, however, increases bleeding risk, with uncertain benefit in reducing thrombosis risk. The What is the Optimal antiplatelet and anticoagulation therapy in patients with oral anticoagulation and coronary StenTing (WOEST) trial sought to address these uncertainties. Patients with an indication for long-term anticoagulation who required PCI were recruited to the trial and randomized to either antiplatelet therapy with clopidogrel (i.e., double therapy), or a combination of aspirin and clopidogrel (i.e., triple therapy) in addition to their anticoagulatin. Triple therapy was considered standard at the time of the study. In summary, patients treated with double therapy had a significantly lower risk of bleeding than those on triple therapy. Moreover, there were no significant differences between the 2 groups in the risk of myocardial infarction, stroke, target vessel revascularization, or stent thrombosis. An important consideration for generalizability is that this trial only involved patients anticoagulated with vitamin K-antagonists, and these results are not reflective of patients taking novel oral anticoagulants.

In-Depth [randomized controlled trial]: This open-label, randomized trial was conducted at 15 sites in the Netherlands and Belgium. Patients were eligible for the study if they were between 18 and 80 years of age, had an indication for long-term anticoagulation (e.g., atrial fibrillation, mechanical heart valve), and had a severe coronary lesion with indication for PCI. Exclusion criteria included a history of intracranial bleeding, cardiogenic shock, a contraindication to aspirin, clopidogrel or both, thrombocytopenia with platelet count < 50 × 10⁹/L, major bleeding in the past 12 months, and pregnancy. Included patients were randomized to either clopidogrel alone (i.e., double therapy) or a combination of aspirin and clopidogrel (i.e., triple therapy) in addition to their anticoagulation with a vitamin K-antagonist. In the case of bare metal stents, antiplatelets were taken for 1 month and up to 1 year, while antiplatelets were administered for at least 1 year in patients with drug-eluting stents. The primary endpoint was any bleeding episode during 1-year follow-up. The composite secondary endpoint included death, myocardial infarction, stroke, target-vessel revascularization and stent thrombosis.

A total of 573 patients underwent randomization. At 1 year, patients in the double therapy group experienced significantly lower risk of overall bleeding compared to the triple therapy group (HR 0.40; 95%CI 0.28-0.58, $p < 0.0001$). The rates of major bleeding, however, were no different between the 2 groups (HR 0.56; 95%CI 0.25-1.27, $p = 0.159$). Patients in the double therapy group also experienced significantly lower risk of the composite secondary endpoint (HR 0.60; 95%CI 0.38-0.94, $p = 0.025$), as they had significantly lower risk of death (HR 0.39; 95%CI 0.16-0.93, $p = 0.027$) than patients on triple therapy. There were no significant differences between the 2 groups in the risk of myocardial infarction, stroke, target vessel revascularization or stent thrombosis.

Dewilde WJ, Oirbans T, Verheugt FW, Kelder JC, De Smet BJ, Herrman JP, et al. Use of clopidogrel with or without aspirin in patients taking oral anticoagulation therapy and undergoing percutaneous coronary intervention: An open-label, randomised, controlled trial. The Lancet. 2013;381(9872):1107-1115.

The RE-ALIGN trial: Dabigatran vs. warfarin for mechanical heart valves

1. In patients with mechanical heart valves, anticoagulation with dabigatran was associated with significantly higher rates of stroke and major bleeding when compared to warfarin.

2. Based on these findings, patients with mechanical heart valves should be anticoagulated with warfarin, as opposed to dabigatran.

Original Date of Publication: September 2013

Study Rundown: Prosthetic heart valve replacement is sometimes recommended for patients with severe valvular heart disease. While mechanical valves are more durable than bioprosthetic ones, they are associated with a higher risk of thromboembolic disease and lifelong anticoagulation is typically needed. Warfarin provides excellent protection against thromboembolic complications in patients with mechanical heart valves, but regular drug monitoring is required. Dabigatran is an oral direct thrombin inhibitor that is effective as an anticoagulant in the treatment of various conditions, including stroke prophylaxis in patients with atrial fibrillation and for the treatment of acute venous thromboembolism, but does not require regular monitoring comparable to warfarin. The Randomized, Phase II Study to Evaluate the Safety and Pharmacokinetics of Oral Dabigatran Etexilate in Patients after Heart Valve Replacement (RE-ALIGN) trial sought to determine whether dabigatran would be effective in preventing thromboembolism in patients with mechanical heart valves, as compared with warfarin. The trial was terminated prematurely due to a significantly higher rate of ischemic or unspecified stroke in the dabigatran group. Moreover, there were significantly higher rates of bleeding in the dabigatran group when compared to those on warfarin. A large proportion of the patients in the dabigatran group discontinued their medications or required dosage adjustments. In summary, the use of dabigatran in patients with mechanical heart valves was linked with significantly higher rates of stroke and bleeding when compared to warfarin therapy. Patients with mechanical heart valves should continue to be anticoagulated with warfarin on the basis of these findings.

In-Depth [randomized controlled trial]: The RE-ALIGN trial was a multicenter, prospective, randomized, phase II, open-label trial with blinded end-point adjudication. Patients were eligible for the trial if they were between 18 and 75 years of age and were undergoing mechanical aortic and/or mitral valve replacement or had undergone mechanical mitral valve replacement > 3 months prior to randomization. Patients were randomized in a 2:1 ratio to treatment with dabigatran and warfarin. For patients in the dabigatran group, starting dose was determined based on creatinine clearance and trough levels were determined at prespecified timepoints; dose adjustments were made to achieve a trough plasma level ≥50 ng/mL. Patients in the warfarin group had their international normalized ratios (INR) checked at prespecified timepoints to ensure they were in target. The primary outcome was the trough level of dabigatran. Efficacy and safety outcomes included rates of stroke, systemic embolism, transient ischemic attack, valve thrombosis, bleeding, venous thromboembolism, and death.

At the interim analysis, 252 patients had undergone randomization, with 168 in the dabigatran group and 84 in the warfarin group. Interim analysis demonstrated that patients being treated with dabigatran had significantly higher risk of bleeding as compared to those on warfarin (RR 2.45; 95%CI 1.23-4.86; p = 0.01). Moreover, 9 patients (5%) experienced stroke and 3 patients (2%) had myocardial infarctions in the dabigatran group, while no strokes or myocardial infarctions were observed in those taking warfarin. The dose of dabigatran was increased in 24% of patients and the drug was discontinued in 8% of patients, as they did not attain trough plasma levels ≥50 ng/mL, despite being on the highest dose.

Eikelboom JW, Connolly SJ, Brueckmann M, Granger CB, Kappetein AP, Mack MJ, et al. Dabigatran versus warfarin in patients with mechanical heart valves. The New England Journal of Medicine. 2013;369(13):1206-1214.

The ICAP trial: Colchicine in acute pericarditis

1. This study demonstrated that colchicine, in addition to standard therapy, significantly reduced the risk of incessant or recurrent pericarditis compared to placebo.

2. There were no significant differences between colchicine and placebo in the risk of gastrointestinal side effects.

Original Date of Publication: October 2013

Study Rundown: Colchicine was originally extracted from the autumn crocus plant, which had been used in ancient times to treat swelling. Colchicine acts by inhibiting mitosis and neutrophil motility and activity, thereby generating an anti-inflammatory effect. It has long been used in the treatment of gout and other inflammatory conditions, with autumn crocus extract first documented as gout therapy in the first century AD. Several trials supported the use of colchicine in treating and preventing acute pericarditis, though these studies were small and nonrandomized.

The Investigation on Colchicine for Acute Pericarditis (ICAP) trial sought to determine the effects of colchicine in treating acute pericarditis. Patients treated with colchicine experienced significantly lower rates of incessant or recurrent pericarditis as compared with those taking placebo. The rates of adverse events and gastrointestinal upset were similar in the 2 groups.

In-Depth [randomized controlled trial]: This randomized controlled trial was conducted at the Maria Vittoria Hospital in Turin, Italy. Patients were eligible if they were > 18 years of age presenting with their first episode of acute pericarditis, diagnosed by observing 2 of typical chest pain, friction rub, suggestive electrocardiogram changes, new/worsening pericardial effusion. Exclusion criteria included tuberculous/neoplastic/purulent pericarditis, severe liver disease or elevated aminotransferase levels, renal dysfunction, hypersensitivity to colchicine, and pregnancy. A total of 240 patients underwent randomization to treatment with colchicine (0.5 to 1 mg daily for 3 months) or placebo, in addition to standard therapy for acute pericarditis (aspirin, ibuprofen, or glucocorticoid therapy with proton-pump inhibitor prophylaxis). The primary outcome was persistent or recurrent pericarditis.

Patients being treated with colchicine experienced significantly lower rates of the primary outcome as compared with those taking placebo (16.7% vs. 37.5%; relative risk reduction 0.56, 95%CI 0.30-0.72, p < 0.001). The recurrence rate was also significantly lower in the colchicine group (9.2% vs. 20.8%; relative risk reduction 0.56, 95%CI 0.13-0.99, p = 0.02). The overall rate of adverse events (p = 0.84) and the incidence of gastrointestinal disturbance (p = 0.67) were similar in the 2 groups.

Imazio M, Brucato A, Cemin R, Ferrua S, Maggiolini S, Begaraj F, et al. A randomized trial of colchicine for acute pericarditis. The New England Journal of Medicine. 2013;369(16):1522-1528.

The PARADIGM-HF trial: Combo angiotensin-neprilysin inhibitor superior to enalapril in heart failure

1. LCZ696 is a novel drug that combines the neprilysin inhibitor, sacubitril, and the angiotensin receptor blocker (ARB), valsartan.

2. In patients with heart failure with reduced ejection fraction, LCZ696 was more effective than enalapril in preventing cardiovascular death and hospitalization.

Original Date of Publication: September 2014

Study Rundown: Over 6 million Americans suffer from heart failure, with half of those from systolic heart failure, or heart failure with reduced ejection fraction, and the other half with heart failure with preserved ejection fraction. The current standard of care consists of an angiotensin converting enzyme (ACE) inhibitor, beta-blocker, and the addition of an aldosterone antagonist as needed. ARBs are used in patients who are unable to tolerate ACE inhibitors. Natriuretic peptides reduce vasoconstriction and sodium retention and are secreted from the heart, kidneys, vasculature, and the central nervous system during heart failure. These natriuretic peptides are degraded by neprilysin. Previous studies have shown that the inhibition of neprilysin leads to an increase of these peptides, thus reducing vasoconstriction and sodium retention. Additionally, the combination of neprilysin and ACE inhibition has been shown in animal studies to be more effective than either therapy alone. However, in clinical trials (OVERTURE and OCTAVE), patients experienced severe angioedema when treated with both drugs together. Promisingly, the combination of an ARB with a neprilysin inhibitor was found to be more effective than ARB alone in treating patients with hypertension and heart failure with preserved ejection fraction. The PARADIGM-HF (Prospective Comparison of ARNI [Angiotensin Receptor–Neprilysin Inhibitor] with ACEI [Angiotensin-Converting–Enzyme Inhibitor] to Determine Impact on Global Mortality and Morbidity in Heart Failure Trial) sought to assess whether the combination of an ARB with neprilysin inhibition was more effective than ACE inhibition alone in class II-IV heart failure patients with reduced ejection fraction. After 27 weeks, the authors found a significant reduction in the rate of cardiovascular death and hospitalizations in patients treated with LCZ696 as compared to the ACE inhibitor, enalapril. This five year phase III trial is the largest trial to date in the evaluation of heart failure therapy. These tremendously positive results suggest that LCZ696 may be a novel therapy in the treatment of heart failure, the first in almost a decade.

In-Depth [randomized control trial]: This randomized, double-blinded trial consisted of 8442 patients with NYHA class II-IV heart failure with an ejection fraction of 35% or less. Patients received either LCZ696 or enalapril treatment daily. The primary outcome was death from cardiovascular causes or hospitalization for heart failure. Prior to randomization, all patients underwent a run-in period where tolerance to both medicines were assessed. The trial was stopped early, after 27 months due to overwhelming benefit of the study drug.

At trial stoppage, death from cardiovascular causes or hospitalization for heart failure occurred in 914 patients (21.8%) in the LCZ696 group and 1117 patients (26.5%) in the enalapril group (hazard ratio 0.8 in the LCZ696 group; $p < 0.001$). Death due to cardiovascular causes was reduced by 20% with LCZ696 treatment, from 16.5% in the enalapril group to 13.3% in the LCZ696 group (hazard ratio 0.80; 95%CI, 0.71 to 0.89; $p < 0.001$). Hospitalizations were reduced by 21% with LCZ696 treatment, from 15.6% in the enalapril group to 12.8% in the LCZ696 group.

Symptomatic hypotension was more present in the LCZ696 group, though cough and hyperkalemia were reduced. Compared to the enalapril group, fewer patients in the LCZ696 group stopped their study medication because of an adverse event (12.3% vs. 10.7%, $p = 0.03$) or because of renal impairment (1.4% vs. 0.7%, $p = 0.002$).

McMurray JJV, Packer M, Desai AS, Gong J, Lefkowitz MP, Rizkala AR, et al. Angiotensin–Neprilysin Inhibition versus Enalapril in Heart Failure. New England Journal of Medicine. 2014 Sep 11;371(11):993–1004.

The DAPT trial: Extended dual antiplatelet therapy after drug eluting stents

1. After 12 months of dual antiplatelet therapy in patients who received drug eluting stents (DES), patients who continued on a thienopyridine in addition to aspirin for 18 months experienced significantly lower rates of stent thrombosis and myocardial infarction compared to those taking placebo.

2. The risk of bleeding was significantly higher in patients who continued on thienopyridine therapy.

Original Date of Publication: December 2014

Study Rundown: Coronary revascularization with DES is increasingly used to treat ischemic heart disease. While DES reduce the risk of restenosis compared to bare metal stents (BMS), they are associated with a higher risk of stent thrombosis, which may result in myocardial infarction and death. After stenting, patients are treated with dual antiplatelet therapy in order to prevent progressive atherosclerosis of the stent itself and potential subsequent plaque rupture. The optimal duration of dual antiplatelet therapy to reduce the risk of stent thrombosis and atherosclerosis, while considering the increased risk of bleeding, is unknown. The purpose of the Dual Antiplatelet Therapy (DAPT) trial was to explore the effects of continuing dual antiplatelet therapy with a thienopyridine and aspirin for an additional 18 months in patients who had already been treated for 12 months.

Researchers concluded that the risk of stent thrombosis and myocardial infarction were significantly reduced in the group continuing dual antiplatelet therapy, compared to those being treated with placebo and aspirin. Patients continuing on dual antiplatelet therapy, however, also experienced significantly higher rates of bleeding. A major limitation of this study was that patients were only eligible for randomization if they were adherent with therapy and did not experience any cardiovascular or cerebrovascular events in the initial 12 month treatment period. As a result, patients who were randomized may be at lower risk of adverse events compared to the general population, thereby limiting generalizability. Notably, the study was funded by 8 companies that manufacture stents and pharmaceuticals.

In-Depth [randomized controlled trial]: A total of 9961 patients from 452 sites in 11 countries were randomized as part of this study. Patients were eligible for the trial if they were > 18 years of age and could be treated with dual antiplatelet therapy after receiving DES (i.e., sirolimus-, zotraolimus-, paclitaxel-, or everolimus-eluting stents) or BMS. In this trial, only data from patients receiving DES were analyzed. All eligible patients were treated with a thienopyridine (i.e., clopidogrel 75 mg daily or prasugrel 10 mg daily) and aspirin for 12 months. Afterwards, patients who did not experience a major adverse cardiovascular or cerebrovascular event were randomized to continue treatment with a thienopyridine or a placebo until the 30 month mark, in addition to daily aspirin. The primary endpoints were the cumulative incidence of stent thrombosis and major adverse cardiovascular and cerebrovascular events (i.e., composite of death, myocardial infarction, and stroke) between months 12 and 30. The primary safety endpoint was the incidence of moderate or severe bleeding. Eight stent and pharmaceutical manufacturers were responsible for funding the study, though they did not have the right to make changes to the manuscript.

Patients who continued thienopyridine therapy experienced significantly lower rates of stent thrombosis when compared to those on placebo (HR 0.29; 95%CI 0.17-0.48). Moreover, the rate of major adverse cardiovascular and cerebrovascular events was also significantly lower in the thienopyridine group (HR 0.71; 95%CI 0.59-0.85). This was driven by significantly lower rates of myocardial infarction in the thienopyridine group (HR 0.47; 95%CI 0.37-0.61), as the rates of death from cardiovascular causes and stroke were similar between the 2 groups. With regards to safety, the risk of bleeding was significantly higher in the group that continued thienopyridine therapy as compared to placebo (HR 1.61; 95%CI 1.21-2.16). Notably, these differences were consistent regardless of the type of stent or thienopyridine used.

Mauri L, Kereiakes DJ, Yeh RW, Driscoll-Shempp P, Cutlip DE, Steg PG, et al. Twelve or 30 months of dual antiplatelet therapy after drug-eluting stents. The New England Journal of Medicine. 2014;371(23):2155-2166.

The BRIDGE trial: Periprocedural bridging in patients with atrial fibrillation

1. Patients with atrial fibrillation are often treated with long-term oral anticoagulation, and may require interruption of their anticoagulation for elective surgeries or invasive procedures.

2. This study demonstrated that periprocedural bridging with dalteparin did not significantly reduce the risk of arterial thromboembolic disease when compared to placebo.

3. Patients treated with bridging dalteparin experienced significantly higher risk of major and minor bleeding.

Original Date of Publication: August 2015

Study Rundown: Patients with atrial fibrillation are at a higher risk of stroke, transient ischemic attack (TIA), and systemic embolism. An important aspect of managing patients with atrial fibrillation involves treating them with long-term oral anticoagulation to reduce this risk. There has long been uncertainty regarding the need for bridging anticoagulation in these patients when their oral anticoagulants are held in preparation for an elective surgery or invasive procedure. The Bridging Anticoagulation in Patients who Require Temporary Interruption of Warfarin Therapy for an Elective Invasive Procedure or Surgery (BRIDGE) trial sought to determine the effects of bridging with dalteparin in patients with atrial fibrillation. In summary, the study demonstrated that there were no significant differences in the rates of arterial embolism (i.e., stroke, TIA, systemic embolism) between those who received bridging therapy and those who did not. The rates of major and minor bleeding were significantly higher, however, in patients who did receive bridging therapy. Based on these findings, periprocedural bridging with low-molecular-weight heparin is not recommended.

One major limitation of the study was that few patients at high-risk of stroke were involved in the study (i.e., CHADS2 score of 5 or 6). Another important note is that patients with mechanical heart valves were not included in this trial. Eisai donated dalteparin to the study, but had no role in the design or conduct of the study, data analysis, or manuscript preparation.

In-Depth [randomized controlled trial]: This randomized trial was conducted at 108 sites in the United States and Canada. Patients were eligible for the trial if they were ≥18 years of age, had permanent or paroxysmal atrial fibrillation or flutter, were on warfarin therapy ≥3 months, were undergoing an elective operation or procedure requiring interruption of their warfarin, and had one of the CHADS2 risk factors (i.e., congestive heart failure, hypertension, age ≥75 years, diabetes mellitus, previous stroke/embolism). Exclusion criteria included having a mechanical heart valve, stroke/systemic embolism/TIA in the previous 12 weeks, major bleeding in the previous 6 weeks, creatinine clearance < 30 mL/minute, platelet count < 100 × $10^3/m^3$, or planned cardiac/intracranial/intraspinal surgery. Eligible patients were randomized in a 1:1 ratio to either bridging with dalteparin (100 IU/kg subcutaneously twice daily) or placebo from 3 days prior to the procedure until 24 hours prior, and then for 5-10 days after the procedure (i.e., until the INR was ≥2). The primary efficacy outcome was the rate of arterial thromboembolism (i.e., stroke, TIA, or systemic embolism), while the primary safety outcome was the rate of major bleeding at 30 days. Minor bleeding was a secondary safety outcome.

Outcomes were assessed for 1813 patients. Very few patients in either group had CHADS2 scores of 5 or 6 (2.7% in the no bridging group, 3.4% in the bridging group). There were no significant differences between the bridging and non-bridging groups in the risk of arterial thromboembolism at 30 days (0.4% vs. 0.3%, respectively; p = 0.01 for non-inferiority, p = 0.73 for superiority). The risk of major bleeding was significantly higher in the bridging group (3.2% vs. 1.3%; p = 0.005). Minor bleeding was also more frequently seen in the bridging group as compared with those on placebo (20.9% vs. 12.0%; p < 0.001).

Douketis JD, Spyropoulos AC, Kaatz S, Becker RC, Caprini JA, Dunn As, et al. Perioperative bridging anticoagulation in patients with atrial fibrillation. The New England Journal of Medicine. 2015;373(9):823-833.

Liraglutide associated with lower incidence of death from CV causes in type 2 diabetics

1. Patients with type 2 diabetes who received liraglutide were observed to have a significantly lower incidence of the composite of death from cardiovascular causes, nonfatal MI, and nonfatal stroke, versus patients who received placebo.

2. The rates of both all-cause mortality and nephropathy were significantly lower for patients who received liraglutide than for patients who received placebo.

Original Date of Publication: July 2016

Study Rundown: Liraglutide is a glucagon-like peptide 1 (GLP-1) analogue, approved for the treatment of type 2 diabetes mellitus (T2DM). While the microvascular benefits of this drug are well characterized through its effect on improving glycemic control, its macrovascular effects are less than certain at this point. In this multicenter, double-blind, placebo-controlled trial, patients were randomized in a 1:1 ratio to receive a once daily liraglutide or placebo subcutaneous injection. The primary outcome in the study was the first occurrence of death from cardiovascular causes, nonfatal MI, or nonfatal stroke. The primary outcome was found to be significantly lower in the liraglutide group than in the placebo group. Additionally, death from CV causes alone was also found to be significantly lower in the liraglutide group than in the placebo group. All-cause mortality was also found to be significantly lower in the liraglutide group than in the placebo group, as well. This study draws strength from strict inclusion and exclusion criteria that made patients, effectively, treatment naïve at baseline: T2DM patients with HbA1c > 7.0% who had not received any medication for this condition previously. Its impact, however, is somewhat limited by the modest follow-up period of 42-60 months.

In-Depth [randomized controlled trial]: This study was a multicenter, double-blind, placebo-controlled trial, that included a total of 9340 patients. The patients were randomized in a 1:1 ratio to receive a once daily liraglutide or placebo subcutaneous injection. The mean follow-up was 3.8 years. The primary composite outcome (first occurrence of death from cardiovascular causes, nonfatal MI, or nonfatal stroke) occurred in fewer patients in the liraglutide group

13.0% than in the placebo group 14.9% (HR 0.87; 95%CI 0.78 to 0.97; p < 0.001 for non-inferiority; p = 0.01 for superiority). Death from CV causes was significantly lower in the liraglutide group 4.7% than in the placebo group 6.0% (HR 0.78; 95%CI 0.66 to 0.93; p = 0.007). The rate of all-cause mortality was also significantly lower in the liraglutide group 8.2% than in the placebo group 9.6% (HR 0.85; 95%CI 0.74 to 0.97; p = 0.02). The rate of nephropathy was significantly lower in the liraglutide group than in the placebo group (1.5 vs 1.9 events per hundred patient-years; HR 0.78; 95%CI 0.67 to 0.92; p = 0.003).

Marso SP, Daniels GH, Brown-Frandsen K, Kristensen P, Mann JFE, Nauck MA, et al. Liraglutide and Cardiovascular Outcomes in Type 2 Diabetes. New England Journal of Medicine. 2016 Jul 28;375(4):311–22.

The FOURIER trial: PCSK9 inhibitor significantly reduces the risk of cardiovascular events

1. In addition to significantly lowering levels of low density lipoprotein cholesterol (LDL-C), evolocumab reduced the composite risk of cardiovascular events in atherosclerotic patients on optimal statin therapy without a significant increase in adverse effects.

2. As individual endpoints, evolocumab did not significantly reduce the rate of either cardiovascular or all-cause mortality relative to placebo.

Original Date of Publication: May 2017

Study Rundown: Through a novel mechanism of decreased LDL-receptor recycling and increased LDL-C clearance, proprotein convertase subtilisin/kexin type 9 (PCSK9) inhibitors have demonstrated powerful and synergistic reductions in LDL-C in conjunction with statin therapy. Yet, no large scale studies have evaluated the efficacy of PCSK9 inhibitors in the prevention of cardiovascular outcomes. This trial evaluated the efficacy of evolocumab, a fully human monoclonal antibody against PCSK9, in reducing cardiovascular outcomes in patients on optimal statin therapy. A significant reduction was found in both the primary (a composite of death, MI, stroke, unstable angina hospitalization, and coronary revascularization) and secondary (death, MI, or stroke) endpoints without an associated increase in adverse events. However, no reduction in cardiovascular or all-cause mortality was found in the analysis of individual outcomes. Given the high cost and unclear mortality benefit, the use of PCSK9 inhibitors will likely remain relegated to select high-risk patients. This was a parallel, double-blinded trial that enrolled a large number of patients with stable atherosclerotic cardiovascular disease and provided the first evidence for the clinical value of PCSK9 inhibitors. While no direct reduction in all-cause death was found, the data supports both the benefit of reducing LDL-C to unprecedented low levels. The major limitation of this study was the short duration of follow-up.

In-Depth [randomized control trial]: This multinational study randomized 27,564 patients with established cardiovascular atherosclerotic disease to treatment with evolocumab (n = 13,784) or matching placebo (n = 13,780) in a 1:1 ratio. All patients had LDL-C of 70 mg/dL (median 92 mg/dL) or non-HDL-

C levels of 100 mg/dL and were on high-intensity (69.3%) or moderate-intensity (30.4%) statin therapy at baseline. Median duration of follow-up was 26 months. The primary end point was major cardiovascular events, defined as the composite of cardiovascular death, MI, stroke, unstable angina hospitalization, or coronary revascularization. The secondary end point was the composite of cardiovascular death, MI, or stroke. Adverse events were collected to assess safety.

At 48 weeks, the mean reduction in LDL-C with evolocumab compared to placebo was 59% (95%CI 58 to 60; p < 0.001), with an absolute reduction of 56 mg/dL (95%CI 55 to 57). This reduction was sustained over time. The primary endpoint occurred in 1344 patients (9.8%) with evolocumab group compared to 1593 patients (11.3%) in placebo (HR 0.85; 95%CI 0.79- 0.92; p < 0.001). The risk reduction in the primary endpoint increased over time (12% in the first year to 19% beyond the first year). The secondary endpoint occurred in 816 (5.9%) with evolocumab compared to 1013 (7.4%) with placebo (HR 0.80; 95%CI 0.73-0.88; p < 0.001). Regarding individual outcomes, there was a 21 to 27% risk reduction in MI, stroke, and coronary revascularization. No significant difference in cardiovascular or all-cause mortality was reported. All data was consistent across major demographic subgroups and quartiles of baseline LDL-C levels. Except for mild injection site reactions (2.1% vs. 1.6% with placebo), no significant difference in adverse events – including new-onset diabetes, antibody development, or neurocognitive adverse events – were associated with evolocumab.

Sabatine MS, Giugliano RP, Keech AC, Honarpour N, Wiviott SD, Murphy SA, et al. Evolocumab and Clinical Outcomes in Patients with Cardiovascular Disease. New England Journal of Medicine. 2017 May 4;376(18):1713–22.

The POET trial: oral antibiotics in stable endocarditis patients noninferior to intravenous treatment

1. Patients with left sided infective endocarditis who switched to oral antibiotics once stable had similar composite adverse event outcomes compared to patients treated with 6 weeks of intravenous antibiotics.

2. Patients in the oral treatment group had hospital stays significantly shorter than those in the intravenous treatment

Original Date of Publication: January 2019

Study Rundown: Left sided infective endocarditis generally requires 6 weeks of closely monitored intravenous antibiotic treatment. Due to the complexity of treatment many patients require extended hospital stays to learn how their treatment should be safely administered. If oral antibiotic therapy was a safe and feasible treatment option, significant treatment adherence issues and costs associated with extended hospital stays could be avoided. The Partial Oral Treatment of Endocarditis (POET) trial sought to evaluate how patients with stable left sided endocarditis responded to intravenous versus oral antibiotic therapy. The primary outcome, a composite of adverse events associated with infective endocarditis, showed oral treatment was noninferior to intravenous treatment at 6 months after treatment randomization. Additionally, hospital stays for patients in the oral treatment group were significantly shorter than in the intravenous group. This pragmatic randomized trial indicates a much more patient friendly oral antibiotic treatment regimen is a viable alternative to the traditional intravenous treatment infective endocarditis patients historically received. The study's strengths include clinician guided choice of antibiotics and extensive subgroup analysis, while its limitations include exclusion of certain infectious organisms and limited generalizability of results as few patients evaluated for trial inclusion ultimately were enrolled in the trial.

In-Depth [randomized control trial]: This noninferiority, Danish, randomized controlled trial enrolled patients between 2011 and 2017. Eligible patients had infectious left sided endocarditis on native or prosthetic valves, had no indications for cardiac surgery, were in a stable clinical condition receiving intravenous antibiotics, and had positive blood culture for streptococcus, *Enterococcus faecalis*, *Staphylococcus aureus*, or coagulase-negative staphylococci. If patients had at least 10 days of antibiotic treatment scheduled, they were eligible for randomization. Patients were randomized to oral (n = 201) or intravenous (n = 199) treatment groups. Patients in the oral group were eligible to receive treatment in in outpatient clinics, while intravenous group patients remained in the hospital. Antibiotics were chosen by the treating physicians. The primary outcome was a composite outcome of mortality, cardiac surgery, clinically relevant embolic events, or relapse of bacteremia within 6 months of trial randomization. Composite outcome events occurred in 12.1% and 9.0% of the intravenously and orally treated patients, respectively (odds ratio [OR], 0.72; 95% confidence interval [CI], 0.37 to 1.36) indicating noninferiority of oral treatment. Incidence of embolic events, cardiac surgery, and bacteremia relapse were similar between the two groups, while incidence of death was greater in the intravenous group. For all subgroups assessed there was no discernable difference outcomes based on treatment received. Pharmacokinetics of orally administered antibiotics were measured, and no oral treatment regimens were changed based on plasma levels.

Iversen K, Ihlemann N, Gill SU, Madsen T, Elming H, Jensen KT, et al. Partial Oral versus Intravenous Antibiotic Treatment of Endocarditis. New England Journal of Medicine. 2019 Jan 31;380(5):415–24.

The PARTNER 3 Trial: Transcatheter aortic-valve replacement versus surgery

1. This study found that composite stroke, mortality, and rehospitalization at one year was lower in aortic stenosis patients receiving transcatheter aortic-valve replacement (TAVR; 8.5%) as compared to surgery (15.1%).

2. The TAVR group also had significantly shorter index hospitalization and reduced risk of 30-day poor treatment outcome.

Original Date of Publication: May 2019

Study Rundown: The Placement of Aortic Transcatheter Valves (PARTNER) 3 Trial demonstrated that in patients with severe aortic stenosis who were classified at low risk for surgery, the one-year composite outcome of stroke, mortality, and rehospitalization was lower in those who received TAVR as compared to surgical aortic-valve replacement. Additionally, secondary endpoints of 30-day stroke, mortality or stroke, atrial fibrillation, and poor treatment outcome were significantly improved in the TAVR group. The major limitation of the was an insufficient follow-up time to determine long-term valve deterioration. Conversely, strengths of trial include large sample size, diversity of study sites, and inclusion of comprehensive secondary endpoints. In summary, the PARTNER 3 Trial demonstrated that in low-risk patients with severe aortic stenosis, TAVR is superior to surgery in reducing one-year composite mortality, stroke, and rehospitalization as well as a variety of secondary outcomes at 30 days. Additionally, those who underwent TAVR had a shorter recovery time as measured by New York Heart Association (NYHA) functional class, 6-minute walk-test distance, and Kansas City Cardiomyopathy Questionnaire score.

In-Depth [randomized control trial]: In the PARTNER 3 Trial, low surgical risk severe aortic stenosis patients were randomized to surgical aortic valve replacement (n = 454) or TAVR (n = 503). Patients were included who had severe calcific aortic stenosis and were deemed low surgical risk by a site heart team and trial case review committee. Primary and secondary endpoints were adjudicated by a clinical events committee. The primary composite endpoint of stroke, mortality, and rehospitalization at one year occurred in 8.5% of the TAVR group as compared to 15.1% of the surgery group (HR 0.54; 95%CI 1.29-2.76). The TAVR group had significantly lower rates than the surgery group of 30-day surgery (p =

0.02), mortality or stroke (p = 0.01), and new-onset atrial fibrillation (p < 0.001) as well as a shorter index of hospitalization (p < 0.001) and lower risk of poor treatment outcome (p < 0.001). The groups did not differ significantly in most safety endpoints at 30 days, including major vascular complications and new permanent pacemaker insertions.

Mack MJ, Leon MB, Thourani VH, Makkar R, Kodali SK, Russo M, et al. Transcatheter Aortic-Valve Replacement with a Balloon-Expandable Valve in Low-Risk Patients. New England Journal of Medicine. 2019 May 2;380(18):1695–705.

The DAPA-HF trial: Dapagliflozin in patients with heart failure

1. This study found that patients with heart failure with reduced ejection fraction (HFrEF) who received dapagliflozin had lower rates of composite cardiovascular death and worsening heart failure (16.3%) compared to controls (21.1%).

2. Presence or absence of diabetes had no significant impact on the outcomes in either group.

Original Date of Publication: November 2019

Study Rundown: The Dapagliflozin and Prevention of Adverse Outcomes in Heart Failure (DAPA-HF) trial evaluated the cardioprotective effects of the sodium–glucose cotransporter 2 (SGLT2) inhibitor dapagliflozin in patents with HFrEF. Composite cardiovascular death and worsening heart failure was significantly lower in those taking dapagliflozin as compared to placebo. Although SGLT2 inhibitors are typically used in diabetic patients, the presence or absence of diabetes did not alter outcomes in either group. The secondary composite outcome of cardiovascular death and hospitalizations for heart failure was also significantly reduced in the dapagliflozin group. The main limitation of the DAPA-HF trail was limited diversity in the study population, possibly impacting generalizability of the results. The DAPA-HF trial was the first study to demonstrate that in HFrEF patients both with and without diabetes, dapagliflozin reduces progression of heart failure, associated hospitalizations, and risk of cardiovascular death.

In-Depth [randomized control trial]: The DAPA-HF trial was conducted on a group of HFrEF patients (n = 4,744) who were randomized into either a dapagliflozin group (2,373) or placebo (n = 2,371) for a median duration of follow-up of 18.2 months. All trial outcomes were adjudicated by a blinded clinical-events committee. The primary composite endpoint of cardiovascular death and worsening heart failure characterized by hospitalization or urgent primary care visit resulting in intravenous therapy was significantly lower in the dapagliflozin group (16.3%) than the placebo group (21.2%) (HR 0.74; 95%CI 0.65-0.85). The dapagliflozin group also had a significantly reduced rate of the composite outcome of cardiovascular death and hospitalization due to heart failure (HR 0.75; 95%CI 0.65-0.85). Both groups were matched at screening for type 2 diabetes (42%) and diabetes status did not have any impact on the primary or the secondary composite outcomes.

McMurray JJV, Solomon SD, Inzucchi SE, Køber L, Kosiborod MN, Martinez FA, et al. Dapagliflozin in Patients with Heart Failure and Reduced Ejection Fraction. New England Journal of Medicine. 2019 Nov 21;381(21):1995–2008.

The VICTORIA trial: Vericiguat in high-risk heart failure

1. This study found that patients with chronic heart failure and reduced ejection fraction who received vericiguat had lower rates of composite cardiovascular death and first hospitalization for heart failure (35.5%) compared to controls (38.5%).

2. Rates of symptomatic hypotension and syncope did not differ between the those on vericiguat as compared to placebo.

Original Date of Publication: May 2020

Study Rundown: The Vericiguat Global Study in Subjects with Heart Failure with Reduced Ejection Fraction (VICTORIA) trial assessed the impact of the novel oral soluble guanylate cyclase stimulator vericiguat on cardiovascular outcomes in patients with chronic heart failure and ejection fraction of less than 45%. The primary outcome of composite cardiovascular death and first hospitalization due to heart failure was significantly lower in patients in the vericiguat group. Syncope and hypotension were slightly higher in the vericiguat group, although results were not statistically significant. The study had a limited follow-up time (median of 10.8 months) although differences between groups were seen starting at three months after baseline. In summary, the VICTORIA trial as the first multinational trial to evaluate the efficacy of vericiguat in reducing cardiovascular mortality and hospitalization in patients with severe heart failure.

In-Depth [randomized control trial]: In the VICTORIA trial, patients with New York Heart Association class II, III, or IV and an ejection fraction of less than 45% were randomized to either receive vericiguat (n = 2,526) or a placebo (n = 2,524). In the VICTORIA trial, patients with New York Heart Association class II, III, or IV, an ejection fraction of less than 45%, and an elevated natriuretic peptide level were randomized to either receive vericiguat (n = 2,526) or a placebo (n = 2,524). The VICTORIA trial was double-blinded, and outcomes were adjudicated by a blinded independent clinical-events committee. The composite endpoint of cardiovascular death and initial hospitalization for heart failure occurred in 35.5% of the vericiguat group as compared to 38.5% of the placebo group (HR 0.90; 95%CI 0.82-0.98). The secondary endpoints did not differ significantly between groups, including symptomatic hypotension (p = 0.12) and syncope (p = 0.30). Although, anemia occurred in a higher proportion of vericiguat patients (7.6%) as compared to placebo (5.7%).

Armstrong PW, Pieske B, Anstrom KJ, Ezekowitz J, Hernandez AF, Butler J, et al. Vericiguat in Patients with Heart Failure and Reduced Ejection Fraction. New England Journal of Medicine. 2020 May 14;382(20):1883–93.

Early rhythm control therapy for atrial fibrillation

1. This study found that in patients with early atrial fibrillation, a composite outcome of cardiovascular death, hospitalization, or stroke was significantly lower in those treated with rhythm control (3.9%) as compared to controls (5.0%).

2. Duration of hospitalization did not vary significantly between groups.

Original Date of Publication: October 2020

Study Rundown: The present study compared long-term outcomes of rhythm control versus therapy as usual in patients diagnosed with early atrial fibrillation. The rhythm control group had a significantly lower rate of first-primary outcome events, including a composite of cardiovascular death, cardiac hospitalization, or stroke. Conversely, duration of hospital stays as well as left ventricular and cognitive function did not differ between the study groups. The major limitation of this study was an open trial design, although assessment of primary outcomes was blinded to reduce bias. This was the first trial to demonstrate that early implementation of rhythm control for atrial fibrillation is associated with long-term reduction in cardiovascular complications and stroke without increasing time admitted to hospital.

In-Depth [randomized control trial]: This study randomized patients who were within a year of atrial fibrillation diagnosis to either rhythm control (n = 1,395) or treatment as usual (n = 1,394) for a median follow-up time of 5.1 years. Adverse events and outcomes were adjudicated by a blinded end-point review committee. The primary outcome was a composite of first-cardiovascular hospitalization, cardiovascular mortality, and stroke which was significantly lower in the rhythm control group (HR 0.79; 96%CI 0.66-0.94). There was no significant difference between groups in left ventricular function, cognitive function atrial fibrillation-related symptoms, or duration of hospitalization. Quality of life as measured by EQ-5D score also did not differ between groups.

Kirchhof P, Camm AJ, Goette A, Brandes A, Eckardt L, Elvan A, et al. Early Rhythm-Control Therapy in Patients with Atrial Fibrillation. New England Journal of Medicine. 2020 Oct 1;383(14):1305–16.

Rivaroxaban noninferior to warfarin in patients with atrial fibrillation and bioprosthetic mitral valves

1. Patients who received rivaroxaban had a statistically significantly longer mean time until occurrence of a major clinical event compared to those who received warfarin.

2. The incidence of secondary-outcome events such as transient ischemic attack (TIA), valve thrombosis, and non-CNS embolism were similar between groups.

Original Date of Publication: November 2020

Study Rundown: Atrial fibrillation is associated with an elevated risk of thromboembolic events that is dramatically exacerbated by the presence of valvular heart disease (VHD). Prophylactic anticoagulant therapy is essential for these individuals, but current recommendations are not easily applicable to this patient population due to their exclusion from participation in several pivotal direct oral anticoagulant (DOAC) versus warfarin trials (i.e. Re-LY, AVERROES, ROCKET-AF). To address this insufficiency of direct evidence, this study specifically investigated the prophylactic effect of rivaroxaban in patients with both atrial fibrillation and a bioprosthetic mitral valve, finding that those who received the DOAC had a significantly longer mean time until a major clinical event compared to those who received warfarin. This effect was consistent across most subgroups, but it was pronounced among patients who were enrolled within 3 months of mitral-valve surgery. In the component breakdown, those who received rivaroxaban had a numerically higher, but not statistically significant, incidence of valve thrombosis versus warfarin at 1 year and a lower incidence of other secondary outcomes such as stroke and death from cardiovascular causes or thromboembolic events. The total number of bleeding events was similar between the two groups, but individual events were generally of lesser severity among those who received rivaroxaban. While these findings cannot be generalized to patients with other types of valvular heart disease, they suggest that rivaroxaban is noninferior to warfarin for thromboembolism prophylaxis in patients with both atrial fibrillation and a bioprosthetic mitral valve.

In-Depth [randomized control trial]: In this multicenter study conducted in Brazil from April 2016 through July 2019, 1005 adults who had atrial fibrillation or flutter and a mitral valve prosthesis and were taking or planning on taking oral anticoagulants for thromboembolism prophylaxis were randomly assigned in a 1:1 ratio to receive either rivaroxaban or warfarin. Rivaroxaban was administered at a dosage of 20 mg per day with the exception of patients with a creatinine clearance of 30-49 mL per minute per 1.73 m^2 of body-surface area, who instead received 15 mg per day; warfarin dosage was adjusted at least every 4 weeks to maintain a target international normalized ratio (INR) of 2.0 to 3.0. The primary outcome was a composite of death, major bleeding, and major cardiovascular events (stroke, TIA, valve thrombosis, systemic embolism unrelated to the central nervous system, or hospitalization for heart failure). The mean time until any of these events was slightly higher in the rivaroxaban group compared to warfarin (347.5 days vs. 340.1 days; restricted mean survival time difference, 7.4 days; 95%CI, −1.4 to 16.3; p < 0.001 for noninferiority and p = 0.10 for superiority). Of the individual components of the composite outcome, valve thrombosis was numerically more frequent in the rivaroxaban group (5 vs. 3), while death from cardiovascular causes or thromboembolic events was slightly more frequent in the warfarin group (3.4% vs 5.1%; hazard ratio [HR], 0.65; 95%CI, 0.35 to 1.20). With the exception of stroke (0.6% vs. 2.4%; HR, 0.25; 95%CI, 0.07 to 0.88), other secondary outcomes were similar between groups at 12 months. Serious adverse events (5.8% vs. 6.9%) and total bleeding events (HR, 0.83; 95%CI, 0.59–1.15) occurred at similar rates in both groups, although the warfarin group had a numerically greater number of major, intracranial, and fatal bleeding incidents.

Guimarães HP, Lopes RD, Silva PGM de B e, Liporace IL, Sampaio RO, Tarasoutchi F, et al. Rivaroxaban in Patients with Atrial Fibrillation and a Bioprosthetic Mitral Valve. New England Journal of Medicine. 2020 Nov 14;

The EARLY-AF Trial: Catheter cryoballoon ablation for atrial fibrillation

1. This study found that in patients with symptomatic paroxysmal atrial fibrillation, patients who received ablation were less likely to experience recurrence of atrial tachyarrhythmia compared to those who received antiarrhythmic drugs (42.9% vs. 67.8%).

2. No significant differs in adverse events were seen between groups.

Original Date of Publication: January 2021

Study Rundown: The Early Aggressive Invasive Intervention for Atrial Fibrillation (EARLY-AF) trial compared catheter cryoballoon ablation to antiarrhythmic drug therapy in patients with symptomatic paroxysmal AF. The ablation group had significantly lower rates of both asymptomatic and symptomatic tachyarrhythmia as compared to those administered antiarrhythmic medications. The main limitation of the EARLY-AF trial was that it did not have the sample size to evaluate cardiovascular outcomes. Although, the primary endpoint of atrial tachyarrhythmia reoccurrence is a significant indicator of recovery from AF. In summary, the EARLY-AF trial demonstrated that individuals who receive catheter cryoballoon ablation following symptomatic paroxysmal AF have lower recurrence of atrial tachyarrhythmia as compared to those who receive antiarrhythmic drugs.

In-Depth [randomized control trial]: In the EARLY-AF trial, patients with symptomatic paroxysmal AF detected on electrocardiography within 24 months of baseline were randomized to either receive antiarrhythmic drug therapy (n = 149) or catheter cryoballoon ablation (n = 154). Although the trial was open-label, end-point adjudication was blinded and conducted by an end-point committee to minimize bias. The primary endpoint of recurrence of atrial tachyarrhythmia 30 seconds or longer was measured by implantable cardiac monitor and occurred less frequently in the ablation group (HR 0.48; 95%CI 0.35-0.66). Symptomatic atrial tachyarrhythmia was also significantly lower in the ablation group (HR 0.39; 95%CI 0.22-0.68). Conversely, serious adverse events did not differ significantly between groups.

Andrade JG, Wells GA, Deyell MW, Bennett M, Essebag V, Champagne J, et al. Cryoablation or Drug Therapy for Initial Treatment of Atrial Fibrillation. New England Journal of Medicine. 2021 Jan 28;384(4):305–15.

The EMPEROR-Preserved trial: Empagliflozin in heart failure

1. The present study demonstrated that in patients with heart failure with preserved ejection fraction (HFpEF) are less likely to experience a composite outcome of cardiovascular death or hospitalization for heart failure if they received empagliflozin (13.8%) as compared to placebo (17.1%).

2. Presence or absence of type 2 diabetes had no impact on the differences in outcomes between groups.

Original Date of Publication: October 2021

Study Rundown: The Empagliflozin Outcome Trial in Patients with Chronic Heart Failure with Preserved Ejection Fraction (EMPEROR-Preserved) trial compared cardiovascular outcomes in individuals with HFpEF who were randomized to empagliflozin or placebo. Participants in the empagliflozin group had significantly lower rates of cardiovascular death or hospitalization related to heart failure, regardless of diabetes status. The number of all-cause hospitalizations were also lower in the empagliflozin group, although mortality rates did not differ. The major limitation of the EMPEROR-Preserved trial was a 23% overall dropout rate, although the rate was not significantly different between groups. Overall, the EMPEROR-Preserved trial demonstrated that in patients with HFpEF, empagliflozin reduces risk of cardiovascular death and heart failure hospitalization.

In-Depth [randomized control trial]: In the double-blinded EMPEROR-Preserved trial, patients with a New York Heart Association class of II to IV and ejection fraction > 40% were randomized to receive either a placebo (n = 2,991) or empagliflozin (n = 2,997). Endpoints were assessed by a blinded clinal events committee. The main composite endpoint of cardiovascular mortality and hospitalization due to heart failure was significantly reduced in participants who were randomized to empagliflozin (HR 0.79; 95%CI 0.69-0.90). Empagliflozin was still superior to placebo in diabetes subgroup analysis. All-cause hospitalization ($p < 0.001$) and glomerular filtration rate decline ($p < 0.001$) were also lower with empagliflozin as compared to placebo. Although, differences in all-cause mortality were not significant between groups (HR 1.00; 95%CI 0.87-1.15).

Anker SD, Butler J, Filippatos G, Ferreira JP, Bocchi E, Böhm M, Brunner–La Rocca HP, Choi DJ, Chopra V, Chuquiure-Valenzuela E, Giannetti N. Empagliflozin in heart failure with a preserved ejection fraction. New England Journal of Medicine. 2021 Oct 14;385(16):1451-61.

III. Critical, Emergent and Pulmonary Care

"Science is built up of facts, as a house is built of stones; but an accumulation of facts is no more a science than a heap of stones is a house."

- Henri Poincaré, PhD

Initial trial of conservative management for splenic injury

1. The conservative, symptomatic management of 16 patients following assumed splenic injury from blunt abdominal trauma resulted in normalization of hemodynamic stability within 2 days of hospital admission. Furthermore, this strategy resulted in complete normalization of clinical examination by 2 weeks post-discharge, and no hospital readmissions.

2. This approach to splenic injury management was supported by subsequent investigations, eventually leading to the acceptance of conservative management as standard of care.

Original Date of Publication: October 1971

Study Rundown: The spleen is particularly susceptible to blunt abdominal trauma and, prior to this study, splenectomy was routine following abdominal injury. However, previous anecdotal evidence of the authors linked nonoperative management to positive outcomes. With the potential for spleen salvage and a reduction in surgical and post-operative risks, this study investigated the outcomes of children who were not treated surgically for their splenic injuries. The small sample size, lack of a control group, and use of descriptive statistics as the only method for analysis limited the study. In addition, conclusions drawn from the study may be inaccurate as patients were assumed to have splenic injury from clinical examination as no method, apart from surgical exploration, could confirm injury.

At the time of its publication, the proposed conservative treatment investigated in the study differed radically from expected surgical intervention. In the present day, conservative management is the preferred method of management for children with splenic injury secondary to blunt trauma. Improved imaging techniques and technology for monitoring patient hemodynamic status now allow for better assessment of the need for surgical intervention. A recent retrospective study of the evolution of splenic injury management found hospital length of stay, transfusion requirements, and mortality decreased as conservative management of splenic injury became widely accepted.

In-Depth [case-series study]: A total of 32 children admitted to the hospital during 1948-1955 following blunt abdominal trauma with potential splenic involvement were included. Six patients underwent splenectomy, 1 patient died from a crush injury, and the remaining 25 underwent nonoperative management. Of these patients, 16 were included in the study (mean age = 10 years, 69% male) as their presentation indicated likely splenic involvement, although this was not confirmed by surgical intervention. Patients underwent standard examinations with researchers reporting close monitoring of patient vitals.

All patients were conscious upon presentation with a complaint of abdominal pain and all had significant abdominal tenderness. Three children had ecchymoses overlying the site of trauma and 3 had potential intraperitoneal fluid detected on physical exam. Patient pulses ranged from 100-140/min and 4 patients had blood pressures < 90/50 mmHg. Complete blood counts included hemoglobin values ranging from 7.9-11.4 g/100 mL (mean = 9.5 g/100 mL) and white blood cell counts ranging from 8000-27 000 mm^3 (mean = 17 000 mm^3). Patient temperatures ranged from 100°F-104°F (mean = 102°F). 9 children received whole blood transfusions for hemodynamic instability and 2 received plasma. All patients received intravenous fluids. Patients were hemodynamically stable within 2 days of admission. Resolution of abdominal tenderness correlated with normalization of heart rate and body temperature. Total length of stay ranged from 4 to 42 days (mean = 16 days). Two weeks after discharge, all patients' physical examinations normalized and no patient underwent readmission.

Douglas GJ, Simpson JS. The conservative management of splenic trauma. Journal of Pediatric Surgery. 1971 Oct 1;6(5):565–70.

Davies DA, Pearl RH, Ein SH, Langer JC, Wales PW. Management of blunt splenic injury in children: evolution of the nonoperative approach. Journal of Pediatric Surgery. 2009 May 1;44(5):1005–8.

Magnesium sulfate in torsade de pointes

1. Intravenous magnesium sulfate was effective at acutely terminating torsade de pointes (TdP).

2. Intravenous magnesium sulfate was not effective in terminating other ventricular tachycardias (VTs) not associated with QT prolongation.

Original Date of Publication: February 1988

Study Rundown: TdP is distinguished from other forms of VT due to its occurrence in patients with marked QT prolongation. Because of this underlying difference, TdP responds to intravenous (IV) magnesium sulfate (MgSO4), while other forms of ventricular tachycardias do not. This article was the first case-series demonstrating the effect of MgSO4 on terminating torsade de pointes. After the publication of this article, MgSO4 became the standard therapy for treatment of TdP. While the study may be considered rudimentary, the researcher's findings were influential as all 12 subjects with TdP responded to MgSO4 and none of the 5 non-TdP VT subjects did. Weaknesses of the study included a low sample size (n = 17) and significant variability in patient demographics, cardiac history and function, baseline electrolyte levels, as well as concurrent therapy. Furthermore, no individual data was shown for the 5 non-TdP subjects. In summary, despite the many weaknesses of the paper by today's standards, this study helped establish MgSO4 as standard practice in treating TdP.

In-Depth [case-series]: A total of 12 patients with TdP and 5 patients with polymorphous VT with normal QT interval were included. These patients were treated with 25% or 50% solutions of MgSO4 and were observed for termination of arrhythmia and recurrence. The mean QT interval was 0.61s in the TdP group (mean QTc of 0.64s) and 0.46s (mean QTc not provided) in the non-TdP VT group. Magnesium levels prior to onset of arrhythmia were available for 8/12 TdP patients and 2/5 non-TdP VT patients and were all within normal limits (1.6-2.5 meq/L). Two out of 12 patients had potassium levels below 3.1 meq/L (both were 2.9 meq/L). No non-TdP VT patient had potassium levels below 3.1 meq/L. Two grams of IV MgSO4 were administered to all 12 TdP and 5 non-TdP subjects as soon as arrhythmia was recognized. Four of the TdP patients received other therapies, which were not effective, prior to MgSO4 therapy. Nine patients responded immediately to the MgSO4. The other 3 patients received a second bolus within 5-15 minutes and were started on a continuous infusion. In 2 patients, the TdP recurred 1-6 hours after infusion was begun and was abolished in both after a third bolus of IV MgSO4. MgSO4 infusion was continued until QT< 0.50s. Two of the 12 patients had elevated magnesium levels (3.5 and 5 meq/L) after treatment with MgSO4. Zero out of the 5 non-TdP VT patients showed improvement with MgSO4 therapy even after 2-3 boluses. Three of the 5 patients responded to other IV antiarrhythmics (2 to lidocaine, 1 to procainamide).

Tzivoni D, Banai S, Schuger C, Benhorin J, Keren A, Gottlieb S, et al. Treatment of torsade de pointes with magnesium sulfate. Circulation. 1988 Feb 1;77(2):392–7.

CT insensitive to mediastinal lymph node metastasis in bronchogenic carcinoma

1. Computed tomography (CT) of the chest is limited in the ability to detect the presence of mediastinal lymph node involvement in patients with bronchogenic carcinoma.

2. This study helped popularize the use of 1 cm (measured in short axis) as the criteria for abnormally enlarged lymph nodes. The rate of positive mediastinal nodal involvement was increased from 13% to 62% for nodes measuring < 1 cm and ≥2 - 2.9 cm, respectively.

Original Date of Publication: February 1992

Study Rundown: Lung cancer is the leading cause of cancer-related death worldwide with over 1.2 million deaths in 2012. Accurate evaluation of mediastinal lymphadenopathy is vital in the staging of a patient with lung cancer to provide prognostic information for patients as well as to direct treatment. CT scans of the chest provide visualization of mediastinal lymph nodes not typically accessible by mediastinoscopy or thoracotomy; however, there have been conflicting reports on the sensitivity and specificity of CT chest to identify lymph node metastases in the mediastinum. The purpose of this landmark prospective trial was to determine the accuracy of CT chest to identify mediastinal lymph node metastases in patients with lung cancer.

The trial prospectively followed over 140 patients with bronchogenic carcinoma that underwent CT chest evaluation with surgical staging correlation. CT evidence of mediastinal metastases was defined as any lymph nodes greater than 1 cm in short axis. At the conclusion of the trial, the sensitivity and specificity of CT examinations for mediastinal metastases were found to be 64% and 62%, respectively. Additionally, the sensitivity for individual nodal stations within the mediastinum was lower at 44%. In particular, there were high rates of false-positive lymph nodes within the right paratracheal group and the aorticopulmonary window. Although larger nodes were associated with increased likelihood of mediastinal metastases, over one-third of all lymph nodes over 2 cm were found to be benign and hyperplastic. The results of this study demonstrated the relative insensitivity of CT to identify mediastinal metastases in patients with lung cancer due to confounding conditions such as atelectasis or pneumonitis leading to hyperplastic and reactive lymph node changes. This landmark trial provides strong evidence for the use of CT chest scans in conjunction with mediastinoscopy or thoracotomy to adequately provide staging information for patients with bronchogenic carcinoma.

In-Depth [prospective cohort]: This was a prospective study of 143 patients with pathologically-confirmed, non-small cell lung cancer from a single institution in the United States. Each patient underwent CT examination of the chest followed by pathological staging of the mediastinum either through mediastinoscopy or thoracotomy. Mediastinal lymph nodes were measured in the short axis and considered abnormal if they measured greater than 1 cm in diameter. The primary outcome of interest was the patient-by-patient accuracy rate of the CT findings correlated with the pathological results from surgical staging. Secondary outcomes included the accuracy of each specific mediastinal nodal station, as defined by the American Thoracic Society mapping scheme, to its pathological correlate. Overall, 401 mediastinal lymph nodes were evaluated, of which 369 (83%) were found to be normal. At the conclusion of the trial, the CT sensitivity for mediastinal metastases for each individual patient was 64% with a specificity of 62%. The sensitivity and specificity for all nodal stations are 44% and 85%, respectively. In the subgroup analysis of each individual lymph node station, groups 4R, 5, and 10R in the right paratracheal and aorticopulmonary window demonstrated the highest false-positive rate. Increase in lymph node size on CT was associated with an increased likelihood of metastatic disease; however, over 33% of the lymph nodes between 2 and 4 cm in size in this cohort demonstrated a benign hyperplastic reaction rather than metastasis. For lymph nodes < 1 cm in short axis diameter, the prevalence of metastases was 13%; for nodes ≥1 – 1.9 cm, the prevalence of metastases was 25%; for nodes ≥2.0 – 2.9 cm, the prevalence of metastases was 62%.

McLoud TC, Bourgouin PM, Greenberg RW, Kosiuk JP, Templeton PA, Shepard JA, et al. Bronchogenic carcinoma: analysis of staging in the mediastinum with CT by correlative lymph node mapping and sampling. Radiology. 1992 Feb 1;182(2):319–23.

The DIGAMI trial: Insulin-glucose infusion in diabetics with acute myocardial infarction

1. In diabetic patients with an acute myocardial infarction (MI), insulin-glucose infusion with subsequent long-term insulin treatment significantly reduced mortality at 1 year.

Original Date of Publication: July 1995

Study Rundown: At the time of the Diabetes Mellitus Insulin-Glucose Infusion in Acute Myocardial Infarction (DIGAMI) study (1995), studies revealed that diabetic patients had higher mortality rates post-MI than non-diabetic patients. This difference remained despite the introduction of new therapeutic measures, such as beta-blockers. Increased fatty acid metabolism in diabetes is theorized to decrease the anaerobic process of glycolysis that is important for the survival of ischemic tissue. The DIGAMI study demonstrated that, in diabetic patients already receiving beta-blockers and thrombolytic treatment, metabolic control via an insulin-glucose infusion and long-term insulin therapy further decreased post-MI mortality after 1 year. It is unclear from the study results whether the immediate insulin-glucose infusion or the subsequent multidose insulin therapy was most responsible for the decrease in post-MI mortality. The lack of free fatty acid measurements also limited the study from clarifying the mechanism of benefit from insulin treatment post-MI. The study only randomized half of the 1240 eligible patients, resulting in a relatively small sample size, wide confidence intervals, and potential bias due to the exclusion of patients unwilling to undergo aggressive insulin therapy. Lastly, > 80% of patients in the study were previously non-insulin dependent, suggesting that the benefits of insulin treatment may be limited to patients with the minimal disease. In summary, the DIGAMI study demonstrated a role for insulin therapy in diabetic patients who experience acute MI.

In-Depth [randomized controlled trial]: This trial involved coronary care units in 19 Swedish hospitals. Inclusion criteria included suspected acute MI within the preceding 24 hours in a patient with previously diagnosed diabetes mellitus (DM), or in a patient with a blood glucose level > 11 mmol/liter without a previous DM diagnosis. All 620 patients received thrombolytic treatment (i.e., streptokinase) and beta-blockade (i.e., metoprolol), and were randomized to additionally receive an insulin-glucose infusion with follow-up multidose insulin therapy, or conventional therapy. At 1 year, the mortality rate in the insulin group was significantly lower than that of the control group (RRR 29%, p = 0.027).

Malmberg K, Rydén L, Efendic S, Herlitz J, Nicol P, Waldenstrom A, et al. Randomized trial of insulin-glucose infusion followed by subcutaneous insulin treatment in diabetic patients with acute myocardial infarction (DIGAMI study): Effects on mortality at 1 year. J Am Coll Cardiol. 1995 Jul 1;26(1):57–65.

Ottawa ankle rules reduce the rate of referral for ankle radiography

1. The Ottawa ankle rules significantly reduced referral for ankle, but not foot, radiography in the emergency department.

2. Patients without fractures spent less time in the emergency department if not referred for radiography without an increased rate of missed fractures.

Original Date of Publication: September 1995

Study Rundown: Ankle and foot injuries are some of the most common complaints evaluated in the emergency department. While relatively few patients sustain a fracture related to their injury, it has long been standard practice to perform plain radiography of the ankle and/or foot on virtually all patients. This, along with unreliable findings made through history taking and physical examination defined the need for decision rules on the use of radiography for acute ankle injuries. The Ottawa ankle rules (Table I) were designed to allow physicians to rapidly identify patients with a negligible risk of fracture based on the assessment of weight-bearing ability and areas of bone tenderness. These decision rules have subsequently been validated and are highly sensitive in identifying fractures.

In the large multicenter trial conducted by Stiell and colleagues, rates of referral for ankle and foot injuries were compared before and after the introduction of the Ottawa ankle rules. The results of this study showed that implementation of the Ottawa ankle rules significantly reduced referral for ankle radiography. Patients without fractures also spent less time in the emergency department if they were not referred for radiography without an increased rate of missed fractures.

In-Depth [non-randomized controlled trial]: This study was conducted across 8 emergency departments in Canada. All adult patients seen at a participating study site with an ankle injury during the 12 month control (before) or intervention (after) periods were included. Before the start of the intervention period, the Ottawa ankle rules were introduced by means of a 1 hour lecture and supported by handouts, pocket cards and posters in each emergency department. The decision to order radiography was left to the discretion of the treating physician. Treating physicians included emergency and family physicians as well as housestaff. Referral for radiography was determined through radiology reports. As part of the intervention, patients deemed to be without fracture were followed up by telephone after 10 days if they did not receive any radiography. Patients that were seen during the first 7 days of each month and received radiography were also followed up.

A total of 12 777 eligible patients (median age 32, range 18-101; 53% men) were seen in a participating emergency department for treatment of an ankle injury. Patients evaluated during the pre-intervention (n = 6288) and intervention (n = 6489) periods did not significantly differ with respect to any baseline patient characteristics. During the pre-intervention period, 82.8% of patients were referred for ankle radiography compared to 60.9% during the intervention period ($p < 0.001$), corresponding to a relative reduction of 26.4%. For 4.9% of cases, radiography was unnecessarily performed according to the Ottawa ankle rules, where only 0.5% of these cases were the result of patient insistence. The proportion of patients referred for ankle imaging was significantly less at all 8 participating hospitals and across all physician subgroups. For foot imaging, however, significant reductions in referral were noted at only 3 of the 8 study sites. Among patients without fracture, those that were not referred for radiography spent less time in the emergency department compared to patients that underwent imaging studies ($p < 0.001$). Of the 2033 patients comprising the follow up group, 10 (0.5%) had a fracture diagnosed after discharge despite no repeat injury, 7 of which had not received radiography (n = 1301). It should be noted, however, that the Ottawa ankle rules were correctly applied in only 1 of the 7 patients from the latter follow-up group. A cost minimization analysis also showed that the mean total expense for patients who had no radiography was less than those who had radiography ($p < 0.001$).

Stiell I, Wells G, Laupacis A, Brison R, Verbeek R, Vandemheen K, et al. Multicentre trial to introduce the Ottawa ankle rules for use of radiography in acute ankle injuries. BMJ. 1995 Sep;311(7005):594-7.

ANKLE series required if:	FOOT series required if:
1) Bone tenderness at posterior edge or tip of lateral malleolus **OR** 2) Bone tenderness at posterior edge or tip or medial malleolus **OR** 3) Inability to bear weight both immediately and in emergency department	1) Bone tenderness at base of 5th metatarsal **OR** 2) Bone tenderness at navicular **OR** 3) Inability to bear weight both immediately and in emergency department

Table I. Ottawa ankle rules.

The NINDS trial: Tissue plasminogen activator in acute ischemic stroke improves functional outcomes

1. Treatment of acute ischemic stroke with tissue plasminogen activator (t-PA) within 3 hours of symptom onset significantly improved functional outcomes 3 months after stroke, when compared with placebo.

2. Tissue plasminogen activator significantly increased the rate of symptomatic intracerebral hemorrhage.

Original Date of Publication: December 1995

Study Rundown: Prior to the National Institute of Neurologic Disorders and Stroke (NINDS) trial, evidence that thrombolytic therapy benefitted patients with ischemic stroke existed, though intracerebral hemorrhage was a frequent complication. Several previous studies found that early treatment (i.e., thrombolytics within 3 hours of symptom onset) was associated with the greatest likelihood of recovery and lower risks of hemorrhage. The NINDS trial was a larger randomized controlled trial that sought to assess the efficacy of using t-PA in treating ischemic stroke within 3 hours of symptom onset. Results showed that the administration of t-PA within 3 hours of symptom onset in patients suffering ischemic stroke significantly improved functional outcomes, as observed at the 3 month mark. Patients treated with t-PA, however, suffered significantly higher rates of symptomatic bleeding. The NINDS trial was the first randomized controlled trial demonstrating that t-PA was beneficial in patients suffering from acute ischemic stroke. While the study used carefully selected sample of stroke cases, the findings of the NINDS trial formed as the basis for approving the use of thrombolytics in the management of acute strokes. It also informed the development of practice guidelines in centers across North America.

In-Depth [randomized controlled trial]: The trial consisted of 2 phases: 1) assessing for improvements in neurologic functioning within 24 hours of symptom onset to measure t-PA activity and 2) assessing for sustained clinical improvement at 3 months. In phase 1, there was no significant difference between the groups in terms of neurologic improvement within the first 24 hours. In phase 2, patients treated with t-PA demonstrated significant improvements on several functional assessment scales (i.e., NIHSS, Barthel, Modified Rankin, Glasgow Outcome) 3 months after the onset of stroke, when compared with patients in the placebo group. There were significantly more symptomatic intracerebral hemorrhages in the t-PA group, though the rate of asymptomatic intracerebral hemorrhages was not different.

The National Institute of Neurological Disorders and Stroke rt-PA Stroke Study Group. Tissue Plasminogen Activator for Acute Ischemic Stroke. New England Journal of Medicine. 1995 Dec 14;333(24):1581–8.

The Rockall score: Risk assessment after acute upper gastrointestinal hemorrhage

1. Age, shock, comorbidity, diagnosis, major stigmata of recent hemorrhage, and rebleeding were independent predictors of mortality following acute upper gastrointestinal hemorrhage.

Original Date of Publication: March 1996

Study Rundown: Acute upper gastrointestinal hemorrhage is a common medical emergency. Risk factors for rebleeding and death were well known at the time of this study's publication but there was previously no clinically useful tool for risk stratifying patients. The Rockall risk scoring system was found to be a good indicator of prognosis following acute upper gastrointestinal hemorrhage. Rebleeding was a particularly important risk factor associated with a 5-fold increase in mortality among middle risk groups. Current treatment protocols specifically target the prevention of rebleeding due to the increased risk of mortality. The Rockall score can be applied in disease management, determining case mix in evaluating outcomes, developing treatment protocols, and selecting patients in clinical trials.

In-Depth [randomized controlled trial]: This study produced a risk scoring system following acute upper gastrointestinal bleeding based on data from 4185 cases identified in 1993 and 1625 cases identified in 1994. In the first phase of data collection, medical staff completed a questionnaire for each identified case, which included risk factors, treatment, endoscopic findings, diagnosis, complications, and mortality. Multiple regression analysis found that the following variables were independent predictors of mortality: age, shock, comorbidity, diagnosis, major stigmata of recent hemorrhage, and rebleeding. The risk scoring system was validated using the second phase of data collection. An integer score was assigned to each category of each significant variable according to its contribution to the logistic regression model. The maximum possible score is 11 with scores of 8 or more considered very high-risk categories. Rebleeding occurred in less than 5% of cases and mortality was close to 0 in patients scoring 0, 1, or 2.

Rockall TA, Logan RF, Devlin HB, Northfield TC. Risk assessment after acute upper gastrointestinal haemorrhage. Gut. 1996 Mar 1;38(3):316–21.

The TRICC trial: Restrictive transfusion in intensive care does not increase mortality

1. Using a restrictive transfusion strategy in critically ill patients did not significantly increase 30-day mortality when compared with a liberal transfusion strategy.

2. Subgroup analyses demonstrated that a restrictive transfusion strategy was associated with a significantly lower mortality in patients with Acute Physiology and Chronic Health Evaluation (APACHE) II score ≤20 and age < 55 years.

Original Date of Publication: February 1999

Study Rundown: The Transfusion Requirements in Critical Care (TRICC) trial sought to explore whether restrictive and liberal red-cell transfusion strategies in critically ill patients resulted in different outcomes. Prior to this study, there were conflicting views about liberal transfusion protocols. Several observational studies suggested that anemia was a risk factor for mortality in critically ill patients, particularly those with cardiovascular disease. It was suggested that anemia may cause excessive stress in severely ill patients, resulting in poorer outcomes. Other studies suggested that the risks of blood transfusion were elevated in the critically ill.

This randomized, controlled trial examined the risks and benefits associated with different transfusion strategies among patients in the intensive care unit (ICU). One strategy was restrictive and sought to maintain lower hemoglobin levels (target between 7.0-9.0 g/dL), while the other was liberal and maintained higher hemoglobin levels (target between 10.0-12.0 g/dL). In summary, there was no difference in 30-day mortality when comparing the groups. Moreover, the study demonstrated that survival was significantly improved when using the restrictive transfusion strategy in subgroups of patients with an APACHE II score ≤20 and age < 55 years ($p = 0.02$). This trial supported the use of a restrictive transfusion strategy in critically ill patients.

In-Depth [randomized controlled trial]: Published in 1999, this study involved 838 critically ill patients recruited from 22 tertiary-level and 3 community ICUs across Canada. Patients were included if they were expected to stay in intensive care for > 24 hours, had a hemoglobin concentration ≤9.0 g/dL within 72 hours of admission, and were considered to be euvolemic by treating physicians. Exclusion criteria included age < 16 years old, inability to receive blood products, active blood loss at the time of enrollment, chronic anemia, pregnancy, brain death, or imminent death. Eligible patients were then randomized to either restrictive (target hemoglobin from 7.0-9.0 g/dL) or liberal transfusion strategies (target hemoglobin 10.0-12.0 g/dL). The primary outcome measure was 30-day mortality. Secondary outcomes included 60-day mortality and mortality in intensive care/during hospitalization. There was no significant difference in 30-day mortality between the groups (ARR 4.7%; 95%CI -0.84-10.2; p = 0.11). The in-hospital mortality rate, however, was significantly lower for patients in the restrictive arm (ARR 5.8%; 95%CI -0.3-11.7; p = 0.05). In the subgroups of patients with a score on the severity-of-disease APACHE II scale of ≤20 and age < 55 years, survival was significantly higher for patients in the restrictive-transfusion group (p = 0.02).

Hébert PC, Wells G, Blajchman MA, Marshall J, Martin C, Pagliarello G, et al. A Multicenter, Randomized, Controlled Clinical Trial of Transfusion Requirements in Critical Care. New England Journal of Medicine. 1999 Feb 11;340(6):409–17.

The ARMA trial: Lower tidal volume ventilation in acute respiratory distress syndrome

1. This trial was terminated early when the data demonstrated that lower tidal volume ventilator settings in acute lung injury (ALI)/acute respiratory distress syndrome (ARDS) patients reduced in-hospital mortality.

2. Low tidal volume ventilation was also associated with an increase in ventilator-free days and a decrease in the number of days with systemic organ failure. There was no significant difference in the incidence of barotrauma between the low and high tidal volume groups.

3. Patients assigned to lower tidal volume ventilator settings initially required a higher positive end-expiratory pressure (PEEP) to maintain arterial oxygenation and were more likely to develop respiratory acidosis, although the difference disappeared by day 7.

Original Date of Publication: May 2000

Study Rundown: In an effort to maintain normal partial pressure of carbon dioxide and arterial pH, patients with ALI or ARDS requiring mechanical ventilation traditionally received higher tidal volumes (10-15 mL/kg) compared to healthy individuals. However, studies in animals showed that higher tidal volumes were associated with increased lung inflammation and injury. This multi-center, randomized, controlled trial compared traditional tidal volume therapy (12 mL/kg) to low tidal volume therapy (6 mL/kg) in mechanically ventilated patients with ALI/ARDS for 28 days. Results revealed that the traditional tidal volume group had significantly increased in-hospital mortality compared to the low tidal volume group. There was no difference in barotrauma between the groups. In summary, this study demonstrated that lower tidal volumes in ALI/ARDS patients reduced in-hospital mortality and the number of days that patients required mechanical ventilation. Of note, patients in the lower tidal volume group required higher PEEP and had a slight, but significant, respiratory acidosis, both of which resolved after 7 days. This suggested that although lower tidal volumes required a higher respiratory rate to maintain adequate ventilation, its benefits on mortality outweighed the transient acid/base and oxygenation imbalances that were effectively managed with higher PEEP and sodium bicarbonate infusion, respectively.

In-Depth [randomized controlled trial]: This trial was conducted at 10 university centers across the United States from 1996-1999. Eligible patients were above the age of 18, intubated, mechanically ventilated, and had an acute decrease to a P/F ratio (i.e., partial pressure of arterial oxygen to fraction of inspired oxygen) of 300 or less with evidence of bilateral lung edema on recent chest radiograph. Patients with chronic lung disease, high pulmonary capillary wedge pressure or evidence of left atrial hypertension, less than 6 months of estimated survival, and other medical problems that would cause poor respiration or oxygenation were excluded. The authors randomized patients to traditional tidal volume therapy of 12 mL/kg or low tidal volume therapy of 6 mL/kg for 28 days. The investigators tracked patients weekly for a total of 180 days. The primary endpoint was in-hospital mortality, with a significant reduction from 39.8% in the traditional group to 31.0% in the low tidal volume group (p = 0.007, 95%CI 2.4-15.3%). There was also a significant decrease in the number of ventilator-free days in the low tidal volume group (p = 0.007) and in the number of days free from organ failure (p = 0.006).

The Acute Respiratory Distress Syndrome Network. Ventilation with Lower Tidal Volumes as Compared with Traditional Tidal Volumes for Acute Lung Injury and the Acute Respiratory Distress Syndrome. New England Journal of Medicine. 2000 May 4;342(18):1301–8.

The CAPRICORN trial: Carvedilol reduces mortality after acute myocardial infarction

1. Carvedilol reduced mortality from cardiovascular causes and recurrent non-fatal infarction after acute myocardial infarction (MI).

2. While carvedilol treatment was associated with a 23% relative risk reduction in all-cause mortality, this did not reach statistical significance.

3. These findings were consistent with previous trials exploring the benefits of beta-blockers in managing acute myocardial infarction.

Original Date of Publication: May 2001

Study Rundown: While previous studies had established the benefits of beta-blockade in managing MI, these trials were conducted prior to widespread use of thrombolysis or angioplasty for reperfusion as well as prior to the introduction of angiotensin converting enzyme (ACE) inhibitors. Thus, the CAPRICORN trial explored the long-term efficacy of carvedilol in patients suffering from acute MI, taking into account recent advances in management. The trial demonstrated that beta-blockers conferred considerable benefits in patients suffering from acute MI. While carvedilol was associated with a relative risk reduction in all-cause mortality of 23%, this did not reach statistical significance due to statistical adjustment partway through the study. However, carvedilol significantly reduced mortality from cardiovascular causes and recurrent non-fatal MI. While previous studies examined beta-blockade prior to the widespread use of reperfusion and ACE inhibitors in managing MIs, the findings from the CAPRICORN trial are consistent with the older data.

In-Depth [randomized controlled trial]: Patients were included if they were 18 years of age, had suffered a definite MI 3-21 days before randomization, had a left ventricular ejection fraction (LVEF) < 40%, and had concurrent treatment with ACE inhibitors for at least 48 hours, unless there was a proven intolerance to ACE inhibitors. They were randomized to either the carvedilol group (maximum dose of 25 mg PO BID) or to placebo. The co-primary endpoints were 1) all-cause mortality and 2) all-cause mortality and cardiovascular hospital admissions. Secondary endpoints were sudden death and hospital admission for heart failure, while other endpoints were recurrent non-fatal MI and all-cause mortality or recurrent non-fatal MI. A total of 1959 patients were recruited from 163 centers in 17 different countries and followed for a mean of 1.3 years. Approximately 46% of patients required reperfusion therapy, largely through thrombolysis, though some did undergo primary angioplasty. Notably, about 98% of patients were taking ACE inhibitors at the time of randomization. While all-cause mortality was reduced by 23% in the carvedilol group, this did not reach statistical significance. There were also no significant differences between the groups in terms of secondary endpoints. Patients in the carvedilol group, however, experienced significantly lower rates of cardiovascular-caused mortality and non-fatal MI.

Dargie HJ. Effect of carvedilol on outcome after myocardial infarction in patients with left-ventricular dysfunction: the CAPRICORN randomised trial. Lancet. 2001 May 5;357(9266):1385–90.

The Canadian CT Head Rule

1. The Canadian CT Head Rule consists of 7 predictor variables to assess the need for computed tomography (CT) imaging in patients with minor head injuries.

2. This study demonstrated that the rule is highly sensitive and may help to reduce the number of CT scans ordered.

Original Date of Publication: May 2001

Study Rundown: First published in The Lancet in 2001, the Canadian CT Head Rule was designed to identify patients who required CT after suffering minor head injuries. The definition of a minor head injury is a history of loss of consciousness, amnesia, or disorientation and a Glasgow Coma Scale (GCS) score of 13-15. At the time, there were conflicting guidelines regarding the use of CT in patients suffering these injuries, and the Canadian CT Head Rule sought to standardize the management of patients while reducing the number of unnecessary CT scans. This study developed the Rule and found it to be a highly sensitive clinical decision rule for patients with minor head injuries. Moreover, the findings suggested that the Rule may help reduce the number of CT scans ordered in assessing patients with minor head injuries.

In-Depth [prospective cohort]: This trial was carried out in 10 Canadian community and academic centers. The primary outcome was the need for neurological intervention (i.e., death within 7 days due to head injury, or need for craniotomy, elevation of skull fracture, intracranial pressure monitoring, or intubation for head injury within 7 days), while the secondary outcome was the presence of clinically important brain injury identified on CT. Patients requiring a CT were identified by standardized physician assessments, which included assessing for pre-determined predictor variables. Patients not requiring a CT were followed-up with a phone call 14 days after their assessment. A total of 3121 patients were enrolled, and 2078 of these patients received CT scans. Logistic regression was carried out to develop a model for identifying cases with clinically important brain injury, and the model was used to generate the 7 predictors in the Canadian CT Head Rule (Figure).

Subsequent analyses demonstrated that the 5 "high risk" factors had a sensitivity of 100% (95%CI 92-100%) and specificity of 68.7% (95%CI 67-70%) for neurological intervention, while CT scans would have been ordered in 32.2% of patients. When all 7 factors were considered, the sensitivity was 98.4% (95%CI

96-99%) and specificity was 49.6% (95%CI 48-51%) for clinically-important brain injury on CT, while CT scans would have been ordered in 54.3% of patients.

Canadian CT Head Rule
CT head is only required for *minor head injury* patients with any of these findings:
High risk (for neurological intervention) 1. GCS score < 15 at 2 hours after injury 2. Suspected open or depressed skull fracture 3. Any sign of basal skull fracture (i.e., hemotympanum, "racoon" eyes, CSF otorrhea/rhinorrhea, battle's sign) 4. Vomiting ≥2 episodes 5. Age ≥65 years
Medium risk (for brain injury on CT) 1. Amnesia before impact ≥30 minutes 2. Dangerous mechanism (i.e., pedestrian struck by motor vehicle, occupant ejected from motor vehicle, fall from elevation ≥3 feet/5 stairs)

Table I. The Canadian CT Head Rule.
Stiell IG, Wells GA, Vandemheen K, Clement C, Lesiuk H, Laupacis A, et al. The Canadian CT Head Rule for patients with minor head injury. Lancet. 2001 May 5;357(9266):1391–6.

The CURE trial: Clopidogrel reduces mortality after acute coronary syndrome

1. The addition of clopidogrel reduced the risk of death from cardiovascular causes, nonfatal myocardial infarction, or other ischemic events in patients with acute coronary syndrome (ACS) without ST elevation.

2. Adding clopidogrel increased the risk of major and minor bleeding, but not life-threatening bleeding.

Original Date of Publication: August 2001

Study Rundown: ACS refers to symptoms attributed to the occlusion of coronary arteries. ST-segment changes help classify ACS, with ST-elevation suggesting a transmural infarct, which typically requires immediate revascularization. Patients suffering ACS without ST-elevation typically do not undergo urgent revascularization. Prior to the Clopidogrel in Unstable Angina to Prevent Recurrent Events (CURE) trial, therapy for ACS without ST-elevation consisted mainly of aspirin and heparin. The purpose of the CURE trial was to explore whether the addition of clopidogrel, a thienopyridine class antiplatelet agent, could further reduce the risk of recurrent ischemic events in patients suffering from ACS without ST-elevation.

Treatment with clopidogrel resulted in a significantly lower risk of death from cardiovascular causes, nonfatal myocardial infarction, or stroke compared to placebo. Of note, the addition of clopidogrel resulted in significantly higher rates of major and minor bleeding complications, though not life-threatening bleeds. Based on the findings of this study, clopidogrel has become widely used in current ACS practice, in addition to aspirin, heparin, and other medications.

In-Depth [randomized controlled trial]: This randomized, controlled trial compared clopidogrel with placebo in addition to aspirin in patients presenting with acute coronary syndromes without ST-segment elevation. Patients were eligible for the trial if they were hospitalized within 24 hours of symptom onset and did not have ST-segment elevation. Patients with contraindications to antithrombotic or antiplatelet therapy, at high risk of bleeding or severe heart failure, taking oral anticoagulants, and those who had revascularization in the past three months or glycoprotein IIb/IIIa inhibitors in the past 3 days were excluded.

The first primary outcome was the composite of death from cardiovascular causes, nonfatal myocardial infarction, or stroke. The second primary outcome was the composite of the first primary outcome with refractory ischemia. Severe ischemia, heart failure and need for revascularization were secondary outcomes and other outcomes were bleeding complications categorized as life threatening, major, or minor.

A total of 12 562 patients from 482 centers in 28 countries were enrolled in the trial. Patients in the clopidogrel group experienced significantly lower rates of the first primary outcome, when compared with patients receiving placebo (RR 0.80; 95%CI 0.72-0.90). The rate of the second primary outcome was also significantly lower in patients treated with clopidogrel (RR 0.86; 95%CI 0.79-0.94). Significantly fewer patients in the clopidogrel group experienced severe ischemia (RR 0.74; 95%CI 0.61-0.90) or recurrent angina (RR 0.91; 95%CI 0.85-0.98). Major bleeding, defined as bleeding requiring transfusion of 2 or more units of blood, was significantly more common in the clopidogrel group (RR 1.38; 95%CI 1.13-1.67).

Yusuf S, Zhao F, Mehta SR, Chrolavicius S, Tognoni G, Fox KK, et al. Effects of clopidogrel in addition to aspirin in patients with acute coronary syndromes without ST-segment elevation. New England Journal of Medicine. 2001 Aug 16;345(7):494–502.

The Rivers trial: Early goal-directed therapy reduces mortality in severe sepsis and septic shock

1. Early goal-directed therapy (EGDT) in patients with severe sepsis and septic shock prior to admission to the intensive care unit was associated with significantly reduced organ dysfunction and mortality rates compared to standard therapy to achieve parameters for hemodynamic support.

Original Date of Publication: November 2001

Study Rundown: Thee systemic inflammatory response syndrome (SIRS) is diagnosed when 2 of the following criteria are present: 1) body temperature < 36ºC or > 38ºC, 2) heart rate > 90 beats/min, 3) respiratory rate > 20 breaths/minute or $PaCO_2$ < 32 mmHg, 4) WBC < 4×10^9/L, WBC > 12×10^9/L, or > 10% bands. Sepsis refers to SIRS that results from infection and this can progress to severe sepsis (i.e., sepsis with organ dysfunction, hypoperfusion, or hypotension) or septic shock (i.e., severe sepsis with hypotension despite adequate fluid resuscitation). In this spectrum of conditions, circulatory changes may arise, resulting in insufficient oxygen delivery to meet metabolic demands. These changes lead to global tissue hypoxia, which may foreshadow multiorgan failure and death. The onset of global tissue hypoxia represents a turning point in the development of sepsis, where intervention may help to avoid poor outcomes.

Commonly referred to as the Rivers trial, this study sought to explore whether EGDT before admission to the intensive care unit (ICU) could reduce the incidence of multiorgan dysfunction, mortality, and the use of health care resources compared to standard therapy in patients with severe sepsis and septic shock. In summary, patients in the standard therapy group had significantly higher APACHE II, SAPS II, and MODS mortality prediction scores compared to patients receiving EGDT. Moreover, the EGDT group experienced significantly lower in-hospital, 28-day, and 60-day mortality rates when compared to patients undergoing standard therapy. The Rivers trial was criticized for being conducted at a single center. Since the trial, numerous multicenter, randomized, controlled trials have been completed comparing EGDT with usual care and have demonstrated no significant difference between the approaches in terms of outcomes.

In-Depth [randomized controlled trial]: This study, conducted at a single tertiary care center in Detroit, randomized 263 patients to either standard therapy or EGDT for 6 hours prior to ICU admission. Patients were included in the trial if they met SIRS criteria and had a systolic blood pressure ≤90 mmHg or a serum lactate ≥4 mmol/L. Exclusion criteria included age < 18 years, pregnancy, or the presence of an acute cerebral vascular event, acute coronary syndrome, acute pulmonary edema, status asthmaticus, cardiac dysrhythmias, contraindication to central venous catheterization, and burn injury, amongst others. Outcome measures included vital signs, resuscitation endpoints, measures of organ dysfunction, and mortality prediction scores (i.e., APACHE II, SAPS II, MODS), and mortality. In the EGDT group, all patients received arterial lines and central venous lines with the ability to monitor central venous oxygen saturation ($ScvO_2$). EGDT involved targeting a series of treatment goals for patients:

1. Central venous pressure (CVP) ≥8-12 mmHg (through crystalloid boluses)
2. Mean arterial pressure (MAP) ≥65 mmHg (through vasopressor administration)
3. Urine output ≥0.5 mL/kg/hour
4. $ScvO_2$ ≥70% (through transfusion of red cells and dobutamine)

After the initial 6-hour period, patients receiving standard therapy had significantly higher APACHE II, SAPS II, and MODS compared to those receiving EGDT ($p < 0.001$ for all comparisons), suggesting higher levels of organ dysfunction in the standard therapy group. Moreover, in-hospital mortality rates (RR 0.58; 95%CI 0.38-0.87), 28-day mortality (RR 0.58; 95%CI 0.39-0.87), and 60-day mortality (RR 0.67; 95%CI 0.46-0.96) were all significantly lower in the EGDT group. There were no significant differences between the groups in terms of measures of health care resource consumption (i.e., mean duration of vasopressor therapy, mechanical ventilation, hospital stay).

Rivers E, Nguyen B, Havstad S, Ressler J, Muzzin A, Knoblich B, et al. Early Goal-Directed Therapy in the Treatment of Severe Sepsis and Septic Shock. New England Journal of Medicine. 2001 Nov 8;345(19):1368–77.

Mild hypothermia improves neurological outcome after cardiac arrest

1. Initiation of a hypothermia protocol for 24 hours after a cardiac arrest significantly improved neurological outcome in surviving patients compared to the normothermia group.

2. Patients who underwent the hypothermia protocol had a significantly lower mortality rate at 6 months.

3. There were no significant differences in adverse outcomes between the groups.

Original Date of Publication: February 2002

Study Rundown: This landmark trial demonstrated that inducing mild hypothermia early in patients who suffered a cardiac arrest reduced permanent neurological damage secondary to global cerebral ischemia. The subjects who underwent cooling within 4 hours of cardiac arrest experienced superior neurological outcomes (according to the Pittsburgh cerebral performance scale) as well as a lower mortality rate 6 months out from the event. There was no difference in adverse outcomes between the groups in the first 7 days after the event, although data showed a trend toward susceptibility to infections in the hypothermia group. The subjects in the normothermia group had a higher prevalence of diabetes mellitus and coronary artery disease compared to the hypothermia group; however, controlling for these baseline differences did not alter the study findings. While the study was not blinded, neurological assessment 6 months after therapy was blinded. The time to initiation of the hypothermia protocol also varied within the group, ranging from 61 to 192 minutes, with a median of 105 minutes. In summary, patients who underwent cooling within 4 hours after a cardiac arrest from ventricular fibrillation experienced a significantly higher rate of favorable neurological outcomes compared to the patients who underwent standard normothermia treatment.

In-Depth [randomized controlled trial]: The trial assigned 275 patients arriving to the ED with a cardiac arrest due to ventricular fibrillation to either standard normothermia or to a mild hypothermia protocol. Eligible subjects were patients between 18-75 years of age who had suffered a cardiac arrest from ventricular fibrillation and had an estimated 5-15 minute delay before cardiac resuscitation was started. Patients with coagulopathies, pregnancy, terminal illness, other causes of cardiac arrest, in a coma state at baseline, or hypotensive or hypoxic for 30 minutes or 15 minutes, respectively, prior to randomization were excluded. The group assigned to mild hypothermia treatment was cooled to a target temperature between 32°C to 34°C with the use of an external cooling device and ice packs, if necessary. Investigators maintained the temperature at 32°C to 34°C for 24 hours, and followed with passive rewarming, which averaged out to an 8-hour period.

The study demonstrated that the group assigned to mild hypothermia treatment experienced a significantly higher rate of favorable neurological outcomes (as assessed blindly 6 months later via the Pittsburgh cerebral performance scale) compared to the group that underwent standard normothermia treatment (55% vs. 39%, RR 1.40; 95%CI 1.08-1.81). The hypothermia group also had a significantly lower 6 month mortality rate compared to the normothermia group (RR 0.74; 95%CI 0.58-0.95). There were no significant differences in complication rates in the first 7 days after randomization between the groups.

Hypothermia after Cardiac Arrest Study Group. Mild Therapeutic Hypothermia to Improve the Neurologic Outcome after Cardiac Arrest. New England Journal of Medicine. 2002 Feb 21;346(8):549–56.

Voriconazole superior to amphotericin B for invasive aspergillosis

1. In immunocompromised patients with invasive aspergillosis, treatment with voriconazole was found to be superior to amphotericin B in achieving successful outcomes.

2. The incidence of serious adverse events was significantly lower in patients in the voriconazole group, as compared with those in the amphotericin B group.

Original Date of Publication: August 2002

Study Rundown: In immunocompromised patients, like those with prolonged neutropenia and previous transplant recipients, invasive aspergillosis is a dangerous and not uncommon complication affecting between 5% to 20% of patients deemed high-risk. For many decades, the standard therapy for invasive aspergillosis infections has been amphotericin B, despite limited success with the treatment and significant risk of toxicity (e.g., fevers/chills, hypotension, kidney injury, hepatotoxicity, cardiac arrhythmias). Prior to this trial, voriconazole had been shown to be somewhat effective in treating invasive aspergillosis, though no randomized trials had been performed. The purpose of this randomized, controlled trial was to compare the effects and safety of voriconazole with amphotericin B in the primary treatment of immunocompromised patients presenting with acute invasive aspergillosis.

At the conclusion of the study, patients treated with voriconazole were significantly more likely than those on amphotericin B to experience a successful outcome. Moreover, while the trial primarily sought to demonstrate non-inferiority, it was able to demonstrate that voriconazole was superior to amphotericin B in the treatment of invasive aspergillosis. Patients in the voriconazole group also experienced significantly fewer adverse events as compared with those in the amphotericin B group. Based on the findings of this study, the Infectious Diseases Society of America currently recommends that voriconazole be the primary treatment of invasive aspergillosis in most patients.

In-Depth [randomized controlled trial]: A total of 277 patients from 95 centers in 19 countries were included in the modified intention-to-treat population, with 144 in the voriconazole group and 133 in the amphotericin B group. Patients were eligible if they were ≥12 years of age, had definite or probable invasive aspergillosis, and were immunocompromised (e.g., allogeneic hematopoietic-cell transplantation, hematologic cancer, aplastic anemia, acquired immunodeficiency syndrome – AIDS, solid-organ transplantation). Exclusion criteria included chronic aspergillosis, aspergilloma, allergic bronchopulmonary aspergillosis, previous systemic therapy with amphotericin B/itraconazole, treatment with interacting drugs (e.g., rifampin), hypersensitivity to azoles or amphotericin B, aminotransferase/bilirubin/alkaline phosphatase level > 5 times the upper limit of normal, serum creatinine > 221 μmol/L (2.5 mg/dL), and pregnancy. Patients in the voriconzole group received 6 mg/kg intravenously twice daily on day 1, followed by 4 mg/kg intravenously twice daily for at least 7 days, and 200 mg orally twice daily afterwards. Those in the amphotericin B group received 1.0-1.5 mg/kg intravenously daily. Planned duration of therapy was 12 weeks, and patients could have been treated with other antifungals should they experience toxicity from treatment or poor response to therapy. The primary aim of the study was to demonstrate non-inferiority of voriconazole as compared with amphotericin B, while the secondary aim was to demonstrate superiority of voriconazole.

At week 12, patients in the voriconazole group were significantly more likely to have a successful outcome than those on amphotericin B (52.8% vs. 31.6%, absolute difference 21.2%, 95%CI 10.4 to 32.9%). Given these findings, voriconazole was found to be superior to amphotericin B for invasive aspergillosis. The survival rate at week 12 was also significantly higher in the voriconazole group (70.8% vs. 57.9%; HR 0.59, 95%CI 0.40-0.88). There were significantly fewer adverse events in patients taking voriconazole as compared with those taking amphotericin B ($p = 0.02$). Although those on voriconazole experienced significantly higher instances of visual disturbances (44.8% vs. 4.3%, $p < 0.001$), all these events resolved without intervention.

Herbrecht R, Denning DW, Patterson TF, Bennett JE, Greene RE, Oestmann JW, et al. Voriconazole versus amphotericin B for primary therapy of invasive aspergillosis. The New England Journal of Medicine. 2002;347(6):408-415.

Canadian C-Spine Rules superior to NEXUS Low-Risk Criteria for detecting cervical-spine injuries

1. The Canadian C-Spine Rule (CCR, Figure I) demonstrated higher sensitivity and specificity for cervical-spine injury compared to the National Emergency X-Radiography Utilization Study (NEXUS) Low-Risk Criteria (NLC, Table I).

Original Date of Publication: December 2003

Study Rundown: According to large trauma registries, approximately 3% of all blunt trauma victims sustain injuries to the spinal column, including injuries to the cervical spine (C-spine). Suspected C-spine fractures are frequently evaluated with radiography; however, there is a lack of consensus among published guidelines with regards to the use of radiography. Two independently validated clinical decision rules are commonly used to determine patient selection of C-spine radiography: the CCR and the NLC. The CCR is a three-step process that evaluates risk factors for serious injury, physical exam findings, and the ability for the patient to rotate their neck. The NLC is made up of five criteria based on patient history (no painful distracting injuries, normal level of consciousness) and physical examination (midline cervical tenderness, focal neurologic deficits, and no evidence of intoxication). The purpose of this landmark prospective trial was to compare the accuracy of both the CCR and the NLC in detecting C-spine injuries.

The prospective trial measured the frequency of clinically important C-spine injuries in over 8000 consecutive patients and reported the accuracy of both the CCR and NLC in detecting these injuries when applied to this cohort. At the conclusion of the trial, the CCR demonstrated a near 100% sensitivity for detecting clinically important C-spine fractures; this was significantly higher than the NLC (90.7%). Additionally, the CCR was also found to be more specific for C-spine injuries compared to NLC. When the sensitivity and specificity were applied to the cohort, the NLC would have missed 1 in 10 clinically important C-spine fractures while requiring a higher radiography rate. Ten percent (10%) of patients were not evaluated for neck range of motion and therefore did not complete the CCR algorithm. However, the sensitivity and specificity of the CCR remained significantly higher than the NLC even if all significant findings in this small subgroup were assumed to be missed by CCR.

The results of this trial demonstrated superior performance of the CCR over the NLC in detecting clinically significant C-spine injuries and supported the use of CCR as the preferred clinical prediction rule. However, the study population was only limited to patients aged greater than 16 years who were alert and in stable condition at the time of assessment. Additionally, the study was performed at institutions where the CCR was developed, precluding validation in alternative clinical settings.

In-Depth [prospective cohort]: This was a prospective study of 8282 consecutive patients with acute trauma to the head and neck for assessment for C-spine injuries in nine tertiary care hospitals in Canada. Patients were included if they were at least 16 years of age and had a Glasgow Coma Scale score of 15 out of 15 at the time of assessment. Patients were excluded if they had penetrating neck trauma, acute paralysis, or were pregnant. All patients were assessed by the CCR and NLC for the study, which was completed by the evaluating emergency physician. Patients underwent plain radiography according to the judgement of the physician independent of the results of the clinical prediction rules. All injuries to the C-spine on radiography were considered significant unless one of the following benign fractures were isolated: transverse process not involving a facet joint, a spinous process not involving lamina, or simple vertebral compression of < 25% of body height. Patients who did not receive radiography were evaluated for C-spine injuries using the Proxy Outcome Assessment Tool, which assessed clinical symptoms 14-days following injury.

At the conclusion of the trial, a total of 169 patients (2%) demonstrated a clinically significant C-spine fracture. The sensitivity for detection of these C-spine fractures was significantly higher in the CCR compared to the NLC (99.4% versus 90.7%; $p < 0.001$). Additionally, the CCR also demonstrated significantly higher specificity for C-spine injuries compared to NLC (40.4% versus 33.0%; $p < 0.001$). In 845 patients (10.2%), the CCR assessment was indeterminate due to the lack of evaluating of neck range of motion. In secondary analysis, if all indeterminate cases were assumed to be negative by the CCR, the sensitivity and specificity was modified to 95.3% and 50.7%, respectively. This remained significantly higher when compared to the NLC.

Stiell IG, Clement CM, McKnight RD, Brison R, Schull MJ, Rowe BH, et al. The Canadian C-Spine Rule versus the NEXUS Low-Risk Criteria in Patients with Trauma. The New England Journal of Medicine. 2003 Dec 25;349(26):2510–8.

Nexus Low Risk Criteria

Cervical spine radiography is indicated for trauma unless the patient exhibits all of the following criteria:

1. No posterior midline cervical tenderness
2. No focal neurological deficit
3. Normal alertness
4. No intoxication
5. No painful distracting injury

Table I. Nexus Low Risk Criteria.

Canadian C-Spine Rule

© 2 Minute Medicine™

For patients with a GCS 15 (alert) & stable trauma patients with concern for cervical spine injury

HIGH RISK FACTORS
Age ≥ 65?
Dangerous mechanism?
Paresthesias in extremities?

Any Yes → **Radiography**

No ↓

LOW RISK FACTORS ALLOWING ASSESSMENT OF RANGE OF MOTION
Simple rearend MVC?**
Sitting position in ED?
Ambulatory?
Delayed neck pain onset?***
Absence of midline c-spine tenderness?

Any Yes ↓   No → **Radiography**

Able to rotate neck 45°?

Yes → **No Radiography**
No → **Radiography**

Figure 1. Canadian C-Spine Rule.

* Dangerous Mechanism
- Fall from ≥ 3 feet/ 5 stairs
- Axial load to head
- High speed motor vehicle accident (MVC) ≥ 100 km/hr, rollover, ejection
- Motorized recreational vehicles
- Bicycle struck or collision

** Simple Rearend MVC Excludes
- Pushed into oncoming traffic
- Hit by bus/large truck
- Rollover
- Hit by high speed vehicle

*** Delayed
- i.e. no immediate onset of neck pain

The SAFE trial: Normal saline vs. albumin for fluid resuscitation

1. There was no significant difference in 28-day mortality when comparing albumin and normal saline for fluid resuscitation in the intensive care unit (ICU) setting.

2. Compared to normal saline, fluid resuscitation with albumin did not yield any significant benefits in terms of secondary outcomes (i.e., length of ICU/hospital stay, duration of supportive treatment measures).

Original Date of Publication: May 2004

Study Rundown: In various types of shock, resuscitation with intravenous fluids helps to maintain circulating pressure and tissue perfusion. A myriad of options are available for fluid resuscitation, including blood products, non-blood products, or a combination. Crystalloid and colloid solutions are classes of fluids that may be used. Crystalloid solutions are composed of sterile water and electrolytes, in concentrations that are similar to human serum. Colloids contain an additional colloidal substance (e.g., albumin, dextran) that does not cross semi-permeable membranes. As a result, colloids are more effective at maintaining intravascular volume. While studies have demonstrated that crystalloids and colloids have different effects on physiological measures, it remains uncertain which may be more beneficial in reducing mortality. This is an important consideration because colloid solutions are more expensive than crystalloids. Moreover, previous systematic reviews reached conflicting conclusions, with studies suggesting albumin-containing solutions were linked with increased mortality and others suggesting there was no significant difference when compared to crystalloids.

The Saline versus Albumin Fluid Evaluation (SAFE) trial was a randomized, controlled trial designed to explore whether the use of 4% albumin led to any significant difference in mortality when compared with 0.9% sodium chloride (i.e., normal saline) in intensive care settings. The trial found no significant difference between the groups in 28-day mortality. Moreover, there were no differences between the groups in length of ICU/hospital stay, duration of mechanical ventilation, or duration of renal replacement therapy.

In-Depth [randomized controlled trial]: This study was conducted in 16 tertiary intensive care units in Australia and New Zealand. Patients were eligible if they were ≥18 years of age, were admitted to intensive care, and required fluid administration. Patients were excluded if they were admitted after cardiac surgery, liver transplantation, or for burns treatment. A total of 6997 patients were randomized to receive either 4 percent albumin or normal saline. Fluids were provided in identical 500 mL bottles. The primary outcome measure was death from any cause in the first 28 days after randomization, while secondary outcomes included the duration of mechanical ventilation, the duration of renal replacement therapy, and the duration of ICU/hospital stay. There was no significant difference between the albumin and saline groups in 28-day mortality (RR 0.99; 95%CI 0.91-1.09). Moreover, there were no significant differences between the groups in terms of length of ICU stay (p = 0.44), length of hospital stay (p = 0.30), duration of mechanical ventilation (p = 0.74), or duration of renal replacement therapy (p = 0.41).

Finfer S, Bellomo R, Boyce N, French J, Myburgh J, Norton R, et al. A comparison of albumin and saline for fluid resuscitation in the intensive care unit. New England Journal of Medicine. 2004 May 27;350(22):2247–56.

The ICTUS trial: Early invasive vs selectively invasive management for acute coronary syndrome

1. There was no significant difference in the composite rate of death, nonfatal myocardial infarction (MI), or rehospitalization for angina in patients with acute coronary syndrome (ACS) treated with early invasive or selectively invasive strategies.

2. Myocardial infarction was significantly more frequent in the early invasive management group but rehospitalization was significantly less frequent in this group.

Original Date of Publication: September 2005

Study Rundown: Guidelines of the American College of Cardiology-American Heart Association and European Society of Cardiology recommend an early invasive strategy for the treatment of ACS without ST-segment elevation. The Invasive versus Conservative Treatment in Unstable Coronary Syndromes (ICTUS) trial suggested that selectively invasive management may be an acceptable alternative approach to treatment. With advances in medical therapy and higher rates of revascularization, patients treated with the selectively invasive strategy showed no difference in the cumulative rate of death, nonfatal MI, or rehospitalization for angina 1 year after randomization. These results suggest that an early invasive strategy may not be superior to a selectively invasive strategy for the treatment of ACS without ST-segment elevation and with elevated cardiac troponin T levels.

In-Depth [randomized controlled trial]: The authors assigned 1200 patients with ACS without ST-segment elevation and with elevated cardiac troponin T levels to management with early invasive strategy or selectively invasive strategies. Both treatment groups received optimized medical therapy. The early invasive strategy involved angiography within 24 to 48 hours of randomization and percutaneous coronary intervention when appropriate. Patients assigned to selectively invasive management were scheduled for angiography and revascularization only if symptoms persisted despite medical therapy or if patients showed hemodynamic or rhythmic instability. A composite of death, recurrent MI or rehospitalization for angina within 1 year was measured as the primary endpoint. There was no significant difference in the cumulative event rate at 1 year between the groups (RR 1.07; 95%CI 0.87-1.33; p = 0.33). Mortality 1 year after randomization was 2.5% in both groups. The risk of MI was significantly higher in the early invasive strategy group (p = 0.005), while rehospitalization was significantly less frequent in this group (p = 0.04).

De Winter RJ, Windhausen F, Cornel JH, Dunselman PHJM, Janus CL, Bendermacher PEF, et al. Early Invasive versus Selectively Invasive Management for Acute Coronary Syndromes. New England Journal of Medicine. 2005 Sep 15;353(11):1095–104.

Fleischner Society Guidelines, 2005 Statement: Limited CT follow-up recommended for small, solitary, pulmonary nodules

1. In patients with a low clinical risk for lung cancer, incidentally-detected small lung nodules (<4 mm) found on computed tomography (CT) scans do not require additional longitudinal imaging follow-up; nodules between 4 to 6 mm require a single follow-up CT in 12 months.

2. In patients with high clinical risk for lung cancer, small lung nodules (<4 mm) require a single follow-up CT at 12 months; nodules between 4 to 6 mm in size require initial follow-up at 6 to 12 months, followed by a repeat follow-up at 18 to 24 months.

Original Date of Publication: November 2005

Study Rundown: Solitary pulmonary nodules are common incidental findings on radiographs or CT scans of the chest, often posing diagnostic difficulties for the radiologist given the wide differential of benign and malignant etiologies. Earlier guidelines recommended up to 5 CT follow-up exams to assess nodules stability, regardless of morphology or size. This often resulted in unnecessary scans and excessive ionizing radiation exposure to patients for nodules with little malignant potential. The purpose of this landmark guideline from the Fleischner Society was to provide expert-consensus guidelines to the follow-up of incidentally found pulmonary nodules on CT.

The guideline article reviewed the results from a number of large international lung cancer screening trials on the outcomes of patients with small pulmonary nodules. The article highlighted the overall low malignancy potential for nodules between 4 and 7 mm in a large lung cancer screening trial as well as the difficulty in accurately measuring small pulmonary nodules to accurately track growth or doubling time. Finally, the article recognized the importance of risk factors (i.e. smoking status, family history, etc.) in assessing small pulmonary nodules. From this data, the Fleischner Society recommended reducing the overall number of CT follow-ups required for small pulmonary nodules.

The Fleischner Society constructed guidelines based on foundational literature demonstrating several key observations:

a. Half of all smokers 50 years of age or older have at least one nodule at screening.

b. Size is a primary determinant of the malignant potential of nodules.

c. Cigarette smoking portends a greater risk of lethal cancers, increasing in proportion to the degree of smoking.

d. Nodules in cigarette smokers grow faster than in nonsmokers.

e. Nodule morphology correlates with malignant likelihood and growth rate (i.e. nonsolid nodules typically carry a lower malignant potential versus solid nodules).

f. Malignant risk of nodules increases with patient age.

Low-risk patients are defined as patients with a minimal or absent smoking history and absence of other known risk factors including a history of lung cancer in a first degree relative and exposure to carcinogenic material (i.e., asbestos, radon, and uranium). Similarly, high-risk patients are defined as patients with a history of smoking or the aforementioned known risk factors. The guidelines do not apply to patient with known or suspected cancers outside of the lungs, patients younger than 35 years of age, or patients with unexplained fever.

The Fleischner Society Guidelines are limited in scope to solitary, solid pulmonary nodules and do not provide follow-up recommendations for subsolid nodules or the presence of multiple nodules. However, the recommendations made by the Fleischner Society have been widely adopted as the imaging follow-up recommendation plan for patients with small, incidentally found pulmonary nodules. A recently published classification system for lung cancer screening, Lung-RADS, by Pinsky et al., was based upon the Fleischner Society criteria. However, this classification system has not yet been prospectively validated.

MacMahon H, Austin JHM, Gamsu G, Herold CJ, Jett JR, Naidich DP, et al. Guidelines for Management of Small Pulmonary Nodules Detected on CT Scans: A Statement from the Fleischner Society. Radiology. 2005 Nov 1;237(2):395–400.

Additional Review:

Pinsky PF, Gierada DS, Black W, Munden R, Nath H, Aberle D, et al. Performance of Lung-RADS in the National Lung Screening Trial A Retrospective Assessment Performance of Lung-RADS in the NLST. Ann Intern Med. 2015 Apr 7;162(7):485–91.

Nodule size	Low-Risk Patient	High-Risk Patient
≤4 mm	– No follow up	– 12 month CT – If stable, no further follow-up
>4 mm - 6 mm	– 12 month CT – If stable, no further follow-up	– 6-12 month CT – If stable, repeat CT at 18-24 months
>6 mm - 8 mm	– 6-12 month CT – If stable, repeat CT at 18-24 months	– 3-6 month CT – If stable, repeat CT at 9-12 months and 24 months
>8 mm	– CT at 3, 9, and 24 months – Consider dynamic contrast-enhanced CT, PET or biopsy	– CT at 3, 9, and 24 months – Consider dynamic contrast-enhanced CT, PET or biopsy

Table I. 2005 Fleischner Society Guidelines for Solid Pulmonary Nodules.

Delayed antimicrobial therapy linked with higher mortality in septic shock

1. Septic shock is a complication of infection with very high mortality rates.

2. This study was one of the first to demonstrate that delaying the provision of effective antimicrobial therapy in septic shock leads to significantly higher mortality rates, supporting recommendations by international guidelines to initiate timely, broad-spectrum, empiric antimicrobial therapy in patients presenting in septic shock.

Original Date of Publication: June 2006

Study Rundown: Sepsis has been defined as a systemic inflammatory response that occurs due to an infectious process. Severe sepsis refers sepsis that is complicated by acute organ dysfunction, while septic shock is a term describing sepsis that is associated with elevated serum lactate levels and persistent hypotension despite appropriate fluid resuscitation. The worldwide incidence of severe sepsis and septic shock has been estimated at 19 million cases yearly. While mortality from severe sepsis and septic shock has decreased considerably over the past few decades, the risk of death remains high and has been estimated at approximately 20-30%, while those who survive often suffer from cognitive deficits and poorer quality of life.

At the time this study was published, numerous international guidelines recommended the initiation of antibiotics within an hour of presentation for patients in severe sepsis and septic shock, though no clinical evidence was available to support this intervention. The purpose of this retrospective, multicenter study was to determine the link between the delay of starting antimicrobial therapy from onset of recurrent or persistent hypotension and mortality in patients with septic shock. This study was the first to provide strong evidence to suggest that delaying antimicrobial therapy in septic shock was associated with higher mortality. The findings supported numerous international guidelines recommending initiation of broad-spectrum, empiric antimicrobial therapy within an hour of presentation of septic shock, as any delays were linked with lower survival.

In-Depth [retrospective cohort]: Researchers studied 3 cohorts of patients ≥18 years of age presenting in septic shock. The first cohort included all cases of septic shock admitted to any intensive care unit (ICU) in Manitoba, Canada from 1999-2004. The second cohort included all cases of septic shock between 1989 and 1999 at a single tertiary care institution in Winnipeg, Manitoba. The third cohort included patients in septic shock during 1999-2004 from 3 academic institutions in the United States. Each case was screened to determine if it met criteria for septic shock as outlined in the 1991 Society of Critical Care Medicine/American College of Chest Physicians Consensus Statement on Sepsis Definitions, with no other evident cause of shock. For each patient, data regarding antimicrobial choice, time of initial parenteral administration, and survival were collected.

A total of 2731 cases of septic shock were identified. The overall mortality rate was 56.2%. A total of 2154 patients received effective antimicrobial therapy after the onset of hypotension, and these patients experienced a mortality rate of 58.0%. A total of 558 received antimicrobials prior to developing hypotension and experienced a mortality rate of 52.2%. Starting effective antimicrobials in the first hour after the onset of hypotension due to septic shock was linked with 79.9% survival to discharge. In the first 6 hours after developing hypotension, each hour of delay resulted in an average survival reduction of 7.6%. On univariate analysis, the delay between recurrent or persistent hypotension and effective antimicrobial therapy was a critical determinant of survival to both ICU and hospital discharge ($p < 0.0001$ for both). Assessing delay of starting antimicrobials as a continuous variable, the adjusted odds ratio of death was 1.119 (95%CI 1.103-1.136, $p < 0.0001$) for each hour of delay, suggesting that each hour of delay in starting antimicrobial therapy was associated with a 12% increase in mortality over the previous hour.

Kumar A, Roberts D, Wood KE, Light B, Parrillo JE, Sharma S, et al. Duration of hypotension before initiation of effective antimicrobial therapy is the critical determinant of survival in human septic shock. Critical Care Medicine. 2006;34(6):1589-1596.

The TORCH trial: Combination of salmeterol and fluticasone in COPD

1. The combination of salmeterol and fluticasone did not significantly reduce all-cause mortality in patients with chronic obstructive pulmonary disease (COPD).

2. When compared with salmeterol alone, fluticasone alone, and placebo, combination therapy significantly reduced the risk of exacerbations and the need for systemic corticosteroids during exacerbations.

Original Date of Publication: February 2007

Study Rundown: The Towards a Revolution in COPD Health (TORCH) trial explored whether combination therapy with salmeterol (a long-acting beta-agonist) and fluticasone propionate (an inhaled corticosteroid) would significantly reduce mortality in patients with COPD as compared with placebo. This landmark study determined that combination therapy was not significantly associated with a reduced all-cause mortality when compared with placebo. Treatment with combination therapy, however, significantly reduced the risk of moderate or severe COPD exacerbations, as well as the likelihood that patients would require systemic corticosteroids during their exacerbations when compared with placebo.

In-Depth [randomized controlled trial]: A total of 6184 COPD patients were randomized to 4 different treatment arms: 1) 1545 were randomized to the placebo group, 2) 1542 were randomized to the salmeterol-only group, 3) 1551 were randomized to the fluticasone-only group, and 4) 1546 were randomized to the combination therapy group (i.e., salmeterol and fluticasone). Eligible patients had at least a 10 pack-year smoking history, were between 40-80 years old, diagnosed with COPD, exhibited a pre-bronchodilator forced expiratory volume in 1 second (FEV1) of less than 60% of the predicted value, showed an increase in FEV1 with use of 400 mcg of albuterol of less than 10% of the predicted value, and had a ratio of pre-bronchodilator FEV1 to forced vital capacity (FVC) of equal to or less than 0.70. Patients were excluded if they had a non-COPD pulmonary condition (e.g., lung cancer, sarcoidosis, asthma), prior lung-volume-reduction surgery or lung transplant, long term supplemental oxygen (i.e., greater than or equal to 12 hours/day), less than 6 weeks of oral corticosteroids, serious uncontrolled disease, received any investigational drugs in the 4 weeks prior to entry, evidence of alcohol or drug abuse, known hypersensitivity to inhaled corticosteroids, bronchodilators, or lactose, or known deficiency of alpha-1 anti-trypsin.

There was no significant difference in all-cause mortality between patients in the combination therapy group compared to the placebo group (HR 0.825; 95%CI 0.681-1.002). While there was no significant difference in all-cause mortality when comparing combination therapy with salmeterol-only therapy (HR 0.932, 95%CI 0.765-1.134), combination therapy was linked to significant reduction in all-cause mortality when compared with fluticasone alone (HR 0.774; 95%CI 0.641-0.934). Combination therapy was also associated with a significantly reduced risk of moderate or severe exacerbation as compared with salmeterol-only (HR 0.88; 95%CI 0.81-0.95), fluticasone-only (HR 0.91; 95%CI 0.84-0.99), and placebo (HR 0.75; 95%CI 0.69-0.81). Moreover, combination therapy was linked to a significant reduction in the risk of exacerbations requiring systemic corticosteroids compared to salmeterol-only (HR 0.71; 95%CI 0.63-0.79), fluticasone-only (HR 0.87; 95%CI 0.78-0.98), and placebo (HR 0.57; 95%CI 0.51-0.64).

Calverley PMA, Anderson JA, Celli B, Ferguson GT, Jenkins C, Jones PW, et al. Salmeterol and Fluticasone Propionate and Survival in Chronic Obstructive Pulmonary Disease. New England Journal of Medicine. 2007 Feb 22;356(8):775–89.

The CORTICUS trial: Hydrocortisone does not reduce mortality in septic shock

1. In patients with septic shock, there was no significant difference in mortality between groups receiving low-dose hydrocortisone compared to placebo.

2. Hydrocortisone therapy was linked to a quicker reversal of shock, but an increased frequency of superinfection.

Original Date of Publication: January 2008

Study Rundown: Recommendations that patients with septic shock be treated with low-dose corticosteroids were based on a limited set of evidence and largely dependent on a single trial. Although insufficiently powered, the Corticosteroid Therapy of Septic Shock (CORTICUS) study was the largest trial to date investigating the use of hydrocortisone in patients with septic shock. The results of the study pointed to a lack of benefit of hydrocortisone therapy in patients with septic shock. It also suggested that response to a corticotropin test is not a useful prognostic factor for response to hydrocortisone. In summary, hydrocortisone therapy did not reduce mortality in this group of patients with septic shock and therapy may be associated with increased incidence of superinfection.

In-Depth [randomized controlled trial]: The authors randomly assigned 499 patients with septic shock to receive low-dose hydrocortisone therapy or placebo. All patients were assessed for a response to a corticotropin test. The primary end point was the rate of death at 28 days in patients without a response to corticotropin. There was no significant difference in the primary outcome between the hydrocortisone and placebo groups (39.2% vs. 36.1%, respectively; $p = 0.69$). There was also no significant difference in the rate of death at 28 days in patients who responded to corticotropin, nor was there a significant difference in overall deaths between the study groups (34.3% vs. 31.5%; $p = 0.51$). Time to reversal of shock was shorter in the hydrocortisone group than the placebo group (3.3 days vs. 5.8 days for all patients). There was a higher incidence of superinfections in the hydrocortisone group, including new episodes of sepsis and septic shock (OR 1.37; 95%CI 1.05-1.79).

Sprung CL, Annane D, Keh D, Moreno R, Singer M, Freivogel K, et al. Hydrocortisone Therapy for Patients with Septic Shock. New England Journal of Medicine. 2008 Jan 10;358(2):111–24.

The ACCORD trial: Intensive glucose control associated with increased mortality

1. Previous studies linked intensive blood glucose control to a reduced risk of microvascular complications. However, questions remained regarding the impact on macrovascular complications and mortality.

2. This study found that targeting HbA1c < 6.0% resulted in a higher risk of cardiovascular and all-cause mortality as compared with standard therapy (i.e., targeting HbA1c between 7.0-7.9%).

Original Date of Publication: June 2008

Study Rundown: The Action to Control Cardiovascular Risk in Diabetes (ACCORD) trial sought to explore whether more intensive glucose control regimens were associated with better outcomes in patients with type 2 diabetes mellitus. Prior to the ACCORD trial, several randomized controlled trials examined blood sugar control in type 2 diabetics. The University Group Diabetes Program (UGDP) study, a randomized controlled trial conducted in 1970, suggested that there was no benefit of glycemic control in new-onset type 2 diabetics. Subsequently, a second randomized trial conducted in Japan demonstrated a reduction in the incidence of microvascular complications with better blood sugar control, while a third demonstrated no significant reduction in cardiovascular events in patients with better blood sugar control. Perhaps the most notable study, however, was the UK Prospective Diabetes Study (UKPDS), a randomized, controlled trial involving 5102 patients with newly diagnosed type 2 diabetes. The study was conducted over a 20 year period (1977-1997) and conclusively demonstrated that microvascular complications were reduced by intensively controlling blood glucose. Despite these studies, however, there was no sufficiently powered, randomized trial explicitly examining the effect of intensive glucose control on cardiovascular outcomes. Thus, the aim of the ACCORD trial was to determine whether intensive therapy to control blood glucose levels (targeting HbA1c < 6.0%) in type 2 diabetics would reduce cardiovascular events, compared to standard therapy (targeting HbA1c from 7.0-7.9%). In summary, this trial demonstrated that intensive glucose lowering significantly increases the risk of cardiovascular and all-cause mortality as compared with standard therapy.

In-Depth [randomized controlled trial]: The study spanned 77 centers across Canada and the United States. Patients were eligible for the trial if they had type 2 diabetes and an HbA1c ≥7.5%. Moreover, eligible patients were either between 40-79 years of age with cardiovascular disease or 55-79 years of age with anatomical evidence of atherosclerosis, albuminuria, left ventricular hypertrophy, or ≥2 additional risk factors for cardiovascular disease (i.e., dyslipidemia, hypertension, current smoker, or obesity). Investigators randomized patients to two different treatment arms: 1) intensive therapy targeting HbA1c < 6.0% or 2) standard therapy targeting HbA1c between 7.0-7.9%. The primary outcome was nonfatal myocardial infarction (MI), nonfatal stroke, or death from cardiovascular causes. Secondary outcomes included all-cause mortality. A total of 10,251 participants were involved in the final analyses. There was no significant difference in the composite primary outcome between the study groups (HR 0.90; 95%CI 0.78-1.04), though the intensive group experienced significantly fewer nonfatal MIs (HR 0.76; 95%CI 0.62-0.92) and significantly more deaths from cardiovascular causes (HR 1.35; 95%CI 1.04-1.76). All-cause mortality was significantly higher in the intensive group (HR 1.22; 95%CI 1.01-1.46). Notably, there were significantly more instances of hypoglycemia in the intensive therapy group as compared with standard therapy (16.2% vs. 5.1%, $p < 0.001$).

Action to Control Cardiovascular Risk in Diabetes Study Group, Gerstein HC, Miller ME, Byington RP, Goff DC, Bigger JT, et al. Effects of intensive glucose lowering in type 2 diabetes. New England Journal of Medicine. 2008 Jun 12;358(24):2545–59.

The UPLIFT trial: Tiotropium improves quality of life in chronic obstructive pulmonary disease

1. Tiotropium did not reduce the mean rate of decline in forced expiratory volume in 1 second (FEV1), a common metric of chronic obstructive pulmonary disease (COPD) progression.

2. Tiotropium significantly improved patient quality of life, mean FEV1, and decreased the incidence of disease exacerbation.

Original Date of Publication: October 2008

Study Rundown: Clinicians can assess COPD by measuring the rate of decline in a patient's FEV1. Previous studies found that at 1 year after initiation, tiotropium, a once-daily, inhaled anticholinergic drug, reduced the decline in FEV1 in contrast to shorter-acting anticholinergic drugs, inhaled corticosteroids, or the mucolytic agent N-acetylcysteine. The Understanding Potential Long-Term Impacts on Function with Tiotropium (UPLIFT) trial assessed the longer-term effects of tiotropium by extending its treatment period to 4 years. The study revealed that in patients with COPD who were permitted to use any respiratory medication concomitantly except other anticholinergic drugs, tiotropium was associated with improved lung function, improved quality of life, and a decreased incidence of disease exacerbation, but ultimately did not slow the rate of decline in FEV1. Study limitations included a relatively high drop-out rate in both the placebo group (44.6%) and tiotropium group (36.2%). Additionally, the study's subjects were predominantly male (75%), limiting generalizability. Tiotropium's main disadvantage is that it is more costly than other alternatives. Given that tiotropium did not affect the rate of disease progression, its use may be better suited to preventing disease exacerbation in patients with moderate or severe cases of COPD. Finally, since patients could not use other inhaled anticholinergics during the study, the study could not compare the efficacy of tiotropium with that of other anticholinergics.

In-Depth [randomized controlled trial]: UPLIFT was a 4-year, randomized, double-blinded trial involving 5993 patients recruited from 490 centers in 37 countries. Of the recruited patients, only 3535 completed the study. Patients with a diagnosis of COPD, age ≥40 years, a smoking history of > 10 pack-years, a post-bronchodilator FEV1 ≤70%, and an FEV1 ≤70% of the forced vital capacity

(FVC) were eligible for the study. Exclusion criteria included a history of asthma, COPD exacerbation, or pulmonary infection. The investigators randomized patients to receive either tiotropium or placebo. All other respiratory medications except inhaled anticholinergic drugs were permitted. The primary endpoint was the rate of decline in the mean FEV1 before and after bronchodilation at day 30. Secondary endpoints include changes in quality of life (as measured by St. George's Respiratory Questionnaire), exacerbations of COPD, and death from any cause. The mean FEV1 values were significantly improved in the tiotropium group at all time points compared to the control, although the mean decline in FEV1 was not significantly different before bronchodilation ($p = 0.95$) or after bronchodilation ($p = 0.21$). The incidence of COPD exacerbation decreased significantly with tiotropium treatment compared to placebo (HR 0.96, $p < 0.001$), while the difference in quality of life also favored tiotropium ($p < 0.001$). However, the incidence of death from any cause was not significantly different between the groups (HR=0.89, $p = 0.09$).

Tashkin DP, Celli B, Senn S, Burkhart D, Kesten S, Menjoge S, et al. A 4-Year Trial of Tiotropium in Chronic Obstructive Pulmonary Disease. New England Journal of Medicine. 2008 Oct 9;359(15):1543–54.

The NICE-SUGAR trial: Intensive glycemic control harmful in the intensive care unit

1. Intensive glycemic control in critically ill patients significantly increased 90-day mortality when compared to conventional glycemic control.

2. The incidence of severe hypoglycemia was significantly higher in patients receiving intensive glycemic control.

Original Date of Publication: March 2009

Study Rundown: In the intensive care unit (ICU), hyperglycemia is a common problem that is associated with increased morbidity and mortality. Previously conducted trials, systematic reviews, and meta-analyses reached conflicting conclusions on the effects of intensive glycemic control. Different groups, however, recommended intensive control for critically ill patients. The Normoglycemia in Intensive Care Evaluation-Survival Using Glucose Algorithm Regulation (NICE-SUGAR) trial sought to determine the impacts of intensive glycemic control on mortality in ICU patients. The trial demonstrated that intensive glucose control to target 81-108 mg/dL (4.5-6.0 mmol/L) was associated with a significantly increased 90-day mortality when compared to conventional glucose control to target ≤180 mg/dL (10.0 mmol/L). Moreover, the risk of severe hypoglycemia was significantly higher in the intensive control group. Based on the findings of this study, intensive glucose control was not recommended for patients in the ICU.

In-Depth [randomized controlled trial]: The study involved 6104 participants recruited from 42 hospitals from across Australia, New Zealand, and Canada. Patients were eligible if they stayed a minimum of 3 consecutive days in the ICU. Investigators randomly assigned patients to either intensive glucose control (target blood glucose between 81-108 mg/dL, or 4.5-6.0 mmol/L) or conventional glucose control (target blood glucose ≤180 mg/dL, or ≤10 mmol/L). Glucose control was achieved through insulin infusion as needed. The intervention was stopped when the patient was eating or discharged from the ICU. The primary outcome was death from any cause within 90 days after randomization. Secondary outcomes included survival time in the first 90 days, cause-specific death, and durations of mechanical ventilation/renal replacement therapy/ICU stay/hospital stay. Intensive glucose control was associated with significantly increased risk of mortality at day 90 when compared to conventional control (OR 1.14; 95%CI 1.02-1.28; ARI 2.6%, NNH 38). The incidence of severe hypoglycemia was significantly higher in patients undergoing intensive glucose control (OR 14.7; 95%CI 9.0-25.9). There were no significant differences between the groups in mechanical ventilation (p = 0.56) or renal replacement therapy requirements (p = 0.39). Moreover, there were no differences between the groups in terms of duration of ICU (p = 0.84) or hospital stay (p = 0.86).

NICE-SUGAR Study Investigators, Finfer S, Chittock DR, Su SY-S, Blair D, Foster D, et al. Intensive versus conventional glucose control in critically ill patients. New England Journal of Medicine. 2009 Mar 26;360(13):1283–97.

Clinical rules accurately predict children at low risk of clinically-important traumatic brain injury

1. This validated clinical prediction tool accurately predicted children at a very low risk of clinically-important brain injury (ciTBI) after head trauma.

2. Two different prediction rules were developed for children over and under 2 years of age.

Original Date of Publication: September 2009

Study Rundown: Traumatic brain injuries are common within the pediatric population resulting in over 500 000 emergency department (ED) visits annually for children under the age of 14. Computed tomography (CT) is the most commonly used imaging modality for assessment of suspected traumatic brain injuries given its widespread availability and accuracy in detecting ciTBI. However, the decision to proceed with CT for children must be balanced with the exposure to ionizing radiation in this young population, particularly in children with apparently minor head trauma. The purpose of this landmark trial was to validate and assess the accuracy of clinical prediction rules to predict children with very low risk ciTBI, which may prevent the need for routine CT scan.

The study prospectively analyzed the clinical outcomes of over 42 000 children who presented to the ED with a minor head trauma and a Glasgow Coma Scale (GCS) of 14 to 15. From the derivation cohort, 2 clinical prediction rules were created for children younger and older than 2 years of age. These prediction rules were validated with a cohort of over 8000 cases of pediatric head trauma. At the conclusion of the trial, for patients younger than two years of age, the clinical prediction tool correctly identified all patients who met the low-risk criteria for ciTBI with a sensitivity and negative predictive value for ciTBI of 100%. For patients older than 2 years of age, the clinical prediction tool demonstrated similar performance with a sensitivity and negative predictive value of 96.8% and 99.9%, respectively, for patients that meet the very low-risk criteria to require neuroimaging. This trial is strengthened by the large sample size and the use of diverse pediatric populations. To date, it is the only clinical prediction tool to be prospectively validated. These clinical prediction rules may help to identify a large group of children presenting with head trauma who meet low-risk criteria for neuroimaging an in whom CT scan could be avoided.

In-Depth [prospective cohort]: This was a prospective observational trial of 42 412 children who presented with a complaint of head trauma across 25 EDs in North America. Key exclusion criteria included known penetrating trauma, neurological disorder, or GCS less than 14 at time of presentation. The primary outcome of interest was the rate of ciTBI, defined as death from traumatic brain injury, neurosurgery, intubation for traumatic brain injury, or hospital admission of two night or more associated with traumatic brain injury. Outcomes for discharged patients were followed up by standardized telephone surveys of parents between 7 and 90 days after ED discharge. Two clinical prediction rules were created from a derivation cohort of 33 875 children. The prediction tool for patients less than 2 years of age included normal mental status, no scalp hematoma except frontal, loss of consciousness for less than 5 seconds, non-severe injury mechanism, no palpable skull fracture, and normal behavior. The prediction tool for patients 2 years of age or older included normal mental status, no loss of consciousness, no vomiting, non-severe injury mechanism, no signs of basilar skull fracture and no severe headache. Patients with altered mental status and signs of fracture were deemed to meet high-risk criteria. Patients meeting criteria other than altered mental status or signs of fracture were considered to be intermediate-risk. Using a validation cohort of 8627 children, the prediction rule for patients younger than 2 years demonstrated a negative predictive value for ciTBI of 100% (95%CI 99.7 to 100%) and sensitivity of 100% (95%CI 86.3 to 100%). The prediction rule for patients older than 2 years of age demonstrated a negative predictive value for ciTBI of 99.9% (95%CI 99.8 to 99.99%) and a sensitivity of 96.8% (95%CI 89 to 99.6%). Patients in the high risk criteria were recommended to undergo neuroimaging. Patients in the intermediate risk criteria were recommended to be considered for neuroimaging in conjunction with clinician experience and parental comfort.

Kuppermann N, Holmes JF, Dayan PS, Hoyle JD, Atabaki SM, Holubkov R, et al. Identification of children at very low risk of clinically-important brain injuries after head trauma: a prospective cohort. The Lancet. 2009 Oct;374(9696):1160–70.

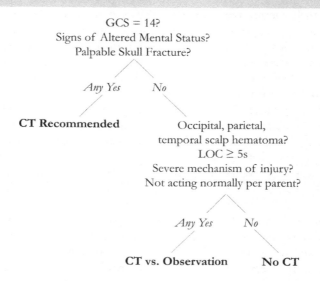

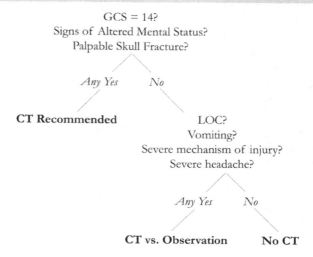

Figure I. Prediction Tool Algorithm. GCS = Glasgow Coma Scale; LOC = Loss of Consciousness.

The SOAP-II trial: First-line vasopressor for shock management

1. There was no significant difference in 28-day, 6 month, or 12 month mortality when comparing dopamine and norepinephrine as first-line vasopressors in managing shock.

2. Dopamine was associated with a significantly higher rate of arrhythmias and severe arrhythmias when compared to norepinephrine.

Original Date of Publication: March 2010

Study Rundown: The Sepsis Occurrence in Acutely Ill Patients II (SOAP-II) trial compared the use of norepinephrine and dopamine as first-line agents in treating patients suffering from circulatory shock. At the time, guidelines and recommendations suggested that either agent may be used as the first-line vasopressor. Some studies, however, had suggested that dopamine use was a predictor of mortality in shock. The SOAP-II trial demonstrated that there were no significant differences in mortality when comparing dopamine and norepinephrine as first-line vasopressors. Dopamine, however, was associated with a significantly higher rate of arrhythmias, as well as severe arrhythmias that led to withholding of the study drug. Moreover, the study demonstrated significantly increased 28-day mortality with dopamine use in a pre-specified subgroup of patients who had cardiogenic shock. These findings challenged the American College of Cardiology-American Heart Association recommendation at the time, which suggested using dopamine as the first-line agent in patients suffering from acute myocardial infarction and hypotension.

In-Depth [randomized controlled trial]: A total of 1679 patients were enrolled from 8 centers in Belgium, Austria, and Spain and randomized to receive dopamine or norepinephrine dosed by body weight. Patients were eligible if they were ≥18 years of age and required a vasopressor for treatment of shock. Shock was defined as a mean arterial pressure < 70 mmHg or systolic blood pressure < 100 mmHg, despite adequate fluid resuscitation, and clinical signs of tissue hypoperfusion (e.g., altered mental state, mottled skin, urine output < 0.5 mL/kg/hour). The primary outcome was 28-day mortality, while secondary outcomes included mortality in the intensive care unit (ICU), in hospital mortality, 6- and 12 month mortality, and days requiring ICU care or organ support. There were no significant differences between the groups in terms of 28-day mortality, mortality in the ICU, or mortality in hospital at 6 and 12 months. There were no significant differences between the groups in terms of number of days requiring ICU care or organ support. The study demonstrated a significantly higher incidence of arrhythmias in the dopamine group compared to the norepinephrine group (24.1% vs. 12.4%, p < 0.001). The dopamine group also experienced a significantly higher incidence of severe arrhythmia, which necessitated stopping the study drug (6.1% vs. 1.6%, p < 0.001). In the pre-specified subgroup of patients suffering cardiogenic shock, 28-day mortality was significantly higher in the dopamine group compared to the norepinephrine group (p = 0.03).

De Backer D, Biston P, Devriendt J, Madl C, Chochrad D, Aldecoa C, et al. Comparison of Dopamine and Norepinephrine in the Treatment of Shock. New England Journal of Medicine. 2010 Mar 4;362(9):779–89.

The CRASH-2 trial: Tranexamic acid reduces mortality in trauma patients

1. Tranexamic acid significantly reduced all-cause mortality in trauma patients with significant hemorrhage, compared to placebo.

2. There were no significant differences in the incidence of vascular occlusive events or the need for transfusion or surgery between the tranexamic acid and placebo groups.

Original Date of Publication: July 2010

Study Rundown: While prior studies demonstrated the benefit of tranexamic acid to manage surgical bleeding, no randomized trials had explored its use in managing trauma patients. The Clinical Randomisation of an Antifibrinolytic in Significant Hemorrhage (CRASH)-2 trial demonstrated that using tranexamic acid in trauma patients suffering from significant hemorrhage reduced all-cause mortality without any significant increase in the incidence of fatal or non-fatal vascular occlusive events. Subsequent analyses of the CRASH-2 trial data demonstrated that tranexamic acid should be delivered as soon as possible, as it is much less effective when given more than 3 hours following the injury. Given its effectiveness and cost-effectiveness, authors of the CRASH-2 trial successfully petitioned for tranexamic acid to be added to the World Health Organization's List of Essential Medicines.

In-Depth [randomized controlled trial]: A total of 20 211 patients were drawn from 274 hospitals in 40 countries and randomized as part of the study. Patients were eligible if they suffered, or were at risk of, significant hemorrhage (i.e., systolic blood pressure < 90 mmHg, or heart rate > 110 beats per minute, or both) within 8 hours of injury. Only patients in which the responsible physician was uncertain about whether to treat with tranexamic acid were eligible; patients with clear indications or contraindications were excluded. Patients were randomized to placebo or tranexamic acid. Those in the tranexamic acid group received a loading dose of 1 g infused intravenously over 10 minutes, followed by 1 g over 8 hours. The primary outcome was death in hospital within 4 weeks of injury, while secondary outcomes included vascular occlusive events, surgical intervention, receipt of blood transfusion, and the number of units of blood products transfused. Tranexamic acid significantly reduced all-cause mortality compared to placebo (RR 0.91; 95%CI 0.85-0.97). In particular, patients in the tranexamic group had a significantly lower risk of death secondary to bleeding (RR 0.85; 95%CI 0.76-0.96). There were no significant differences between the groups in the risk of fatal or non-fatal vascular occlusive events or need for transfusion of blood products or surgery.

CRASH-2 trial collaborators, Shakur H, Roberts I, Bautista R, Caballero J, Coats T, et al. Effects of tranexamic acid on death, vascular occlusive events, and blood transfusion in trauma patients with significant haemorrhage (CRASH-2): a randomised, placebo-controlled trial. Lancet. 2010 Jul 3;376(9734):23–32.

The ACURASYS trial: Neuromuscular blockade in early acute respiratory distress syndrome

1. In patients with severe acute respiratory distress syndrome (ARDS), treatment with neuromuscular blockade in the first 48 hours significantly reduced 90-day and 28-day mortality, compared to placebo.

2. The treatment group experienced significantly lower rates of barotrauma.

3. There were no differences between the groups in the rate of intensive care unit (ICU)-acquired paresis.

Original Date of Publication: September 2010

Study Rundown: ARDS is characterized by hypoxemic respiratory failure, bilateral chest infiltrates, and high mortality. While the ARMA trial had demonstrated that lung-protective mechanical ventilation was effective, no other measures had convincingly reduced mortality from ARDS at the time of this study. The ARDS et Curarisation Systematique (ACURASYS) trial was conducted to evaluate if early treatment of ARDS with cisatracurium besylate, a neuromuscular blocker, would significantly improve outcomes. In summary, treating patients with severe ARDS with neuromuscular blockade in the first 48 hours of onset significantly reduced 90- and 28-day mortality. Patients receiving neuromuscular blockade also experienced significantly lower rates of barotrauma, while there were no significant differences between the groups in the rate of ICU-acquired paresis. One criticism of the study is that the authors did not use train-of-four stimulation to assess the extent of neuromuscular blockade, and based their dosing solely on a previous smaller study.

In-Depth [randomized controlled trial]: A total of 340 patients from 40 ICUs across France enrolled in the trial. Patients were eligible for the trial if they were receiving invasive mechanical ventilation, had acute hypoxemic respiratory failure, and met severe ARDS criteria (i.e., $PaO_2:FiO_2$ ratio $<$ 150 with positive end-expiratory pressure $\geq$5 cm H_2O, tidal volumes between 6-8 mL/kg, bilateral pulmonary infiltrates, non-cardiogenic edema) for $\leq$48 hours. Exclusion criteria included age $<$ 18 years, treatment with neuromuscular blockade at enrollment, known pregnancy, increased intracranial pressure, severe chronic liver disease, bone-marrow transplantation or chemotherapy-induced neutropenia, and pneumothorax, amongst others. Investigators randomized patients to receive cisatracurium besylate (15 mg rapid infusion, followed by continuous infusion of 37.5 mg/hour) or a placebo infusion. The primary outcomes were in-hospital and 90-day mortality. The secondary outcomes included 28-day mortality, the rate of barotrauma, and the rate of ICU-acquired paresis.

The only baseline difference between the groups was a significantly lower $PaO_2:FiO_2$ ratio in the cisatracurium group compared to the placebo group (p = 0.03). After adjusting for baseline $PaO_2:FiO_2$, treatment with cisatracurium significantly reduced 90-day mortality compared to placebo (HR 0.68; 95%CI 0.48-0.98). Moreover, 28-day mortality was also significantly lower in the cisatracurium group (ARR -9.6%; 95%CI -19.2 to -0.2%). Patients in the cisatracurium group also had significantly lower rates of barotrauma (RR 0.43; 95%CI 0.20-0.93) and ICU-acquired paresis (p = 0.51) compared to patients receiving placebo.

Papazian L, Forel J-M, Gacouin A, Penot-Ragon C, Perrin G, Loundou A, et al. Neuromuscular Blockers in Early Acute Respiratory Distress Syndrome. New England Journal of Medicine. 2010 Sep 16;363(12):1107–16.

The LACTATE trial: Early lactate-guided therapy in intensive care patients

1. Therapy aimed at reducing lactate levels by 20% every 2 hours during the first 8 hours of intensive care unit (ICU) admission reduced in-hospital mortality and decreased ICU stays.

2. Patients in the early lactate-guided therapy group received more fluids and started on vasopressors earlier than in the control group, but did not have a faster reduction rate of lactate levels.

Original Date of Publication: September 2010

Study Rundown: Elevated blood lactate levels are a known prognostic factor for morbidity and mortality in the ICU. This multi-center, open-label, randomized controlled trial compared standard early goal-directed therapy (EGDT) to EGDT combined with early lactate-guided therapy in patients admitted to the ICU with increased lactate levels. The goal of early lactate-guided therapy was to reduce the lactate level by at least 20% every 2 hours during the first 8 hours of admission in hopes of reducing end-organ damage and improving outcomes in the ICU. The trial found that lactate-guided therapy significantly reduced in-hospital mortality, mechanical ventilation, and ICU stay. There was no difference in the time to stopping vasopressors or in the initiation of renal replacement therapy. In summary, this study demonstrated that frequent monitoring of lactate levels (every 2 hours), with the goal of reducing levels by 20% per 2 hours, during the initial 8 hours of admission to the ICU was beneficial to patients. Of note, there was no significant difference in the rate of lactate reduction between the groups, despite more aggressive fluid and vasopressor resuscitation in the lactate group. This suggested that trending lactate levels early on may be useful as an indicator of improvement, or lack thereof, in a patient undergoing aggressive resuscitation in the ICU.

In-Depth [randomized controlled trial]: This trial was conducted at 4 ICUs across the Netherlands between 2006 and 2008. Eligible patients were all ICU patients above the age of 18 with a lactate level at or above 3.0 mEq/L on admission. The study excluded patients with liver failure or post-liver surgery, recent epileptic seizures, a contraindication for a central venous catheterization, an evident aerobic cause of hyperlactatemia, or those with a do-not-resuscitate status. Patients were randomized into 2 groups: 1) the experimental group where therapy was aimed to decrease lactate levels by at least 20% every 2 hours or 2) the control group with standard therapy, where the team only had the admission lactate level. Treatment period was first 8 hours of ICU admission. Patients were followed to hospital discharge or death. The primary endpoint was in-hospital mortality, with significant reduction in-hospital mortality observed in the lactate-guided therapy group after adjustment for age, sex, and initial assessment of organ failure by APACHE and SOFA scores (HR 0.61; 95%CI 0.43-0.87). There was also a decrease in ICU stay in the lactate-guided therapy group (HR 0.65; 95%CI 0.50-0.85) compared to the standard therapy group.

Jansen TC, van Bommel J, Schoonderbeek FJ, Sleeswijk Visser SJ, van der Klooster JM, Lima AP, et al. Early Lactate-Guided Therapy in Intensive Care Unit Patients. Am J Respir Crit Care Med. 2010 Sep 15;182(6):752–61.

Fleischner Society Guidelines, 2013 Update: Frequent CT follow-up recommended for subsolid pulmonary nodules

1. In patients with incidentally-detected, solitary, pure ground-glass nodules (GGNs) > 5 mm on computed tomography (CT), initial follow-up is recommended at 3 months, followed by annual CT surveillance. Nodules ≤5 mm require no follow-up.

2. In patients with multiple incidentally-detected pure GGNs ≤5 mm, follow-up CT scans at 2 and 4 years is recommended.

3. In patients with incidentally-detected multiple pure GGNs > 5 mm without a dominant lesion, follow-up at 3 months with annual CT surveillance is recommended.

4. Solitary part-solid or multiple nodules with a dominant lesion require extended follow-up.

Original Date of Publication: January 2013

Study Rundown: The original Fleischner Society Guidelines for pulmonary nodules published in 2005 provided guidance for follow-up of solitary pulmonary nodules found incidentally on CT. However, they did not provide specific considerations for a special subset of subsolid or GGNs, nor the presence of multiple nodules. A previous study by Henschke et al. demonstrated that subsolid nodules have an increased risk of malignancy compared to pure solid nodules. The purpose of this landmark guideline from the Fleischner Society was to provide recommendations for imaging follow-up of this unique subset of nodules.

The position statement provided six recommendations for the management of subsolid pulmonary nodules found on CT, detailed in the schematic on the following page. Three are related to solitary subsolid nodules. Specifically, the statement recommends no follow-up for solitary subsolid nodules less than 5 mm in size.

For subsolid nodules greater than 5 mm or for any solitary nodules with both subsolid and solid components, more frequent CT imaging follow-up is required starting at 3 months, followed by yearly CT surveillance for three years. The remaining three recommendations are related to multiple subsolid nodules. For patients with multiple subsolid nodules which are smaller than 5 mm in size, CT follow-up is recommended only at 2 and 4 years. Patients with multiple nodules as well as a dominant lesion (>5 mm) require more frequent follow-up starting at 3 months followed by annual CT surveillance for three years. Finally, in patients with a dominant lesion which contains both subsolid and solid components, increased frequency of follow-up is recommended starting at 3 months, with recommendation for surgical biopsy or resection if the lesion persists and especially if it features a solid component > 5 mm.

In addition to the six recommendations, the position statement highlights the importance of using contiguous thin sections (i.e. 1 mm slices) with mediastinal and lung windows to determine the presence of a non-solid component of pulmonary nodules. Additionally, the position statement clarified the use of position emission tomography (PET) in this subgroup as valuable only in the assessment of nodules with both solid and non-solid components greater than 10 mm in size. The recommendations are strengthened by the grading of each specific recommendation based on the quality of the evidence. The updated Fleischner Society Guidelines provide expert opinion based on currently available evidence and has been widely adopted as the imaging follow-up recommendation plan for the management of subsolid pulmonary nodules.

Naidich DP, Bankier AA, MacMahon H, Schaefer-Prokop CM, Pistolesi M, Goo JM, et al. Recommendations for the Management of Subsolid Pulmonary Nodules Detected at CT: A Statement from the Fleischner Society. Radiology. 2013 Jan 1;266(1):304–17.

Additional Review:

Henschke CI, Yankelevitz DF, Mirtcheva R, McGuinness G, McCauley D, Miettinen OS. CT Screening for Lung Cancer. Am J Roentgenol. 2002 May 1;178(5):1053–7.

The PROSEVA trial: Proning in severe ARDS

1. In patients with severe acute respiratory distress syndrome (ARDS), prone-positioning significantly reduced 28- and 90-day mortality when compared to patients who remained in supine position only.

2. Proned patients were also successfully extubated at higher rates and required fewer days of ventilation when compared to supine patients.

Original Date of Publication: June 2013

Study Rundown: ARDS is characterized by the 4 following criteria: 1) lung injury of acute onset (i.e., within 1 week of a clinical insult), 2) bilateral opacities on chest imaging, 3) lung infiltrates not cardiogenic in nature, and 4) $PaO_2:FiO_2$ ratio < 300. ARDS can be caused by pneumonia, sepsis, blood transfusions, trauma, aspiration, pancreatitis, medications, and chemical inhalation. Previously, the ARMA trial demonstrated that lower tidal volume ventilation significantly reduced in-hospital mortality, while the ACURASYS trial revealed that neuromuscular blockade early in severe ARDS also led to reduced mortality. In the Proning Severe ARDS Patients (PROSEVA) trial, patients with severe ARDS were randomized to either prone-positioning for 16 hours or left in supine position. In summary, proning significantly reduced 28- and 90-day mortality compared to leaving patients in the supine position. Proned patients also experienced significantly higher rates of successful extubation and fewer days requiring ventilation compared to those in the supine group. Notably, all of the centers involved in this study had considerable experience with proning patients.

In-Depth [randomized controlled trial]: This trial was conducted at 27 intensive care units (ICUs) across France and Spain, all of which had at least 5 years of experience with prone positioning. Of the 3449 patients admitted with ARDS, 474 patients were randomized as part of this trial to either sessions consisting of 16 consecutive hours of prone positioning or remaining in the supine position. The inclusion criteria were ARDS (i.e., as defined using the American-European Consensus Conference criteria), endotracheal intubation and mechanical ventilation for ARDS < 36 hours, and severe ARDS (i.e., PF ratio < 150 mmHg, FiO2 > 0.60, PEEP > 5 cm H2O, tidal volume 6 mL/kg). The primary endpoint was 28-day mortality, while the secondary endpoints included 90-day mortality, rate of successful extubation, and the number of ventilator-free days.

In the majority of patients, the cause of ARDS was pneumonia. The average number of proning sessions per patient was 4±4, while the mean duration per session was 17±3 hours. All patients in the prone positioning group underwent at least 1 session. The risk of 28-day mortality was significantly lower in patients who underwent proning compared to those who remained in the supine position (aHR 0.42; 95%CI 0.26-0.66). This difference remained significant at 90 days (aHR 0.48; 95%CI 0.32-0.72). Moreover, patients in the prone group experienced significantly higher rates of successful extubation at day 90 (HR 0.45; 95%CI 0.29-0.70) and significantly higher numbers of ventilation-free days at day 28 and 90 ($p < 0.001$ at both time points). With regards to complications, patients in the supine group experienced significantly more cardiac arrests compared to the prone group ($p = 0.02$).

Guérin C, Reignier J, Richard J-C, Beuret P, Gacouin A, Boulain T, et al. Prone Positioning in Severe Acute Respiratory Distress Syndrome. New England Journal of Medicine. 2013 Jun 6;368(23):2159–68.

INPULSIS: Nintedanib for Idiopathic Pulmonary Fibrosis

1. In this report of two randomized, placebo-controlled trials, nintedanib reduced force vital capacity decline in patients with idiopathic pulmonary fibrosis versus control over 52 weeks.

2. Nintedanib was relatively safe, with its most frequent adverse event being diarrhea.

Original Date of Publication: May 2014

Study Rundown: The INPULSIS 1 and 2 trials sought to evaluate the efficacy of nintedanib, an intracellular tyrosine kinase inhibitor, in the treatment of idiopathic pulmonary fibrosis. Overall, the rate of decline of forced vital capacity (FVC), a surrogate for disease progression, was significantly reduced in those receiving nintedanib ($P < 0.001$ in both trials). The INPULSIS-2 trial additionally found a significant increase in the time to first disease exacerbation in the treatment group ($P = 0.005$), however INPULSIS-1 did not. Diarrhea was the most frequently reported adverse event in both groups, usually mild to moderate in intensity, leading to discontinuation for less than 5% of participants in both trials. The rate of serious adverse events did not differ significantly versus placebo for both trials. Although this is a well-designed trial offering convincing support for the use of nintedanib in idiopathic pulmonary fibrosis, it has several limitations. It failed to show a clear effect of nintedanib on improved time to first acute exacerbation of disease, an important endpoint given its high association with morbidity and mortality.

In-Depth [randomized, controlled trial]: The INPULSIS-1 and 2 trials randomized 1066 and 515 patients, respectively, between May 2011 and September 2012 at 205 sites internationally. All patients were 40 years or older with a diagnosis of idiopathic pulmonary fibrosis in the past 5 years. Patients were randomized to receive either 150mg of nintedanib twice daily or placebo for a total of 52 weeks, with spirometric testing for FVC performed periodically during this period. Overall, the adjusted annual decline in FVC was significantly reduced in the treatment group for both trials ($P < 0.001$ for both). Time to first acute exacerbation was similar between treatment groups for INPULSIS-1 ($P = 0.67$), however was significantly lower in the nintedanib group for INPULSIS-2 ($P = 0.005$). There was no significant difference in deaths from any cause in either trial. Over 90% of patients in both trials reported mild to moderate diarrhea when using nintedanib. Serious adverse events did not differ significantly between groups.

Richeldi L, du Bois RM, Raghu G, Azuma A, Brown KK, Costabel U, et al. Efficacy and Safety of Nintedanib in Idiopathic Pulmonary Fibrosis. New England Journal of Medicine. 2014 May 29;370(22):2071–82.

The SEPSISPAM trial: Mean arterial pressure targets in septic shock

1. This trial demonstrated that mortality did not differ with a mean arterial pressure (MAP) target of 80-85mmHg (36.6%) as compared to 65-70mmHg (34.0%) in septic shock patients.

2. Incidence of new atrial fibrillation was significantly increased in the 80-85mmHg MAP threshold group.

Original Date of Publication: April 2014

Study Rundown: The Sepsis and Mean Arterial Pressure (SEPSISPAM) trial compared a resuscitation target MAP of 80-85mmHg to a target of 65-70mmHg in septic shock patients. The primary end point measured was all-cause mortality measured at 28 days after resuscitation, which did not differ significantly between groups. Secondary outcomes of 90-day mortality and serious adverse events also did not differ between groups. Although, new onset atrial fibrillation and need for renal-replacement in chronic hypertension patients was increased in the 80-85mmHg target group. The limitations of the present study included variations in MAP during treatment as well as differential use of glucocorticoids between patients. Although, MAP fluctuation was not significant enough to warrant a protocol violation. The SEPSISPAM trial was the first to demonstrate that low versus high MAP targets in septic shock patients do not impact mortality following resuscitation.

In-Depth [randomized control trial]: The SEPISPAM trial included patients who required resuscitation for septic shock, randomizing participants into a target MAP of 80-85mmHg (n = 142) as compared to 65-70mmHg (n = 132). The primary outcome of all-cause mortality at 28 days did not differ in the high target group as compared to the low target group (HR 1.07; 95%CI 0.84-1.38), which was sustained at 90 days (HR 1.04; 95%CI 0.83-1.30). Conversely, the high threshold groups had significantly higher rates of new atrial fibrillation (p = 0.02) and need for renal-replacement therapy in participants with chronic hypertension (p = 0.04). Serious adverse events did not differ between groups (p = 0.64).

Asfar P, Meziani F, Hamel J-F, Grelon F, Megarbane B, Anguel N, et al. High versus Low Blood-Pressure Target in Patients with Septic Shock. New England Journal of Medicine. 2014 Apr 24;370(17):1583–93.

The TRISS trial: Transfusion thresholds in septic shock

1. This study found that patients with chronic heart failure and reduced ejection fraction who received vericiguat had lower rates of composite cardiovascular death and first hospitalization for heart failure (35.5%) compared to controls (38.5%).

2. Rates of symptomatic hypotension and syncope did not differ between the those on vericiguat as compared to placebo.

Original Date of Publication: May 2020

Study Rundown: The Transfusion Requirements in Septic Shock (TRISS) trial compared outcomes in septic shock patients who either received transfusions at a lower or higher hemoglobin threshold. The primary outcome measure of all-cause mortality at 90 days did not differ significantly between groups. Although, the secondary outcome of units of blood transfused during hospitalization was lower in the low hemoglobin threshold group. Other secondary outcomes did not differ between groups, including ischemic events, adverse reactions to transfusion, need for life support, as well as days alive without vasopressor or inotropic therapy, mechanical intervention, or renal-replacement therapy. Major limitations of the TRISS trial included that it was not blinded, and no adjustment was made for concomitant interventions. Although, due to the size of a trial and use of stratified randomization these limitations likely did not impact the final outcomes. The TRISS trial demonstrated in a large cohort of septic shock patients that a lower hemoglobin transfusion threshold reduced the units of blood used but did not impact 90-day mortality.

In-Depth [randomized control trial]: The TRISS trial group randomized septic shock patients into either a low hemoglobin transfusion threshold group of ≤ 7g per deciliter (n = 503) or a high hemoglobin threshold group of ≤ 9g per deciliter (n = 497). The primary outcome of 90-day all cause mortality did not differ significantly (p = 0.44) between the higher and lower threshold groups (RR 0.94; 95%CI 0.78-1.09). The majority of the secondary outcomes did not differ between groups, including use of life support (p = 0.14), ischemic events in the intensive care unit (p = 0.64), serious adverse reactions (p = 1.00), as well as days alive without vasopressor or inotropic therapy (p = 0.93), without mechanical ventilation (p = 0.49), and without renal-replacement therapy (0.54). Conversely, a significantly lower amount of blood transfusions were performed in the lower threshold group as compared to the higher threshold group (p< 0.001).

Holst LB, Haase N, Wetterslev J, Wernerman J, Guttormsen AB, Karlsson S, et al. Lower versus Higher Hemoglobin Threshold for Transfusion in Septic Shock. New England Journal of Medicine. 2014 Oct 9;371(15):1381–91.

RE-VERSE AD trial: Idarucizumab for the Reversal of Anticoagulation by Dabigatran

1. This study determined that idarucizumab is effective in reversing anticoagulation by the direct thrombin inhibitor Dabigatran.

2. Idarucizumab had an onset of action within minutes, supporting its use in emergency situations.

Original Date of Publication: June 2015

Study Rundown: The Reversal Effects of Idarucizumab on Active Dabigatran (RE-VERSE AD) trial demonstrated that Idarucizumab could be used to rapidly reverse anticoagulation from dabigatran in patients with acute bleeding events or who required emergent surgery or other invasive intervention. Because of its inclusion of acutely ill patients, this study is more applicable to real clinical scenarios wherein rapid reversal of anticoagulation is required. However, this study is significantly limited by its small sample size, lack of a control group, and its use of laboratory tests as primary outcomes as opposed to more clinically relevant patient outcomes. This study was among the first to demonstrate the efficacy of idarucizumab, and subsequent larger-scale studies have since confirmed its efficacy. Idarucizumab is currently FDA-approved for the urgent reversal of the anticoagulant effects of dabigatran.

In-Depth [randomized controlled trial]: The RE-VERSE AD study aimed to determine if idarucizumab, a monoclonal antibody that binds and neutralizes thrombin-bound dabigatran, was effective in reversing dabigatran's anticoagulant effects. This interim analysis included patients from 35 countries taking dabigatran who either required rapid reversal of anticoagulation for life-threatening bleeding, or who required it for urgent surgery or invasive procedures (n = 90). All patients were administered 5g of intravenous idarucizumab total, given as two 2.5mg bolus infusions, and blood samples were collected at various time points from baseline to 24 hours after the second bolus. The primary end point of this study was the maximum percent reversal of anticoagulation by dabigatran, as measured by dilute thrombin time and ecarin clotting time. Patients with normal values prior to their first idarucizumab dose were excluded from subsequent analysis. Secondary outcomes included the proportion of patients with complete normalization of these values, reduction in unbound dabigatran serum concentration, and clinical outcomes. Overall, the median maximum percentage reversal of anticoagulation was 100% in both groups, and reversal was evident within minutes (95%CI 100-100). The vast majority of patients had normal dilute thrombin time and ecarin clotting times after administration (between 88-98%), and at 4-hours after treatment, nearly all had unbound dabigatran concentrations near the lower limit of quantification (96%). A total of 21 patients had serious adverse clinical events, including 18 deaths.

Pollack CV, Reilly PA, Eikelboom J, Glund S, Verhamme P, Bernstein RA, et al. Idarucizumab for Dabigatran Reversal. New England Journal of Medicine. 2015 Aug 6;373(6):511–20.

ANNEXA-A and ANNEXA-R Trials: Andaxanet Alfa for Reversal of Apixaban and Rivaroxaban

1. This study determined that andaxanet alfa is effective in reversing anticoagulation by the direct factor Xa inhibitors apixaban and rivaroxaban.

2. No significant thrombotic or bleeding events were associated with andaxanet alfa use.

Original Date of Publication: December 2015

Study Rundown: The ANNEXA-A and ANNEXA-R trials demonstrated the efficacy of andaxanet alfa as a reversal agent for the direct factor Xa inhibitors apixaban and rivaroxaban. Andaxanet was rapid in onset and offset of action, making it ideal for use when urgent reversal of anticoagulation is required. Furthermore, there were no adverse thrombotic or bleeding events in patients receiving andaxanet, thereby supporting its safety profile. This study is strengthened by its inclusion of older participants, who are often excluded from such trials, and as a result more closely approximates clinical practice. Analysis of various biomarkers and measurements of anticoagulation was also very thorough. This study is limited by its small sample size and by its population of only healthy volunteers without significant comorbidities or urgent indications for reversal of anticoagulation. Further study regarding the efficacy and safety of andaxanet is needed in these excluded populations. In summary, the ANNEXA-A and ANNEXA-R trials were among the earliest to demonstrate the efficacy and safety of andaxanet in reversing anticoagulation, and further study could solidify its use as a universal antidote for direct factor Xa inhibitors.

In-Depth [randomized control trial]: The ANNEXA-A and ANNEXA-R trials sought to evaluate the efficacy and safety of andaxanet alfa, a recombinant human factor Xa protein, in reversing anticoagulation by the direct factor Xa inhibitors apixaban and rivaroxaban. All participants in both trials were healthy volunteers aged 50-75 and were administered direct factor Xa inhibitors until steady state plasma levels were achieved. The ANNEXA-A trial and ANNEXA-R trials randomized participants to receive either andexanet or placebo for reversal of apixaban (n = 62), and reversal of rivaroxaban (n = 80) respectively. The primary endpoint for both trials was the percent change in anti-factor Xa activity, measured via chromogenic assay of enzyme activity. Secondary end points included the proportion of participants with > 80% reduction in anti-factor Xa activity, changes in biomarkers such as thrombin, and clinical outcomes such as thrombosis and bleeding. Overall, administration of andexanet was associated with a significant reduction in anti-factor Xa activity compared with placebo for both the apixaban (mean [±SD] reduction, 94±2% vs. 21±9%; $p < 0.001$) and the rivaroxaban (92±11% vs. 18±15%, $p < 0.001$) groups. All participants receiving the full dose of andexanet had > 80% reversal of anti-factor Xa activity, whereas none receiving placebo did ($p < 0.001$). Thrombin generation also increased more rapidly in the andexanet group. The duration of anticoagulation reversal was relatively short, with biomarkers returning to placebo levels within 1-3 hours after cessation of andexanet. There were no significant thrombotic or bleeding events.

Siegal DM, Curnutte JT, Connolly SJ, Lu G, Conley PB, Weins BL, et al. Andexanet Alfa for the Reversal of Factor Xa Inhibitor Activity. New England Journal of Medicine. 2015 Dec 17;373(25):2413-24.

SALT-ED: Normal Saline versus Balanced Crystalloids in Noncriticaly Ill Adults

1. This trial found no difference in a composite measurement of in-hospital death and length of stay between normal saline and balanced crystalloids in noncritically ill adults.

2. Major adverse renal events were lower in incidence at 30 days in the balanced crystalloids group.

Original Date of Publication: March 2018

Study Rundown: The SALT-ED study was a landmark trial demonstrating no difference in hospital-free days at day 28 (a composite measurement of in-hospital death and length of stay) in noncritically ill adults when receiving normal saline versus balanced crystalloids (Ringer's Lactate or Plasma-Lyte A). Eligible adults had received at least 500mL of fluid in the emergency department before being admitted to hospital outside of the intensive care unit (ICU). The median hospital-free days was 25 and did not differ significantly between the two groups. Of note was the significant difference in major renal adverse events at 30 days between balanced crystalloid (4.7%) versus normal saline (5.6%), with a corresponding number needed to treat of 111. As balanced crystalloids are largely similar to normal saline in availability and cost, the authors present this paper as support for the use of the former in general fluid resuscitation. A major strength of this study was high adherence to the assigned fluid group; likewise, from a pragmatic standpoint, the unblinded trial design facilitated the use of the assigned fluid group immediately in acute situations. Limitations of the study included its single center design, limiting its generalizability. Likewise, its pragmatic design prevented the collection of detailed patient data to further stratify participants by characteristics. Finally, a major shortcoming was that fluid administration was recorded only in the emergency department before admission into hospital, despite outcome measurements lasting 4 weeks.

In-Depth [Multiple-crossover trial]: The SALT-ED trial was conducted between January 2016 and April 2017 in a high-volume, tertiary-care, academic, hospital-based emergency department in the United States. Eligible patients were adults in the emergency department having received at least 500mL of intravenous fluid and subsequently admitted to hospital outside of the ICU.

Given that this was a crossover trial, the fluid used was swapped each month for all patients over the study period. Overall, 13 347 patients were eligible for inclusion over this 16 month period. No significant difference was found in hospital-free days between the two groups, with a median of 25 days (p = 0.41). Importantly, patients in the balanced crystalloid group did have a lower incidence of major renal adverse events at 30 days (4.7% *vs.* 5.6%; p = 0.01). These events included new renal-replacement therapy, significantly elevated serum creatinine, or stage 2 or higher acute kidney injury.

Self WH, Semler MW, Wanderer JP, Wang L, Byrne DW, Collins SP, et al. Balanced Crystalloids versus Saline in Noncritically Ill Adults. New England Journal of Medicine. 2018 Mar 1;378(9):819–28.

TRAPS: Rivaroxaban vs. Warfarin for Secondary Prevention in Antiphospholipid Syndrome

1. This study was halted prematurely due to an excess of thromboembolic and bleeding events in patients treated with rivaroxaban compared to warfarin.

2. There were no deaths from thromboembolic or bleeding events in either group.

Original Date of Publication: September 2018

Study Rundown: The Trial on rivaroxaban in AntiPhospholipid Syndrome (TRAPS) was halted early as data showed that secondary prevention with rivaroxaban in high-risk triple-positive patients with antiphospholipid (aPL) syndrome was associated with an excess of thromboembolic and bleeding events compared to warfarin. Thus, this trial showed that treatment with rivaroxaban in these patients was inferior to treatment with warfarin. Strengths of this study include the completeness of its dataset, with no patients lost to follow-up, and its characterization of thromboembolic and bleeding outcomes. However, this study is limited by its relatively small sample size, the fact that it was not blinded, and of course, its early termination. Furthermore, as this study was restricted to a very specific subset of high-risk patients with aPL syndrome, future research is needed to determine if these results are generalizable to all patients with aPL syndrome. Ultimately, warfarin remains the standard of treatment in high-risk patients with aPL syndrome, as rivaroxaban is associated with increased adverse clinical outcomes.

In-Depth [randomized controlled trial]: The Trial on Rivaroxaban in AntiPhospholipid Syndrome (TRAPS) sought to test whether rivaroxaban is non-inferior to warfarin for prevention of thromboembolic events in high-risk patients with aPL syndrome. The study included participants aged 18-75 who were triple positive for all 3 aPL tests (lupus anticoagulant, anti- cardiolipin antibodies, and anti– b2-glycoprotein I antibodies) and had a history of a previously documented thrombotic event (n = 120). Participants were randomized to receive rivaroxaban (n = 59) or warfarin (n = 61) and were followed for incidence of thromboembolic events, major bleeding, and vascular death. The trial was stopped prior to completion for an excess of events in the patients treated with rivaroxaban compared to warfarin (11 vs. 2, respectively, HR 6.7; 95%CI 1.5-30.5; p = .01). Events included ischemic stroke, myocardial infarction, and major bleeding. There were no venous thromboembolism events nor any deaths in the 'as treated' population for either the rivaroxaban nor the warfarin group.

Pengo V, Denas G, Zoppellaro G, Jose SP, Hoxha A, Ruffatti A, et al. Rivaroxaban vs warfarin in high-risk patients with antiphospholipid syndrome. Blood. 2018 Sep 27;132(13):1365–71.

IV. Gastroenterology

"Science is a field which grows continuously with ever expanding frontiers. Further, it is truly international in scope…Science is a collaborative effort. The combined results of several people working together is often much more effective than could be that of an individual scientist working alone."

- John Bardeen, PhD

The Child-Pugh score: Prognosis in chronic liver disease and cirrhosis

1. The Child-Pugh score was developed in 1973 to predict surgical outcomes in patients presenting with bleeding esophageal varices.

2. Presently, the score is used with the Model for End-Stage Liver Disease (MELD) to determine priority for liver transplantation.

Original Date of Publication: August 1973

Study Rundown: Originally developed in 1973, the Child-Pugh score estimated the risk of operative mortality in patients with bleeding esophageal varices. It has since been modified, refined, and become a widely used tool to assess prognosis in patients with chronic liver disease and cirrhosis. The score considers 5 factors, 3 of which assess the synthetic function of the liver (i.e., total bilirubin level, serum albumin, and international normalized ratio, or INR) and 2 of which are based on clinical assessment (i.e., degree of ascites and degree of hepatic encephalopathy). Critics of the Child-Pugh score have noted its reliance on clinical assessment, which may result in inconsistency in scoring. Others have suggested that its broad classifications of disease are impractical when determining priority for liver transplantation; nevertheless, it remains widely used. The MELD is a newer scoring system that has been developed to address some of the concerns with the Child-Pugh score, and both systems are often used in conjunction to determine liver transplantation priority.

In-Depth [case series study]: Thirty-eight consecutive cases of bleeding esophageal varices requiring surgery were included in the study. The severity of liver disease was assessed in each patient based on five clinical features: 1) total bilirubin level, 2) serum albumin, 3) prothrombin time (now measured as the INR), 4) the degree of ascites, and 5) the grade of hepatic encephalopathy. The total point score was used to determine the patient's Child-Pugh class (Figure). Class A patients (n = 7) experienced a 29% operative mortality rate, while Class B (n = 13) and Class C (n = 18) patients had operative mortality rates of 38% and 88%, respectively. Since its publication, the Child-Pugh score has undergone modifications and is currently used to assess the severity and prognosis of chronic liver disease and cirrhosis. It is often used together with the MELD to determine the priority for liver transplantation. The current Child-Pugh scoring system is outlined below.

Pugh RNH, Murray-Lyon IM, Dawson JL, Pietroni MC, Williams R. Transection of the oesophagus for bleeding oesophageal varices. Br J Surg. 1973 Aug 1;60(8):646–9.

Child-Pugh Score			
Factor	1 point	2 points	3 points
Total bilirubin (μmol/L)	< 34	34-50	> 50
Serum albumin (g/L)	> 35	28-35	< 28
PT INR	< 1.7	1.71-2.30	> 2.30
Ascites	None	Mild	Moderate to Severe
Hepatic encephalopathy	None	Grade I-II (or suppressed with medication)	Grade III-IV (or refractory)
	Class A	Class B	Class C
Total points	5-6	7-9	10-15
1-year survival	100%	80%	45%

Table I. Child-Pugh score.

The Harvey-Bradshaw Index is a practical alternative to the Crohn's Disease Activity Index in measuring disease severity

1. The Crohn's Disease Activity Index (CDAI) is accurate in quantifying disease severity in patients with Crohn's disease, but is cumbersome in practice.

2. The Harvey-Bradshaw Index (HBI) is a practical alternative that is simpler and has been statistically validated.

Original Date of Publication: March 1980

Study Rundown: Crohn's disease in a disorder of unidentified etiology characterized by inflammation of the gastrointestinal tract. The course tends to follow a chronic pattern of remissions and exacerbations with significant variability of organ distribution, yielding a broad spectrum of clinical presentations. The CDAI was developed as a research tool in an attempt to quantify the degree of illness. It gives a score based on a diary of symptoms kept by the patient for 7 days, taking into account other measurements such as the patient's weight and hematocrit. While the CDAI has been shown to be accurate in assessing disease severity and avoiding a single 'good or bad day' bias, it is criticized as too burdensome for routine practice.

The HBI was devised as a simpler version of the CDAI. It consists of only clinical parameters, does not require biochemical tests, and is far simpler to use than the CDAI. Best, a contributor to the CDAI, drew statistically significant correlations between the HBI and CDAI using prediction limits. Vermeire et al. further validated these correlations using statistical analysis of 2 large multicenter prospective cohort studies (PEGylated antibody fragment evaluation in Crohn's disease: safety and efficacy – PRECiSE 1 and 2). Both indicated that the HBI is a good – though imperfect – substitute for the CDAI in evaluating disease severity. These results support the use of the HBI for routine practice, reserving the CDAI for clinical trials requiring high accuracy.

In-Depth [prospective cohort]: The CDAI is based on 8 parameters, each adjusted using a weighting factor (indicated in parentheses), as follows: number of liquid or soft stools each day for seven days (x2), abdominal pain each day for seven days (x5), general well-being each day for seven days (x7), presence of complications (x20), taking Lomotil or opiates to control diarrhea (x30), presence of an abdominal mass (x10), hematocrit of under 0.47 in men and 0.42 in women (x6), and percentage deviation from standard weight (x1). Points are added for clinical findings of arthritis, uveitis, fistulae or abscesses, fevers, and other complications. Remission of disease is defined as a score below 150 and severe disease is defined as a value greater than 450. The HBI uses only 5 items: general well-being, abdominal pain, number of liquid stools per day, abdominal mass, and complications. The first three of these are scored from the previous day to reduce bias.

112 patients attending a gastroenterology clinic were assessed with both the CDAI and the HBI on the same visit. The results were then plotted and regression analysis was run to assess the correlation between the two methods of data collection. The results indicated a positive correlation of 0.93 ($p < 0.001$). The results of PRECiSE 1 and 2 indicated a pooled correlation of 0.800 (0.780 – 0.819 confidence interval). This is in close agreement with Best's finding of a 27-point change in the CDAI for every point change in the HBI.

Harvey RF, Bradshaw JM. A Simple Index of Crohn's-Disease Activity. The Lancet. 1980 Mar 8;315(8167):514.

Additional Review:

Vermeire S, Schreiber S, Sandborn WJ, Dubois C, Rutgeerts P. Correlation between the Crohn's disease activity and Harvey–Bradshaw indices in assessing Crohn's disease severity. Clinical Gastroenterology and Hepatology. 2010 Apr 30;8(4):357-63.

Best WR. Predicting the Crohn's disease activity index from the Harvey-Bradshaw index. Inflammatory bowel diseases. 2006 Apr 1;12(4):304-10.

Harvey-Bradshaw Index	
Symptom	Severity score
General well-being	0 = very well 1 = slightly below par 2 = poor 3 = very poor 4 = terrible
Abdominal pain	0 = none 1 = mild 2 = moderate 3 = severe
Number of liquid stools daily	1 per occurrence
Abdominal mass	0 = none 1 = dubious 2 = definite 3 = definite and tender
Complications	1 per item: – Arthralgia – Uveitis – Erythema nodosum – Aphthous ulcer – Pyoderma gangrenosum – Anal fissure – New fistula – Abscess

Table I. Harvey-Bradshaw Index. The index is based on five variables that are added to give a total score. Evaluation is done over a single day. General well-being, abdominal pain, and number of liquid stools daily are in based on the previous day.

Crohn's Disease Activity Index		
Variable	Scale	Weight
Liquid or very soft stool	Daily stool count summed for 7 days	2

Abdominal pain	Sum of 7 days of daily ratings as:
	    0=none
	    1=mild
	    2=moderate
	    3=severe
		5

General well-being	Sum of 7 days of daily ratings as:
	    0=generally well
	    1=slightly below par
	    2=poor
	    3=very poor
	    4=terrible
		7

Features of extraintestinal disease	Presence of any of the following in the previous 7 days:
	  – Arthritis or arthralgia
	  – Skin or mouth lesions
	  – Iritis or uveitis
	  – Anal fissures, fistulas, perianal abscess
	  – Other external fistulas
	  – Fever > 100°F
		20 each

Opiates for diarrhea	0=no 1=yes	30
Abdominal mass	0=none 2=questionable 5=definite	10
Hematocrit	Men 47% hematocrit Women 42% hematocrit	6
Body weight	100 x [1-(body weight/standard weight)]	1

Table II. Crohn's Disease Activity Index. Compared to the HBI, three additional variables are evaluated (opiate use, hematocrit, and body weight). Each variable is given a relative weight. the index also is tracked over a week-long period.

CT evaluation in pancreatitis strongly correlates with patient outcomes

1. Among patients with acute pancreatitis, the presence and degree of pancreatic necrosis correlated with average hospital length of stay, complications, and mortality.

2. By combining existing an existing acute pancreatitis grading system with computed tomography (CT) evaluation of pancreatic necrosis, the authors generated a CT Severity Index that strongly correlated with patient outcomes.

Original Date of Publication: February 1990

Study Rundown: Acute pancreatitis is a common condition involving inflammation of the pancreas. Though most patients have a benign course without associated complications, some develop severe disease associated with high rates of morbidity and mortality. Numerous attempts have been made to estimate patient prognosis in acute pancreatitis, including attempts to correlate imaging findings with patient outcomes using CT. Due to limitations in early CT technology, however, pancreatitis grading scales suffered from poor sensitivity and specificity and were not widely used. In this trial, the study authors attempted to build on these prior works by using contrast-enhanced CT to evaluate the presence and degree of pancreatic necrosis as a prognostic indicator in acute pancreatitis. Using a prospective patient cohort at a single institution, the study authors demonstrated a strong, positive relationship between pancreatic necrosis and patient outcomes. Compared to those with a normal-appearing pancreas by CT, patients with necrosis had significantly longer hospital lengths of stay and higher rates of complications. All deaths in the study cohort were in patients with pancreatic necrosis. Combining this information with previously-described rating scales, the authors were then able to generate the CT Severity Index (CTIS), a numeric scale to predict the risk of complications and death. Applying this scale to the study cohort, morbidity and mortality strongly correlated with CTIS score. Primary limitations of this study included modest sample size and the associated low mortality rate. Subsequent work in pancreatitis imaging has expanded upon this landmark trial, the results of which remain in modern clinical practice as the modified CTIS.

In-Depth [prospective cohort]: Eighty-eight patients (mean age, 52 years) with signs and symptoms of acute pancreatitis were enrolled. All patients were initially managed with standard medical therapy, including nasogastric suction, analgesia, and intravenous fluids. Surgical intervention was pursued in patients with sepsis refractory to medical management. All patients underwent CT imaging of the abdomen with intravenous and oral contrast for evaluation of pancreatic necrosis at the time of admission, and a subset of patients received additional, subsequent CT imaging (mean number of CTs/patients, 2.9). Scans were interpreted blindly and assessed for two specific features: the patient's five-point pancreatitis grade, based on previously published data; and the qualitative degree of decreased pancreatic parenchymal enhancement. This latter variable was taken to represent the presence of pancreatic necrosis, and was reported as one of four possible severities. Additional collected data included Ranson's score, hospital length of stay, morbidity—defined as pancreatic abscess or pseudocyst formation—and mortality.

At the end of the trial, 66 (75.0%) patients had uncomplicated courses and recovered with medical therapy alone, while 22 (25.0%) patients required surgical intervention. Five (5.7%) patients died. In total, pancreatic necrosis was detected in 18 (20.5%) patients. Average length of stay was 109 days among patients with > 50% necrosis, as compared to 25 days among those without evidence of necrosis at presentation. The average Ranson's score (a marker of severity, maximum score 11) was 1.9 among those without necrosis and 5.5 among those with > 50% necrosis. Patients with CT evidence of necrosis had morbidity and mortality rates of 82% and 23%, respectively, as compared with respective rates of 6% and 0% among those without necrosis. The positive predictive value for abscess formation of 77% among patients with necrosis, and the negative predictive value of abscess formation among those without necrosis was 97%. By combining pancreatitis grade and CT extent of pancreatic necrosis, a CT Severity Index was created with a maximum score of 10 (highest severity). Among study patients with a CTSI 0-3, there was 3% mortality and 8% morbidity; among patients with CTSI 7-10, mortality and morbidity were 17% and 92%, respectively.

Balthazar EJ, Robinson DL, Megibow AJ, Ranson JH. Acute pancreatitis: value of CT in establishing prognosis. Radiology. 1990 Feb 1;174(2):331–6.

Endoscopic biliary drainage in acute cholangitis

1. For patients with severe acute cholangitis due to choledocholithiasis, endoscopic biliary drainage reduced hospital mortality compared to surgical decompression.

2. Endoscopic biliary drainage was associated with fewer post-treatment complications, although the decrease was not statistically significant for all types of complications.

Original Date of Publication: June 1992

Study Rundown: At the time of this study, surgical decompression was the conventional treatment for severe acute cholangitis arising from choledocholithiasis. Surgery, however, was associated with significant morbidity and mortality. Several uncontrolled studies had shown that endoscopic biliary drainage was a safe therapeutic alternative for acute cholangitis that reduced the mortality rate. This study was the first randomized, controlled trial that sought to determine the benefits of endoscopic biliary drainage compared to surgical decompression for patients with severe acute cholangitis. Results demonstrated that endoscopic biliary drainage was associated with significantly lowered hospital mortality rates compared to surgical decompression. Endoscopic intervention also significantly reduced the rates of certain complications, including the rates of ventilator support and residual stones after procedure.

A potential study limitation was that patients randomized to receive surgical decompression experienced longer wait times before undergoing treatment compared to patients randomized to receive endoscopic biliary drainage. The treatment delay for the surgery group, on the order of a couple hours, was due in part to the limited number of immediately available operating rooms. This delay could have resulted in worsened cholangitis in the surgery group specifically, and may have potentially biased the study's results in favor of endoscopic biliary drainage. However, these delays reflect the challenges in arranging emergent surgery that occur in practice. In summary, the findings of this study support the use of endoscopic biliary drainage as a safe and effective treatment for severe acute cholangitis due to choledocholithiasis.

In-Depth [randomized controlled trial]: This trial enrolled 82 patients from the Queen Mary Hospital in Hong Kong. Eligible patients included those diagnosed with acute cholangitis due to choledocholithiasis based on the presence of septic shock or progressive biliary sepsis manifesting as mental confusion or antibiotic-refractory fever. All patients underwent emergency diagnostic endoscopic retrograde cholangiopancreatography (ERCP) prior to randomization for endoscopic biliary drainage or surgical decompression. A total of 41 patients were randomized to each treatment group. All patients received definitive therapy following biliary drainage. Mortality was defined as death within 48 hours after biliary drainage, in the absence of other contributory causes. Morbidity included any complications that arose after treatment. Cholangitis was considered to have resolved once body temperature and blood pressure were normalized for at least 8 hours.

The mortality rate was significantly lower for patients undergoing endoscopic biliary drainage compared to patients undergoing surgical decompression (10% versus 32%; $p < 0.03$). The rate of complications was not significantly different between the groups (34% versus 66%; $p > 0.05$). Only the rates of residual calculi and ventilator support were significantly lower for patients receiving endoscopic drainage compared to surgery. The time needed to normalize body temperature and blood pressure was not different between patients receiving endoscopic biliary drainage and surgical decompression.

Lai ECS, Mok FPT, Tan ESY, Lo C, Fan S, You K, et al. Endoscopic Biliary Drainage for Severe Acute Cholangitis. The New England Journal of Medicine. 1992 Jun 11;326(24):1582–6.

Prednisolone vs. placebo in severe alcoholic hepatitis

1. Compared to placebo, patients with severe alcoholic hepatitis treated with 28 days of prednisolone had significantly improved short-term survival.

2. There remains significant controversy surrounding the use of glucocorticoids in managing severe alcoholic hepatitis, as numerous other trials have demonstrated no mortality benefit, but significantly higher infection risk with glucocorticoid therapy.

Original Date of Publication: February 1992

Study Rundown: Alcoholic hepatitis is a form of acute liver disease that may develop in individuals with prolonged, heavy alcohol intake. In patients with alcoholic hepatitis, conventional management consists of abstinence from alcohol, correction of dietary deficiencies, and supportive care. Maddrey discriminant function is a prognostic tool that is used to assess the severity of alcoholic hepatitis. Patients with scores ≥32 are termed severe alcoholic hepatitis and experience significantly higher rates of morbidity and mortality than those with less severe disease. Prior to this study, several randomized trials had explored using glucocorticoids in managing alcoholic hepatitis, though results were conflicting. Meta-analyses of these trials suggested that there may be a benefit of using glucocorticoids in patients with severe disease. Thus, the purpose of this trial was to determine whether treating patients with severe alcoholic hepatitis with glucocorticoids would significantly reduce mortality as compared with placebo. Researchers found that corticosteroid therapy was associated with significantly reduced mortality in patients with severe alcoholic hepatitis, as characterized by Maddrey discriminant function ≥32 or hepatic encephalopathy. Subsequent studies of glucocorticoids have continued to produce conflicting results, and there remains controversy surrounding their use in managing alcoholic hepatitis, as other studies have demonstrated significantly higher rates of infection with prednisolone therapy. While pentoxifylline has also been studied in severe alcoholic hepatitis, the results describing their effects have also been conflicting.

In-Depth [randomized controlled trial]: A total of 65 participants were selected from 2 hospitals in France and randomized to treatment with prednisolone 40 mg daily or placebo for 28 days. Patients unable to take oral medications received intravenous infusions of prednisolone or placebo. Patients were eligible for the trial if they had biopsy-proven alcoholic hepatitis and severe alcoholic hepatitis (i.e., spontaneous hepatic encephalopathy or Maddrey discriminant score ≥32). Exclusion criteria included gastrointestinal bleeding or bacterial infection that could not effectively be treated within the first 48 hours. The primary endpoint was mortality within 2 months.

The 2 groups did not differ with regards to sex, age, duration of hospitalization before entry into the study, the presence of ascities, spontaneous hepatic encephalopathy, or esophageal varices. Survival in the prednisolone group was 88±5% and 88±5% at 1 and 2 months, respectively, compared to 62±9% and 45±8% in the placebo group for the same timepoints. Survival was significantly better in patients treated with corticosteroid than those taking placebo, regardless of the presence or absence of encephalopathy (adjusted log-rank test 9.9; $p = 0.0017$). The cumulative 6 month survival rates were 84±6% in the prednisolone group and 45±9% in the placebo group (low-rank test 9.5; $p = 0.002$).

Ramond MJ, Poynard T, Rueff B, Mathurin P, Théodore C, Chaput JC, et al. A randomized trial of prednisolone in patients with severe alcoholic hepatitis. The New England Journal of Medicine. 1992;326(8):507-512.

Transjugular intrahepatic portosystemic shunt effective in preventing recurrent variceal hemorrhage

1. In patients with recurrent variceal bleeding secondary to portal hypertension, the use of transjugular intrahepatic portosystemic shunt (TIPS) demonstrated high efficacy in preventing variceal re-bleeds.

2. The major complications associated with TIPS are stent occlusion and stenosis as well as an increased incidence of hepatic encephalopathy.

Original Date of Publication: January 1994

Study Rundown: In patients with advanced liver disease and cirrhosis, variceal bleeding resulting from increased portal pressure is a potentially-life threatening complication. Each variceal bleeding episode is associated with a 30% mortality rate and a 70% risk of recurrent bleeding within 1 year. In patients refractory to medical and endoscopic management, surgical portacaval shunts were historically the mainstay of therapy in selected patients. The advent of TIPS, which involves creating a low-resistance channel between the hepatic and portal vein via percutaneous vascular access, provided a less invasive alternative to reducing portal hypertension. The purpose of this landmark prospective trial was to report the safety and efficacy of TIPS in the treatment of recurrent variceal bleeds secondary to liver cirrhosis.

The prospective trial reported the outcomes of 100 patients with cirrhosis and recurrent variceal bleeding. The majority of patients had failed previous endoscopic sclerotherapy. Outcomes of interest included frequency of technical success, evidence of decreased portal pressure via duplex sonography, variceal re-bleeding rates post-procedure, and rates of complication. At the conclusion of the trial, TIPS was successfully performed in nearly all patients in the cohort resulting in a significant reduction of portal venous pressure gradient. Subsequently, over 90% of patients were free of variceal bleeds at 6 month follow-up. The major complications included stent restenosis and occlusion, which occurred in 30% of patients. All patients experiencing complications were successfully managed with re-stent or dilatation. TIPS was associated with an increase in hepatic encephalopathy, although this was comparable to the rates observed in surgical shunts. This trial is limited by the observational nature of the trial and the lack of comparison groups to endoscopic sclerotherapy or surgical shunts. However, this was the first large trial to describe the successful use of TIPS. Future randomized trials have confirmed the conclusions of this trial and have established TIPS as a viable treatment method for patients with recurrent variceal bleeds

In-Depth [prospective cohort]: This was a prospective study of 112 consecutive patients that underwent TIPS for recurrent variceal bleeding secondary to liver cirrhosis. Twelve patients were excluded due to the presence of either portal vein thrombosis, severe hepatic encephalopathy, stenosis of celiac trunk, or another primary liver malignancy. Overall, 90 patients in the cohort had TIPS inserted electively while 10 patients were treated emergently for acute variceal bleeds. The majority (92%) of patients had previous unsuccessful endoscopic sclerotherapy treatment. After insertion of TIPS, patients were followed at 1 month and then at 3 month intervals for sonographic assessment of stent patency and clinical assessment of hepatic encephalopathy. At the conclusion of the trial, TIPS were successfully inserted in 93 of 100 patients in the cohort. The mean duration of each procedure was 1.2 hours (range 30 minutes to 3 hours). There was significant reduction of portal pressure gradient associated with a significant elevation of portal blood flow post-TIPS. Major complications occurred in 15 patients and consisted of intraperitoneal and biliary hemorrhage as well as hematoma of the liver capsule. Two patients had migration of the stent to the pulmonary arteries.

At clinical follow-up, the proportion of patients that remained free of variceal bleeding at 6 months and 1 year post-TIPS was 92% and 85%, respectively. The 1-year survival in this cohort was 85%. The incidence of hepatic encephalopathy increased from 10% to 25% post-treatment. Older patients and larger diameter of shunt used were significantly associated with development of hepatic encephalopathy. Additionally, 31 patients developed stent occlusion or stenosis. Of these, 10 patients developed recurrent variceal bleeding at 1-year follow-up. Smaller stent diameter was a significant risk factor for stent occlusion/stenosis. All patients experiencing stent occlusion/stenosis were successfully treated with re-stent, thrombolysis, or stent dilation.

Rossle M, Haag K, Ochs A, Sellinger M, Noldge G, Perarnau J-M, et al. The Transjugular Intrahepatic Portosystemic Stent-Shunt Procedure for Variceal Bleeding. New England Journal of Medicine. 1994 Jan 20;330(3):165–71.

Omeprazole vs placebo for bleeding peptic ulcer

1. Patients presenting with upper gastrointestinal bleeds experienced a significantly lower risk of continued bleeding and need for surgery when treated with omeprazole compared to placebo.

2. There was no significant difference in mortality between the groups, though the omeprazole group had significantly lower red cell transfusion requirements.

Original Date of Publication: April 1997

Study Rundown: Upper gastrointestinal bleeding is a common cause of hospitalization. While endoscopy has long been an important component of managing upper gastrointestinal bleeds, there were no well-studied medical therapies at the time this trial was conducted. It had been shown that platelet function is poorer in low pH, thus, it was thought that reducing gastric acidity would help control bleeding. Prior studies with H2-receptor antagonists demonstrated mixed results, as intravenous famotidine was not shown to be effective. The purpose of this trial was to explore whether treatment with a proton pump inhibitor would improve mortality and need for surgery in patients presenting with upper gastrointestinal bleeds. In summary, patients treated with omeprazole had significantly lower rates of continued bleeding and surgery for ongoing bleeding compared to those being treated with placebo. There was no significant difference between the groups in bleeding-related mortality 30 days after admission.

In-Depth [randomized controlled trial]: This trial was conducted at a single tertiary care center in India. A total of 220 patients were randomized to either treatment with oral omeprazole 40 mg every 12 hours for 5 days or matching placebo. After appropriate resuscitation, all patients underwent upper endoscopy within 12 hours after admission. Patients with duodenal, gastric or stomal ulcers and stigmata of recent hemorrhage (i.e., arterial spurting, visible vessel, oozing from ulcer, adherent clot to ulcer) were considered eligible for the trial. Exclusion criteria were severe terminal illness that made endoscopy dangerous or undesirable, profuse hemorrhage with persistent shock necessitating emergent surgical intervention, or bleeding from a Mallory-Weiss tear/varices/erosion/tumors/unknown source. Endpoints studied were continued bleeding, recurrent bleeding, surgery, and mortality within 30 days after admission from causes related to bleeding or treatment. The risk of continued bleeding was significantly higher in the placebo group compared to the omeprazole group (OR 4.7; 95%CI 2.7-7.4). The risk of surgery to control bleeding was also significantly higher in the placebo group (OR 3.9; 95%CI 1.7-8.5). There was no significant difference between the 2 groups in terms of the risk of mortality. Patients in the omeprazole group required significantly fewer units of blood transfused per patient ($p < 0.001$).

Khuroo MS, Yattoo GN, Javid G, Khan BA, Shah AA, Gulzar GM, et al. A Comparison of Omeprazole and Placebo for Bleeding Peptic Ulcer. New England Journal of Medicine. 1997 Apr 10;336(15):1054–8.

Magnetic resonance based preoperative evaluation for perianal fistulas superior to traditional clinical method and improve surgical outcomes

1. Preoperative magnetic resonance imaging (MRI) requiring no patient preparation has excellent concordance with surgical findings in perianal fistula and aids in surgical planning.

2. MRI is better than initial surgical exploration in the prediction of patient outcomes.

Original Date of Publication: May 2000

Study Rundown: A perianal fistula is an abnormal connection between a primary opening inside the anal canal to a secondary opening in the perianal skin, often from a draining anorectal abscess. The management of perianal fistulas is a challenging issue in colorectal surgery. Surgery is the primary treatment with the aim of draining local infection, removing the fistulous tract, and protecting sphincter function. In addition to preoperative sphincter function, surgical outcome relies on fistula location, type, and duration. Thus, a thorough understanding of anorectal anatomy is imperative before performing surgery.

Perianal fistulas traditionally are classified by location in relation to the external anal sphincter proposed by Park et al. using only the coronal axis (Table I). Clinical examination based on this classification proved superior to many prior tested imaging techniques, including fistulography, anal endosonography, and computed tomography. However, radiologists at the St. James's University Hospital recommended a classification that applies Parks surgical classification to MR imaging findings in both the axial and coronal planes (Table II). This provided a more accurate description of the fistula's relationship to the anatomy of the anal canal and sphincter complex. The St. James's University Hospital classification thus increases the chance of accurate indication for surgery and avoidance of adverse side effects from inaccurate treatment.

In-Depth [classification system based on prospective data]: This prospective study used gradient-echo T1 dynamic contrast material-enhanced MR imaging to demonstrate and classify perianal fistulas into five grades that were based on Parks's surgical classification. The grades expand on Parks's classification by classifying anatomy based on the axial and coronal planes. Using both planes, MR imaging clearly shows the anatomical location and course of "high" perianal fistulas that are often misdiagnosed by clinical examination. T2-weighted and short-inversion-time inversion recovery (STIR) show pathologic fistulas, secondary fistulous tracks, and fluid collection. STIR imaging occasionally failed to indicate secondary fistulous tracks and small edematous changes.

The St. James's University Hospital classification system was based on 300 patients with surgically proven fistulas. Fistulas were organized into five grades based on increasing severity: grade 1, simple linear intersphincteric fistula; grade 2, intersphincteric fistula with abscess or secondary tract; grade 3, trans-sphincteric fistula; grade 4, trans-sphincteric fistula with abscess or secondary tract within the ischiorectal fossa; grade 5, supralevator and translevator disease. Patient outcome was predicated on whether further surgery was indicated after MR imaging. Use of this classification indicated a significant correlation with patient outcome ($p < 0.001$). MR imaging grades 1 and 2 were associated with no indication for surgery and MR imaging grades 3-5 were associated with indication for surgery. The study concluded that any tract or abscess in the ischiorectal fossa is related to a complex fistula indicating the need for surgery (grades 3-5).

Morris J, Spencer JA, Ambrose NS. MR Imaging Classification of Perianal Fistulas and Its Implications for Patient Management. RadioGraphics. 2000 May 1;20(3):623–35.

Parks AG, Gordon PH, Hardcastle JD. A classification of fistula-in-ano. Br J Surg. 1976 Jan 1;63(1):1–12.

Type	Description and subtypes
I	Intersphincteric - Simple low track - High track - High track with rectal opening - Extra rectal extension
II	Trans-sphincteric - Uncomplicated - High track
III	Suprasphincteric - Uncomplicated - High track
IV	Extrasphincteric - Secondary to trauma - Secondary to anorectal disease - Secondary to pelvic inflammation

Table I. Parks Classification. Underneath each major classification are subtypes. Unlike the St. James classification, complications are associated with each type.

Grade	Description
1	Simple linear intersphincteric fistula
2	Intersphincteric fistula with abscess or secondary track
3	Trans-sphincteric fistula
4	Trans-sphincteric fistula with abscess or secondary track within the ischiorectal fossa
5	Supralevator and translevator disease

Table II. St. James's Classification. Grades 1 and 2 were strongly correlated with no subsequent surgery, while grades 3-5 strongly correlated with surgical intervention.

Intravenous omeprazole after endoscopy reduces rebleeding in patients with peptic ulcers

1. After endoscopic treatment, intravenous omeprazole significantly reduced the risk of rebleeding in patients with peptic ulcers at 3, 7, and 30 days when compared with placebo.

Original Date of Publication: August 2000

Study Rundown: Previous research had demonstrated that proton pump inhibitors in upper gastrointestinal bleeding prior to upper endoscopy significantly reduced the risk of rebleeding and need for surgery to control bleeding. The purpose of this trial was to explore whether continuing proton pump inhibitors after endoscopy would provide any benefits. The findings of this trial demonstrated the value of intravenous proton pump inhibitor after endoscopy in reducing the risk of rebleeding in patients with peptic ulcers. The fact that this study was carried out at a single center in a predominantly Chinese population may limit the generalizability of the study. Moreover, the use of intravenous omeprazole is another concern, as it may not be available in certain other practice settings. Other studies, however, have demonstrated similar benefits with using orally administered proton pump inhibitors. In summary, intravenous omeprazole is associated with reduction in the risk of rebleeding in patients with bleeding peptic ulcers after endoscopic treatment.

In-Depth [randomized controlled trial]: The trial was conducted at the Chinese University of Hong Kong. Patients were eligible for the trial if they were > 16 years of age and if endoscopic treatment of ulcers was successful. A total of 240 patients were randomized to receive either intravenous omeprazole (i.e., 80 mg bolus, then 8 mg/hour for 72 hours) or placebo after endoscopic treatment for bleeding peptic ulcers. Patients receiving placebo had significantly higher risk of recurrent bleeding at 3 days (RR 4.80; 95%CI 1.89-12.2; $p < 0.001$), 7 days (RR 3.71; 95%CI 1.68-8.23), and 30 days (RR 3.38; 95%CI 1.60-7.13) compared to those receiving omeprazole. Moreover, omeprazole significantly reduced the length of hospitalization ($p = 0.006$) and blood transfusion requirements ($p = 0.04$), though there were no significant differences in mortality between the 2 groups at 30 days (RR 2.40; 95%CI 0.87-6.60).

Lau JYW, Sung JJY, Lee KKC, Yung M, Wong SKH, Wu JCY, et al. Effect of Intravenous Omeprazole on Recurrent Bleeding after Endoscopic Treatment of Bleeding Peptic Ulcers. New England Journal of Medicine. 2000 Aug 3;343(5):310–6.

Decrease in symptom severity linked to infliximab Crohn's treatment

1. The severity of Crohn's disease as assessed by the Pediatric Crohn's Disease Activity Index (PCDAI) in patients recruited from 3 pediatric specialty centers decreased significantly over the course of a 12-week treatment regimen with infliximab.

2. All patients were on corticosteroids at the start of the study; however, steroid administration decreased significantly over the course of the investigation.

Original Date of Publication: August 2000

Study Rundown: Crohn's disease is an inflammatory bowel disease (IBD) often diagnosed in adolescence and young adulthood and results from an immune-mediated, inflammatory process with the potential to affect any portion of the gastrointestinal tract. Knowing that tumor necrosis factor -α (TNF-α), a cytokine involved in the modulation of the inflammatory responses, is increased in patients with Crohn's and that the drug infliximab (Remicade) acts to neutralize TNF-α, this study built upon encouraging research in adult patients in investigating the potential utility of infliximab in the pediatric population. In this study, 19 patients with poor response to other therapies were started on varying infliximab dosing schedules. All patients were on daily prednisone at baseline. Crohn's disease symptom status was assessed at baseline, 1 month, and 3 months into the study through physician assessment and use of the PCDAI.

Over the study period, the severity of Crohn's symptoms by PCDAI score and the doses of steroids used to treat disease decreased significantly. This study was limited by the variation in infliximab dosing schedules, lack of a control group, and small sample size. However, it stands as one of the first studies to investigate the use of infliximab in a pediatric population with Crohn's and indicated many potential positive outcomes. Following Food and Drug Administration approval in 2006, infliximab was, and still is, used in pediatric patients with moderate to severe Crohn's who have not responded adequately to other therapies. While only 3 of the 19 patients in this study experienced any type of adverse reactions, adverse effects from long-term use, including lymphoma, are of major concern in patients. The risk of malignancy along with other severe reactions continues to be investigated. In addition, many patients with Crohn's are on combined therapies, the efficacy and adverse effects of these regimens are also under investigation.

In-Depth [prospective cohort]: Pediatric patients with Crohn's disease, treated at 3 IBD specialty centers, and who had responded poorly or not at all to previously treatment strategies or depended entirely on corticosteroids, were eligible to participate. A total of 19 patients were recruited (average age 14.4 years, with a mean 3.5 years since diagnosis) to receive infliximab administered intravenously at a dose of 5 mg/kg over 2 hours. The number of treatments varied among participants. Treatment outcomes were assessed by physician assessment and the PCDAI, a physician-completed health evaluation, filled out prior to infliximab treatment and then 4 and 12 weeks after initiation. Patients were followed for an additional 3 to 9 months following the 12-week evaluation. At the time of treatment initiation, all patients had moderate to severe disease as measured by the evaluation tool and all were on daily corticosteroids with 14 participants on an additional agent.

Over the course of treatment, all patients experienced symptomatic improvement. After 4 weeks of therapy, 9 patients were asymptomatic and PCDAI values significantly decreased from 42.1 ± 13.7 to 10.0 ± 5.6 ($p < 0.0001$). Over the 12-week study period, patients became increasingly symptomatic, but the 12-week PCDAI still remained significantly lower than the score at the time of treatment initiation at 26.8 ± 16.4 ($p < 0.01$). Prednisone dosing decreased over the course of the study with doses at both 4 weeks and 12 weeks significantly lower than at baseline (28 ± 14 mg at baseline vs. 20 ± 12 mg at 4 weeks and 8 ± 12 mg at 12 weeks, $p < 0.01$) and 9 participants on no corticosteroids at the study's conclusion. At final follow-up, 3 patients had inactive disease, 9 had mild disease, and 4 had moderate disease. Three patients experienced adverse reactions such as dyspnea and rash which were controlled in 2 who received pretreatment with diphenhydramine prior to administration of infliximab.

Hyams JS, Markowitz J, Wyllie R. Use of infliximab in the treatment of Crohn's disease in children and adolescents. The Journal of Pediatrics. 2000 Aug 1;137(2):192–6.

The MELD score: Predicting survival in end-stage liver disease

1. The Model for End-Stage Liver Disease (MELD) is a reliable tool for predicting short-term survival in patients with advanced liver disease.

2. The score is generalizable to diverse etiologies and a wide range of disease severity.

Original Date of Publication: February 2001

Study Rundown: The MELD was originally developed to predict outcomes in patients after a transjugular intrahepatic portosystemic shunt (TIPS) procedure. This study assessed whether the model could reliably predict short-term survival in patients with chronic liver disease. The investigators found that MELD scores were a good predictor of 1-week, 3 month and 1-year survival, which had important implications for the model's use in the allocation of donor livers. Previously, the Child-Turcotte-Pugh (CTP) system was used to rank patients according to urgency and medical need, however the broad classifications made it difficult to rank patients according to severity of disease. Another issue with CTP scores was the subjectivity involved in some of the criteria (e.g., assessment of ascites and encephalopathy). The MELD criteria were an improvement on these aspects of CTP scores as patients were assigned a numerical score based on objective measures.

In-Depth [cohort study]: This study evaluated the validity of the MELD score for predicting survival in patients with end-stage liver disease. The model used measures of serum creatinine, total serum bilirubin, International Normalized Ratio (INR) for prothrombin time and etiology of cirrhosis to assess disease severity. The model was assessed in 4 independent samples, which included patients hospitalized with advanced end-stage liver disease, ambulatory patients with noncholestatic cirrhosis, ambulatory patients with primary biliary cirrhosis (PBC) and a historical group of cirrhotic patients from a period when liver transplantation was not widely available. The primary outcome measure was 3 month survival and validity was also assessed for predicting 1-week and 1-year survival. The C statistics for 3 month mortality in the hospitalized, ambulatory noncholestatic, ambulatory PBC and historical groups respectively were 0.87, 0.80, 0.87 and 0.78. These values changed minimally when etiology of disease was excluded from the model. The MELD score was found to be a reliable tool to predict survival in patients with chronic liver disease.

Kamath PS, Wiesner RH, Malinchoc M, Kremers W, Therneau TM, Kosberg CL, et al. A model to predict survival in patients with end-stage liver disease. Hepatology. 2001 Feb 1;33(2):464–70.

Ceftriaxone vs. norfloxacin for prophylaxis in patients with cirrhosis and gastrointestinal bleeding

1. In cirrhotic patients who presented with gastrointestinal bleeding, patients treated with ceftriaxone were significantly less likely to develop proved or possible infections when compared to those treated with norfloxacin.

2. The ceftriaxone group was also significantly less likely to developed proved infections or spontaneous bacteremia and bacterial peritonitis.

3. There were no significant differences between the 2 groups in 10-day or hospital mortality.

Original Date of Publication: October 2006

Study Rundown: Patients with cirrhosis are at elevated risk of developing gastrointestinal bleeding. Cirrhotic patients who present with gastrointestinal bleeding are also at significant risk of bacterial infection, with large proportions of patients either presenting with bacterial infections or developing them during their hospitalization. Previous efforts had shown that antibiotic prophylaxis in these patients significantly reduced the risk of infection, though questions remained regarding the best antibiotic choice. While norfloxacin was commonly used, rising prevalence of quinolone resistance was rendering this less effective. The purpose of this trial was to compare the effects of oral norfloxacin with intravenous ceftriaxone when used in prophylaxis for cirrhotic patients presenting with gastrointestinal bleeding.

In summary, patients with cirrhosis presenting with gastrointestinal bleeding were significantly less likely to develop proved or possible infections when treated with ceftriaxone as compared with norfloxacin. Those on ceftriaxone were also significantly less likely to develop proved infections and spontaneous bacteremia or spontaneous bacterial peritonitis. There were no significant differences between the groups in 10-day or hospital mortality, and there were no drug-related adverse events noted during the study period.

In-Depth [randomized controlled trial]: This randomized trial was conducted at 4 hospitals in Spain. Patients were included if they were between 18-80 years of age, had hematemesis and/or melena in the 24 hours prior to enrollment, and advanced cirrhosis (i.e., ≥2 of severe malnutrition, serum bilirubin > 3 mg/mL, ascites, hepatic encephalopathy). Exclusion criteria were allergy to cephalosporin or quinolones, signs of infection (i.e., fever > 37.5°C, white cell count > 15 000/mm^3, immature neutrophils > 500/mm^3, ascitic polymorphonuclear cell count > 250/mm^3, > 15 leukocytes/field in urine sediment, pneumonia on chest x-ray), treatment with antibiotics 2 weeks before bleed, known advanced hepatocellular carcinoma, and human immunodeficiency virus infection. Eligible patients were randomized in a 1:1 ratio to norfloxacin 400 mg orally every 12 hours or ceftriaxone 1 g intravenously daily for 7 days. The primary outcome was the development of proved or possible infection in the 10 days after enrollment.

A total of 124 patients were randomized, with 111 being considered in the final analysis. Patients in the ceftriaxone group were significantly less likely to develop proved or possible infection when compared with those on norfloxacin (11% vs. 33%, p = 0.01). Patients in the ceftriaxone group were also significantly less likely to develop proved infection (11% vs. 26%, p = 0.03) or spontaneous bacteremia or bacterial peritonitis (2% vs. 12%, p = 0.03). There were no significant differences between the 2 groups in 10-day or hospital mortality. No adverse effects related to norfloxacin or ceftriaxone were observed during the study period.

Fernandez J, Ruiz del Arbol L, Gomez C, Durandez R, Serradilla R, Guarner C, et al. Norfloxacin vs ceftriaxone in the prophylaxis of infections in patients with advanced cirrhosis and hemorrhage. Gastroenterology. 2006;131(4):1049-1056.

Omeprazole before endoscopy in patients with gastrointestinal bleeding

1. Compared to placebo, treating patients with omeprazole bolus and infusion prior to endoscopy significantly reduced the need for endoscopic therapy, reduced the rate of post-endoscopy active bleeding, and reduced the length of hospitalization.

2. Treating patients with omeprazole pre-endoscopy did not significantly reduce the need for emergency surgery and did not reduce 30-day mortality as compared with placebo.

Original Date of Publication: April 2007

Study Rundown: In patients with upper gastrointestinal bleeding, infusion of a high-dose proton-pump inhibitor (PPI) after hemostasis via endoscopy was known to reduce recurrent bleeding and improved clinical outcomes. The adjuvant use of high-dose PPIs in endoscopic therapy has also been endorsed and confirmed in 2 meta-analyses. Clot formation over arteries is a pH-dependent process; a gastric pH > 6 is thought to be critical for platelet aggregation. Prior to this study, treatment with PPIs was often initiated before endoscopy in patients presenting with upper gastrointestinal bleeding. However, there was a lack of evidence to support such an approach. This trial demonstrated that omeprazole bolus and infusion before endoscopy accelerated the resolution of bleeding in ulcers and reduced the need for endoscopic therapy. Moreover, omeprazole treatment prior to endoscopy was associated with reduced active bleeding post-endoscopy and led to shorter hospital stays. There were no significant differences between the groups in the rate of recurrent bleeding within 30 days, need for emergency surgery, or 30-day mortality.

In-Depth [randomized controlled trial]: Participants in the trial were randomized to 2 treatment groups: 1) patients received an intravenous infusion of omeprazole or 2) a placebo. Each patient received an 80-mg intravenous bolus injection followed by continuous infusion of 8 mg per hour until endoscopic examination the following morning. Patients were eligible for the trial if they had hypotensive shock with a systolic blood pressure ≤90 mmHg or pulse ≥110 beats per minute was stabilized after their initial resuscitation. Exclusion criteria included long-term aspirin use, unstable condition requiring urgent endoscopy, a moribund state, and a known PPI allergy. A total of 188 of those evaluated were excluded for other reasons that were not mentioned. The primary study endpoint was the need for endoscopic therapy at the first endoscopic examination. Secondary endpoints included signs of bleeding, need for urgent endoscopy, duration of hospital stay, need for transfusion, need for emergency surgery to achieve hemostasis, and rates of recurrent bleeding and death from any cause within 30 days after randomization.

A total of 638 patients underwent randomization. Compared to patients treated with placebo, patients in the omeprazole group required significantly less endoscopic treatment (RR 0.67; 95%CI 0.51-0.90). Moreover, patients treated with omeprazole also required less endoscopic therapy for bleeding peptic ulcers (RR 0.61; 95%CI 0.44-0.84) and had less post-endoscopy active bleeding (RR 0.44; 95%CI 0.23-0.83) compared to those treated with placebo. Notably, a larger proportion of omeprazole-treated patients had hospital stays < 3 days compared to those on placebo (RR 1.23; 95%CI 1.07-1.42). There were no significant differences between the groups in the rate of recurrent bleeding within 30 days, need for emergency surgery, or 30-day mortality.

Lau JY, Leung WK, Wu JCY, Chan FKL, Wong VWS, Chiu PWY, et al. Omeprazole before Endoscopy in Patients with Gastrointestinal Bleeding. New England Journal of Medicine. 2007 Apr 19;356(16):1631–40.

Early transjugular intrahepatic portosystemic shunt in cirrhosis and variceal bleeding

1. In patients with severe liver disease and variceal bleeding, early transjugular intrahepatic portosystemic shunt (TIPS) significantly reduced rates of treatment failure, length of hospitalization, and mortality compared to control.

2. There were no significant differences between the two groups in the rates of adverse events.

Original Date of Publication: June 2010

Study Rundown: Variceal bleeding is a major cause of death for patients with liver cirrhosis and portal hypertension. Guidelines at the time of this study recommended treatment consisting of vasoactive drugs (e.g., octreotide), prophylactic antibiotics, and endoscopic techniques such as variceal ligation for dealing with variceal bleeding. When standard treatment failed, TIPS had been shown to be effective, though was associated with substantial mortality due in large part to hepatic encephalopathy. Previous studies suggested that the earlier use of TIPS can decrease mortality for patients with severe liver disease who are at a high risk of treatment failure. This trial was the first to compare the use of early TIPS with the current standard of care for acute variceal bleeding.

Results showed that early use of TIPS was associated with a significant decrease in the rate of rebleeding and failure to control bleeding. Early TIPS also significantly reduced mortality and led to shorter stays in the intensive care unit (ICU). Notably, early TIPS use was not associated with a significantly higher rate of adverse events, such as hepatic encephalopathy. A major limitation of the study was its small size (only 63 patients were randomized), meaning it was insufficiently powered for subgroup analyses. Thus, for example, the study could not determine whether early TIPS had greater benefit for the study's more severe cases of liver disease (those classified as Child-Pugh class C) in comparison to the study's less severe cases (those classified as Child-Pugh class B). In summary, results of this study supported the early use of TIPS for the treatment of patients with severe liver disease and variceal bleeding. Importantly, the results suggested that use of early TIPS was not associated with an increased risk of hepatic encephalopathy.

In-Depth [randomized controlled trial]: Sixty-three patients from 9 centers in Europe were enrolled in this trial. Eligible patients had liver disease classified as Child-Pugh class B (i.e., moderately severe) or class C (i.e., most severe), had liver cirrhosis with acute bleeding of esophageal varices, and were already receiving treatment in the form of vasoactive drugs (e.g., octreotide), antibiotics, and endoscopic band ligation (EBL). Patients with age > 75 years, pregnancy, hepatocellular carcinoma, previous TIPS, portal-vein thrombosis, or heart failure were excluded. Within 24 hours of admission, 31 patients were randomized to the "early TIPS" group, where they received treatment with a polytetrafluoroethylene-covered stent within 72 hours after randomization. The remaining 32 patients were randomized to the "pharmocotherapy-EBL" group, where they continued to receive vasoactive drug therapy followed treatment with nonspecific beta-blockers (e.g., propranolol and nadolol) and EBL-TIPS was provided as a rescue therapy. The primary endpoint was the composite outcome of failure to control bleeding and the failure to prevent rebleeding in the next year. Secondary endpoints included mortality at 6 weeks and 1 year, the development of sequelae associated with portal hypertension, and the number of days spent in the ICU.

Results demonstrated that 97% of the early-TIPS group avoided occurrence of the primary endpoint, compared to 50% in the pharmacotherapy-EBL group ($p < 0.001$). At 1 year, the survival rate was 86% in the early-TIPS group compared to 61% in the pharmacotherapy-EBL group ($p < 0.001$). Patients in the pharmacotherapy-EBL group spent a higher proportion of their follow-up time in the ICU ($p = 0.01$). There was no difference in the rate of adverse rates for both treatment groups, including for hepatic encephalopathy ($p = 0.13$), and development of ascites ($p = 0.11$).

García-Pagán JC, Caca K, Bureau C, Laleman W, Appenrodt B, Luca A, et al. Early Use of TIPS in Patients with Cirrhosis and Variceal Bleeding. The New England Journal of Medicine. 2010 Jun 24;362(25):2370–9.

The COGENT: Omeprazole with antiplatelet therapy in upper gastrointestinal bleeding

1. In patients treated with dual antiplatelet therapy, the addition of omeprazole significantly reduced the rate of gastrointestinal events compared to placebo.

2. The addition of omeprazole to clopidogrel and aspirin did not significantly change the rate of cardiovascular events compared to placebo.

Original Date of Publication: November 2010

Study Rundown: Antiplatelet therapy is commonly prescribed to people who suffer from cardiovascular disease, including myocardial infarctions, transient ischemic attacks, and stroke. A common complication of antiplatelet therapy, however, is gastrointestinal bleeding and this risk is increased when patients are being treated with dual antiplatelet agents. Moreover, evidence from observational studies were inconsistent with regards to a potential interaction between clopidogrel, a commonly prescribed antiplatelet agent, and proton pump inhibitors (PPIs). Thus, the purpose of the Clopidogrel and Optimization of Gastrointestinal Events Trial (COGENT) was to assess the efficacy and safety of clopidogrel and PPIs in patients with coronary artery disease. The trial revealed that treatment with omeprazole in patients on dual antiplatelet therapy reduced the rate of gastrointestinal events without a significant difference in the rate of cardiovascular events. Notably, this trial was stopped prematurely, as there was an unexpected loss of funding. As a result, the intended study enrollment and event rates were not achieved. Nevertheless, this study provided evidence in support of the use of proton pump inhibitors in patients on dual antiplatelet therapy to reduce the rate of gastrointestinal events.

In-Depth [randomized controlled trial]: Originally published in NEJM in 2010, this randomized, controlled trial assessed the risk of gastrointestinal bleeding in patients receiving dual antiplatelet therapy with and without concomitant omeprazole. A pharmaceutical company was involved in the design of the study. A total of 3761 patients from 393 sites in 15 countries being treated with aspirin (75-325 mg daily) and clopidogrel (75 mg daily) were randomized to receive either omeprazole (20 mg daily) or placebo in addition. Patients were eligible for the study if they were ≥21 years of age and it was anticipated that they would require clopidogrel and aspirin therapy for the next 12 months. The primary endpoint was a composite of upper gastrointestinal events, including upper gastrointestinal bleeding, symptomatic uncomplicated gastroduodenal ulcers, obstruction, and perforation. The primary cardiovascular safety endpoint was a composite of death from cardiovascular causes, nonfatal myocardial infarction, coronary revascularization, or ischemic stroke. The trial was stopped prematurely when the sponsor suddenly lost financial backing. At 180 days, the omeprazole group had a significantly lower rate of gastrointestinal events when compared to the placebo group (HR 0.34; 95%CI 0.18-0.63). The omeprazole group also experienced significantly less overall gastrointestinal bleeding as compared with placebo (HR 0.30; 95%CI 0.13-0.66). There was no significant difference between the 2 groups in terms of the rate of cardiovascular events (HR 0.99; 95%CI 0.68-1.44).

Bhatt DL, Cryer BL, Contant CF, Cohen M, Lanas A, Schnitzer TJ, et al. Clopidogrel with or without Omeprazole in Coronary Artery Disease. New England Journal of Medicine. 2010 Nov 11;363(20):1909–17.

Weekly semaglutide effective for decreasing body weight in obesity

1. Once-weekly treatment of semaglutide was associated with meaningful body weight reduction at 68 weeks compared to placebo in patients with obesity.

2. Semaglutide treatment was associated with more gastrointestinal and hepatobiliary adverse events.

Original Date of Publication: March 2021

Study Rundown: Obesity is increasing in North America and remains significant comorbidity leading to increased metabolic disorders, cardiovascular disease, and malignancies. Semaglutide, a glucagon-like peptide-1 (GLP-1) analog, is approved for type 2 diabetes. This study evaluated the efficacy and safety of semaglutide to reduce body weight in patients with obesity and without diabetes. The study determined a clinically meaningful change in the baseline weight compared to placebo. Furthermore, there was greater cardiovascular risk factor reduction in the group treated with semaglutide. Patient physical function scores were also better with semaglutide treatment. Gastrointestinal side effects such as nausea and diarrhea were more common in the treatment group. The study was limited by males being underrepresented, which limited the generalizability of the study. Nonetheless, the study's results are significant, showing semaglutide and lifestyle intervention compared to lifestyle alone led to a greater reduction in body weight.

In-Depth [randomized control trial]: This was a multicenter, randomized, double-blind placebo-controlled trial of 1,961 patients. Patients with a body mass index (BMI) $\geq$ 30 or BMI $\geq$ 27 with one of the following weight-related comorbidities: hypertension, dyslipidemia, obstructive sleep apnea, or cardiovascular disease were included in the study. Patients with known diabetes or a glycated hemoglobin level of 6.5% or greater, previous obesity surgical treatment, or use of antiobesity medication within 90 days of enrollment were excluded from the study. Patients were randomized in a 2:1 ratio of either semaglutide and lifestyle intervention or placebo and lifestyle intervention, respectively. The primary endpoints were percentage change in body weight from baseline to week 68 and reduction in body weight of five percent or more in the same time period. The mean change in body weight was -14.9% in the semaglutide group compared to -2.4% in the control group (95% confidence interval [CI] -13.4 to -11.5, P < 0.001). The semaglutide group had more patients with at least 5%

weight reduction (86.4%) compared to the placebo group (31.5%) (P < 0.001). Gastrointestinal side effects were more common in the semaglutide group (74.2%) compared to the placebo group (47.9%). Finally, 7.0% in the semaglutide group and 3.1% in the control group stopped treatment owing to adverse events. In summary, this trial demonstrates promising data on the use of semaglutide for obesity management.

Wilding JPH, Batterham RL, Calanna S, Davies M, Gaal LFV, Lingvay I, et al. Once-Weekly Semaglutide in Adults with Overweight or Obesity. New England Journal of Medicine. 2021 Feb 10;

V. Hematology/Oncology

"Everything is theoretically impossible, until it is done."

- Robert A. Heinlein

The Milan Criteria: Liver transplantation is effective for treating cirrhotic patients with unrespectable hepatocellular carcinomas

1. Patients with cirrhosis and unresectable hepatocellular carcinomas (HCC), either 1 tumor less than 5 cm or no more than 3 tumors less than 3 cm (Milan Criteria), who received orthotopic liver transplants (OLTs) had a 75% 4-year actuarial survival rate and an 83% rate of recurrence-free survival.

2. Patients who's excised livers showed their HCCs were accurately staged and met Milan Criteria had statistically better survival rates than patients whose tumors where mistakenly staged too low and included in the study.

Original Date of Publication: March 1996

Study Rundown: HCC is a primary liver malignancy that often occurs in patients with chronic liver disease and cirrhosis. The development of cirrhosis and subsequent HCC is closely associated with liver damage by causes such as chronic hepatitis infections, alcohol abuse, or genetic causes. Symptoms of advanced HCC include upper right quadrant abdominal pain, an enlarged abdomen, and weight loss. Screening of known cirrhotic patients using imaging or the alpha-fetoprotein (AFP) blood biomarker now allows many HCCs to be diagnosed early. Prognosis for patients with HCC has been poor, with 5-year survival rates ranging from approx. 20-40%.

Retrospective studies have suggested OLT may be a beneficial treatment compared to liver resection, especially for early stage HCC. In this small study of 48 patients with unrespectable, early stage HCC as defined by the size and number of tumors present were given orthotopic liver transplants and followed up to assess survival and recurrence. Results showed patients meeting the criteria of the study as verified by pathological examination of the liver had significantly better 4-year survival and recurrence outcomes than patients with more advanced cancers. The Milan criteria established in this study indicating OLT for early-stage

HCC has good prognosis has been used in policy by insurers and organ networks to help select patients most likely to benefit from the procedure. A larger prospective cohort by Duffy and colleagues indicated that HCC at a later stage, defined by UCSF criteria as 1 tumor less than 6.5 cm in diameter, a maximum of 3 total tumors with none greater than 4.5 cm in diameter, and cumulative tumor size less than 8 cm, did not have statistically different 5-year post transplant survival rates.

In-Depth [prospective cohort]: This prospective trial was conducted at The National Cancer Institute in Milan, Italy. Patients with unresectable HCC due to multifocality, inoperable location, or causing hepatic insufficiency were evaluated for inclusion in this study (n = 295). Histologic confirmation of cirrhosis and histologic or serum confirmation of early stage HCC deemed 60 patients eligible for the study. Eligible patients were assessed via hepatic angiography and liver CT scans to confirm there was 1 tumor less than 5 cm in diameter or no more than 3 tumors each less than 3 cm in diameter. Suspicion or evidence of tumor invasion into blood vessels or lymph nodes excluded patients from the study. The study followed 48 patients (38 male, median age 52, age range 39-60) who met these criteria. Cirrhosis was caused by hepatitis infection in 45 patients. Liver function was assessed using Child-Pugh classification. Most patients classified as having intermediate or poor hepatic function (Child-Pugh class A or B) received anticancer treatment prior to transplantation (n = 26). All patients with normal liver function (n = 15) and some with intermediate or poor function (n = 5) were not pretreated with anticancer regimens. Liver transplantations were performed when a compatible liver became available. Tumor stage follow-up using ultrasound, chest radiography, and serum AFP was performed every 3 months after transplantation, abdominal and chest CT scans were performed every 6 months, and radionuclide bone scans were performed every 8 months.

Follow-up time for patients in this study was a median of 26 months (range 9-54). Death following transplantation occurred in 8 patients, and 2 patients required retransplantation due to recurrent viral hepatitis. Cancer recurrence occurred in 4 patients at a median of 4 months following transplantation. For all patients who underwent liver transplantation, the survival rate at 4 years was 75% and recurrence-free survival was 83%. Survival was statistically not affected by patient age, sex, preoperative anticancer treatment, or common markers of chronic liver disease (T stage, number of tumors, serum AFP levels, and presence of a capsule). Pathological examination of excised livers indicated 13 patients (27%) had tumors that did not meet the study criteria regarding size/number of tumors. For patients who were preoperatively staged accurately, the 4-year overall survival rate was 85% and recurrence freed survival rate was 92%. Those mistakenly understaged had 4-year overall and recurrence free survival rates of 50 and 59%, respectively.

Mazzaferro V, Regalia E, Doci R, Andreola S, Pulvirenti A, Bozzetti F, et al. Liver Transplantation for the Treatment of Small Hepatocellular Carcinomas in Patients with Cirrhosis. New England Journal of Medicine. 1996 Mar 14;334(11):693–700.

Additional Review:

Duffy JP, Vardanian A, Benjamin E, Watson M, Farmer DG, Ghobrial RM, et al. Liver Transplantation Criteria For Hepatocellular Carcinoma Should Be Expanded. Ann Surg. 2007 Sep;246(3):502–11.

Vena caval filters in pulmonary embolism prophylaxis

1. Permanent vena caval filter placement in addition to anticoagulant therapy reduced the short-term occurrence of pulmonary embolism (PE), but increased the long-term risk of recurrent deep vein thrombosis (DVT).

2. There was no significant difference in efficacy between low molecular-weight heparin (LMWH) and unfractionated heparin (UFH) as early anticoagulant therapy for PE prophylaxis.

Original Date of Publication: February 1998

Study Rundown: In patients who are at high-risk for PE and have a contraindication to anticoagulation, a vena caval filter is a potential option to reduce the risk of PE. This multicenter study in France is the only randomized, controlled trial that evaluated whether filter placement decreases the incidence of PE, as well as DVT both in short-term and long-term follow-up. The study demonstrated that the use of a permanent vena caval filter in addition to heparin therapy reduced the occurrence of a PE in the short-term. The data, however, also showed that in long-term follow-up of 2 years, there was a significant increase in recurrent DVTs in patients who received a filter. This most likely relates to thrombosis at the filter site, but it may counteract the benefits gained earlier with the reduction in PE occurrence. In summary, this study showed that filters lower the risk of PE in the short-term, but later increase the risk of recurrent DVT. It also confirmed the results of previous studies that showed no difference in effectiveness between LMWH and UFH for early anticoagulant therapy. Overall, the evidence in this study does not support the use of inferior vena cava (IVC) filters in addition to anticoagulant therapy to prevent PE's and recurrent DVT's. Of note, this study excluded patients with DVT who had a contraindication to anticoagulation, which is one of the commonly cited indications for filter placement.

In-Depth [randomized controlled trial]: This study was a multicenter, non-blinded, 2x2, randomized-controlled trial that randomized 400 patients to vena caval filter placement or no placement, and to receive LMWH or UFH as a bridge to warfarin. Patients over 18 years of age with confirmed DVT with or without concomitant symptomatic PE, and whose physicians believed they were at high risk for a PE, were eligible for the study. Patients with history of IVC filter placement, contraindication to anticoagulant therapy, or likelihood of noncompliance were excluded. Two hundred patients were assigned to receive vena caval filters. One hundred ninety-five of the 400 patients were assigned to LMWH while the other 205 were assigned to UFH for the first 8-12 days of anticoagulant therapy. The subjects underwent a baseline V/Q scan and/or pulmonary angiography to evaluate for a PE. All subjects were transitioned to warfarin therapy after 8-12 days for a duration of 3 months or maintained on UFH if oral anticoagulation was not possible. Patients were followed for 2 years. The primary outcome was occurrence of a symptomatic PE within the first 12 days of anticoagulant therapy. The secondary outcome was occurrence of symptomatic PE, DVT, major filter complication, and/or major bleeding during the follow-up period.

Filter vs. No Filter

The study demonstrated that there were significantly fewer patients (2 vs. 9 patients) in the filter group compared to the non-filter group who had had a PE in the first 12 days of anticoagulation therapy (OR 0.22; 95%CI 0.05-0.90). Results were similar when analysis was adjusted for heparin therapy and presence of PE at enrollment. In the 2-year follow-up, there was a significantly higher number of recurrent DVTs in the filter group compared to the no-filter group (OR 1.87; 95%CI 1.10-3.20). There was no significant difference in PE incidence, mortality, or major bleeding between the groups at the 2-year mark.

LMWH vs. UFH

There was no significant difference in incidence of PE or DVT between the anticoagulant groups during the first 12 days as well as at the 2-year mark. There was also no statistical significance in mortality or adverse effects between the groups. There was no evidence of statistically significant interaction between filter and heparin anticoagulant therapy for both primary and secondary outcome events.

Decousus H, Leizorovicz A, Parent F, Page Y, Tardy B, Girard P, et al. A Clinical Trial of Vena Caval Filters in the Prevention of Pulmonary Embolism in Patients with Proximal Deep-Vein Thrombosis. New England Journal of Medicine. 1998 Feb 12;338(7):409–16.

Arterial chemoembolization improves survival in non-resectable hepatocellular carcinoma

1. In patients with unresectable hepatocellular carcinoma (HCC), arterial chemoembolization with doxorubicin demonstrated significant survival benefit compared to control group.

2. The randomized controlled trial had strict inclusion criteria and only included patients with Child-Pugh Class A/B with no evidence of end-stage tumoral disease, portal vein obstruction, or encephalopathy.

Original Date of Publication: May 2002

Study Rundown: HCC is the most common primary liver cancer and the second-leading cause of cancer mortality worldwide. While the mainstay of treatment is surgical resection, many patients do not meet the eligibility criteria for curative resection due to large disease burden. Alternative treatment modalities for patients with non-resectable HCC such as arterial chemoembolization of the feeding hepatic artery were developed; however, early trials evaluating the use of arterial chemoembolization demonstrated conflicting evidence on the survival benefit of these procedures.

The purpose of this landmark randomized controlled trial was to determine the effectiveness of arterial chemoembolization in a study population most likely to benefit from this procedure. The trial randomized over 100 patients with non-resectable HCC to chemoembolization with doxorubicin or symptomatic control. The trial excluded all patients with advanced disease (Child-Pugh Score C), extra-hepatic disease, or portal vein thrombosis. The trial was stopped early due to the significant survival benefit observed in the patient group randomized to arterial chemoembolization. Additionally, the use of chemoembolization was associated with a significantly lower rate of tumor invasion of portal vein at two years of follow-up. The results of this trial demonstrated a significant survival benefit of arterial chemoembolization in a stringently selected patient population with non-resectable HCC.

In-Depth [randomized controlled trial]: This was a single-blind, multi-center randomized controlled trial evaluating the survival benefit of arterial chemoembolization in patients with non-resectable HCC. All adult patients (n = 903) with a biopsy- or imaging-confirmed diagnosis of HCC were consecutively screened for enrollment over four years across three centers in Barcelona, Spain. The inclusion criteria were patients with HCC that were deemed not suitable for curative treatment. Key exclusion criteria included patients with Child-Pugh class C disease, evidence of extra-hepatic disease, presence of vascular invasion, renal failure, or end-stage tumoral disease. Overall, 112 patients with non-resectable were recruited and randomized to either chemoembolization with gelatin sponge and doxorubicin, arterial embolization alone, or symptomatic treatment. Arterial embolization with or without doxorubicin was performed at baseline, 2 months, 6 months, and every 6 months thereafter. Treatment was halted if the patient developed any of the exclusion criteria. Treatment response was monitored by contrast-enhanced spiral computed tomography at 6 months post-recruitment. The primary end-point was overall survival with a secondary endpoint of treatment response.

Overall, 40 patients were randomized to chemoembolization, 37 patients were randomized to arterial embolization only, and 35 patients were randomized to symptomatic treatment. There were no significant differences in the baseline characteristics between each group with the exception of serum bilirubin, which was significant higher in the control group. The trial was stopped early due to significant survival benefit in the chemoembolization group compared to control (HR: 0.47; 95%CI 0.25-0.91; p = 0.025). At the conclusion of the trial, the mean survival for the chemoembolization group was significantly longer compared to control group (25.3 months versus 17.9 months; p < 0.009). There were no direct survival comparisons between the chemoembolization group and the embolization group; however, only chemoembolization was associated with a decreased risk of portal-vein thrombosis compared to control at two-year follow-up (17% versus 58%; p = 0.005). The mean number of chemoembolization treatment sessions was 3.08 (95%CI: 2.4-3.5). Eleven patients had treatment-related complications and there was only one treatment-related death. Common complications included cholecystitis, leukopenia, and spontaneous bacterial peritonitis.

Llovet JM, Real MI, Montaña X, Planas R, Coll S, Aponte J, et al. Arterial embolisation or chemoembolisation versus symptomatic treatment in patients with unresectable hepatocellular carcinoma: a randomised controlled trial. The Lancet. 2002 May 18;359(9319):1734–9.

No survival difference between lumpectomy and mastectomy for breast cancer

1. In women with stage I or II breast cancer, there was no significant difference in overall survival in women treated with total mastectomy compared to breast-conserving surgery.

2. Adjuvant radiation therapy was associated with reduced ipsilateral recurrence in lumpectomy-treated women.

Original Date of Publication: October 2002

Study Rundown: Breast cancer is the most common type of cancer affecting women. These cancers arise from tissues in the breast, with the 2 most common types being ductal and lobular carcinomas. Risk factors for developing breast cancer include increasing age, being female, having a family history of breast cancer, certain genetic defects (i.e., BRCA1 and BRCA2), and early menarche/late menopause. While the incidence of breast cancer has increased steadily over the past decades, mortality rates have declined significantly since the 1980s. This may be attributed to increased screening, more effective screening programs, and better treatment amongst numerous other factors. Breast cancer treatment consists of a combination of local and systemic therapy, depending on the cancer characteristics and staging. In the 1970s, several studies were conducted to address lingering questions regarding the surgical management of breast cancer. Several randomized controlled trials were conducted to assess the efficacy of breast-conserving therapy.

One particular study explored whether lumpectomy, a procedure where the tumor was resected with clean margins, with or without radiation therapy was comparable to radical mastectomy. Previous analyses suggested that there were no significant differences in survival between the study groups. This study reported the 20 year findings of this randomized controlled trial. Lumpectomy followed by radiation therapy was not associated with not reduced survival or reduced recurrence of breast cancer in the ipsilateral breast when compared to radical mastectomy and lumpectomy alone, respectively. Currently, systemic therapy is used routinely as adjuvant treatment after surgery to reduce the risk of distant micrometastases.

In-Depth [randomized controlled trial]: This trial followed 1851 women diagnosed with invasive breast tumors with positive or negative axillary lymph nodes (i.e., stage I or II). Participants were randomized to treatment total mastectomy, lumpectomy or lumpectomy followed by breast irradiation. These findings were reported after 20 years of follow-up. Breast irradiation was associated with reduced recurrence in the ipsilateral breast in women treated with lumpectomy and who had tumor-free margins on surgical specimens. The benefit of radiation therapy was independent of nodal status. At 20 year follow-up after surgery, 14.3% of women who underwent lumpectomy with radiation had a recurrence in the ipsilateral breast compared to 39.2% in women who underwent lumpectomy alone ($p < 0.001$). No significant difference was found in disease-free survival or overall survival among the 3 treatment groups.

Fisher B, Anderson S, Bryant J, Margolese RG, Deutsch M, Fisher ER, et al. Twenty-Year Follow-up of a Randomized Trial Comparing Total Mastectomy, Lumpectomy, and Lumpectomy plus Irradiation for the Treatment of Invasive Breast Cancer. New England Journal of Medicine. 2002 Oct 17;347(16):1233–41.

OPTN and UNOS update policy regarding hepatocellular carcinoma

1. Administrators overseeing the national liver transplantation network approved new policy to standardize radiologic imaging criteria for patients with hepatocellular carcinoma (HCC) to qualify for exemption points. Radiologists in US liver transplantation centers asked to implement this policy.

2. This new policy recommends various technical and procedural standards for CT and MR imaging, diagnosis, and classification criteria of HCC. It also seeks to standardize reporting requirements of HCC assessment to transplant networks.

Original Date of Publication: February 2013

Study Rundown: In the United States today, there are approximately three times more patients awaiting liver transplants than those who actually receive a liver. In order to distribute livers to patients determined to be most in need, the Organ Procurement and Transplantation Network (OPTN) and United Network for Organ Sharing (UNOS) set policy in 2002 giving priority to patients most ill and most likely to benefit from transplantation. Patients with early stage HCC have very good prognosis if able to receive a transplant. Therefore, the 2002 OPTN policy was designed to be favorable to patients reported to have early stage HCC and gave exemption points to early-stage HCC patients moving them higher on the Model for End-Stage Liver Disease (MELD) scale of 6 (less ill) to 40 (gravely ill) used to guide which patients received livers. However, the 2002 OPTN/UNOS policy had little structure guiding how HCCs should be diagnosed and reported to the networks. Assessment of UNOS data in 2006 indicated radiologic and pathologic assessment of HCCs only matched for 44.1% of cases. This prompted interest in creating new policy that would enhance imaging accuracy, diagnosis, and reporting of HCC to the transplant networks in order to better distribute liver transplants to HCC patients most likely to benefit.

The new liver allocation policy was approved by OPTN/UNOS in 2011. This policy outlines various technological and procedural standards for imaging, classifying, and reporting HCC studies to OPTN. Under the OPTN classification system there are two broad categories of classes, Class 0 and class 5. Class 0 imaging studies are not of sufficient standard to qualify for exception points, and

Class 5 studies may qualify for exemption points. Based on characteristics of the tumor upon imaging, the HCC may be reported as Class 5A, 5A-g, 5B, 5T, or 5X, each of which may change the number of exemption points a patient may receive and change their likelihood of receiving a liver transplant.

In-Depth [policy update]: To increase the likelihood that patients with early-stage HCC receive a liver transplant, as their post transplant survival rates are high but current severity of illness is relatively low, these patients are given exception points on OPTN/UNOS transplant lists. New OPTN/UNOS recommendations aim to verify that patients receiving exemption points do indeed have early-stage HCC and outline technological and procedural standards to be met for imaging studies. Such standards include type of CT or MR scanner and contrast to be used. If a liver imaging study reported to OPTN/UNOS does not meet these recommended specifications, it is assigned as Class 0 and no exemption points can be applied. For Class 0 studies it is recommended that the imaging study be redone meeting stated standards.

If the imaging study meets these standards, it is Class 5 and further categorized. If the nodule in question is 1-2 cm in diameter and meets qualitative imaging criteria for HCC it is Class 5A. If a nodule appears arterially hyperenhanced, is at least 10 mm in diameter at diagnosis, and has grown 50+% in diameter over a period of 6 months or less is Class 5A-g. A patient having 2-3 Class 5A or 5A-g lesions would qualify them for exemption points. Arterially enhanced 2-5 cm nodules with at least one of two venous phase features (washout or pseudocapsule), or arterially enhanced 2-5 cm nodules displaying 50+% growth in diameter over a period of 6 months or less is Class 5B. Exemption points may be individually requested for Class 5B nodules. Arterially enhanced 5+cm nodules with at least one of two venous features, is Class 5X and typically not eligible for liver transplant. Nodules categorized as Class 5 or confirmed as HCC upon biopsy which were subsequently treated are Class 5T. Class 5T nodules may receive exemption points based on the prior treatment and size. Reports to OPTN seeking exemption points for HCC must use the described classification system. A summary at the end of the report listing number, location, and size of nodules is strongly encouraged.

Wald C, Russo M, Heimbach J, Hussain H, Pomfret E, Bruix J. New OPTN/UNOS Policy for Liver Transplant Allocation: Standardization of Liver Imaging, Diagnosis, Classification, and Reporting of Hepatocellular Carcinoma. Radiology. 2013;266(2):376-382.

The CLOT trial: Dalteparin vs warfarin for venous thromboembolism in malignancy

1. Dalteparin, a low-molecular-weight heparin (LMWH), was superior to warfarin in preventing recurrent venous thromboembolism (VTE) in the setting of malignancy.

2. There was no significant difference in risk of major bleeding with dalteparin as compared to warfarin.

Original Date of Publication: July 2003

Study Rundown: Prior to the Randomized Comparison of Low-Molecular-Weight Heparin versus Oral Anticoagulant Therapy for the Prevention of Recurrent Venous Thromboembolism in Patients with Cancer (CLOT) trial, patients with VTE in the setting of malignancy were treated similarly to patients with other high-risk hypercoagulable states. That is, these patients were treated with long-term oral anticoagulation, like warfarin, with initial bridging with subcutaneous heparin or LMWH. There were questions as to whether the more predictable pharmacokinetics and drug interactions of LMWH could offer benefits compared to oral anticoagulants in the setting of cancer, given that these patients are often undergoing complex treatment regimens and are frequently further burdened with degrees of liver dysfunction and malnutrition. The CLOT trial sought to address whether long-term anticoagulation with subcutaneous dalteparin offered benefit compared to oral anticoagulation in the cancer population in preventing recurrent VTE. The study demonstrated that dalteparin was superior in preventing recurrent VTEs in the setting of malignancy when compared to oral anticoagulation with warfarin. There was no significant difference between the therapies in terms of bleeding risk. Given these results, in the setting of acute VTE associated with malignancy without active bleeding, it is reasonable to initiate treatment with a LMWH as opposed to oral vitamin K antagonists for up to 6 months to prevent recurrent VTEs.

In-Depth [randomized controlled trial]: The study included 676 patients from 48 clinical centers in 8 countries. Patients were eligible for the trial if they were adult patients with active cancer and newly diagnosed, symptomatic proximal deep vein thrombosis, pulmonary embolism, or both. Patients were excluded from the trial if they weighed ≤40 kg, had an Eastern Cooperative Oncology Group performance status of 3 or 4, had been treated with therapeutic heparin for > 48 hours before randomization, had active or serious bleeding in the 2 weeks prior, had platelet count < 75,000/mm³, had contraindications to heparin treatment or contrast medium, had creatinine ≥3 times the upper limit of normal, were pregnant, or could not return for follow-up. Patients were randomized to 2 groups: 1) warfarin with initial bridging using dalteparin and 2) dalteparin only. The study lasted for 6 months. The primary outcome was the first episode of objectively documented, symptomatic recurrent DVT and/or PE during the study period. Secondary outcomes studied included any bleeding event. The incidence of recurrent thromboembolism in the dalteparin only group was significantly lower than the oral anticoagulation group (HR 0.48; 95%CI 0.30-0.77). There was no significant difference in bleeding detected between the groups, with 6% of patients in the dalteparin group and 4% in the oral anticoagulation group experiencing bleeding (p = 0.27). The mortality rates were 39% and 41% in the dalteparin and oral anticoagulation groups (p = 0.53), respectively, and it was noted that 90% of these deaths were attributed to progression of malignancy.

Lee AYY, Levine MN, Baker RI, Bowden C, Kakkar AK, Prins M, et al. Low-Molecular-Weight Heparin versus a Coumarin for the Prevention of Recurrent Venous Thromboembolism in Patients with Cancer. New England Journal of Medicine. 2003 Jul 10;349(2):146–53.

Finasteride significantly reduces the incidence of prostate cancer

1. Finasteride therapy significantly reduced the incidence of prostate cancer compared to placebo.

2. Patients treated with finasteride were significantly more likely to have high-grade prostate cancers in a sample healthy population.

3. Patients treated with finasteride experienced significantly higher rates of sexual side effects, including erectile dysfunction, loss of libido, and gynecomastia.

Original Date of Publication: July 2003

Study Rundown: While some evidence at the time suggested that finasteride, which inhibits the conversion of testosterone to dihydrotestosterone, reduced the risk of prostate cancer, there were no large, randomized, controlled trials to support this observation. In this landmark study, patients with a prostate-specific antigen (PSA) of ≤3.0 ng/mL and normal rectal examination were randomized into 2 groups. In the first group patients received finasteride 5 mg daily and in the second group patients were given placebo. Over the 7-year trial period, this study demonstrated that patients treated with finasteride experienced a significantly lower incidence of prostate cancer than those in the placebo group. Patients in the finasteride group also had significantly higher likelihood of developing high-grade prostate cancer. The finasteride group experienced increased sexual side effects such as decreased potency, libido, and ejaculate volumes, but also decreased urinary problems such as incontinence, frequency, and urinary tract infections. Nevertheless, in the final analysis, mortality from prostate cancer was low in both groups (5 prostate cancer-related deaths in each group).

In-Depth [randomized controlled trial]: This double-blinded, randomized, controlled trial included participants ≥55 years of age, who had a normal rectal examination, and had a PSA level of ≤3.0 ng/mL. A total of 18 882 men were randomized to receive either finasteride 5 mg daily or placebo and followed for 7 years. The primary outcome measured was prevalence of prostate cancer over the course of the study. Secondary outcomes were prostate cancer mortality and tumor grade (specifically, Gleason grade ≥7) based on prostate biopsies. At the end of the study, all participants not diagnosed with prostate cancer were offered a prostate biopsy at 7 years ±90 days after randomization. The study was terminated 15 months prior to its anticipated completion - at this time, 81.3% of participants had completed the 7-year follow-up.

In the final analysis of 9060 participants, the rate of prostate cancer diagnosis was significantly lower in the finasteride group compared to placebo (RRR 24.8%; 95%CI 18.6-30.6; p < 0.001). A total of 48.4% of prostate cancer diagnoses were made based on end-of-study prostate biopsies, while the others were made based on cause-driven biopsies or interim procedures. Finasteride treatment was associated with higher rates of high-grade prostate cancer, defined as tumors of Gleason grade 7 or higher (37.0% vs. 22.2%, p < 0.001). The use of finasteride was also associated with higher rates of various sexual side effects, including reduced ejaculate volume (60.4% vs. 47.3%), erectile dysfunction (67.4% vs. 61.5%), loss of libido (65.4% vs. 59.6%), and gynecomastia (4.5% vs. 2.8%, p < 0.001 for all comparisons). Urinary urgency/frequency (12.9% vs. 15.6%), urinary retention (4.2% vs. 6.3%), and prostatitis (4.4% vs. 6.1%) rates were all significantly higher in the placebo group (p < 0.001 for all comparisons). There was no significant difference in mortality from prostate cancer in the two groups (5 deaths per group).

Thompson IM, Goodman PJ, Tangen CM, Lucia MS, Miller GJ, Ford LG, et al. The Influence of Finasteride on the Development of Prostate Cancer. New England Journal of Medicine. 2003 Jul 17;349(3):215–24.

Radiofrequency thermal ablation superior to percutaneous ethanol injection in hepatocellular carcinoma

1. In patients with hepatocellular carcinoma (HCC) not eligible for surgical resection, the use of radiofrequency thermal ablation (RFA) demonstrated significantly higher local recurrence-free survival compared to percutaneous ethanol injection (PEI).

Original Date of Publication: July 2003

Study Rundown: HCC is the second-leading cause of cancer mortality worldwide and often occurs in the setting of cirrhosis and chronic liver disease. Curative treatment can be obtained with surgical resection or liver transplantation; however, a large proportion of patients are poor candidates for curative treatment due to poor underlying liver function. Both PEI and RFA are alternative modalities that induce local tumor necrosis in patients with HCC with underlying cirrhosis who are not eligible for surgical intervention. The purpose of this randomized controlled trial was to compare the effectiveness of PEI and RFA in patients with HCC.

The trial randomized over 100 patients with HCC ineligible for surgical resection or liver transplantation to either RFA or PEI, both performed with ultrasound guidance. Patients were excluded if they had advanced liver disease (Child Pugh class C) or evidence of extra-hepatic disease or vascular invasion. At the conclusion of the trial, there was a significantly higher rate of local recurrence-free survival at 1- and 2-years in the RFA group compared to PEI. Additionally, there was a trend towards the RFA group for improved overall survival, which did not reach statistical significance. The mean number of treatment sessions was significantly lower in the RFA group with no significant increase in the complication rate compared to PEI. The results of this study demonstrate a superiority of RFA compared to PEI and support the use of RFA as the optimal alternative modality in HCC patients ineligible for curative surgical intervention. However, this study does not provide data for survival beyond two-year follow-up; as such, the long-term benefit of RFA over PEI is unknown.

In-Depth [randomized controlled trial]: This was an open-labeled, multi-center randomized controlled trial analyzing the effectiveness of RFA to PEI in patients with HCC not eligible for curative surgical interventions. The inclusion criteria included all adult patients with cirrhosis and a concurrent single HCC < 5 cm in diameter or as many as 3 HCCs with a maximum dimension of < 3 cm in diameter. Patients must be ineligible for surgical intervention or liver transplantation. Key exclusion criteria included presence of extrahepatic disease or evidence of tumor vascular invasion. Patients were also excluded if the HCCs were located less than 1 cm away from the hepatic hilum or gallbladder. The primary outcome was overall survival with a secondary endpoint of local recurrence-free survival rate. Each RFA or PEI procedure was standardized and supervised by a trial co-investigator. Follow-up for evaluation of local recurrence was done by serum α_1-fetoprotein and abdominal ultrasound at three-month intervals and dual phase spiral computed tomography at 6 month intervals.

Overall, 50 patients were randomized to the PEI group and 52 patients were randomized to the RFA group. There were no statistically significant differences in baseline characteristics in each treatment group, with the exception of patient age and albumin concentration. Patients were followed up for mean period of 22.9 months and 22.4 months for the RFA and PEI group, respectively. At the conclusion of the trial, the 1- and 2-year local recurrence survival rate was significantly higher in the RFA group compared to the PEI group (RR: 0.17; 95%CI 0.06-0.51; p = 0.002). There was a trend towards increased 1- and 2-year overall survival in the RFA group compared to PEI, which did not reach statistical significance (RR: 0.20; 95%CI 0.02-1.69; p = 0.138). Patients in the PEI group had an average of 5.4 (+/- 1.6) PEI sessions while the RFA group had an average of 1.1 (+/- 0.5) sessions. There was no significant difference in the frequency of adverse events such as post-procedural pain and fever. There were no procedure-related deaths, hemorrhage, or infection noted in either treatment group.

Lencioni RA, Allgaier H-P, Cioni D, Olschewski M, Deibert P, Crocetti L, et al. Small Hepatocellular Carcinoma in Cirrhosis: Randomized Comparison of Radio-frequency Thermal Ablation versus Percutaneous Ethanol Injection. Radiology. 2003 Jul 1;228(1):235–40.

Dexamethasone effective as an initial therapy for immune thrombocytopenic purpura

1. Of 125 patients with newly diagnosed immune thrombocytopenic purpura (ITP), 106 (85%) had an initial response to high-dose dexamethasone therapy.

2. Half of the 106 patients with an initial response to high-dose dexamethasone had a sustained response after 6 months of follow-up.

Original Date of Publication: August 2003

Study Rundown: This study assessed the effectiveness of high-dose dexamethasone as an initial therapy for newly diagnosed ITP. The results were promising as 85% of patients showed an initial response to therapy and half of these patients had a sustained response after six months of follow-up. This demonstrated that a short course (i.e., four days) of high-dose glucocorticoids could be effective as an initial treatment for ITP, avoiding the numerous and potentially severe complications associated with longer courses of prednisone, which was the standard therapy at the time. The high-dose dexamethasone was well-tolerated. No patients discontinued treatment due to side effects in this study. This prospective case-series involved a relatively large sample of patients; however, the study lacked a control group to compare its performance to a placebo or treatment with prednisone.

In-Depth [case series study]: This study recruited consecutive adult patients who presented with a new diagnosis of ITP. Of 157 consecutive patients, 125 met eligibility criteria – a platelet count of less than 20 000 per mm^3, or a platelet count of less than 50 000 per mm^3 and clinically significant bleeding. The exclusion criteria were relapsed ITP, treatment with corticosteroids in the previous 6 months, a history of clinically significant adverse effects from previous corticosteroid treatment (e.g., psychosis, avascular necrosis), uncontrolled hypertension or diabetes mellitus, and pregnancy. Patients were treated with 40 mg daily of oral dexamethasone for 4 days. Initial treatment response was defined as an increase in platelet count of at least 30 000 per mm^3, a platelet count greater than 50 000 per mm^3 by day 10 after treatment was started, and bleeding cessation. A sustained response was defined as a platelet count above 50 000 per mm^3 after 6 months of follow-up. Of the 125 patients included, 106 (85%) had an initial response to high-dose dexamethasone. Of the 19 patients who did not have a treatment response, 14 responded to either intravenous immune globulin or anti-D immune globulin. The remaining patients underwent splenectomy or received cytotoxic therapy. The median follow-up period was 30.5 months. Of the 106 patients with an initial response to dexamethasone therapy, 53 (50%) had a sustained response and required no further treatment. The remaining 53 patients had a relapse but responded to a second course of high-dose dexamethasone. No patient discontinued treatment due to adverse effects.

Cheng Y, Wong RSM, Soo YOY, Chui CH, Lau FY, Chan NPH, et al. Initial Treatment of Immune Thrombocytopenic Purpura with High-Dose Dexamethasone. New England Journal of Medicine. 2003 Aug 28;349(9):831–6.

The Wells DVT criteria: A clinical prediction model for deep vein thrombosis

1. The Wells DVT criteria estimated the pre-test probability of deep vein thrombosis (DVT).

2. D-dimer testing in outpatients informed the need for venous ultrasonography in the diagnosis of DVT.

Original Date of Publication: September 2003

Study Rundown: DVT is a condition where blood clots form in the deep venous system. While DVTs most frequently occur in the lower extremities, they may also develop in the upper extremities and other deep veins, such as the portal vein. Patients with DVT often present with pain, swelling, and erythema in the affected extremity. Pulmonary embolism is a concerning and potentially life-threatening complication of DVT, as pieces of thrombus may embolize to the lungs. As a result, patients with DVT are often treated with anticoagulants or, in certain circumstances, mechanical vena caval filters. Originally developed in 1995, the Wells DVT criteria help determine a patient's pre-test probability of having a DVT. These criteria have been subsequently refined and included in an algorithm to guide diagnostic evaluation for DVT using D-dimer testing and venous ultrasonography. This study was published in 2003 and helped elucidate the role of D-dimer in evaluating patients with suspected DVT. The trial found that the D-dimer test had a negative predictive value of 99.1% (95%CI 96.7-99.9) in patients with low pre-test probability of DVT. In patients likely to have a DVT, its negative predictive value was 89.0% (95%CI 80.7-94.6). Thus, D-dimer testing was deemed useful to rule out DVT in patients with low likelihood of thrombus based on clinical assessment.

In-Depth [randomized controlled trial]: In this study, 1096 outpatients who presented with a suspected DVT were first assessed using the clinical model to determine their pre-test probability of DVT (i.e., likely or unlikely). Investigators then randomized patients to the control group (i.e., ultrasonography) or to the intervention group (i.e., D-dimer and ultrasonography). There were no significant differences between the groups in terms of thromboembolic events encountered in follow-up at 3 months. The D-dimer group was associated with significantly lower use of venous ultrasonography, compared to the control group. In patients unlikely to have DVT, the D-dimer test had a negative predictive value of 99.1% (95%CI 96.7-99.9). In patients likely to have DVT, the D-dimer test had a negative predictive value of 89.0% (95%CI 80.7-94.6).

The Wells DVT criteria (Figure)

≥2 indicates that the probability of DVT is likely; < 2 indicates that the probability of DVT is unlikely.

Wells PS, Anderson DR, Rodger M, Forgie M, Kearon C, Dreyer J, et al. Evaluation of D-Dimer in the Diagnosis of Suspected Deep-Vein Thrombosis. New England Journal of Medicine. 2003 Sep 25;349(13):1227–35.

Criteria	Points
Active cancer	1
Bedridden recently > 3 days or major surgery within 4 weeks	1
Calf swelling > 3 cm compared to the other leg (measured 10 cm below tibial tuberosity)	1
Collateral (nonvaricose) superficial veins present	1
Entire leg swollen	1
Localized tenderness along deep venous system	1
Pitting edema, greater in symptomatic leg	1
Paralysis, paresis, or recent plaster immobilization of the lower extremity	1
Previously documented DVT	1

Table I. The Wells DVT Criteria. ≥2 indicates that the probability of DVT is likely; < 2 indicates that the probability of DVT is unlikely.

Hepatocellular carcinoma screening reduces mortality in high risk patients

1. Patients at a high risk for hepatocellular carcinoma (HCC) who underwent biannual screening with serum alpha-fetal protein (AFP) levels and liver ultrasound were much more likely to be diagnosed with cancer in the earlier stages and receive curative treatment.

2. Biannual screening for hepatocellular carcinoma led to a significant reduction in 5-year mortality.

Original Date of Publication: July 2004

Study Rundown: Since the 1970s, it has been common practice to screen for HCC in high-risk patients with AFP levels and ultrasound. However, this trial was the first randomized controlled trial to demonstrate a reduction in mortality with biannual combined screening. Compared to the control group, the group who received screening (at least once) during the course of the study had HCC diagnosed at earlier stages than the control group. More subjects in the screening group were able to undergo resectable surgery than in the control group. Five-year survival was 46.4% in the screening group and 0.00% in the control group. In summary, biannual screening with AFP levels and ultrasound significantly improved survival in patients with hepatitis B virus (HBV) who were found to have HCC. Biannual screening was shown to detect cancers at an earlier stage that allowed for more effective and curative therapy. Of note, the study only included patients with known chronic hepatitis infections. In addition, the majority of the participants was male and under the age of 50. Currently, the HCC screening guidelines do not discriminate by age, but it is important to know that these results may not be as accurate for an older population.

In-Depth [randomized controlled trial]: This study was conducted in primary care centers across Shanghai, China from 1993 to 1997. Eligible patients were all patients 35-59 years of age who either had a history of chronic hepatitis or serum evidence of a hepatitis B infection. Patients with a known history of HCC, other malignant diseases, or serious illnesses were excluded. Investigators randomized patients to screening vs no screening groups. Screening included a biannual serum AFP level and liver ultrasound. A subject's participation at least once in the screening was required for inclusion in the screening group. The median number of screenings a subject participated in was 5. Serum AFP levels above 20 mcg/L were considered abnormal. Any abnormality found on screening was re-evaluated by screening a 2nd time to reduce false-positives. Patients were followed for 5 years.

The primary end-point was mortality from HCC, with a significant reduction observed in the screening group (83.2 per 100 000) compared to the no-screening group (131.5 per 100 000 with a rate ratio of 0.63, 95%CI 0.41-0.98). Patients in the screening group were also more likely to be diagnosed with HCC at earlier stages (60.5% were diagnosed with Stage I HCC in the screening group compared to 0.0% in the no-screening group). Forty-six percent of HCC patients in the screening group were able to undergo surgical resection while 50.7% in the no-screening group were treated conservatively. Five-year survival was 46.4% in the screening group and 0.00% in the control group (X^2 35.50, p < 0.01).

Zhang B-H, Yang B-H, Tang Z-Y. Randomized controlled trial of screening for hepatocellular carcinoma. J Cancer Res Clin Oncol. 2004 Mar 20;130(7):417–22.

Intraperitoneal chemotherapy improves advanced ovarian cancer survival

1. Women with advanced-stage (≥Stage III) ovarian cancer randomized to intraperitoneal chemotherapy achieved an increase in overall survival compared to controls.

Original Date of Publication: January 2006

Study Rundown: Ovarian cancer is the deadliest gynecologic malignancy. Due to nonspecific presenting symptoms and disease predilection for early intraabdominal spread via peritoneal lymphatics, the majority of patients present with advanced-stage disease. As of the early 2000s, the standard of care for women with advanced disease involved optimal tumor reductive surgery, defined as resection of all disease > 1 cm, followed by adjuvant intravenous chemotherapy. The most common chemotherapy regimen involved 6 cycles of paclitaxel and a platinum analogue, such as cisplatin. The peritoneal cavity is the primary site of disease in ovarian cancer, which triggered researchers to postulate that applying chemotherapy locally to the peritoneal cavity might improve disease response and decrease toxicities associated with intravenous chemotherapy. Previous trials comparing intravenous only (IV) versus intravenous plus intraperitoneal (IV/IP) chemotherapy produced mixed results: one demonstrated a significant survival advantage in the IV/IP group while another showed an improvement in the progression-free interval but not survival.

This landmark Phase 3 clinical trial compared the standard of care, IV cisplatin/paclitaxel, to IV paclitaxel with IP cisplatin/paclitaxel and found that the IV/IP regimen was associated with increase in both progression-free survival and overall survival. However, the minority (<50%) of patients in the IV/IP group completed 6 cycles of treatment due to toxicities including fatigue, pain and neurologic side effects. Findings changed clinical practice such that patients with advanced-stage ovarian cancer who seek to maximize survival at the cost of an increased risk of treatment-associated toxicities are now offered IP chemotherapy. Strengths included parsimonious, multicenter, randomized controlled trial through the Gynecologic Oncology Group (GOG). Central review of the complete medical record by GOG physician-scientists permitted adherence to strict inclusion and exclusion criteria. Findings are limited by a low completion rate of IV/IP regimen due to toxicities, which may bias results toward the null.

In-Depth [randomized controlled trial]: A total of 415 women with Stage III ovarian carcinoma or primary peritoneal carcinoma who underwent optimal tumor reductive surgery (no residual mass greater than 1.0 cm) were randomized to receive intravenous cisplatin/paclitaxel ("IV," n = 210) or intravenous paclitaxel followed by intraperitoneal cisplatin/paclitaxel ("IV/IP," n = 205) for 6 cycles of chemotherapy occurring every three weeks at one of the Gynecologic Oncology Group (GOG) clinical centers across the United States (Columbus, New York, Irvine, Philadelphia, Oklahoma, Baltimore). Primary outcome was duration of overall survival. Secondary outcomes included progression-free survival, quality of life and treatment-associated toxicities.

Among women with Stage III ovarian cancer who underwent optimal tumor reductive surgery, those randomized to IV/IP chemotherapy experienced an increased duration of overall survival (67 versus 50 months, p = 0.03) and a longer progression-free survival (24 versus 18 months, p = 0.05) compared to those randomized to IV chemotherapy. Compared to women receiving standard IV chemotherapy alone, women in the IV/IP group were more likely to report toxicities including fatigue, pain and neurologic side effects but experienced a similar quality of life 1 year after treatment.

Armstrong DK, Bundy B, Wenzel L, Huang HQ, Baergen R, Lele S, et al. Intraperitoneal cisplatin and paclitaxel in ovarian cancer. The New England Journal of Medicine. 2006;354(1):34-43.

The RAPTURE trial: Radiofrequency ablation effective and safe in lung cancer

1. Percutaneous radiofrequency ablation (RFA) demonstrated robust levels of efficacy and safety in patients with malignant lung cancers who are poor candidates for surgery.

2. RFA was only performed in lung tumors less than 3.5 cm in diameter in this cohort.

Original Date of Publication: July 2008

Study Rundown: Primary lung cancer is the leading cause of death in the United States with over 160 000 deaths annually. Lungs are also a frequent site of metastasis from colorectal, breast, and renal cancers. Traditional treatment of malignant lung cancers primarily involved surgical resection. However, this excluded a large group of patients with reduced pulmonary reserve or comorbid conditions who were deemed poor surgical candidates. A previous retrospective review by Simon et al. demonstrated in a cohort of 153 patients that CT-guided RFA of lung tumors were associated with robust rates of safety and promising long-term survival rates. The purpose of this landmark prospective trial was to determine the safety and efficacy of RFA in malignant lung cancers.

The trial prospectively followed over 100 patients with either non-small cell lung cancer (NSCLC) or lung metastasis that was deemed ineligible for other curative treatments. The trial only included patients with up to three tumors per lung with no tumor larger than 3.5 cm in diameter. The primary outcome was technical success, safety, and confirmed response as determined by a 1 month follow-up CT scan. At the conclusion of the trial, technical success was achieved in 99% of patients with no significant changes to pulmonary function or procedure-related deaths within the study group. Complete clinical response was maintained in 88% of patients at 1-year post procedure, with no difference in responsiveness between tumor subtypes. The study is limited by the relatively small sample size and the lack of efficacy data for masses greater than 3.5 cm due to the technical size limitations of the ablation sphere. Additionally, Simons et al. and others have shown poorer clinical outcome for patients with tumor greater than 3 cm in size. Given the lack of current randomized controlled trials in this population, this was one of the first trials to demonstrate prospectively the robust technical feasibility and safety profile of RFA in the treatment of malignant lung cancers.

In-Depth [prospective cohort]: This study was a prospective, intention-to-treat, multi-center clinical trial of 106 patients from seven centers in Europe, United States, and Australia. Patients with pathology-proven NSCLC (n = 33), or metastasis from other primary cancers (n = 73) were included. All patients were deemed a non-surgical candidate or unfit for additional radiotherapy or chemotherapy. Key exclusion criteria included patients with greater than three tumors per lung, tumor size of 3.5 cm or greater, or patients with previous pneumonectomy. RFA was performed by a 150-200 W generators with a deployment device with a maximum ablation sphere of 5 cm in diameter. Post-procedure, patients were schedule for follow-up at 3 months intervals for up to two years. The primary outcome of interest was the technical success, safety, and rate of confirmed clinical response. Clinical response was defined as a reduction in tumor size of at least 30% with no evidence of tumor growth or contrast enhancement on follow-up CT scan. Secondary outcomes were overall and cancer-specific survival. At the conclusion of the trial, technical success was achieved in 105 of 106 (99%) patients. With respect to complications, 20% of patients experienced symptomatic pneumothorax requiring chest tube drainage, however, there were no procedural-related deaths or worsening of pulmonary function performance post-RFA. Confirmed clinical response of treated lesions was demonstrated in 88% of the patient cohort. There were no differences noted in tumor response between cancer subtypes. Overall, the two-year cancer-specific survival rate for patients with NSCLC, colorectal metastases, and other primary metastases were 73% (95%CI 0.54 to 0.86), 68% (95%CI 0.54 to 0.80), and 67% (95%CI 0.48 to 0.84), respectively.

Lencioni R, Crocetti L, Cioni R, Suh R, Glenn D, Regge D, et al. Response to radiofrequency ablation of pulmonary tumors: a prospective, intention-to-treat, multicentre clinical trial (the RAPTURE study). Lancet Oncol. 2008 Jul;9(7):621–8.

Additional Review:

Simon CJ, Dupuy DE, DiPetrillo TA, Safran HP, Grieco CA, Ng T, et al. Pulmonary Radiofrequency Ablation: Long-term Safety and Efficacy in 153 Patients. Radiology. 2007 Apr 1;243(1):268–75.

The RECIST 1.1 trial: Measuring tumor burden to assess response to therapy

1. Response to tumor therapy can be assessed by defined target lesions from a subset of measurable lesions.

2. Disease can be classified as demonstrating complete response (CR), partial response (PR), progressive disease (PD), or stable disease (SD) based on the radiographic evaluation of target lesions.

Original Date of Publication: January 2009

Study Rundown: The development of anticancer agents has also necessitated adequate methods to measure tumor response to therapy. In 1979, the World Health Organization (WHO) came together and published a set of criteria to standardize the research definitions of tumor response. Subsequently, researchers continued to disagree on certain definitions, including what constituted a measurable lesion, what the minimum size or number of lesions were to be recorded, how to define disease progression, and how to integrate cross-sectional imaging into response evaluation. These limitations led to modifications of the original WHO criteria, but adoption of these modified criteria remained nonuniform amongst researchers. This heterogeneity in the criteria led to development of new guidelines in 2000, described as the Response evaluation criteria in solid tumors (RECIST), which sought to unify and standardize many of the previously addressed limitations, and provide a consistent framework for the further evaluation of anticancer therapies. The original RECIST guidelines established the conditions for a measurable versus non-measurable lesion, the differences between a target and non-target lesion, and the definitions for therapy response, which included CR, PR, SD and PD.

Since the initial RECIST guidelines, subsequent difficulties and challenges were raised with the defined criteria. Specifically, there was disagreement in the maximum number of lesions to assess in order to measure tumor burden response, how to incorporate pathological lymph nodes into the therapy response, the type of confirmation needed for response in different types of trials, defining disease progression and unequivocal progression, and managing the detection of new lesions. These issues led to development of a RECIST working group to update the original guidelines. A combination of researchers, imaging specialist, and statisticians developed a database of prospective data in order to develop revisions of the original guidelines, named RECIST 1.1. These revised guidelines remained tied to the anatomical evaluation of disease rather than newer assessment tools (e.g. functional or hybrid anatomical/functional assessments of disease).

The RECIST 1.1 guidelines incorporated a large prospective dataset from numerous trials and determined that the maximum number of lesions required to assess tumor burden was 5, reduced from a prior maximum of 10, with a maximum of 2 per organ (down from 5 per organ). Additionally, lymph nodes with a short axis of > 15 mm were considered pathological and measurable. These could be defined as target lesions and the short axis measurement were included in the sum of lesions in the overall calculation for tumor response. Another revision of the prior guidelines was that randomized studies with a control arm for comparison did not require confirmation of response, as the control arm allowed for a comparative mechanism to measure response to therapy. Conversely, confirmation of progression is required in non-randomized trials in which the objective response rate is the key endpoint. RECIST 1.1 also updated the definition of disease progression. In addition to the original definition of a 20% increase in sum of the target lesions, it now also required a 5 mm absolute increase in the sum of target lesions (to prevent overcalling progression). Unequivocal progression in a patient with non-target and measurable disease was defined as the substantial worsening of non-target disease, despite stable or responsive disease, that would merit discontinuation of therapy. The use of FDG-PET was also addressed, incorporating it in the assessment of disease progression and/or the identification of new disease. Lastly, while CT and MRI could be used for the assessment of disease, ultrasound was excluded for the use of assessing therapy response.

In-Depth [prospective cohort]: This prospective cohort incorporated data from > 6500 patients, including simulation studies and literature reviews. This dataset prospectively documented the change in measurements of solid tumors, which included > 18 000 target lesions. Using these data, researchers defined a measurable lesion as one that could be accurately measured, and that the measurement taken was the largest dimension in the plane of measurement, with a minimum size of 10 mm by CT scan (obtained by a CT scanner with a slice thickness no greater than 5 mm). Additionally, a 10 mm caliper measurement by clinical exam can be used, or a 20 mm minimum by chest radiograph to measure index lesions. Lymph nodes were defined as pathological when they measured greater than or equal to 15 mm in the short axis (assessed by CT scan with slice thickness no greater than 5 mm). Lesions that did not meet these criteria are deemed non-measurable. Lesions must have measured > 20 mm if non-spiral CT or MRI is used. Lytic bone lesions were confirmed with PET, bone scan, or plain film, but only measured with CR or MRI, and only if they met the prior measurable requirements. Cystic lesions that were thought to represent metastases were measured if they met measurability requirements, but non-cystic lesions were preferred as target lesions. Lesions that have either coalesced into one lesion or broken up into smaller lesions could be measured, but lesions that have broken into smaller ones were treated individually and measured in their respective largest diameters. Lesions that were too small to measure reproducibly but were present on follow up should be assigned a value of 5 mm.

The response to therapy was obtained by assessing the baseline overall tumor burden, and was only be established in patients with at least one measurable lesion. In patients with more than one measurable lesion, a maximum of five measurable target lesions were recorded as representative lesions, with a maximum of two per organ site. RECIST guidelines delineated that these target lesions should be the largest lesions within their respective organs and should have measurements that are reproducible on subsequent measurements. Tumor burden was defined as the sum of the diameters of the target lesions, with the initial measurement taken as the baseline sum diameter. Once target lesions were identified, they should be used in subsequent evaluation studies. All other lesions identified are labeled as non-target lesions.

CR was defined as the disappearance of all target lesions, with the reduction of all pathological lymph nodes to < 10 mm. PR was defined as at least 30% decrease in the sum of the target lesions, in comparison to the baseline sum diameter. PD was defined as a 20% increase in the sum of the diameters in comparison to the smallest sum of diameters with an absolute increase of at least 5 mm. In addition, any new lesion was considered progressive disease. SD was defined as meeting neither the criteria for partial response nor for progressive disease, in comparison to the smallest sum of diameters.

These guidelines allow for the assessment of therapy response in patients undergoing antitumor therapy, but they rely on the assumption that all disease response is manifested as a steady decline in tumor burden. Subsequent research in novel treatment modalities, such as immune therapy, has suggested that positive disease response may not follow a linear decline in tumor burden, but in fact may have a small period of tumor burden increase or even new lesions on a short-term basis. However, with continued therapy, the overall disease burden may improve or continue to be stable over a long period of time, and suggests that the RECIST criteria may not encompass all types of therapy response, in particular with new targeted therapies.

Eisenhauer EA, Therasse P, Bogaerts J, Schwartz LH, Sargent D, Ford R, et al. New response evaluation criteria in solid tumours: Revised RECIST guideline (version 1.1). European Journal of Cancer. 2009 Jan 1;45(2):228–47.

Additional Review:

Therasse P, Arbuck SG, Eisenhauer EA, Wanders J, Kaplan RS, Rubinstein L, et al. New Guidelines to Evaluate the Response to Treatment in Solid Tumors. JNCI J Natl Cancer Inst. 2000 Feb 2;92(3):205–16.

Response Category	RECIST 1.1 Definition
CR	- Resolution of all known disease - Malignant nodes < 10 mm
PR	- Measurable target lesions - 30% decrease in the sum of longest diameter - No evidence of progression of other disease
SD	- Nonsufficient shrinkage to qualify of PR OR Nonsufficient increase to qualify for PD - Reference: smallest sum of diameters
PD	- Measurable target lesions - 20% increase in sum of longest diameter - Minimum absolute increase of 5 mm - Reference: smallest sum in study or appearance of new lesions

Table I. Recist 1.1 criteria. CR = complete response; PR = partial response; SD = stable disease; PD = progressive disease.

- Measurable lesion: longest diameter measurement of tumor lesions ≥10 mm (CT or skin caliper); ≥20 mm if by chest radiograph.
- Measurable node: ≥15 mm in short axis.
- Baseline sum: sum of diameters of target lesions, nodes, and longest diameters of other lesions.
- Disease burden assessed at baseline: measurable target lesions, up to 5 total (2 per organ); other lesions nontarget..

The PLCO trial 1: PSA and digital rectal examination in prostate cancer screening

1. Subjects who underwent annual prostate-specific antigen (PSA) testing for 6 years and annual digital rectal examination (DRE) for 4 years had a significantly increased incidence of prostate cancer compared to usual care.

2. Screening with PSA testing and DRE did not significantly reduce mortality from prostate cancer compared to usual care.

Original Date of Publication: March 2009

The Prostate, Lung, Colorectal, and Ovarian (PLCO) Cancer Screening Trial is a large population-based randomized trial sponsored by the National Cancer Institute (NCI) to explore the effects of screening on cancer mortality. The trial has been conducted at 10 different centers across the U.S. Participants randomized to the intervention group receive active screening for PLCO cancers (i.e., chest x-ray, flexible sigmoidoscopy, CA-125, transvaginal ultrasound, PSA, digital rectal examination) in the first 6 years of the trial and are subsequently followed for another 7 years. Participants randomized to the usual care group are managed with usual medical care and are followed for 13 years. The trial began in 1993 and the screening phase of the trial was completed in 2006, though follow-up will continue until 2015. We report below on the findings regarding prostate cancer screening using PSA testing and digital rectal examination.

Study Rundown: The combination of PSA testing and DRE was been the standard screening approach for prostate cancer for several decades. While many clinicians used this approach, there was significant uncertainty regarding the benefits and harms of prostate cancer screening. This led to the release of conflicting guidelines from different organizations, such as the American Cancer Society and the U.S. Preventative Task Force (USPSTF). The prostate component of the PLCO trial assessed the effect of annual PSA testing for 6 years and annual DRE for 4 years on mortality rates from prostate cancer. The study revealed that screening with PSA testing and DRE was associated with an increased incidence of prostate cancer, but not with a significant reduction in mortality when compared with usual care. Thus, the concern was that prostate cancer screening may expose patients to the risks of overdiagnosis and overtreatment of prostate cancer, with no actual benefit in survival.

The limitations of this study included a relatively high PSA testing and DRE rate in the control group, ranging from 40%-52% for PSA testing and 41%-46% for DRE. This rate of screening in the control group may have reduced the relative difference in prostate cancer mortality between the control and screening groups. Secondly, about 44% of subjects in both groups had undergone 1 or more PSA tests at baseline, which may have excluded more easily detectable cancers prior to the enrollment in the study, thereby also potentially leading to a reduction in the observed difference in prostate cancer mortality. Finally, it is possible that improvements in prostate cancer therapy equally reduced death from prostate cancer in both experimental groups, thereby dampening the survival benefits of early cancer detection from screening. In summary, the prostate component of the PLCO trial found that screening with PSA testing and DRE was not associated with significant decreases in prostate cancer mortality.

In-Depth [randomized controlled trial]: The PLCO trial was a randomized, controlled trial that enrolled 154 900 participants between 55-74 years of age from 10 study centers in the U.S. The exclusion criteria were a history of PLCO cancer, current cancer treatment, and more than one instance of PSA testing in the 3 years prior to enrollment. Of the enrolled participants, 38 343 were assigned to the screening group that received annual PSA testing for 6 years and annual DRE for 4 years, while 38 350 were assigned to the control group. Follow-up remains planned for all subjects for at least 13 years, but the results of this study were released with at least 7 years of follow-up for all patients and 10 years of follow-up for 67% of the patients due to public health considerations raised by the study's results. At 7 years, more subjects in the screening group were diagnosed with prostate cancer than in the control group (rate ratio 1.22; 95%CI 1.16-1.29). This difference persisted for patients with 10 years of follow-up (rate ratio 1.17; 95%CI 1.11-1.22). There was, however, no significant difference in mortality from prostate cancer between the screening and control groups at 7 years (rate ratio 1.16; 95%CI 0.76-1.76) or 10 years of follow-up (rate ratio 1.09; 95%CI 0.76-1.76).

Andriole GL, Crawford ED, Grubb RL, Buys SS, Chia D, Church TR, et al. Mortality Results from a Randomized Prostate-Cancer Screening Trial. New England Journal of Medicine. 2009 Mar 26;360(13):1310–9.

Stereotactic body radiotherapy as a state of the art treatment option in inoperable non-small cell lung cancer

1. Stereotactic body radiotherapy (SBRT) achieved a 3-year local tumor control rate of 92% with limited toxicity, making SBRT a valuable treatment option in inoperable (and potentially even operable) patients

Original Date of Publication: July 2009

Study Rundown: Lung cancer is the most common cancer worldwide, and non-small cell lung cancer (NSCLC) accounts for the majority of cases. Surgical resection remains the mainstay of treatment for patients with stage I NSCLC approved for surgery. Historically, medically inoperable patients with NSCLC were managed with radiation therapy (RT) and showed poor five-year survival rates, presumably from insufficient doses. Phase II trials, however, have shown that SBRT – a method using precise targeted radiation to minimize radiation to adjacent tissue – produces tumor control rates even higher than surgical intervention. SBRT can thus administer biologic doses up to twice as high as RT without harmful affects to normal tissue.

Though studies have shown good rates of local tumor control and toxicity for SBRT, the vast majority have been retrospective. Given the paucity of prospective trials and the lack of long-term follow-up data, application of SBRT remains limited. This multicenter prospective phase II study assessed the 36 month survival of NSCLC and evaluated tumor control, survival, and toxicity based on SBRT. The results indicate a tumor control rate similar to surgery in operative cases, a favorable 3-year cancer specific-survival rate, and minimal toxicity. The later Radiation Therapy Oncology Group (RTOG) 0236 trial from Timmerman et al. reported an even high rate of primary tumor control with minimal toxicity. It is noted that the optimal dose and schedule for SBRT is still undefined for treating NSCLC.

In-Depth [prospective cohort]: This prospective phase II study recruited 60 patients with medically inoperable stage I NSCLC, mainly due to COPD (60%) or cardiovascular disease (25%) across 7 centers in Nordic countries. Patients with prior malignancy or a primary tumor next to the trachea, main bronchus, or esophagus were excluded to ensure safety. After patients were referred to RT units, two were excluded based on insufficient radiation dose and one was lost to follow-up. The remaining 57 patients with NSCLC (70% T1N0M0 and 30% T2N0M0) were treated with SBRT using 6 MV from a linear accelerator, after defining the gross tumor volume (GTV, the size of the macroscopic tumor), clinical target volume (CTV, the volume of microscopic and gross malignant tissue), and planning target volume (PTV, the CTV plus a margin of safety around the tumor). CT was performed before each treatment to verify target reproducibility. Patients were then assessed with toxicity grading and chest CT or x-ray at 6 weeks, every 3 months for the first 18 months, and at 24 and 36 months following treatment. Lung function was measured at 3, 9, and 18 months using the Karnofsky performance score.

After the study's conclusion at 36 months, the Kaplan-Meier estimated progression-free survival rate was 52%. The lung cancer-specific survival rates at 1, 2, and 3 years were 93%, 88%, and 88%, respectively. The Kaplan-Meier estimated local tumor control at 3 years was 92%. Four patients (7%), all with T2N0M0 tumors, showed local tumor progression. No patient was lethally affected by SBRT and 14 patients (25%) had no pulmonary adverse effects.

Baumann P, Nyman J, Hoyer M, Wennberg B, Gagliardi G, Lax I, et al. Outcome in a Prospective Phase II Trial of Medically Inoperable Stage I Non–Small-Cell Lung Cancer Patients Treated With Stereotactic Body Radiotherapy. JCO. 2009 Jul 10;27(20):3290–6.

Additional Review:

Timmerman R, Paulus R, Galvin J, Michalski J, Straube W, Bradley J, et al. Stereotactic Body Radiation Therapy for Inoperable Early Stage Lung Cancer. JAMA. 2010 Mar 17;303(11):1070–6.

Immune-related response criteria captures tumor response to therapy

1. Immune-related response criteria should be used to capture the effects of immunotherapeutic agents as they more accurately capture the variable antitumor response seen after their use.

2. Ipilimumab monotherapy resulted in distinct response patterns that are not captured by the existing guidelines for tumor response described by Response Evaluation Criteria in Solid Tumors (RECIST) or other similar guidelines.

Original Date of Publication: November 2009

Study Rundown: The development of anticancer therapies spurred the development of novel methods for measuring therapy response. From early World Health Organization (WHO) criteria to more recent RECIST and RECIST 1.1 criteria, the development of a common language for the description of tumor response has been important for clinical and basic research. Importantly, these criteria have also established the guidelines for defining progressive disease (PD). However, the development of immunotherapeutic agents led to the clinical observation that the response criteria delineated by the WHO or RECIST guidelines did not seem to capture the response of these new, targeted therapies. Specifically, the original paradigm defined stable disease (SD) as a subset that had either not reached a definition for partial response (PR) or PD, and importantly, it was not viewed as an endpoint indicative of therapy response. In the immunotherapy trials however, stable disease has been used as a marker for improved clinical outcome. Another key difference observed in immunotherapy was that patients would often experience an increase in tumor burden before seeing an overall complete response, PR, or SD. Under the RECIST guidelines, a substantial increase in tumor burden would have represented PD, and led to the cessation of therapy, preventing researchers from demonstrating long-term therapeutic effects that may have occurred after this short-term increase in tumor burden.

In 2004 and 2005, an expert panel of over 200 oncologists, immunotherapists, and industry experts convened to develop new guidelines that adequately accounted for these observed clinical differences in patients undergoing immunotherapy. This expert panel used the results obtained from a large clinical trial program of patients with advanced melanoma undergoing immunotherapy. They concluded that the appearance of antitumor activity may take longer for immune therapy than for cytotoxic therapy, and that the response to therapy may occur after PD. They also provided a definition for clinically insignificant PD and suggested that SD durability may represent true antitumor activity. Additionally, new criteria were established for the assessment of tumor response, named the immune-related response criteria (irRC), which allowed for new lesions to be included into tumor burden without necessarily signaling progressive disease.

In-Depth [expert opinion] An expert panel used the clinical observations obtained from the use of ipilimumab (an immunotherapy agent that directs human monoclonal antibodies to block CTLA-4 receptor) in patients with advanced melanoma. These clinical observations were obtained from phase II clinical trials that included a total of 487 patients from 3 centers and recorded the patterns of clinical response to immunotherapy. Patients were treated with induction therapy followed by maintenance therapy, and an independent committee used the original WHO criteria and irRC to evaluate tumor response. Patients were expected to experience an increase in tumor burden before a response was obtained, and continued immunotherapy if they had not developed clinical deterioration. About 30% of patients who were treated in the phase II trials had CR, PR, or SD at week 12. Patients with SD at week 12 also demonstrated a slow response (PR and CR) after week 12. Additionally, patients who had PD at week 12 also demonstrated a response to therapy or SD after week 12 with the continuation of immunotherapy. Four distinct patterns of tumor response were obtained: response in baseline lesions by week 12 with no new lesions, stable disease, response after an initial increase in total tumor burden, and a reduction of total tumor burden concurrent with the appearance of new lesions after week 12. WHO or RECIST guidelines had previously not described the latter two criteria.

The irRC guidelines define tumor burden as the sum of diameters of index lesions and of new measurable lesions. Index lesions are defined as the two largest perpendicular diameters of all index lesions (with index lesions defined as up to five lesions per organ, 10 visceral lesions, and five cutaneous lesions). New lesions are limited to those that are greater than 5 mm, up to 5 new lesions per organ, 5 per cutaneous lesions, and 10 visceral lesions. For complete response (irRC), disappearance of a lesions must be confirmed by a consecutive evaluation no less than 4 weeks from the date of first documented complete disappearance. For partial response (irPR), a decrease in tumor burden must be greater than or equal to 50% relative to baseline and confirmed at least 4 weeks after documentation. For stable disease (irSD), response does not meet criteria for irCR or irPR, and there must be no evidence of disease progression. For disease progression (irPD), there must be an increase in tumor burden greater than or equal to 25% relative to the minimum recorded burden and must be confirmed by consecutive assessment at least 4 weeks from the date of first documentation. Patients could have irPR or irSD even in the presence of new lesions as long as they met the definitions of irPR or irSD. These new guidelines for measuring the response to immunotherapies allows for the incorporation of clinical criteria and flexible time points that were previously not captured by the guidelines set forth by RECIST 1.1.

Wolchok JD, Hoos A, O'Day S, Weber JS, Hamid O, Lebbé C, et al. Guidelines for the Evaluation of Immune Therapy Activity in Solid Tumors: Immune-Related Response Criteria. Clin Cancer Res. 2009 Dec 1;15(23):7412–20.

The RE-COVER trial: Dabigatran non-inferior to warfarin in treating acute venous thromboembolism

1. The RE-COVER trial demonstrated that treating acute venous thromboembolism (VTE) with 6 months of dabigatran 150 mg twice daily was non-inferior to dose-adjusted warfarin to an INR of 2-3.

2. Though dabigatran therapy does not require international normalized ratio (INR) monitoring, it is considerably more expensive than warfarin.

Original Date of Publication: December 2009

Study Rundown: Prior to the publication of the RE-COVER trial, dabigatran, an oral, direct thrombin inhibitor, had been shown to be as effective as enoxaparin in the prevention of venous thromboembolism after elective hip and knee arthroplasty. Another study had demonstrated that dabigatran was as effective as warfarin when used for stroke prophylaxis in patients with atrial fibrillation, while also having a similar safety profile and not requiring periodic INR monitoring. The purpose of the RE-COVER trial was to determine whether or not dabigatran could be used as an alternative to warfarin in the treatment of acute VTE. The findings demonstrated that in patients with acute VTE, dabigatran was non-inferior to warfarin in preventing symptomatic VTE or death associated with VTE. A larger number of patients in the dabigatran group discontinued their medication due to an adverse effect, and the incidence of dyspepsia was also higher in the dabigatran group. One common criticism of the study is that a pharmaceutical company played a large part in designing and conducting the trial. It is also important to note that treatment with dabigatran is considerably more expensive than warfarin, and that dabigatran should only be considered in patients with sufficient renal function.

In-Depth [randomized controlled trial]: The RE-COVER trial, published in NEJM in 2009, was a randomized, double-blind, non-inferiority trial comparing dabigatran with warfarin in the treatment of acute VTE. A total of 2564 patients were randomized to receive either 6 months of dabigatran 150 mg twice daily or dose-adjusted warfarin with a target INR of 2-3. Patients in both groups were treated with at least 5 days of parenteral anticoagulation prior to starting on their oral anticoagulants. Notably, the study was funded, designed, and conducted by the manufacturer of dabigatran in conjunction with the study steering committee.

The primary efficacy endpoint was a composite of symptomatic VTE or death associated with VTE in the 6 month period after randomization. Patients were assessed at 7 days after randomization, and then monthly for 6 months. Patients were recruited from 228 different centers in 29 countries. Parenteral anticoagulation was given for a mean of 10 days in both groups.

Dabigatran was demonstrated to be to be non-inferior to warfarin in the primary efficacy outcome. There were no significant differences between the groups in terms of the incidence of major bleeding, though patients in the warfarin group experienced a significantly higher rate of any bleeding event. Significantly more patients in the dabigatran group experienced an adverse event that led to discontinuation of the study drug (HR 1.33; 95%CI 1.01-1.76). Patients in the dabigatran group also experienced significantly higher incidence of dyspepsia compared to the warfarin group (2.9% in dabigatran group, 0.6% in warfarin group).

Schulman S, Kearon C, Kakkar AK, Mismetti P, Schellong S, Eriksson H, et al. Dabigatran versus Warfarin in the Treatment of Acute Venous Thromboembolism. New England Journal of Medicine. 2009 Dec 10;361(24):2342–52.

The EINSTEIN-DVT trial: Rivaroxaban in acute deep vein thrombosis

1. Rivaroxaban was non-inferior to standard therapy of enoxaparin and vitamin K antagonist (VKA) in treating acute, symptomatic deep vein thrombosis (DVT).

2. The risk of major and clinically relevant nonmajor bleeding was not significantly different when comparing rivaroxaban with standard therapy.

Original Date of Publication: December 2010

Study Rundown: The EINSTEN-DVT trial demonstrated that rivaroxaban is non-inferior to standard therapy (i.e., enoxaparin and warfarin) in treating acute, symptomatic DVT and preventing the recurrence of symptomatic venous thromboembolism (VTE). Moreover, this study demonstrated that there was no significant increase in the risk of bleeding with rivaroxaban, when compared to standard therapy. The new oral anticoagulants have shown much promise in randomized controlled trials thus far, particularly in treating acute VTE, VTE prophylaxis, and stroke prophylaxis in atrial fibrillation. Compared with low molecular weight heparins and VKA, these new oral agents are much easier to administer and also far less cumbersome with regards to monitoring. Concerns remain, however, regarding the lack of effective reversal agents for these medications, as numerous studies have demonstrated increased risk of clinically relevant bleeding. In summary, rivaroxaban was non-inferior to standard therapy, consisting of enoxaparin and warfarin, in treating acute, symptomatic DVT. Given the lack of a reversal agent, however, physicians should exercise caution in selecting the appropriate patients for treatment with the new oral anticoagulants.

In-Depth [randomized controlled trial]: The EINSTEN-DVT trial consisted of two studies carried out in parallel. The first was an open-label, non-inferiority study that compared the effects of rivaroxaban with standard therapy (i.e., subcutaneous enoxaparin followed by a VKA) in treating acute, symptomatic DVT (the Acute DVT study). In the rivaroxaban group, patients received 15 mg BID for 3 weeks, followed by 20 mg OD for the remainder of the treatment time (3, 6, or 12 months). Patients in the standard therapy group were managed with enoxaparin until international normalized ratios (INR) exceeded 2, and their VKA dose was titrated to an INR of 2-3. The second was a double-blind, superiority study that compared 6-12 months of treatment with rivaroxaban with placebo after patients had completed 6-12 months of treatment for venous thromboembolism (the Extension study). Patients in the rivaroxaban group received 20 mg OD. In both studies, the primary outcome was the recurrence of symptomatic venous thromboembolism (i.e., DVT, non-fatal or fatal pulmonary embolism). Notably, patients were excluded from both studies if they had creatinine clearance < 30 mL/min. or clinically significant liver disease (i.e., acute hepatitis, chronic active hepatitis, cirrhosis).

A total of 3449 patients were randomized to as part of the Acute DVT study, while 1197 were enrolled in the Extension study. In the Acute DVT study, there were no significant differences between the two groups in terms of the primary outcome (HR 0.68; 95%CI 0.44-1.04). Moreover, there were no significant differences in terms of major bleeding (HR 0.63; 95%CI 0.33-1.30). In the Extension study, the rivaroxaban group experienced significantly lower rates of the primary outcome, as compared to the placebo group (HR 0.18; 95%CI 0.09-0.39). Patients in the rivaroxaban group, however, did experience significantly higher rates of major and clinically relevant nonmajor bleeding (HR 5.19; 95%CI 2.3-11.7).

EINSTEIN Investigators, Bauersachs R, Berkowitz SD, Brenner B, Buller HR, Decousus H, et al. Oral rivaroxaban for symptomatic venous thromboembolism. New England Journal of Medicine. 2010 Dec 23;363(26):2499–510.

The NLST trial: CT screening reduces lung cancer mortality

1. Low-dose computed tomography (CT) screening significantly reduced lung cancer mortality when compared to screening with chest radiography.

2. Screening for lung cancer with either modality resulted in very high false positive rates.

Original Date of Publication: August 2011

Study Rundown: Prior studies have shown that lung cancer screening using chest radiography does not decrease lung cancer mortality. The use of molecular markers in screening is also under study, but currently unsuitable for clinical application. In contrast, observational studies have suggested that low-dose helical CT may be superior to chest radiography in detecting early-stage lung cancer. The National Lung Screening Trial (NLST) was a randomized, controlled study that compared 3 annual low-dose CTs with chest radiography in lung cancer screening. In summary, this study demonstrated that low-dose CT screening significantly reduced lung cancer-related mortality when compared with chest radiography. Additionally, low-dose CT screening detected more lower-stage cancers than chest radiography and low-dose CT significantly decreased all-cause mortality.

Strengths of the study include the participants' high adherence rate. Approximately 95% of participants adhered to the three rounds of screening in the low-dose CT group, while 93% adhered in the radiography group. Advancements in CT scanners since the time of the study may lead to further reductions in lung cancer mortality, though may also contribute to higher rates of false positives. The major limitations of this study are the limited follow-up and the very high false-positive rates in both the CT and radiography groups. Recently, the United States Preventive Services Task Force issued a draft statement recommending screening high-risk individuals with low-dose CT on an annual basis based on the results of the NLST trial, though there remains controversy in this area. The American Cancer Society, for example, recommends discussing screening with low-dose CT, while cautioning patients about the high likelihood of false positives and potential further investigation.

In-Depth [randomized controlled trial]: The NLST was a randomized trial that enrolled 53 454 patients. Eligible patients were between 55-74 years of age, had at least a 30 pack-year smoking history, and, if former smokers, had stopped smoking within the last 15 years. The exclusion criteria were a previous diagnosis of lung cancer, having a chest CT in the previous 18 months, hemoptysis, or unexplained weight loss in the previous year. In the end, 26 722 patients were randomized to screening through 3 annual low-dose CTs and 26 732 to 3 annual chest radiographs. Chest radiography, rather than community care, was chosen for the control group because the concomitant Pancreatic, Lung, Colorectal, and Ovarian (PLCO) cancer trial was evaluating the effect of chest radiography versus community care for lung cancer. Data analysis was conducted according to the intention-to-screen principle. For low-dose CT, any non-calcified nodule larger than 4 mm in diameter was classified as a positive finding. For chest radiography, any non-calcified nodule was classified as a positive finding. Results showed that low-dose CT was associated with a significant 20.0% relative reduction in lung cancer mortality (95%CI 6.8-26.7%, $p = 0.004$). Low-dose CT was also associated with significantly higher incidence of lung cancer (RR 1.13; 95%CI 1.03-1.23). All-cause mortality was significantly lower in the low-dose CT group by 6.7% (95%CI 1.2-13.6%, $p = 0.02$).

National Lung Screening Trial Research Team, Aberle DR, Adams AM, Berg CD, Black WC, Clapp JD, et al. Reduced lung-cancer mortality with low-dose computed tomographic screening. The New England Journal of Medicine. 2011 Aug 4;365(5):395–409.

The EINSTEIN-PE trial: Rivaroxaban to treat pulmonary embolism

1. Rivaroxaban, an oral factor Xa inhibitor, was non-inferior to standard anticoagulation therapy (i.e., low-molecular weight heparin [LMWH] and a vitamin K antagonist) in the prevention of recurrent thromboembolism following a pulmonary embolism (PE).

2. The rate of major bleeding was significantly lower with rivaroxaban than with standard anticoagulant therapy.

Original Date of Publication: April 2012

Study Rundown: For many years, standard therapy for PE consisted of LMWH followed by a vitamin K antagonist, such as warfarin. Although effective, treatment with warfarin requires frequent blood tests and is thus burdensome for patients. The EINSTEIN-PE trial found that treatment with rivaroxaban alone was non-inferior to standard therapy in preventing recurrent thromboembolism. It also demonstrated that rivaroxaban, an oral factor Xa inhibitor, did not require laboratory monitoring for the prevention of recurrent thromboembolism following an acute PE. The rivaroxaban group also had significantly fewer major bleeding events when compared with standard therapy. A major limitation of the EINSTEIN-PE trial was its open-label design, which increased the risk of bias. Notably, 5% of patients participating in the study had cancer. Previous studies, including the CLOT trial, have helped establish guidelines recommending the use of LMWH in treating thromboembolism in the context of malignancy, and this recommendation has not changed in light of the findings of the EINSTEIN-PE trial. The study was funded by 2 pharmaceutical companies.

In-Depth [randomized controlled trial]: Originally published in 2012, the EINSTEIN-PE trial was a randomized, open-label, non-inferiority trial involving 4832 patients. Eligible patients were those who had an acute, symptomatic PE with or without symptomatic deep vein thrombosis (DVT). Investigators randomized patients to receive rivaroxaban or standard therapy (i.e., enoxaparin with either warfarin or acenocoumarol). The primary efficacy outcome was recurrent venous thromboembolism (i.e., PE and/or DVT), and the primary safety outcome was clinically relevant nonmajor bleeding or major bleeding (defined as bleeding in critical sites). Rivaroxaban was non-inferior to standard therapy in preventing recurrent venous thromboembolism post-PE (HR 1.12; 95%CI 0.75-1.68). The rate of major bleeding was also lower in the rivaroxaban group, as compared to standard therapy (HR 0.49; 95%CI 0.31-0.79).

EINSTEIN–PE Investigators, Büller HR, Prins MH, Lensin AWA, Decousus H, Jacobson BF, et al. Oral rivaroxaban for the treatment of symptomatic pulmonary embolism. New England Journal of Medicine. 2012 Apr 5;366(14):1287–97.

The PLCO trial 2: Flexible sigmoidoscopy in colon cancer screening

1. Compared to usual care, screening with flexible sigmoidoscopy significantly reduced the incidence of colon cancer in the distal and proximal colon.

2. Screening with flexible sigmoidoscopy significantly reduced mortality cancers of the distal colon only when compared with usual care.

Original Date of Publication: June 2012

The Prostate, Lung, Colorectal, and Ovarian (PLCO) Cancer Screening Trial is a large population-based randomized trial sponsored by the National Cancer Institute (NCI) to explore the effects of screening on cancer mortality. The trial has been conducted at 10 different centers across the U.S. Participants randomized to the intervention group receive active screening for PLCO cancers (i.e., chest x-ray, flexible sigmoidoscopy, CA-125, transvaginal ultrasound, PSA, digital rectal examination) in the first 6 years of the trial and are subsequently followed for another 7 years. Participants randomized to the usual care group are managed with usual medical care and are followed for 13 years. The trial began in 1993 and the screening phase of the trial was completed in 2006, though follow-up will continue until 2015. Here, we report on the findings regarding colorectal cancer screening using flexible sigmoidoscopy.

Study Rundown: Colon cancer screening with fecal occult blood testing (FOBT) was previously reported to reduce colon cancer incidence and mortality. Flexible sigmoidoscopy is an endoscopic procedure where the most distal segment of the colon is examined. Previous studies conducted in Europe suggested that sigmoidoscopy was associated with reductions in both colon cancer incidence and mortality. The colorectal component of the PLCO trial assessed the effect of screening with two flexible sigmoidoscopies, spaced 3 or 5 years apart, on the incidence of and mortality from colon cancer in patients from the U.S. This study demonstrated that screening with flexible sigmoidoscopy was associated with a significant reduction in incidence of both distal and proximal colon cancer, regardless of the stage of the cancer, when compared to the usual-care group. Screening was also associated with a significant reduction in mortality independent of cancer stage, but only for distal colon cancer. For proximal colon cancer, screening resulted in reduced mortality for cancers staged I, II, or III, but not IV.

Study limitations included a substantial rate of endoscopy use in the usual-care group during the time the intervention group was undergoing screening - 46.5% of the usual-care group underwent either a flexible sigmoidoscopy or colonoscopy. This use may have dampened the difference in incidence and mortality between the usual-care and screening groups. In summary, the colorectal component of the PLCO trial found that screening with flexible sigmoidoscopy was associated with decreased colon cancer mortality and incidence. The study results support routine screening with flexible sigmoidoscopy followed by colonoscopy for cases of abnormal screening results.

In-Depth [randomized controlled trial]: The PLCO cancer trial was a randomized, controlled trial that enrolled 154 900 participants between 55-74 years of age from 10 study centers in the U.S. The primary exclusion criteria were a history of PLCO cancer, ongoing cancer treatment, and lower endoscopy (i.e., flexible sigmoidoscopy, colonoscopy, or barium enema) in the previous 3 years. Of the enrolled participants, 77 445 were randomized to receive flexible sigmoidoscopy at baseline and again after 3 or 5 years, while the other 77 455 were assigned to receive usual care. The primary endpoint was death from colon cancer, while secondary endpoints included colorectal cancer incidence, cancer stage, survival, harms of screening, and all-cause mortality. The primary analysis was an intention-to-screen comparison of mortality between the two experimental groups.

At a median follow-up of 11.9 years, the intervention group experienced a significant 21% reduction in colon cancer incidence compared to the usual care group (RR 0.79; 95%CI 0.72-0.85). This reduction was observed for both distal colon cancer (RR 0.71, 95%CI 0.64-0.80) and proximal colon cancer (RR 0.86; 95%CI 0.76-0.97). Additionally, there was a 26% reduction in colon cancer mortality due to screening (RR 0.74; 95%CI 0.63-0.87). This reduction was only significant for distal colon cancer (RR 0.50; 95%CI 0.38-0.64), but not proximal colon cancer (RR 0.97; 95%CI 0.77-1.22).

Schoen RE, Pinsky PF, Weissfeld JL, Yokochi LA, Church T, Laiyemo AO, et al. Colorectal-Cancer Incidence and Mortality with Screening Flexible Sigmoidoscopy. New England Journal of Medicine. 2012 Jun 21;366(25):2345–57.

The ATLAS trial: Duration of adjuvant tamoxifen in estrogen receptor-positive breast cancer

1. Among women with early estrogen receptor (ER)-positive breast cancer, continuing adjuvant tamoxifen for 10 years significantly reduced breast cancer recurrence, breast cancer mortality, and overall mortality when compared with stopping at 5 years after diagnosis.

2. Patients treated with adjuvant tamoxifen for 10 years had significantly higher risk of endometrial cancer and pulmonary embolism.

Original Date of Publication: March 2013

Study Rundown: In women with ER-positive breast cancer, previous trials had demonstrated that treatment with adjuvant tamoxifen for 5 years significantly reduced the risk of recurrence both during the treatment time and for 10 years after. During this 15-year period, mortality from breast cancer was also significantly reduced. Tamoxifen treatment, however, is linked with significantly increased risk of certain side effects, including endometrial cancer and thromboembolic disease. The Adjuvant Tamoxifen: Longer Against Shorter (ATLAS) trial compared the effects of 10 years of adjuvant tamoxifen treatment with 5 years of adjuvant tamoxifen treatment on outcomes in patients with ER-positive breast cancer. Over the duration of follow up, 10 year treatment significantly reduced breast cancer recurrence, breast cancer mortality, and overall mortality compared to the standard 5-year course of tamoxifen. However, this increased benefit came at the expense of significantly increased rates of endometrial cancer and pulmonary embolism. The study remains ongoing and future data will help elucidate the longer-term effects of prolonged tamoxifen treatment in patients with early ER-positive breast cancer.

In-Depth [randomized controlled trial]: This multinational study included 12 894 women with early breast cancer, 6454 of whom were randomized to continue tamoxifen for 10 years (i.e., the intervention group) after diagnosis and 6440 of whom were randomized to stop tamoxifen use at 5 years (i.e., the control group). While all 12 894 were included in the analysis for side effects, only women with ER-positive disease were included in the main analysis for breast cancer recurrence and mortality - 6846 women. Patients were eligible for inclusion if they had early breast cancer (i.e., completely resectable disease), they had subsequently received tamoxifen and were still on it (or had stopped in the past year and could resume treatment quickly), they were clinically free of disease (i.e., local recurrence resected, no distant recurrence), follow-up was practicable, and there was uncertainty between the patient and her physician regarding whether to continue tamoxifen treatment. There were no restrictions based on patient age, the type of initial surgery or histology, hormone receptor status, nodal status, or other treatments. Patients were not eligible if they had any contraindications to continuing tamoxifen (e.g., pregnancy, breastfeeding, retinopathy, endometrial hyperplasia).

In women with ER-positive disease, continuing tamoxifen treatment for 10 years significantly reduced the risk of breast cancer recurrence (RR 0.84; 95%CI 0.76-0.94), breast cancer mortality (RR 0.83; 95%CI 0.72-0.96), and overall mortality (RR 0.87; 95%CI 0.78-0.97) when compared to 5 years of treatment. Notably, during years 5-14 after diagnosis, the absolute recurrence reduction was 3.7% with extended tamoxifen treatment (21.4% vs. 25.1%). The relative risk of pulmonary embolus (RR 1.87; 95%CI 1.13-3.07) and endometrial cancer (RR 1.74; 95%CI 1.30-2.34) were significantly higher in women who continued tamoxifen compared to the control group, while the risk of ischemic heart disease was significantly reduced (RR 0.76; 95%CI 0.60-0.95).

Davies C, Pan H, Godwin J, Gray R, Arriagada R, Raina V, et al. Long-term effects of continuing adjuvant tamoxifen to 10 years versus stopping at 5 years after diagnosis of oestrogen receptor-positive breast cancer: ATLAS, a randomised trial. Lancet. 2013 Mar 9;381(9869):805–16.

The AMPLIFY trial: Apixaban for treatment of venous thromboembolism

1. Apixaban was found to be non-inferior to conventional therapy (i.e., enoxaparin followed by warfarin) in the treatment of acute venous thromboembolism (VTE).

2. Major bleeding was found to be significantly less common in patients treated with apixaban as compared with conventional therapy.

Original Date of Publication: August 2013

Study Rundown: New oral anticoagulants are being increasingly used for a number of different indications, including stroke prophylaxis in patients with atrial fibrillation and treatment of venous thromboembolic disease. The purpose of the Apixaban for the Initial Management of Pulmonary Embolism and Deep vein thrombosis as First-Line Therapy (AMPLIFY) trial was to determine if apixaban, an oral factor Xa inhibitor, was non-inferior to conventional therapy (i.e., enoxaparin followed by warfarin) for the treatment of acute VTE disease. In summary, apixaban was found to be non-inferior to conventional therapy in preventing recurrent venous thromboembolism or death from venous thromboembolism. The rate of major bleeding was significantly lower in patients treated with apixaban as compared with conventional therapy. Of note, the study was funded and partially designed by two pharmaceutical companies.

In-Depth [randomized controlled trial]: This randomized, non-inferiority trial was conducted at 358 centers in 28 countries. A total of 5400 patients were enrolled and randomized to treatment with apixaban or conventional therapy (i.e., enoxaparin for 5 days and warfarin for 6 months with target INR between 2-3). Patients were included in the trial if they were > 18 years of age, had objectively confirmed proximal deep vein thrombosis (DVT) and/or pulmonary embolism. Exclusion criteria included active bleeding, a high risk of bleeding, other contraindications to anticoagulation, cancer, provoked venous thromboembolic disease, dual antiplatelet therapy, and creatinine clearance < 25 mL/min. The primary efficacy outcome was a composite of recurrent symptomatic venous thromboembolism or death from venous thromboembolism. Secondary outcomes included each component of the primary outcome, in addition to cardiovascular mortality and all-cause mortality. The primary safety outcome was major bleeding. There was no difference in the rate of the primary outcome in the two groups (RR 0.84; 95%CI 0.60-1.18) and the findings met criteria for non-inferiority. Moreover, there were no significant differences between the groups in terms of the risk of cardiovascular or all-cause mortality. Major bleeding occurred significantly less frequently in patients treated with apixaban compared to those on conventional therapy (RR 0.31; 95%CI 0.17-0.55).

Agnelli G, Buller HR, Cohen A, Curto M, Gallus AS, Johnson M, et al. Oral Apixaban for the Treatment of Acute Venous Thromboembolism. New England Journal of Medicine. 2013 Aug 29;369(9):799–808.

The SOME trial: Screening for occult malignancy in unprovoked venous thromboembolism

1. There were no significant differences between the 2 strategies in the number of occult malignancies diagnosed, and the number of occult malignancies missed by the initial screen.

Original Date of Publication: August 2015

Study Rundown: Venous thromboembolism is a common class of disease characterized by the formation of clots in the deep veins. These clots can be classified as being provoked, or unprovoked in the absence of a known risk factor (e.g., overt active cancer, current pregnancy, thrombophilia, previous clot, recent immobilization, recent major surgery). Unprovoked venous thromboembolism has been identified as an early sign of cancer, as previous studies had demonstrated that up 10% of patients were diagnosed with malignancy in the year afterwards. Thus, clinicians have struggled with how to investigate potential malignancy in patients with unprovoked venous thromboembolism. The Screening for Occult Malignancy in Patients with Idiopathic Venous Thromboembolism (SOME) trial sought to address this question.

The trial randomized individuals with unprovoked venous thromboembolism to either limited-screening for occult malignancy or to limited-screening plus comprehensive CT of the abdomen and pelvis. There were no significant differences between the 2 groups in the number of occult malignancies identified. There were also no significant differences between the 2 strategies in the number of malignancies initially missed on screening, but subsequently discovered. Based on these findings, a strategy of conducting limited-screening for occult malignancy may be appropriate for individuals who present with a first unprovoked venous thromboembolism.

In-Depth [randomized controlled trial]: A total of 854 patients from 9 participating Canadian centers were included in the intention-to-test analysis. Patients were eligible if they had a new diagnosis of first unprovoked symptomatic venous thromboembolism (i.e., proximal lower extremity deep-vein thrombosis, pulmonary embolism, or both). Exclusion criteria included age < 18 years, refusal or inability to provide informed consent, allergy to contrast media, creatinine clearance < 60 mL/minute, weight > 130 kg, ulcerative colitis, and glaucoma.

Included patients were randomized in a 1:1 fashion to receive either limited occult-cancer screening (i.e., basic bloodwork, chest radiography, and recommended sex-specific screening) or limited occult-cancer screening plus comprehensive CT scan of the abdomen and pelvis. The primary outcome was newly diagnosed cancer during the 1-year follow-up period in patients with negative screen for occult malignancy. Secondary outcomes were the number of occult malignancies diagnosed, the number of early cancers diagnosed in screening and during follow-up, the incidence of recurrent venous thromboembolism, 1-year cancer-related mortality, and 1-year overall mortality.

There were no significant differences between the 2 groups in the number of occult cancers diagnosed. A total of 14 patients (3.2%; 95%CI 1.9 to 5.4%) in the limited-screening group and 19 patients (4.5%; 95%CI 2.9 to 6.9%) in the limited-screening plus CT group received diagnoses of occult cancers (p = 0.28). In both groups, several occult malignancies were missed by the initial screening strategies, with 4 (29%; 95%CI 8 to 58%) missed in the limited-screening group and 5 (26%; 95%CI 9 to 51%) missed in the limited-screening plus CT group (p = 1.0). Kaplan-Meier analysis showed that there was no significant difference in time to detection of missed occult cancers between the 2 groups (p = 0.87). There were no significant differences between the groups in the incidence of recurrent venous thromboembolism (p = 1.0), cancer-related mortality (p = 0.75), or overall mortality (p = 1.0).

Carrier M, Lazo-Langner A, Shivakumar S, Tagalakis V, Zarychanski R, Solymoss S, et al. Screening for occult cancer in unprovoked venous thromboembolism. The New England Journal of Medicine. 2015;373(8):697-704.

VI. Imaging

"In science the credit goes to the man who convinces the world, not to the man to whom the idea first occurs."

- Sir William Osler

Bosniak classification system differentiates benign renal cysts from cystic carcinoma

1. The presence of calcification, septa, irregularities or thickness in cyst walls on ultrasound (US) or computed tomography (CT) can be used to identify potentially malignant lesions requiring surgery.

2. Hyperdense cysts can be considered benign without further imaging if they demonstrate a specific appearance (smooth, round, sharply marginated, and homogeneous), lack of enhancement, and size < 3 cm.

Original Date of Publication: January 1986

Study Rundown: Renal cysts are a common incidental finding on imaging studies done to evaluate potential abdominal or pelvic pathologies. Most often, renal cysts are discovered through US or CT. While many simple or uncomplicated cysts do not pose any difficulty in diagnosis, the management of complicated cystic lesions has often been met with a difference of clinical opinion.

Bosniak proposed an approach towards the diagnosis of renal cysts using US and CT imaging. This includes a classification system for renal cysts and cystic lesions. Category I lesions include simple benign cysts of the kidney diagnosed definitively by sonography and/or CT. Category II lesions are minimally-complicated cysts that are benign but have some concerning radiologic findings (i.e. septa, minimal calcification, infection or high density). Category III lesions are complicated cystic lesions exhibiting some but not all radiologic features of malignancy, and therefore require surgical exploration. Category IV lesions are malignant cystic carcinomas.

In-Depth [review]: Bosniak provides a detailed diagnostic algorithm towards the radiological imaging of renal cysts. For masses first identified through urography without clear characteristics of malignancy (i.e. fat or calcification within the mass, increased tissue density, irregularity of margins, or invasion of collection system), US should be performed with results of previous imaging available for review. If the mass does not meet all criteria for a simple cyst on US, CT examination including contrast-enhanced and non-contrast-enhanced scans should be performed. Non-contrast-enhanced scans allow for evaluation of a lesion's contrast enhancement, which is of particular value in identifying vascular renal masses. The Bosniak classification system (Table I) was made on the basis of the most common and pertinent radiological findings made through US and/or CT with respect to renal cysts. This includes calcification seen within a renal lesion, which should always be interpreted as a sign of possible malignancy. However, if all other US and CT criteria for a cyst are present, a small amount of calcium or lining in the wall or septa of a lesion may indicate a complicated cyst without malignancy (category II lesion). However, extensive calcification in the wall of the lesion warrants category III classification requiring surgical exploration to rule out malignancy. Calcification associated with an enhancing soft-tissue mass indicates malignancy (category IV) and necessitates radical nephrectomy.

In addition, while many benign cysts have fine septa, lesions with numerous septa, irregular septal walls, septa over 1 mm in thickness, or with associated solid elements at attachment sites should be explored surgically (category III). If very irregular and numerous septa are present and associated with solid areas, a cystic carcinoma (category IV) can be diagnosed. Thickening or irregularity of the wall of a lesion also excludes benignity, placing such lesions in categories III or IV, depending on the severity of findings.

Bosniak also states the importance of assessing fluid density in cysts. Hyperdense renal cysts, usually containing old blood and often seen in patients with polycystic kidney disease, have a higher attenuation than surrounding renal parenchyma on non-contrast-enhanced CT scans. Following intravenous (IV) administration of contrast material, these lesions appear either isodense or hypodense when compared to the renal parenchyma, and can be considered benign if all of the following criteria are met: a) the lesion is smooth, round, sharply marginated and homogeneous, b) the lesion does not enhance with IV administration of contrast material and does not change in configuration, and c) the lesion is 3 cm or less in size. Lesions over 3 cm in size may still be benign, though US should be used to characterize it as a fluid-filled cyst. Lesions meeting all of the above criteria do not require surgical exploration or removal but should be monitored carefully through CT surveillance.

Bosniak MA. The current radiological approach to renal cysts. Radiology. 1986 Jan;158(1):1-10.

Additional Review:

Bosniak, MA. The Bosniak Renal Cyst Classification: 25 Years Later. Radiology. 2012 Mar;262(3):781-5.
Israel GM, Bosniak MA. How I do it: evaluating renal masses. Radiology. 2005 Aug;236(2):441-50.

Table I. Bosniak classification system.

Bosniak Category	Characteristics	Management
I	Water attenuation, nonenhancing	Benign; no follow-up
I	No septa, calcifications, or solid components	Benign; no follow-up
II	Few hairline-thin septa in which slight enhancement may be perceptible but not measurable	Essentially always benign: no follow-up
II	Fine calcification or short segment of slightly thicker calcification may be present in wall or septa	Essentially always benign: no follow-up
II	Hyperdense lesions: homogeneous, sharply marginated, nonenhancing, size < 3 cm	Essentially always benign: no follow-up
IIF	Multiple septa which can be minimally thickened, with slight enhancement that can be perceptible but not measurable	Usually benign; follow-up required to prove stability
IIF	Calcification of the wall or septa may be thick and nodular	Usually benign; follow-up required to prove stability
IIF	Hyperdense lesions: homogeneous, sharply marginated, nonenhancing, size > 3 cm	Usually benign; follow-up required to prove stability
III	Thick and/or irregular wall of lesion with measurable enhancement	Cannot exclude neoplasm; need surgical intervention for histologic diagnosis
IV	Distinct enhancing soft tissue components independent of wall or septa	Definitely malignant; need to be surgically removed

Ultrasound sensitive for appendicitis, improves outcomes

1. Among patients with signs and symptoms consistent with acute appendicitis (AA), ultrasound demonstrated a sensitivity and specificity of 80% and 100%, respectively.

2. The use of ultrasound led to an appropriate change in patient management in 26.1% of cases.

Original Date of Publication: September 1987

Study Rundown: AA is a common cause of abdominal pain in both children and adults, and can be challenging to diagnose by physical examination alone. By the mid-1980s a number of small, retrospective studies had been performed suggesting a diagnostic role for graded-compression ultrasound (GCUS), a technique that involves the application of pressure to abdominal wall with the ultrasound probe to minimize obscuring bowel gas. However, the results were felt to be equivocal, and GCUS was not widely adopted. In the present trial, the question of GCUS as a diagnostic tool in the evaluation of patients with suspected AA was addressed prospectively in a large cohort of patients at a single academic medical center. All enrolled patients were imaged after initial assessment by a surgeon, and changes in planned patient management were recorded alongside the diagnostic performance of GCUS. Results showed a high sensitivity and specificity for AA as well as a favorable trend toward improved patient care, with changes in management made for over one-quarter of patients. Notably, GCUS was not able to visualize the appendix in a significant minority of cases, in part reflecting limitations in ultrasound technology at the time of the study's publication.

In-Depth [prospective cohort]: A total of 111 consecutive patients (mean age 29 years, range 8-86 years) with a clinical presentation concerning for AA were prospectively enrolled at a single academic medical center over a 5 month period. All enrolled patients were first clinically evaluated by a member of the surgical staff using a combination of physical examination, laboratory studies, and plain x-ray images. Immediately following this, patients then received comprehensive abdominal ultrasound using graded compression for optimization of bowel visualization. All ultrasound studies were performed by radiologists and evaluated on several parameters, including appendiceal visualization, certainty of appendiceal visualization, and the presence imaging findings consistent with complications such as appendiceal perforation. After a maximum period of 6 hours of patient observation and prior to being informed of ultrasound findings, the evaluating surgeon was then asked to provide recommendations for operative or non-operative management. Imaging findings were then provided alongside an opportunity to alter management plans. The final diagnosis was determined using surgical pathology, intraoperative findings, or clinical diagnosis in combination with radiology and other supporting data.

An unequivocal ultrasound diagnosis was rendered in 83 (74.8%) patients. Among these patients, the overall sensitivity and specificity for the diagnosis of AA were 80% and 100%, respectively. When considering only those patients with non-perforated AA, the sensitivity remained essentially unchanged at 80.5% but decreased to 28.5% for patients with perforated AA. This was felt to be related to obscuration of the bowel wall by free intra-abdominal fluid and difficult patient examination secondary to peritonitis. In 29 (26.1%) patients, GCUS led to an appropriate change in management, including 16 (14.4%) patients originally triaged to conservative management who instead underwent surgical intervention. Among 4 of the 28 (14.3%) patients without a definitive final diagnosis, the appendix was unequivocally visualized but the patients did not undergo surgery because of symptom resolution.

Puylaert JBCM, Rutgers PH, Lalisang RI, de Vries BC, van der Werf SDJ, Dörr JPJ, et al. A Prospective Study of Ultrasonography in the Diagnosis of Appendicitis. New England Journal of Medicine. 1987 Sep 10;317(11):666–9.

Compression ultrasound identifies proximal deep venous thrombosis with high sensitivity and specificity

1. Vein compressibility assessed with ultrasonography (US) was highly sensitive and specific for the diagnosis of proximal-vein deep vein thrombosis (DVT) when compared to contrast venography.

2. Isolated calf-vein thrombosis could not be reliably detected through compression US.

Original Date of Publication: February 1989

Study Rundown: DVT refers to the formation of a blood clot within a deep vein, most commonly at or above the knee, such as the popliteal, femoral and iliac veins. If left untreated, patients are at risk for fatal pulmonary embolism. Diagnosis based on clinical signs and symptoms, however, is unreliable, necessitating the use of more objective testing. Historically, this has included contrast material phlebography, a technique that was later replaced by non-invasive tests such as phleborheography and impedance plethysmography. Impedance plethysmography reliably identifies occlusive thrombi in the proximal veins (popliteal, femoral or iliac veins), but is less reliable in the detection of non-occlusive proximal DVT and thrombi found in the calf. As such, other methods of DVT detection emerged, including US. While many different US diagnostic criteria had been initially proposed, Cronon and colleagues demonstrated that vein compressibility assessed through US could be used with high sensitivity and specificity in detecting DVT.

In this larger prospective study later conducted by Lensing and colleagues, gold standard contrast venography was compared to real-time B-mode US using the single criterion of vein compressibility. The results of this study showed that US had high sensitivity and specificity in the detection of proximal-vein thrombosis. Isolated calf-vein thrombosis, however, was not reliably detected through US, limiting its sensitivity for thrombi in this location. The study also found visualization of an echogenic band in the proximal veins to be a highly sensitive but non-specific criterion for proximal-vein thrombosis. Changes in vein diameter during the Valsalva maneuver were neither sensitive nor specific.

In-Depth [prospective cohort]: All outpatients with suspected DVT were referred for evaluation and consecutively screened for enrollment (n = 233). Key exclusion criteria included anticoagulant treatment for more than 48 hours before referral, known allergy to contrast material, or a recent episode of DVT in the past year. Following screening and consent, each patient underwent US of the symptomatic leg, where only the common femoral and popliteal veins were scanned. Compressibility of both veins was considered a negative test result, while non-compressibility of one or more veins was considered positive for venous thrombosis. Contrast venography was subsequently performed within 2 hours of US and interpreted by a radiologist blinded to the results of US. In a subset of 45 patients, US was repeated by an independent examiner to determine interobserver agreement on compressibility.

Contrast venography and US was successfully performed in a total of 220 patients (median age 56 years, range 17-86; 56% women). Based on the reference standard (venography), 66 patients were found to have proximal-vein thrombosis. Calf-vein thrombosis was confirmed in 11 patients. On US, all 66 cases with proximal-vein thrombosis were found to have non-compressible common femoral veins, popliteal veins or both. Therefore, the sensitivity of US in detecting proximal-vein thrombosis through non-compressibility was 100% (95%CI 95-100%). Of the 143 patients without DVT on venography, 142 had fully compressible proximal veins on US, yielding a specificity of 99% (95%CI 97-100%). The sensitivity of US in detecting calf-vein thrombosis, however, was limited to only 36% (95%CI 11-70%). Interobserver agreement on compressibility was 100% (kappa = 1). The study also found visualization of an echogenic band in the proximal veins to be highly sensitive (99%) but not specific (52%) in DVT detection. The percent change in vein diameter during Valsalva maneuver proved to be of limited use in detecting DVT with a sensitivity and specificity of 55% and 67%, respectively.

Lensing AW, Prandoni P, Brandjes D, Huisman PM, Vigo M, Tomasella G, et al. Detection of deep-vein thrombosis by real-time B-mode ultrasonography. The New England Journal of Medicine. 1989 Feb;320(6):342-5.

Additional Review:

Cronan JJ, Dorfman GS, Scola FH, Schepps B, Alexander J. Deep venous thrombosis: US assessment using vein compression. Radiology. 1987 Jan;162(1):191-4.

Fewer adverse drug reactions occur with nonionic than ionic contrast media

1. The prevalence of adverse drug reactions (ADRs) with the use of intravenous high-osmolar, ionic contrast media was over four-fold greater compared to low-osmolar, nonionic contrast.

2. Severe reactions, including dyspnea, hypotension, cardiac arrest and syncope occurred in over five times as many patients administered ionic media as compared to those administered nonionic media.

Original Date of Publication: June 1990

Study Rundown: Contrast agents, like any intravenously administered drug, pose a significant risk of immediate ADRs ranging from mild nausea, vomiting, pruritus or urticaria to severe and life-threatening reactions such as anaphylaxis or cardiac arrest. Prior to the widespread introduction of nonionic contrast agents in the 1980s, ionic agents were the only available contrast media for contrast-enhanced examinations or angiography, and the value of transitioning to the newer, unqualified agents was questioned on the basis of cost versus a potentially marginal safety benefit. The present study sought to determine if the use of nonionic over ionic agents would improve the safety of contrast-enhanced examinations through a large-scale prospective cohort during a transition period in Japan in which both agents would be in active use.

Including 330 000 cases over three years, the prevalence of any ADRs with the use of intravenous high-osmolar, ionic contrast media was 12.66% as opposed to 3.13% for low-osmolar, nonionic contrast media. Severe ADRs requiring immediate treatment occurred in 0.22% of patients administered ionic contrast media versus 0.04% of those administered nonionic agents. The most significant risk factors for the occurrence of ADRs included young age (less than 30), a history of atopy or other allergy, and a history of cardiac disease. These findings corroborated, on a large-scale, prior findings that the use of nonionic over ionic contrast agents posed a significant improvement in patient safety with regard to the occurrence of all ADRs, and even more importantly, the occurrence of severe and life-threatening ADRs at any level of baseline patient risk. Notably, this study did not examine the risk of contrast-induced nephropathy with these agents, instead focusing primarily on anaphylactic and anaphylactoid reactions.

In-Depth [prospective cohort]: This trial was conducted at 198 institutions across Japan over a period of three years and included 337 647 cases, during which both ionic (50.1% of cases) and nonionic (49.9% of cases) contrast agents were available and in current use in the country. The study was restricted to examinations utilizing intravenous contrast administration only. Cases were excluded if patients underwent examinations other than contrast-enhanced CT, intravenous urography or intravenous digital subtraction angiography, or if records of the ADR or contrast medium were incomplete. ADRs were recorded using a standardized event reporting form by the examining physician at each institution, and were reported at an average rate of 67.8% (range 59.1%-82.3%) independent of patient criteria. ADRs were defined as the acute onset of nausea, vomiting, sensation of heat, urticaria, flushing, vascular pain, hoarseness, coughing, sneezing, chest or abdominal pain, palpitations, rigors, or facial edema. Severe ADRs were defined by dyspnea, sudden hypotension, cardiac arrest or loss of consciousness.

The overall prevalence of all ADRs was significantly lower for ionic (12.66%) versus nonionic (3.13%) contrast agents ($p < 0.01$). An even greater difference was appreciated for severe reactions, at 0.22% for ionic (n = 367) versus 0.04% (n = 70) for nonionic media ($p < 0.01$). A single fatality occurred in each group, but they were not clearly causally associated with contrast administration. Over 70% of ADRs occurred within 5 minutes of contrast administration in either group. Subgroup analysis revealed that no significant differences in the prevalence of ADRs occurred according to sex or mode of injection. Groups with the greatest prevalence of severe ADRs included those with a history of prior reaction to contrast media (0.73% for ionic versus 0.18% for nonionic agents), a history of general allergy (0.53% for ionic versus 0.10% for nonionic agents) or atopy (0.49% for ionic versus 0.11% for nonionic agents), a history of cardiac disease (0.53% for ionic versus 0.10% for nonionic agents), and those aged 20-29 (0.24% for ionic versus 0.06% for nonionic agents.) Premedication with steroids, antihistamines or sedatives had a positive effect only on the prevalence of severe reactions for ionic agents, but not for nonionic agents. Lastly, subgroups receiving more than 80 mL of ionic contrast showed the lowest prevalence of ADRs (9.9-11.32%), while among those receiving nonionic contrast, the prevalence of ADRs was lowest for the subgroup receiving 81-100 mL (2.50%).

Katayama H, Yamaguchi K, Kozuka T, Takashima T, Seez P, Matsuura K. Adverse Reactions to Ionic and Nonionic Contrast Media, A Report from the Japanese Committee on the Safety of Contrast Media. Radiology. 1990 Jun 175:621–28.

Visualization of noncystic masses on transvaginal ultrasound sensitive and specific for ectopic pregnancy

1. Sonographic demonstration of any non-cystic adnexal mass is both sensitive and specific for in the diagnosis of ectopic pregnancy (EP) by transvaginal ultrasonography (TVUS).

2. Visualization of a non-cystic adnexal mass is comparably specific to direct imaging of a living extrauterine pregnancy or gestational sac, but significantly more sensitive for EP.

Original Date of Publication: April 1994

Study Rundown: EP is life threatening obstetric emergency in which gestation occurs outside the uterus, often presenting as an acute onset of pelvic pain with vaginal bleeding. The majority of EPs occur within the fallopian tube, but the embryo may also implant within the cervix, ovaries, or abdomen, and may require emergent laparoscopic removal in any of these locations. Accurate diagnosis includes both the measurement of serum human chorionic gonadotropin levels to confirm pregnancy and ultrasonographic visualization of ectopic products of conception, as confirmed by the works of Shalev et al., Condous et al., and Gracia and Barnhart. Once multiple studies confirmed the appropriateness of TVUS as the first-line study in the diagnosis of EP, the question arose regarding what must specifically be visualized at the threshold of positivity to most sensitively and specifically diagnose EP. The referenced study reviewed and meta-analyzed the contemporary literature to determine which of four criteria, in descending order of stringency, was most appropriate to use as the broad threshold for TVUS positivity in the diagnosis of EP. The four criteria reviewed were, at the most stringent, (1) direct visualization of a living extrauterine pregnancy, followed by (2) an extrauterine gestational sac with yolk sac or embryo, (3) an empty tubal ring, or extrauterine fluid collection with a surrounding hyperechoic ring, or (4) any adnexal mass other than a simple cyst, allowing inclusion of visualized hematoma in addition to any products of conception. The authors found that while the more stringent criteria were most specific (99-100%), they were highly insensitive (20-65%), and bore only moderate negative predictive values (78-89%). The least stringent criterion traded a minimally decreased specificity (98.9%) for a significant improvement in sensitivity (84%) and negative predictive value (95%). By these criteria, TVUS interpretation in the diagnosis of EP was simplified, thereby reducing failures to diagnose a potentially fatal condition while improving early recognition of EP and increasing opportunities for medical management with methotrexate over laparoscopic intervention. Notably, this study did not evaluate the effect on visualization of free fluid within the peritoneum, which may occur following rupture of an EP, but nonetheless established the most sensitive and specific criterion by which to interpret TVUS in the diagnosis of EP.

In-Depth [systematic review and meta-analysis]: This systematic review and meta-analysis pooled data from studies published between 1986 and 1993 examining the use of TVUS in the diagnostic workup of patients with suspected EP. A total of 2216 patients (1651 with EP, and 565 without) spanning 10 studies were included in which all enrolled patients were assessed by TVUS in the workup for EP with subsequent surgical confirmation of all cases. Sensitivity, specificity, positive and negative predictive values were calculated using Bayes' theorem for each of four different positivity criteria used as the diagnostic threshold in TVUS assessment. Given that EPs may be visualized as anything ranging from an intact extrauterine pregnancy to an adnexal hematoma or other complex adnexal mass, the four tested criteria sought to encompass a stepwise progression in sonographic specificity as follows: the most stringent criterion required visualization of an extrauterine embryo with a heartbeat (20.1% sensitivity, 100% specificity, NPV 78.5%); followed by an extrauterine gestational sac with yolk sac or embryo (36.6% sensitivity, 100% specificity, NPV 82.2%); an adnexal mass with a central anechoic region or hyperechoic rim, known as an "empty tubal ring" (64.6% sensitivity, 99.5% specificity, NPV 89.1%); or the least stringent criterion, any adnexal mass other than a simple cyst or intraovarian lesion (84.4% sensitivity, 98.9% specificity, NPV 94.8%). As the threshold for positivity became less stringent, the sensitivity dramatically increased, yet with minimal decrease in overall specificity, finding that TVUS performed best using the most lax threshold when EP is suspected. This study established the simplest and most effective interpretation strategy for TVUS in the diagnosis of EP for both presurgical and medical management, and created an interpretative baseline for comparison to alternative diagnostic techniques.

Brown DL, Doubilet PM. Transvaginal sonography for diagnosing ectopic pregnancy: positivity criteria and performance characteristics. JUM. 1994 Apr 1;13(4):259–66.

Additional Review:

Shalev, E, Yarom I, Bustan M, Weiner E, Ben-Shlomo I. Transvaginal sonography as the ultimate diagnostic tool for the management of ectopic pregnancy: experience with 840 cases. Fertility and Sterility. 1998 Jan 1;69(1)62–5.

Condous G, Okaro E, Khalid A, Lu C, Van Huffel S, Timmerman D, Bourne T. The accuracy of transvaginal ultrasonography for the diagnosis of ectopic pregnancy prior to surgery. Human Reproduction. 2005 Feb 3;20(5):1404-09.

Gracia CR, Barnhart KT. Diagnosing ectopic pregnancy: decision analysis comparing six strategies. Obstetrics & Gynecology. 2001 Mar 1;97(3)464-70.

MRI reveals lumbar intervertebral disk herniations are common in asymptomatic individuals

1. Magnetic resonance imaging (MRI) of the lumbar spine in individuals without back pain revealed that at least a single intervertebral disk bulge was prevalent in over half of those imaged, while over a quarter showed at least a single disk protrusion.

2. Other abnormalities were common, including Schmorl's nodes, defects of the annulus fibrosis, and facet arthropathy, without significant differences in the prevalence of any given abnormality between the sexes.

Original Date of Publication: July 1994

Study Rundown: Low back pain remains a difficult management dilemma given the chronicity of most complaints and poor symptomatic response to intervention, leading to a great deal of unnecessary spinal imaging at significant cost to the medical system. Even in light of positive findings on imaging, clinicians have had difficulty correlating symptoms to imaging findings. Prior to this study, the term "herniation" was used to describe the spectrum of intervertebral disk abnormalities seen on MRI ranging from small bulges, to larger protrusions or even complete extrusions without differentiation. The authors here showed that among individuals without back pain, the prevalence of at least a single disk bulge was 52% on MRI of the lumbar spine, with an age-dependent association demonstrated for both the number of disks affected and the prevalence of bulges seen. Disk protrusions were evident in 27% of asymptomatic individuals, while extrusions were found in only 1% of those imaged. The vast majority of disk abnormalities were found at the L4-5 and L5-S1 spaces, and least commonly at the L1-2 space. Similarly, findings of Schmorl's nodes, or disk herniation into an adjacent vertebral body end plate, annular defects, and facet arthropathy were seen in 19%, 14%, and 8% of asymptomatic subjects, respectively. These findings, in light of the more specific terminology introduced, demonstrated that disk bulges and protrusions, but not extrusions, were highly prevalent in the population and could not reliably predict symptoms of back pain, and in fact may be purely coincidental.

In-Depth [prospective cohort]: This prospective trial enrolled 98 volunteers without back pain symptoms (mean age 42.3 years; 49% female) at a community hospital in California. Exclusion criteria included a history of back pain lasting greater than 48 hours or any history of lumbosacral radiculopathies. Each subject underwent 1.5T MRI of the lumbar spine in both the axial and sagittal planes, and completed a survey to score their level of baseline physical activity from 0 (no exercise) to 4 (five or more workouts per week). In addition to the 98 MRIs produced for these subjects, 27 abnormal studies of the lumbar spine were randomly intermixed to reduce interpretation bias. All studies were interpreted independently by a pair of experienced neuroradiologists at an outside academic medical center blinded to the clinical status of the study subjects, and results of the two readings were averaged for final summary of the data. The specific nomenclature used to describe intervertebral disk findings was described as follows: Normal (without disk extension beyond the interspace), bulge (with symmetric extension of the disk beyond the interspace), protrusion (with asymmetric extension of the disk beyond the interspace), or extrusion (with the extruding disk material larger in diameter than the remaining disk in the interspace).

Among the asymptomatic individuals imaged, 52% had a disk bulge at at least one level, 27% demonstrated at least one protrusion, and only 1% demonstrated an extrusion, for a total of 64% of those without back pain demonstrating a disk abnormality at one level and 38% with abnormalities at more than one level. Abnormalities of the intervertebral disks were most prevalent at the L5-S1 and L4-5 levels, with a decreasing prevalence toward the L1-2 level. There were no differences in the prevalence of disk abnormalities between the sexes, but an increase in the prevalence of disk bulges was seen with increasing age ($p < 0.001$) at every disk level. Age also predicted an increase in the prevalence of multiple disk abnormalities ($p < 0.001$). The physical activity score did not correlate significantly to the number of visualized disk abnormalities. A variety of other, non-intervertebral disk spinal abnormalities were noted among those imaged: Most commonly, Schmorl's nodes were noted in 19% of subjects, defects of the annulus fibrosis in 14%, facet arthropathy in 8%, and spondylolysis, spondylolisthesis, central canal stenosis, and neural foraminal stenosis were each seen in 7% of imaged subjects.

Jensen MC, Brant-Zawadzki MN, Obuchowski N, Modic MT, Malkasian D, Ross JS. Magnetic Resonance Imaging of the Lumbar Spine in People Without Back Pain. The New England Journal of Medicine. 1994 Jul 14;331(2):69–73.

Breast ultrasound sensitive for cancer, carries a low false positive rate

1. In a large cohort of women referred for evaluation of one or more solid breast lesions, ultrasound (US) showed a sensitivity of 98.4% for malignancy and was associated with a negative predictive value of 99.5%.

Original Date of Publication: July 1995

Study Rundown: US is a powerful medical imaging tool. It is portable, quickly generates clinically-relevant data, and is not associated with ionizing radiation exposure. The technology has found applications in nearly every area of medicine, and has been particularly beneficial in the area of breast imaging. At the time of this study, US was used to help identify simple breast cysts, a common and benign finding that can generate initial concern when identified on mammography. Given the success of US in this area, numerous attempts were made to expand the technology's use to include other indeterminate breast lesions, particularly solid masses. Initial studies were unsupportive, however, and multiple guideline sets were published explicitly recommending against the use of US for solid breast mass evaluation.

Given dramatic improvements in the resolution and functional capabilities of US, however, this issue was revisited in 1995 with publication of this prospective trial. A large cohort of women with suspicious breast lesions referred for breast US were evaluated over several years. Only women with solid lesions were considered. All women underwent biopsy following their US, and biopsy and imaging results were compared to determine the diagnostic performance of US. Results revealed that, contrary to prior data, US was highly sensitive for malignancy in solid breast masses. Conversely, in the absence of concerning imaging features, US appropriately excluded malignancy with few diagnostic errors. Strengths of the trial included its prospective methodology, the large number of patients successfully enrolled, and the low attrition rate. The primary limitations of the trial included heterogeneous biopsy methods and the inherent variability associated with subjective rating scales. Today, breast US remains a substantial component of the breast imager's toolkit, and is routinely used for solid breast mass evaluation.

In-Depth [prospective cohort]: A total of 662 patients (mean age 47 years) with suspicious breast lesions were prospectively enrolled over an approximately 4-year period following referral for breast US. The most common reason for referral was an antecedent abnormal mammogram. A total of 750 solid nodules were evaluated by US. Studies were blindly interpreted by 5 breast radiologists and findings were classified as "benign" or "malignant" based on the presence or absence of several previously-published imaging features. When no features were present, a classification of "indeterminate" was made. When available, initial mammograms and their interpretations were also reviewed. All enrolled patients subsequently underwent either core needle or excisional biopsy for definitive pathologic diagnosis. These final diagnoses were compared with imaging results to determine the diagnostic performance of US in the evaluation of suspicious solid breast lesions.

Pathologic examination revealed 625 (83%) benign nodules and 125 (17%) malignant nodules. The most common malignant lesion was infiltrating ductal adenocarcinoma, and the most common benign lesion was fibroadenoma. One hundred (73%) of the 137 malignant nodules were correctly diagnosed by US. The overall sensitivity and specificity for breast US in the detection of malignancy were 98.4% and 67.8%, respectively. Due to a high false positive rate, the positive predictive value was 38%, while the negative predictive value was 99.5%, with only 2 false positive examinations. Twenty-seven nodules that were interpreted as malignant or indeterminate by US had been previously interpreted as definitively or probably benign by mammography. An additional 44 nodules accurately interpreted as malignant by US were interpreted as indeterminate by mammography. The US features most strongly associated with malignancy were speculation (OR 5.5), taller-than-wider shape (OR 4.9), and angular margins (OR 4.0).

Stavros AT, Thickman D, Rapp CL, Dennis MA, Parker SH, Sisney GA. Solid breast nodules: use of sonography to distinguish between benign and malignant lesions. Radiology. 1995 Jul 1;196(1):123–34.

Magnetic resonance cholangiopancreatography diagnoses bile duct obstruction with high sensitivity and specificity

1. Magnetic resonance cholangiopancreatography (MRCP) diagnosed bile duct obstruction with high sensitivity and specificity when compared to invasive endoscopic retrograde cholangiopancreatography (ERCP).

2. MRCP was highly specific but less sensitive in identifying causes of bile duct obstruction such as malignancy or choledocholithiasis.

Original Date of Publication: October 1995

Study Rundown: Ultrasound and computed tomography have long been used in the noninvasive diagnosis of biliary obstruction, though are limited by their low sensitivity in detecting common bile duct (CBD) stones. ERCP involves endoscopically accessing the pancreatic ducts and biliary tree and directly visualizing them via injection of iodinated contrast, allowing sensitive detection of stones and other pathology as well as the capability for direct therapeutic intervention if necessary. Its invasive nature, however, remains a limitation. MRCP was created to allow noninvasive evaluation of the biliary tree using magnetic resonance imaging.

In the study conducted by Guibaud and colleagues, MRCP was compared to ERCP in the diagnosis of bile duct obstruction. The results of this study demonstrated that MRCP can be used in diagnosing bile duct obstruction with high specificity and sensitivity, with few false negative results. MRCP was also able to correctly identify choledocholithiasis or malignancy as causes of obstruction with high specificity and acceptable sensitivity, informing its subsequent increasing use as a reliable noninvasive tool in the workup of biliary obstruction.

In-Depth [prospective cohort]: All patients with clinically suspected bile duct obstruction were referred for evaluation and consecutively screened for enrollment (n = 206). Patients were excluded if direct cholangiographic, histopathological or surgical proof of bile duct obstruction could not be obtained, ERCP was unsuccessful, MRCP could not be performed due to claustrophobia, or if the results of either technique were inadequate. All patients included in the study underwent MRCP with heavily T2-weighted fast spin-echo sequences. All MR images were evaluated by 2 reviewers without knowledge of clinical parameters or results of other imaging studies. The final diagnosis and, where applicable, the cause of bile duct obstruction, was determined through ERCP. The following diagnoses were considered causes of obstruction: CBD stones, malignant obstruction, chronic pancreatitis, intrahepatic stones and distal obstruction from an undetermined cause.

ERCP and MRCP were successfully performed in a total of 126 patients (mean age 57 years, range 12-91 years; 40% male). Based on the reference standard, 79 patients (63%) were found to have bile duct obstruction. Among these patients, MRCP correctly diagnosed bile duct obstruction in 72 patients, yielding a sensitivity of 91% (95%CI 85-100%) and specificity of 100%. In addition, MRCP correctly diagnosed malignancy as a cause of obstruction in 12 out of 14 patients, corresponding to a sensitivity of 86% (95%CI 67-100%) and specificity of 98% (95%CI 96-100%). In diagnosing choledocholithiasis as a cause of obstruction, the sensitivity of MRCP was less at 81% (95%CI 68-95%), with a specificity of 98% (95%CI 95-100%).

Guibaud L, Bret PM, Reinhold C, Atri M, Barkun AN. Bile duct obstruction and choledocholithiasis: diagnosis with MR cholangiography. Radiology. 1995 Oct;197(1):109-15.

Chemical shift and gadolinium-enhanced MRI identifies adrenal adenomas with high specificity and acceptable sensitivity

1. The relative change in mass-liver signal intensity (SI) ratio on opposed-phase versus in-phase magnetic resonance (MR) imaging was highly specific and sensitive in characterizing adrenal masses as adenomas.

2. Adenomas and nonadenomas could not be effectively differentiated with maximum SI after contrast administration or maximum washout.

Original Date of Publication: November 1995

Study Rundown: Adrenal masses are common incidental findings seen on computed tomography and encompass a spectrum of benign and malignant causes. For patients with extra-adrenal primary malignancy, deciphering the nature of concurrent adrenal lesions is critical given that the adrenal glands are in some instances the only site of metastatic disease. In attempting to differentiate adenomas from malignant adrenal masses using MR, the SI ratio of the adrenal mass to liver or fat on T1-weighted (T1W) and T2-weighted (T2W) spin-echo images generated with low- and medium-field strength magnets was initially proposed. However, with significant overlap in ratios for adenomas and nonadenomas, this MR technique proved to be of limited use in identifying malignant adrenal masses. This was until Mitchell and colleagues established that lipid-sensitive chemical shift techniques could be used to identify adrenal adenomas. This was on the basis that benign adrenocortical masses often contain high lipid content, while metastases and pheochromocytomas do not. Adenomas and nonadenomas also have different patterns of gadolinium enhancement on fast gradient-echo (GRE) images.

The present study by Korobkin and colleagues evaluated the use of chemical shift and dynamic gadolinium-enhanced MR imaging in characterizing adrenal masses. Definitive diagnoses were made on the basis of other clinical imaging and pathologic criteria. The results of this study found that a decrease in the relative SI ratio on opposed-phase chemical shift images could be used to identify adenomas with high specificity and acceptable sensitivity. Visual assessment of adrenal masses with maximum SI after gadolinium enhancement did not allow for effective differentiation between adenomas and nonadenomas, and did not improve with washout.

In-Depth [prospective cohort]: Patients with adrenal masses detected through abdominal CT were consecutively enrolled into this study and further evaluated with chemical shift MR imaging, dynamic gadolinium-enhanced MR imaging, or both. Adrenal masses were assessed and defined as either adenomas or nonadenomas on the basis of other non-MR imaging and pathologic criteria. This included NP-59 scintigraphy, which was used to evaluate clinically suspected hyperfunctioning adenomas and some suspected non-hyperfunctioning adenomas. Percutaneous biopsy was performed when the adrenal mass was the only suspected metastatic site from an extra-adrenal primary neoplasm. Quantitative and qualitative review of the MR images was performed, assessing mass-liver SI ratios for T1W and T2W images. The relative change in mass-liver and mass-paraspinal muscle SI ratios on opposed-phase versus in-phase GRE imaging, the relative change in mass-liver SI ratio on fat-saturated T1W versus conventional T1W imaging, and the maximum SI of adrenal masses on gadolinium-enhanced images were also compared to unenhanced images. Comparing SI at maximum enhancement to that on the final 10-minute image allowed for the assessment of maximum gadolinium washout for each evaluated mass. Qualitative review was conducted using a 5-point scale and carried out by 2 investigators blinded to the clinical history and results of previous non-MR imaging. A single investigator blinded to the clinical data and qualitative results was responsible for quantitative review.

A total of 43 patients with 51 adrenal masses participated in this study. Of the 51 adrenal masses evaluated, 35 (n = 28, mean age 57 years, range 35-78 years) were diagnosed as adenomas using non-MR imaging and/or pathology. The remaining 16 masses (n = 15, mean age 51 years, range 19-72) were diagnosed as nonadenomas.

Based on the results of qualitative review comparing adenomas and nonadenomas, the relative change in mass-liver ratio SI on opposed-phase versus in-phase GRE images was able to characterize adenomas with 100% specificity and 81% sensitivity. Adenomas were also identified with 100% specificity using the relative change in mass-muscle SI ratio on opposed-phase versus in-phase images (77% sensitivity) and the relative change in mass-liver SI ratio on fat-saturated T1W versus conventional T1W images (30% sensitivity). However, the maximum SI of an adrenal mass after contrast administration and following maximum contrast washout were of little to no diagnostic value, with 100% overlap in SI for adenomas and nonadenomas.

Korobkin M, Lombardi TJ, Aisen AM, Francis IR, Quint LE, Dunnick NR, Londy F, Shapiro B, Gross MD, Thompson NW. Characterization of adrenal masses with chemical shift and gadolinium-enhanced MR imaging. Radiology. 1995 Nov;197(2):411-8.

Additional Review:

Mitchell DG, Crovello M, Matteucci T, Petersen RO, Miettinen MM. Benign adrenocortical masses: diagnosis with chemical shift MR imaging. Radiology. 1992 Nov;185(2):345-51.

Hepatic arterial phase imaging more sensitive than portal venous phase in the detection of hepatic lesions and arterioportal shunting

1. Hepatic arterial phase imaging detected more hepatic lesions than portal venous phase (PVP) imaging, as well as arterioportal shunting not seen on PVP images.

2. PVP imaging was more sensitive in the detection of portal vein thrombosis due to hepatic tumor invasion.

Original Date of Publication: May 1996

Study Rundown: The administration of contrast has improved the imaging of malignant liver lesions using computed tomography (CT). Some tumors, however, are more difficult to visualize despite the use of contrast, including primary hepatocellular carcinoma (HCC), metastases from renal cell carcinoma, pancreatic islet cell tumors and breast carcinoma. This can be explained by the increased vascularity of these lesions, which allows for rapid enhancement and attenuation, similar to background liver parenchyma. In recognizing that the visualization of morphologic CT contrast patterns is largely influenced by techniques of contrast administration, Freeny and colleagues found that benign hepatic hemangiomas could be differentiated from malignant hepatic neoplasms using bolus dynamic scanning. In a later study, Heiken and colleagues established that CT imaging of hepatic tumors could be further improved by performing CT during arterial portography (CTAP) via the superior mesenteric or splenic arteries. This technique allowed for the enhancement of the portal vein and intrahepatic vessels, which proved to be useful in predicting tumor behavior when Matsui and colleagues observed that intranodular portal blood flow decreased with increasing tumor grade. The same study also found that hepatic angiography could be used to identify HCCs as the arterial blood flow to these lesions exceeds that of the surrounding liver. As such, these lesions can be seen early during contrast administration through the aorta or hepatic artery, otherwise known as the hepatic arterial-dominant phase (HAP) of contrast delivery.

In the study conducted by Baron and colleagues, hepatic arterial-dominant phase (HAP) imaging was compared to portal venous-dominant phase (PVP) imaging in the evaluation of HCC. The results of this study showed that considerably more lesions were detected during HAP than PVP, including lesions not seen with PVP imaging. HAP imaging was also able to identify arterioportal shunting, which was not evident in any of the images produced during PVP. Both techniques were able to identify portal venous thrombosis, however, some cases were missed with HAP imaging when compared to PVP imaging. Therefore, the use of both HAP and PVP imaging optimizes the evaluation of patients with or at risk of HCC.

In-Depth [retrospective cohort]: All patients with a proven diagnosis of HCC visualized with biphasic helical CT between 1993 and 1994 were assessed for inclusion in the study (n = 78). HCC was confirmed through needle core biopsy, fine-needle aspiration or surgical resection. Patients were excluded if they had received prior iodized oil infusion, or if any technical failures encountered during scanning prohibited the acquisition of PVP images within the required time. Patients eligible for inclusion in the study received either 150 mL of ionic contrast material (iothalamate meglumine 60%) at a rate of 2.5 mL/sec, or nonionic contrast material (ioversol 68%) at a rate of 3-5 mL/sec. As all patients had proven HCC, all lesions with a similar appearance to the lesion sampled for biopsy without meeting CT criteria for hemangiomas, cyst or confluent fibrosis, were also considered tumor nodules. Three investigators retrospectively reviewed all CT scans, and consensus was reached for all cases.

A total of 66 patients (mean age 58 years) were included in this study. Based on the results of both PVP and HAP imaging, 326 lesions were detected with an average of 5 lesions per patient. Of these 326 lesions, PVP images depicted 268 (82%) compared to 309 (95%) on HAP images. For 7 patients, lesions were seen only on HAP images, and not depicted in PVP imaging. However, in 13 patients, PVP images showed additional lesions not seen on HAP imaging. PVP imaging was also more sensitive in the detection of portal venous thrombosis due to tumor invasion, detecting 21 cases compared to 17 on HAP imaging, but not arterioportal shunting. Based on HAP imaging, arterioportal shunting was evident in 11 patients, while no cases were identified through PVP imaging.

Baron RL, J H Oliver r, G D Dodd r, Nalesnik M, Holbert BL, Carr B. Hepatocellular carcinoma: evaluation with biphasic, contrast-enhanced, helical CT. Radiology. 1996 May;199(2):505-11.
Additional Review:

Freeny PC, Marks WM. Patterns of contrast enhancement of benign and malignant hepatic neoplasms during bolus dynamic and delayed CT. Radiology. 1986 Sep;160(3):613-8.

Heiken JP, Weyman PJ, Lee JK, Balfe DM, Picus D, Brunt EM, et al. Detection of focal hepatic masses: prospective evaluation with CT, delayed CT, CT during arterial portography, and MR imaging. Radiology. 1989 Apr;171(1):47-51.

Matsui O, Kadoya M, Kameyama T, Yoshikawa J, Takashima T, Nakanuma Y, Unoura M, Kobayashi K, Izumi R, Ida M. Benign and malignant nodules in cirrhotic livers: distinction based on blood supply. Radiology. 1991 Feb;178(2):493-7.

CT-guided percutaneous lung biopsies more effective for larger pulmonary nodules

1. Computed tomography (CT)-guided percutaneous lung biopsies demonstrated a significantly higher accuracy for pulmonary nodules greater than 1.5 cm in diameter compared to small pulmonary nodules (<1.5 cm).

2. There were no significant differences in the rates of complications for either large or small pulmonary nodules.

Original Date of Publication: July 1996

Study Rundown: CT-guided percutaneous needle aspiration lung biopsy provides a minimally-invasive method of distinguishing benign and malignant lung lesions. However, this procedure may be associated with an increased risk of complications, including pneumothorax, air embolism, and inadequate sampling leading to false-negative results. The purpose of this landmark retrospective review was to explore the differences in diagnostic accuracy as well as the complication rates for CT-guided percutaneous needle aspiration biopsies between small (<1.5 cm) versus large (>1.5 cm) lung nodules.

This trial retrospectively reviewed the outcomes of 97 consecutive patients that underwent CT-guided percutaneous needle aspiration of a lung mass. At the conclusion of the trial, the diagnostic accuracy of needle aspiration was high for both small and large pulmonary nodules; however, percutaneous biopsies of larger nodules demonstrated significantly higher diagnostic accuracy and overall sensitivity compared to small nodules. Furthermore, small pulmonary nodules had a higher false-negative rate compared to large nodules. With respect to procedural complications, there were no significant differences in the rates of pneumothorax between patients with small and large lung nodules, with an overall low number requiring chest tube placement.

This trial demonstrated that CT-guided percutaneous needle aspiration was safe and had an acceptable accuracy for both large and small pulmonary nodules; however, biopsy of small nodules resulted in a significantly lower accuracy. Additionally, the high false-negative rate for small nodules indicates that a negative result may be of limited clinical value. The results of this trial support the use of additional biopsy procedures for negative percutaneous results. Furthermore, although the size cut-off in this trial was 1.5 cm, most large pulmonary nodules in the study were larger than 3 cm. The majority of subsequent studies on percutaneous lung biopsies have used 3 cm as the cut-off for small pulmonary nodules.

In-Depth [retrospective cohort]: This study included 97 consecutive patients that underwent CT-guided percutaneous needle aspiration lung biopsy in a single center. The primary outcome was the diagnostic accuracy and safety of CT-guided lung biopsies. All biopsies were performed by chest radiologists, chest radiology fellows, or radiology residents under the supervision of attending radiologists. Overall, 27 small nodules (mean size: 1.15 cm; range: 0.4 to 1.5 cm) and 70 large nodules (mean size: 3.17 cm; range: 1.6 to 8.2 cm) were biopsied. All biopsy specimens were correlated with pathologic findings from surgery. At the conclusion of the trial, 23 of 27 (85%) small nodules and 62 of 70 (89%) large nodules were found to be malignant. Biopsy of large pulmonary nodules demonstrated a significantly higher sensitivity (94% versus 72%; $p < 0.05$) and accuracy (96% versus 74%; $p < 0.05$) compared to small nodules. There were no differences between specificity between large and small nodule biopsy. There were similar rates of pneumothorax for patients with both small and large pulmonary nodules. There were no post-procedural fatalities in either group.

Li H, Boiselle PM, Shepard JO, Trotman-Dickenson B, McLoud TC. Diagnostic accuracy and safety of CT-guided percutaneous needle aspiration biopsy of the lung: comparison of small and large pulmonary nodules. Am J Roentgenol. 1996 Jul 1;167(1):105–9.

Percutaneous ethanol injection safe and effective in hepatocellular carcinoma

1. In a large prospective cohort of patients with hepatocellular carcinoma (HCC) and contraindications to surgical management, the use of percutaneous ethanol injection (PEI) was associated with favorable survival outcomes and few adverse events at five years.

Original Date of Publication: October 1995

Study Rundown: First described in the mid-1980s, the use of PEI for the treatment of HCC generated significant interest in the oncology community. Though surgical resection or liver transplant have historically been the preferred means of managing HCC patients, PEI was among the first in a subset of minimally-invasive treatment modalities to show promise for patients with contraindications to surgical treatment. Advantages of PEI over surgery include the low cost, short treatment time, lack of need for general endotracheal anesthesia, and the ability to perform the procedure in the outpatient setting. The majority of early PEI trials suggested treatment efficacy and improved patient survival; however, these trials were generally small in size and tracked patient outcomes for only short post-treatment intervals, and thus their validity remained uncertain.

This trial was the first to enroll a large, prospective cohort and follow them over several years after PEI with the goal of more definitively defining the procedure's outcomes among HCC patients. Conducted at multiple clinical sites in Italy, the trial included patients with absolute or relative contraindications to surgical management and followed them for an average of three years following PEI. Given the large but highly heterogeneous population within the trial, the authors were able to generate survival data stratified according to discrete clinical factors such as tumor size, multiplicity, and Child class. The results showed overall survival trends comparable to surgical resection, and outlined in particular how survival after PEI varied as a function of patient-specific factors, most notably Child class. The rate of major complications was low, and only one death was attributable to the procedure. With these data published, PEI became the de facto standard of care for patients with contraindications to surgery and ushered in, alongside transarterial chemoembolization, the modern era of minimally-invasive HCC therapies.

In-Depth [case series study]: A total of 746 patients (76% men; mean age 64 years) were prospectively enrolled from nine academic medical centers in Italy. Primary enrollment criteria included a pre-enrollment diagnosis of HCC and either tumor inoperability (as defined by factors such as multiple tumor foci and advanced patients age), patient refusal of surgical intervention, or referral for non-operative management at the request of the primary treating physician. Prior to PEI, all enrolled patients underwent ultrasound and contrast-enhanced computed tomography (CT) to assess disease burden. PEI was performed without general anesthesia in the outpatient setting under ultrasound guidance in one or more sessions. Treatment efficacy was assessed at one month by ultrasound, CT, and serum alpha fetoprotein, and then by imaging at 3-6 month intervals thereafter. Kaplan-Meier survival curves were generated and stratified according to factors such as tumor size, tumor number, and Child class.

The mean follow-up time was 36 months (range 12-90 months). Cumulative five-year survival varied from 26-40% among patients with one or more HCC lesions without extrahepatic involvement, and was 47% and 29% for Child class A and B patients, respectively. Among those patients with extrahepatic disease or Child class C cirrhosis, cumulative five-year survival was 0%. Local recurrence at the site of prior PEI was noted in 17% of lesions, the majority of which were treated with repeat PEI. The 30-day mortality rate was 0%, and the overall procedure-specific mortality rate was 0.1%. Major complications such as significant bleeding occurred in 1.3% of patients. Though not formally evaluated, the average cost of PEI at the participating centers was approximately $1,000 USD, as compared to $30,000 USD for surgical resection.

Livraghi T, Giorgio A, Marin G, Salmi A, de Sio I, Bolondi L, et al. Hepatocellular carcinoma and cirrhosis in 746 patients: long-term results of percutaneous ethanol injection. Radiology. 1995 Oct 1;197(1):101–8.

Rapid CT contrast washout differentiates adrenal adenomas from nonadenomas

1. The mean percentage of computed tomography (CT) contrast washout was significantly greater for adenomas compared to nonadenomas in all delayed scans.

2. Delayed enhanced CT scans discriminated adenomas from nonadenomas with high sensitivity and specificity at various time points, as early as 5 to 15 minutes after enhancement.

Original Date of Publication: March 1998

Study Rundown: Adrenal mass lesions are incidentally discovered in up to 5% of patients subjected to CT for indications unrelated to adrenal disease. In patients without a known history of cancer, most of these lesions are benign. For patients with a diagnosed extra-adrenal malignancy, the likelihood that an incidentally discovered adrenal lesion is malignant increases considerably. On unenhanced CT scans, benign adrenal adenomas are characterized by low attenuation. On contrast-enhanced CT, however, attenuation values cannot differentiate between benign and malignant lesions. As such, other imaging modalities or repeat imaging have been historically used to differentiate between benign and malignant adrenal masses. This was until several studies noted that intravenous (IV) contrast medium tended to "wash out" faster from adenomatous lesions than non-adenomatous lesions, and therefore, CT attenuation measurements could be used after a variable delay period to characterize adrenal lesions. Given that delayed CT attenuation measurements are dependent on the type, total dose and injection rate of IV contrast material, however, measures of absolute attenuation on delayed scans were found not found to be useful. In response, the use of enhancement washout curves was proposed to differentiate adrenal adenomas from nonadenomas.

In this study conducted by Korobkin and colleagues, contrast enhancement washout curves were generated following delayed contrast-enhanced CT scans of adrenal adenomas and nonadenomas. The results of this study showed that the mean percentage of enhancement washout for adrenal adenomas far exceeded that observed in nonadenomas. The authors also demonstrated that delayed enhanced CT scans could discriminate adenomas from nonadenomas with high sensitivity and specificity at various time points, as early as 5 to 15 minutes after enhancement. Pena and colleagues later confirmed in their study that the relative percentage washout on dynamic and delayed enhanced CT scans could be used to characterize adrenal masses.

In-Depth [prospective cohort]: Patients with adrenal masses identified through abdominal or chest CT were consecutively enrolled into this study. Adrenal adenoma diagnoses were confirmed through various means, including percutaneous biopsy, stable appearance on follow-up CT examinations and an attenuation value of < 10 Hounsfield Units (HU) on unenhanced CT. Nonadenoma diagnoses were confirmed through surgery, percutaneous biopsy, substantial growth or shrinkage at short-term follow-up, and stable CT for 1 case of myelolipoma. Unenhanced and standard enhanced scans were obtained for all adrenal masses, and delayed enhanced CT values were studied in 2 groups of patients. In the first group, delayed scans were obtained at 15, 30 and 45 minutes following the initial enhanced CT. In the second group, delayed scans were obtained at 5, 10 and 15 minutes after the initial enhanced CT. From these scans, percentages of initial enhancement at these time points were calculated and used to generate washout curves for adrenal adenomas and nonadenomas. Calculations of sensitivity and specificity for the diagnosis of adenoma using delayed enhanced CT were made after selecting an optimal threshold value.

A total of 66 patients with 76 adrenal masses were evaluated. The masses consisted of 52 adenomas (n = 45; mean age 64 years, range 43-80 years; 53% men) and 24 nonadenomas (n = 21; mean age 60 years, range 31-76 years; 71% men). Consistent with previous studies, there was no significant difference in mean CT attenuation at initial enhancement for adenomatous versus nonadenomatous masses. However, a statistically significant difference in mean CT attenuation between adenomas and nonadenomas was observed for unenhanced ($p < 0.001$) and all delayed enhanced ($p < 0.001$) scans. For unenhanced scans, an optimal threshold of 10 HU corresponded to a sensitivity of 87% and specificity of 100%. For the 15-minute delayed enhanced scan, the sensitivity and specificity were both 96% at a threshold of 37 HU. Differences in mean percentages of initial enhancement were also found to be statistically significant between the adenoma and nonadenoma groups at all delayed times ($p < 0.001$). The mean percentage of enhancement washout for adrenal adenomas was 51% at 5 minutes and 70% at 15 minutes, compared to 8% and 20% for nonadenomas, respectively. On the 15-minute delayed enhanced scans, an optimal threshold for adenoma diagnosis was established at 60% contrast enhancement washout, associated with a sensitivity of 88% and specificity of 96%.

Korobkin M, Brodeur FJ, Francis IR, Quint LE, Dunnick NR, Londy F. CT time-

attenuation washout curves of adrenal adenomas and nonadenomas. American Journal of Roentgenology. 1998 Mar;170(3):747-52.

Additional Review:

Blake MA, Cronin CG, Boland GW. Adrenal imaging. American Journal of Roentgenology. 2010;194(6):1450.

Boland GWL, Blake MA, Hahn PF, Mayo-Smith WW. Incidental Adrenal Lesions: Principles, Techniques, and Algorithms for Imaging Characterization. Radiology. 2008 Dec;249(3):756-75.

Peña CS, Boland GWL, Hahn PF, Lee MJ, Mueller PR. Characterization of Indeterminate (Lipid-poor) Adrenal Masses: Use of Washout Characteristics at Contrast-enhanced CT. Radiology. 2000 Dec;217(3):798-802. BI-RADS study identifies mammography features with high positive predictive values for carcinoma

Breast cancer is the second leading cause of cancer death in women. Given that many early breast cancers are asymptomatic and elude detection by physical exam, mammography was developed as a screening tool to uncover breast cancers at an earlier stage, thereby improving prognosis. The American Cancer Society currently recommends that women of average breast cancer risk begin obtaining annual screening mammograms between the ages of 40 and 45 depending on preference, with the option to switch to biennial screening after age 55. Modified screening protocols starting at an earlier age are employed in patients with higher risk on the basis of family history or genetic risk modifiers.

Mammograms can reveal a spectrum of findings, some of which prompt suspicion for malignancy but many of which are benign. The growth of mammography in the 1980s resulted in a compelling need to craft a standardized reporting system for describing these findings and translating them into management recommendations. In response, the American College of Radiology (ACR) developed the Breast Imaging-Reporting and Data System (BI-RADS) system, which comprises a lexicon for describing mammographic findings, a structure for mammography reports, a set of final assessment categories with management guidelines, and technical recommendations for performing mammographic studies. The first edition of BI-RADS was released in 1993 with the intent of allowing periodic updates as new data and clinical experience emerged. Subsequent iterations built upon the original BI-RADS structure, with the fourth edition in 2003 introducing analogous reporting constructs for breast ultrasound and breast MRI. Currently, BI-RADS is in its fifth edition (2013) and remains the standard reporting paradigm in breast imaging. Please see Tables I-III for the current BI-RADS classification and lexicon.

As an early effort to characterize the performance of the first edition of BI-RADS and inform future modification of the reporting terminology, the following study by Liberman et al. evaluated the positive predictive value of the various BI-RADS terms used for mammographic interpretation. Findings revealed that several features pertaining to masses (spiculated margins, irregular shape) and calcifications (linear morphology, segmental or linear distribution) were highly associated with malignancy, demonstrating positive predictive values ranging from 68-81%.

1. **Lesions observed in mammography with spiculated margins, linear calcification morphology, irregular shape, segmental calcification distribution, or linear calcification distributions have high positive predictive values (81%, 81%, 73%, 74%, 68%, respectively).**

2. **Using the BI-RADS lexicon (Table I), radiologists had very comparable positive predictive values for detecting carcinoma in lesions categorized as a 4 or 5.**

Original Date of Publication: July 1998

Study Rundown: Seeking to better standardize characterization and reporting of mammography readings, the ACR developed BI-RADS nomenclature. This study sought to evaluate the positive predictive value of the various descriptive terms BI-RADS offers for mammogram interpretation. Results showed that among lesions that would typically be followed up by physicians, several lesional features were highly associated with cancerous biopsies, with positive predictive values for carcinoma ranging from 68-81%. Utilization of BI-RADS terminology also showed different radiologists characterized lesions into various final assessment categories describing the suspicion of cancerous lesions at statistically similar rates.

In-Depth [prospective cohort]: Patients at Memorial-Sloan Kettering with impalpable breast lesions seen upon initial mammographic interpretation were referred for surgical tissue biopsy. Prior to surgery, 1 of 5 academic radiologists evaluated the mammographic lesion images. Lesions that had already undergone a prior biopsy were excluded from the study and image interpretation. In total, 492 lesions from 466 women (median age 52, range 27-92) were included in the study, with 73 (16%) of the women having had breast cancer previously. Lesions were characterized using BI-RADS terminology describing mass margins and shape, and calcification morphology and distribution. The most worrisome descriptor in the radiologist's interpretation was used to give the lesion a final classification on a scale of 1 (normal mammography) to 5 (highly suggestive of malignancy).

Carcinoma was confirmed in 225 (46%) of the lesions. Within subcategories of lesions, 50% (79/158) of noncalcified masses, 86% (12/14) of calcified masses, and 42% (134/320) of calcifications without mass were carcinomas. BI-RADS final assessments by reading radiologists placed 26% (129/492) of lesions in category 5, 72% (355/492) in category 4, and 2% (8/492) in category 3. Carcinoma was confirmed in 81% (105/129) of category 5, 34% (120/355) of category 4, and 0% (0/8) of category 3 lesions. Amongst the BI-RADS features used to assign final assessment grades to lesions, high positive predictive values were found in 5 of them: spiculated margins (81%), linear calcification morphology (81%), irregular shape (73%), segmental calcification distribution (74%), or linear calcification distribution (68%).

Liberman L, Abramson A, Squires F, Glassman J, Morris E, Dershaw D. The breast imaging reporting and data system: positive predictive value of mammographic features and final assessment categories. American Journal of Roentgenology. 1998;171(1):35-40.

Additional Review:

ACR. ACR BI-RADS® Atlas - American College of Radiology [Internet]. 2016. Available from: http://www.acr.org/Quality-Safety/Resources/BIRADS.

BI-RADS Framework

Category	Descriptor	Management	Cancer Probability
0	Incomplete – Need additional imaging evaluation and/or prior mammograms for comparison	Further imaging needed	N/A
1	Negative	Routine screening	0%
2	Benign	Routine screening	0%
3	Probably benign	Short interval follow-up	< 2%
4	Suspicious	Consider biopsy	4a. Low suspicion (≥ 2 to $\leq 10\%$) 95% 4b. Moderate suspicion (> 10 to $\leq 50\%$) 4c. High suspicion (> 50% to < 95%)
5	Highly suggestive of malignancy	Biopsy or surgery	$\geq 95\%$
6	Known biopsy-proven malignancy	Appropriate action (i.e. surgery)	N/A

Table I. BI-RADS classification.
Table compiled using information from www.acr.org/Quality-Safety/Resources/BIRADS.

BI-RADS 5th Edition Mammography Lexicon

Breast composition	a. Entirely fatty b. Scattered areas of fibroglandular density c. Heterogeneously dense, which may obscure masses d. Extremely dense, which lowers sensitivity		
Mass	shape	oval / round / irregular	
	margin	circumscribed / obscured / microlobulated / indistinct / spiculated	
	density	fat / low / equal / high	
Asymmetry	asymmetry / global / focal / developing		
Architectural distortion	Distorted parenchyma with no visible mass		
Calcifications	morphology	typically benign	skin / vascular / coarse "popcorn like" / large rod-like / round / rim / dystrophic / milk of calcium / suture
		suspicious	amorphous / coarse heterogenous / fine pleiomorphic / fine linear or fine linear branching
	distribution	diffuse / regional / grouped / linear / segmental	
Associated features	skin retraction / nipple retraction / skin thickening / trabecular thickening / axillary adenopathy / architectural distortion / calcifications		
Location	laterality / quadrant and clock face / depth / distance from the nipple		

Table II. Updated BI-RADS fifth Edition (2013) mammography lexicon. Table compiled using information from www.acr.org/Quality-Safety/Resources/BIRADS.

BI-RADS 5th Edition Ultrasound Lexicon		
Tissue composition (screening only)	a. homogenous - fat b. homogenous - fibroglandular c. heterogenous	
Mass	shape	oval / round / irregular
	margin	a. circumscribed b. not circumscribed (indistinct, angular, microlobulated, spiculated)
	orientation	parallel / not parallel
	echo pattern	anechoic / hyperechoic / complex cystic and solid / isoechoic / heterogenous
	posterior features	no features / enhancement / shadowing / combined pattern
Calcifications	in mass / outside mass / intraductal	
Associated features	architectural distortion / duct changes / skin changes (thickening, retraction) / edema / vascularity (absent, internal, rim) / elasticity (soft, intermediate, hard)	
Special cases	simple cyst / clustered microcysts / complicated cyst / mass in or on skin / foreign body including implants / intramammary or axillary lymph nodes / AVMs / Mondor disease / postsurgical fluid collection / fat necrosis	

Table III. Updated BI-RADS fifth Edition (2013) ultrasound lexicon. Table compiled using information from www.acr.org/Quality-Safety/Resources/BIRADS.

Endovaginal ultrasound highly sensitive screen for endometrial cancer

1. Endovaginal ultrasound (EVUS) revealing an endometrial stripe of 5 mm or greater was 96% sensitive for endometrial cancer and 92% sensitive for other endometrial disease, allowing for noninvasive screening and subsequent determination of candidacy for endometrial biopsy.

2. EVUS was less specific among postmenopausal women utilizing hormone replacement therapy (HRT) than among those who refrained from HRT, and this overall low sensitivity necessitated endometrial biopsy in all women with an abnormal EVUS.

Original Date of Publication: November 1998

Study Rundown: Endometrial cancer is the third most common cancer of the female reproductive tract after ovarian and cervical cancers, but has a low mortality rate if brought to early medical attention. It typically presents with painless, abnormal uterine bleeding among postmenopausal women, particularly those who are obese or utilizing HRT without progesterone supplementation, as unopposed estrogens promote endometrial hyperplasia. Prior to the widespread use of EVUS in screening symptomatic women for endometrial abnormalities, endometrial biopsy was the only diagnostic tool used in the workup of at-risk women with abnormal uterine bleeding. However, endometrial biopsy is invasive, painful, and can be nondiagnostic or inaccurate in over a quarter of attempts. The referenced study reviewed the literature from 1966 to 1996 regarding the use of EVUS as the first-line screening tool among women with suspicion of endometrial cancer in an effort to determine if a negative screening EVUS could obviate the need for endometrial biopsy. Utilizing an endometrial thickness threshold of 5 mm for positivity on any given EVUS examination, the authors found a pooled sensitivity of 96% for the detection of endometrial cancer and 92% for other endometrial disease, including atypical endometrial hyperplasia or endometrial polyps. Additionally, no significant sensitivity difference was found between women using HRT and those not. However, specificity for the detection of endometrial cancer varied significantly between women who did and did not use HRT, finding almost three times as many women on HRT to have an abnormal EVUS despite normal histology on biopsy. Of note, this analysis did not include studies involving women using tamoxifen, which may markedly thicken the endometrium, and also did not evaluate the use of EVUS as a screening tool in asymptomatic women due to the rarity of endometrial cancer. The variability and overall low-to-moderate specificity of EVUS demonstrated it to be an improper tool for the ultimate diagnosis of an endometrial abnormality, but it displayed excellent sensitivity characteristics in the initial workup of at-risk women presenting with abnormal uterine bleeding concerning for malignancy. A negative EVUS result was shown to reduce the pretest odds of cancer by roughly 90% regardless of HRT status, therefore effectively ruling out cancer and preventing unnecessary invasive biopsies.

In-Depth [systematic review and meta-analysis]: This systematic review and meta-analysis pooled data from 35 studies published between 1966 and 1996 examining the use of EVUS in the diagnostic workup of primarily postmenopausal patients with suspected endometrial cancer, all of which were confirmed by endometrial biopsy. A total of 5892 women (mean age 61 years; 471 women using HRT) were included, with 94% presenting with vaginal bleeding. The sensitivity, specificity, and positive and negative predictive values were calculated for EVUS in the detection of both endometrial cancer and other endometrial abnormalities (polyps or atypical hyperplasia), and among women who were and were not utilizing postmenopausal HRT. Within the sampled group, the prevalence of endometrial cancer was calculated to be 13%, while that of endometrial polyps or hyperplasia was 40%. Women with normal endometrial histology displayed a mean endometrial thickness of 4±1 mm, while women with endometrial polyps, hyperplasia and cancer displayed mean thicknesses of 10±3 mm, 14±4 mm and 20±6 mm, respectively. A 5 mm threshold for EVUS positivity was selected as it displayed the best overall sensitivity and specificity characteristics. Regardless of HRT status, the sensitivity of EVUS in testing for endometrial cancer was 96% (95%CI 94-98%), while it was 92% (95%CI 90-93%) in testing for other endometrial abnormalities. This lack of variation despite HRT status and high sensitivity demonstrated that EVUS is highly accurate in the exclusion of endometrial disease, with a negative likelihood ratio of 0.05-0.12. Therefore, in a woman with a 10% pretest probability of endometrial disease, typical for that of postmenopausal women presenting with abnormal uterine bleeding, a negative EVUS reduced her risk of disease to 1%. Regarding specificity, the study found that EVUS cannot accurately distinguish between endometrial cancers, polyps or hyperplasia, necessitating a subsequent endometrial biopsy in all women with an abnormal EVUS. This study definitively established EVUS as an effective first-line tool in the diagnostic workup of women with suspected endometrial cancer while providing the baseline, evidence-based threshold for examination positivity used in current practice.

Smith-Bindman R, Kerlikowske K, Feldstein V, Subak L, Scheidler J, Segal M, Brand R, Grady D. Endovaginal ultrasound to exclude endometrial cancer and other endometrial abnormalities. Journal of the American Medical Association. 1998 Nov 4;280(17):1510–17.

Breast MRI most sensitive screening modality in high-risk patients

1. Among patients with a familial or genetic predisposition to the development of breast cancer, magnetic resonance imaging (MRI) of the breast was significantly more sensitive than either clinical exam or mammography for the detection of invasive breast cancer.

2. Invasive breast cancers detected by MRI were more frequently less than one centimeter in diameter and displayed a lower incidence of axillary nodal metastases or micrometastases than those detected by mammography or clinical breast exam.

Original Date of Publication: July 2004

Study Rundown: Breast cancer screening for women aged 50 to 70 has been shown to significantly reduce cancer-related mortality. However, for women with a strong family history of early breast cancer or known germline oncogenic mutations such as the *BRCA1* or *BRCA2* mutations, screening at an earlier age may be warranted due to their high lifetime cancer risk. Screening of the general population at younger ages has been of unclear value due to increased breast density among premenopausal women potentially reducing the sensitivity of mammography. Among those with genetic predispositions to breast cancer, mammography has been further limited, demonstrating a low sensitivity for cancer detection due in part to rapid tumor growth and an increased incidence of atypical historadiological characteristics of the tumors in these women. Contrast-enhanced breast MRI had been suggested as an alternative screening modality for high-risk women given its high sensitivity and the relative indifference of the modality to breast density. In the referenced article, yearly mammography and serial clinical breast examinations were prospectively compared to yearly screening breast MRI in younger women with an established predisposition to breast cancer. In nearly 3 years of screening high-risk women with a mean age of 40 years, contrast-enhanced breast MRI was by far the most sensitive modality at 79.5%, performing significantly better than either mammography or clinical breast exam at 33.3% and 17.9%, respectively. However, the specificity and positive predictive value of MRI was the lowest of the three methods at 89.8% and 7.1%, as compared to mammography at 95.0% and 8.0%, respectively. Notably, tumors detected by breast MRI were significantly more likely to be of lower stage, with more tumors found at sizes less than 10 mm in diameter, and fewer tumors with micrometastases or axillary nodal metastases, suggesting earlier detection in the natural course of the disease. No differences in disease-free or overall survival could be determined as no mortalities were recorded during the course of the study. These findings demonstrated that MRI had significantly better overall discriminating capacity than either mammography or clinical breast exam in screening women at high-risk for breast cancer.

In-Depth [prospective cohort]: This prospective trial enrolled 1909 women (mean age 40 years; range 19-72 years, 75% premenopausal) at multiple centers across Europe who were known to be at high risk for breast cancer (greater than 15% lifetime risk) due either to a strong family history of early breast cancer or known genetic mutation. Women were excluded from the study if they had symptoms suggestive of current breast cancer or a personal history of breast cancer. All subjects were screened by twice yearly clinical breast exam and yearly mammography and contrast-enhanced breast MRI over a median follow-up period of 2.9 years (mean 2.7, range 0.1-3.9 years). Results from each modality were blinded such that no examination could influence another. Radiologic studies were scored on the BI-RADS system, with the threshold for positivity set to category 3 ("probably benign or uncertain result") for both statistical analysis and further investigation by ultrasonography, fine-needle aspiration or biopsy as necessary. Results of these further investigations were used to diagnose a tumor as benign or malignant, and formed the basis for subsequent determinations of specificity and positive predictive value for each screening modality. The overall sensitivity of MRI for the detection of invasive breast cancers (excluding ductal carcinoma in situ) among high-risk women was 79.5% using BI-RADS 3 or higher as the cutoff for positivity, as compared to 17.9% for clinical breast exam and 33.3% for mammography. The specificity of clinical examination was the highest at 98.1%, while mammography and breast MRI were 95.0% and 89.8%, respectively. The positive predictive value of MRI was 7.1% as compared to 9.6% for clinical exam and 8.0% for mammography. Based on the area under the receiver operator curves for both MRI and mammography, MRI showed a significantly better discriminating capacity than mammography (Difference in AUC 0.141, 95%CI 0.020-0.262; $p < 0.05$). Tumors detected by MRI were generally of a lower stage than those detected by alternative methods, with 43.2% found at a diameter of less than 10 mm, versus only 12.5% and 14.0% in each respective average risk control group ($p < 0.001$ and $p = 0.04$). Additionally, the incidence of either positive axillary lymph node metastases or micrometastases was 21.4% as compared to 52.4% and 56.4% in each control group ($p < 0.001$ and $p = 0.001$, respectively.) During the median 2.9 years of follow up, none of the patients with breast cancer died, therefore no difference of disease-free or overall survival could be assessed.

Kriege M, Brekelmans CT, Boetes C, Besnard PE, Zonderland HM, Obdeijn IM, et al. Efficacy of MRI and Mammography for Breast-Cancer Screening in Women with a Familial or Genetic Predisposition. The New England Journal of Medicine. 2004 Jul 29;351(5):427–37.

MRI enhances diagnostic certainty of ovarian cancer following indeterminate ultrasound

1. In women with an indeterminate ovarian mass on ultrasonography, magnetic resonance imaging (MRI) provided a significantly higher change in post-test probability compared to computed tomography (CT) or Doppler ultrasound.

Original Date of Publication: July 2005

Study Rundown: Ovarian cancer is the second most common gynecological malignancy with a world-wide incidence of 11.9 cases per 100 000 women. Accurate diagnosis of patients presenting with adnexal masses is crucial to allow timely surgical diagnosis and intervention. Although ultrasound is the first-line imaging modality in women for assessment of a suspicious adnexal mass, at the time of this study there was no evidence-based consensus on the management options for patients following an indeterminate adnexal mass on ultrasonography. The purpose of this landmark meta-analysis was to determine the optimal second-line imaging modality to assess an indeterminate ovarian mass on ultrasound for both pre- and post-menopausal women.

The trial performed a literature review to determine the prevalence of ovarian cancer in patients presenting with an adnexal mass as well as the sensitivity and specificity of Doppler ultrasound, CT, and MRI in the characterization of adnexal masses following ultrasonography. The change in pre- and post-test probabilities was calculated for each imaging modality. At the conclusion of the trial, the use of any additional imaging modalities was associated with a significant increase in post-test probability for both pre- and post-menopausal women. However, MRI demonstrated significantly higher diagnostic certainty in post-test probability for ovarian cancer compared to Doppler US or CT in both pre- and post-menopausal women. The positive likelihood ratio for contrast-enhanced MRI was 10-fold higher than Doppler US and approximately 7-fold higher than CT. The results of this trial demonstrate that in both pre- and post-menopausal women with an indeterminate ovarian mass on ultrasonography, second-line imaging is warranted to improve diagnostic certainty for ovarian cancer. Additionally, MRI is the ideal second line imaging modality and provides a significantly higher level of diagnostic certainty in comparison to Doppler US or CT.

The study was limited by the absence of integration of serum CA-125 into the diagnostic algorithm of adnexal masses, which may have improved diagnostic certainty. Nevertheless, this study served to inform the use of MRI as the second line imaging modality to determine the need for surgical evaluation of suspected ovarian cancer in both pre- and post-menopausal women.

In-Depth [meta-analysis]: The authors performed a literature review of English-language studies using MEDLINE database to determine the pre-test probability of ovarian cancer in pre- and post-menopausal women. The authors performed a literature review of 83 articles which met the following inclusion criteria: 1) presence of adnexal mass not detected during screening; 2) availability of histopathological information. Two experienced readers abstracted data from each article and disagreements were resolved with consensus. A similar methodology was utilized for a literature review of 12 articles to determine the sensitivity and specificity of ovarian mass characterization by Doppler US, CT, and MRI. Positive and negative likelihood ratios were calculated from the average weighted means of sensitivity and specificity. At the conclusion of the trial, the post-test probability following an indeterminate US result was 25% and 63% for pre- and post-menopausal women, respectively. Robust negative LR following initial indeterminate US result were seen for Doppler US (0.19), CT (0.22), and contrast-enhanced MRI (0.2). With respect to positive LR, contrast-enhanced MRI (44.2) was significantly more robust compared to Doppler US (4.69) and CT (6.81). This effect was seen in both pre- and post-menopausal women.

Kinkel K, Lu Y, Mehdizade A, Pelte M-F, Hricak H. Indeterminate Ovarian Mass at US: Incremental Value of Second Imaging Test for Characterization—Meta-Analysis and Bayesian Analysis. Radiology. 2005 Jul 1;236(1):85–94.

MRI effective for the assessment of acute appendicitis in pregnancy

1. In pregnant patients with suspected acute appendicitis and equivocal abdominal ultrasound, magnetic resonance imaging (MRI) demonstrated high accuracy, sensitivity, and negative predictive value for acute appendicitis.

Original Date of Publication: March 2006

Study Rundown: Acute appendicitis is a common cause of lower abdominal pain during pregnancy, with an incidence of 1 case per 1500 pregnancies. Ultrasonography is the initial imaging modality of choice to evaluate patients with acute right lower quadrant pain in pregnancy. However, due to the anatomical changes associated with the large gravid uterus, the sensitivity and specificity of identifying the appendix on ultrasonography is significantly lower compared to the general population. In cases of an equivocal ultrasound examination, MRI may be used to assess the appendix while avoiding ionizing radiation. The purpose of this landmark retrospective cohort was to determine the accuracy of MRI in the assessment of acute appendicitis during pregnancy.

This trial retrospectively reviewed 51 consecutive pregnant patients who were clinically suspected of having acute appendicitis that underwent MRI examinations of the abdomen with oral contrast. Positive appendicitis findings included a dilated appendix with high-signal intensity luminal fluid on T2-weigted imaging or periappendiceal fat stranding. At the conclusion of the trial, MRI demonstrated positive findings in all four patients that had confirmed acute appendicitis. No cases of appendicitis were missed by MRI. Additionally, in patients with no appendicitis, MRI demonstrated an alternate diagnosis for acute abdominal pain in 25% of patients. This study was the one of the first to demonstrate the high accuracy and negative predictive value to rule-out acute appendicitis in pregnant patients and highlighted the value of MRI in detecting periappendiceal findings as well as other potential etiologies of acute abdomen pain in pregnancy. Limitations included a small sample size and the fact that cases in which the appendix could not be visualized (16% of all patients) were classified as true negatives for statistical calculations rather than indeterminate. A number of other small retrospective reviews by Cobben et al., Brichard et al., and Israel et al., have confirmed the accuracy of MRI to be able to visualize the appendix in addition to determining other potential causes of acute abdominal pain.

In-Depth [retrospective cohort]: This study reviewed 51 consecutive pregnant patients (mean age: 28.3 years; range: 15-37, mean gestational age: 19.8 weeks; range: 4-38 weeks) that underwent oral-contrast enhanced MRI imaging of the abdomen for assessment of acute appendicitis in a single institution in the United States. 94% (48/51) of patients had ultrasound prior to MRI examination. All MRI examinations were performed on a 1.5-T coil with T1- T2-, Half-Fournier single-shot fast spin echo, and transverse time-of-flight gradient echo sequences. Interpretation of a positive finding of acute appendicitis was based on the presence of a dilated (>7 mm in diameter) appendix with high signal intensity luminal fluid on T2-weight images. Positive appendicitis was also noted if periappendiceal fat stranding was observed. The primary outcome was the accuracy, sensitivity, specificity, as well as positive and negative predictive values for appendicitis. At the conclusion of the study, MRI imaging demonstrated positive findings of appendicitis in all four cases with three inconclusive cases. All four patients with positive MRI findings had pathologically or CT-confirmed acute appendicitis. The appendix could not be visualized in 8 of the remaining 47 patients (17%) without acute appendicitis. As the study classified these nonvisualized cases as negatives rather than indeterminate, this translated into a prevalence-adjusted accuracy of 94% and a sensitivity, specificity, and negative predictive value of 100%, 93.6%, and 100%, respectively. Additionally, in patients with no evidence of acute appendicitis, MRI imaging provided an additional 58 alternative diagnoses related to the patient's acute abdominal pain, including an enlarged right gonadal vein (n = 11), right hydronephrosis (n = 25), degenerated fibroids (n = 6), and sub-chorionic hemorrhage (n = 11).

Pedrosa I, Levine D, Eyvazzadeh AD, Siewert B, Ngo L, Rofsky NM. MR *Imaging Evaluation of Acute Appendicitis in Pregnancy.* Radiology. 2006 Mar 1;238(3):891–9.

Additional Review:

Cobben LP, Groot I, Haans L, Blickman JG, Puylaert J. *MRI for Clinically Suspected Appendicitis During Pregnancy.* Am J Roentgenol. 2004 Sep 1;183(3):671–5.

Birchard KR, Brown MA, Hyslop WB, Firat Z, Semelka RC. *MRI of Acute Abdominal and Pelvic Pain in Pregnant Patients.* Am J Roentgenol. 2005 Feb 1;184(2):452–8.

Israel GM, Malguria N, McCarthy S, Copel J, Weinreb J. *MRI versus ultrasound for suspected appendicitis during pregnancy.* J Magn Reson Imaging. 2008 Aug 1;28(2):428–33.

The PIOPED II trial: CT sensitive and specific for pulmonary embolism

1. Multidetector computed tomographic angiography (CTA) was highly sensitive and specific for the diagnosis of pulmonary embolism (PE) when compared to a composite reference standard.

2. When combined with computed tomographic venography (CTV), sensitivity was increased without a significant increase in the specificity, positive predictive value, or negative predictive value.

Original Date of Publication: June 2006

Study Rundown: PE refers to the blockage of one or more arteries within the lung by a blood clot or other substance that originated within another part of the body. It is a commonly considered diagnosis among patients presenting to the emergency department with shortness of breath and chest pain, and failure to diagnose PE is associated with significant mortality. Historically, the diagnosis was made by the introduction of contrast material directly into the pulmonary arteries by a catheter. This technique was replaced by ventilation-perfusion (VQ) scanning, which compares patterns of blood flow and oxygenation in the lung using a radioactive tracer. Though significantly less invasive, VQ scanning was often difficult to interpret and was itself replaced by CTA beginning in the 1980s and 1990s.

Early reports of the diagnostic performance of CTA were generally positive but mixed, and the optimal method for evaluating patients with suspected PE initially remained uncertain. In the second Prospective Investigation of Pulmonary Embolism Diagnosis (PIOPED II) trial, CTA with and without concomitant lower extremity CTV was compared with a composite reference standard including both VQ scanning and conventional angiography. The results of this trial showed that both CTA and combined CTA-CTV were highly sensitive and specific for the diagnosis of PE, and that the combination of clinical judgment with the results from CTA or CTA-CTV evaluation was sufficient to accurately rule-in and rule-out PE in the vast majority of patients.

In-Depth [prospective cohort]: This prospective trial was conducted at 8 clinic sites throughout North America. All adult patients with signs and symptoms concerning for acute PE who were referred for evaluation were consecutively screened for enrollment (n = 7284). Both inpatients and outpatients were considered. Key exclusion criteria included anticoagulant use, hemodialysis, critical illness, patients on ventilators, and recent myocardial infarction. Following screening and consent, all enrolled patients (n = 1090) underwent combined CTA-CTV, as well as one or more of the components that together formed the composite reference standard. This included VQ scanning, lower extremity venous ultrasonography with Doppler imaging, and, when necessary, digital subtraction angiography (DSA) of the pulmonary arteries. All imaging studies were reviewed by 2 blinded radiologists unaffiliated with the clinical sites, with additional radiologists serving as arbiters in the event of discordant interpretations. Patients were considered to have a positive CTA if there was any partial or complete filling defect identified within one or more pulmonary arteries, and a positive CTV if there was any partial or complete filling defect identified within one of the lower extremity veins. Using the composite reference standard, patients were diagnosed with PE if any of the following conditions were met: high probability VQ scan in a patient without a history of PE; filling defect on pulmonary DSA; or visualized lower extremity clot by ultrasound.

A total of 824 patients (mean age 51.7 ± 17.1 years; 62% women; 89% outpatient) successfully completed both CTA-CTV and the composite reference standard. Among this cohort, 192 PEs were diagnosed. For those with diagnostic-quality CTA alone (773 patients, 94%), the sensitivity was 83% and the specificity was 96%, while the positive and negative predictive values were 86% and 95%, respectively. Considering those patients with diagnostic-quality combined CTA-CTV (737 patients, 89%) separately, the sensitivity was 90% and the specificity was 95%, while the positive and negative predictive values were 85% and 97%, respectively. The results varied substantially by clinical suspicion, with a positive predictive value of 96% among those with a high pre-test probability of PE and a positive predictive value of 58% among those with a low-pretest probability. Complications associated with CTA-CTV were rare and included mild allergic reactions and transiently increased creatinine.

Stein PD, Fowler SE, Goodman LR, Gottschalk A, Hales CA, Hull RD, et al. Multidetector Computed Tomography for Acute Pulmonary Embolism. New England Journal of Medicine. 2006 Jun 1;354(22):2317–27.

Breast density increases the risk of cancer and hinders mammographic detection

1. Women with mammographic density obscuring more than 75% of the imaged breast demonstrated a significantly increased risk of breast cancer detected either by screening or within 12 months of a negative screening examination, compared to those with density in less than 10% of the mammogram.

2. The increase in risk of breast cancer in women with dense breasts was greatest in younger women. In this demographic, 25% of all detected cancers were attributable to density in at least 50% of the mammogram.

Original Date of Publication: January 2007

Study Rundown: Mammography is an X-ray based modality, visualizing the various tissues of the breast based on their inherent attenuation properties. Fat appears radiolucent, while epithelial and stromal tissues appear radiodense. As the relative proportion between these tissues shifts away from fat, the breast becomes increasingly "dense" on mammography. As many tumors may also appear radiodense, they may be hidden by the predominance of stroma within a dense breast, subsequently hindering early detection, while that increased density may itself be a risk factor for oncogenesis. Unfortunately, this interaction between breast density and the ability to detect cancers on screening previously confounded research regarding the risks associated with mammographic density. Cancer risk would be underestimated if based solely on those tumors detected at screening due to an omission of those masked by breast density, while risk would be overestimated if based solely on cancers detected by alternate means, as it would focus only on those missed at screening.

The present study attempted to better estimate the true risk of mammographic density as it relates to breast cancer by determining the risk both at the time of screening and thereafter among women with quantified breast density from three large national case-control studies. Women with density in 75% or more of the mammogram demonstrated a significantly increased risk of breast cancer compared to those with density in 10% or less of the mammogram both at the time of screening or by alternate means. This risk was found to persist for up to 8 years after initial screening. The attributable risk of cancer to breast density was most marked in younger women, for whom 26% of all detected cancers, and 50% of those detected within 1 year of a negative examination were attributable to density in at least 50% of the mammogram. This study established an accurate estimate of the incidence of breast cancers attributable to increased breast density by combining those data for those detected at screening and those detected up to 12 months after a negative screening examination, representing cancers likely present at the time of initial screening but obscured by mammographic density.

In-Depth [case-control study]: This retrospective case-control study pooled data from three large mammographic screening programs in Canada, the National Breast Screening Study (NBSS), the Ontario Breast Screening Program (OBSP), and the Screening Mammography Program of British Columbia (SMPBC.) A total of 1114 case-control pairs were included (mean age 56.7±9.1 years). Case subjects had histologically verified invasive breast cancer, excluding those with cancers detected within 12 months of their first screening mammogram, while up to 10 control subjects were matched to each index case on the basis of age, body-mass index, pregnancy and menopause history, hormone-replacement use, family history of breast cancer, and quantification of mammographic density. Mammograms from each subject were submitted and independently classified into one of six quantified degrees of breast density (0%, < 10%, 10 to < 25%, 25 to < 50%, 50 to < 75%, and ≥75%) by two radiologists and a single observer using a computer-assisted technique.

Notably, the average percentage of mammographic density was 5.8% higher among case subjects than control subjects at baseline. Women below the median age of 56 years were 3 times more likely to have breasts with a mammographic density of ≥50%. The combined odds ratio for the detection of breast cancer among women with ≥75% mammographic density was 4.7 (95%CI 3.0-7.4) as compared to those with ≤10% density. For those cancers detected at screening, the odds ratio was 3.5 (95%CI 2.0-6.2), while it was 17.8 (95%CI 4.8-65.9) for those cancers detected within 12 months of a negative screening mammogram. For cancers detected over a year after the last negative screening mammogram, the odds ratio was 5.7 (95%CI 2.1-15.5). These increased risks were significantly associated with percentage of breast density at all time periods, up to 8 years after entry into the study ($p < 0.001$). The attributable risk of breast cancer for a mammographic density of ≥50% was 16% for all cancers, much of which was limited to the 12 months following screening, suggesting that tumor masking was the principal mechanism of risk, rather than rapid tumor growth.

Boyd NF, Guo H, Marin LJ, Sun L, Stone J, Fishell E, et al. *Mammographic Density and the Risk and Detection of Breast Cancer*. The New England Journal of Medicine. 2007 Jan 18;356(3):227–36.

Detection of advanced colorectal neoplasia by CT colonography comparable to optical colonoscopy

1. Computed tomographic colonography (CTC) and optical colonoscopy (OC) screening strategies resulted in similar detection rates of advanced neoplasia.

2. Rates of positive screening based on polyp size were achieved through CTC with significantly fewer adverse events compared to OC.

Original Date of Publication: October 2007

Study Rundown: Advanced neoplasia of the colon consists of adenocarcinomas and advanced adenomas, the latter of which are associated with a high risk of progression to cancer. Due to their potential to transform into invasive lesions, the early detection and removal of advanced adenomas represent key steps in reducing colorectal cancer mortality. Historically, fecal occult blood testing and sigmoidoscopy were used as primary screening tools. However, it was later found that over a third of colonic polyps are located proximal to the splenic flexure, rendering these methods inadequate in screening the entire colon. It was not until years later that single contrast barium enema (SCBE), and then double contrast barium enema (DCBE) emerged as the first radiologic imaging tests allowing for the detection of colonic neoplasms. Owing to the technically demanding and time-consuming nature of these imaging studies, the barium enema was later replaced by CTC as the primary imaging test used in colorectal cancer screening. In a prior prospective cohort conducted by Yee and colleagues, in which 300 patients underwent CTC followed by standard colonoscopy, CTC had a high sensitivity in the detection of clinically important polyps.

In the present study conducted by Kim and colleagues, CTC was compared to OC in the detection of advanced adenomas and adenocarcinomas. The results of this study showed that the total number of advanced neoplasms detected through CTC was similar to that detected by primary OC, with CTC requiring significantly fewer polypectomies to achieve these outcomes. While the rate of colonic perforations in the primary OC group was within an expected range, no serious complications were reported as a result of CTC.

In-Depth [non-randomized trial]: The results of a CTC screening program were compared to those of an OC screening program. Patients in each study group were consecutively enrolled, with partially overlapping time periods, from the same general screening population and geographic region. Key exclusion criteria included polyp surveillance, history of a bowel disorder (i.e. inflammatory bowel disease), polyposis syndromes, and hereditary nonpolyposis colorectal cancer (HNPCC) syndrome. Polyps were defined as large if measuring at least 10 mm in size, small if between 6-9 mm, and diminutive if 5 mm or less. As part of CTC preparation, 250 mL of 2% barium and 60 mL of diatrizoate were administered to tag residual stool and fluid, respectively. Colon distention was achieved through automated delivery of carbon dioxide. All CTC imaging studies were reviewed by 1 of 5 gastrointestinal radiologists and, where present, polyps were measured with electronic calipers. For all polyps > 6 mm, same-day therapeutic OC was offered unless contraindicated. Patients with only 1-2 polyps measuring between 6-9 mm were also given the option of CTC surveillance only. Polyps identified through OC were measured through in vivo OC estimation and removed with standard techniques.

A total of 3120 (mean age 57 years, SD 7.2 years; 44% male) and 3163 patients (mean age 58.1 years, SD 7.8. years; 44% male) underwent primary CTC and primary OC, respectively. Following primary CTC, 246 patients (7.9%) were referred for therapeutic OC. The total number of polyps removed in patients that underwent primary OC was 2434, far exceeding the 561 that were removed in patients who underwent primary CTC ($p < 0.001$). However, there were no statistically significant differences between groups with respect to the number of large ($p = 0.92$) or small ($p = 0.14$) advanced adenomas removed. The two screening strategies also had similar rates of positive screening results based on size threshold for polyps measuring ≥10 mm ($p = 0.06$) and ≥ 6 mm ($p = 0.59$). While there were no perforations or serious complications related to CTC or subsequent therapeutic OC, colonic perforation occurred in 7 (0.2%) patients in the primary OC screening group, of which 4 required surgical repair.

Kim DH, Pickhardt PJ, Taylor AJ, Leung WK, Winter TC, Hinshaw JL, et al. CT colonography versus colonoscopy for the detection of advanced neoplasia. The New England Journal of Medicine. 2007 Oct;357(14):1403-12.

Additional Review:

Levine MS, Yee J. History, Evolution, and Current Status of Radiologic Imaging Tests for Colorectal Cancer Screening. Radiology. 2014 Nov;273(2S):S160-S80.

Yee J, Akerkar GA, Hung RK, Steinauer-Gebauer AM, Wall SD, McQuaid KR. *Colorectal Neoplasia: Performance Characteristics of CT Colonography for Detection in 300 Patients 1*. Radiology. 2001 Jun;219(3):685-92.

MRI offers an alternative to endoscopic assessment of disease activity and severity in ileocolonic Crohn's disease

1. Magnetic resonance imaging (MRI) offers an effective alternative to endoscopy for quantifying disease severity in Crohn's disease.

2. MRI required 3T field strength, both oral and rectal contrast, IV antiperistalsis medication, and IV contrast administration.

Original Date of Publication: January 2009

Study Rundown: Appropriate therapy of Crohn's disease depends on disease severity and complications. The variable lifelong clinical course therefore necessitates frequent and accurate evaluation of disease activity. Historically, the diagnostic gold standard for Crohn's disease is based on endoscopic findings coupled with biochemical markers (such as faecal calprotectin (fC) and C-reactive protein (CRP)) and clinical scores (Harvey-Bradshaw Index (HBI) and Crohn's disease activity index (CDAI)). Endoscopy, however, only can access the proximal small bowel or terminal ileum. Imaging modalities have consequently been tested. Computed tomography (CT) enterography is limited use due to exposure to ionizing radiation. Transabdominal ultrasound lacks sensitivity and specificity and has high interobserver variability and is limited by overlying bowel gas. Magnetic resonance (MR) imaging lacks radiation exposure, has validated sensitivity and specificity, high soft-tissue resolution, and is therefore being increasing utilized in the diagnosis of Crohn's disease.

There was previously a lack of definitive criteria to evaluate Crohn's disease based on MR parameters. In a 2008 cross-sectional study done at the Hospital Clinic de Barcelona, a Magnetic Resonance Index of Activity (MaRIA) using wall signal intensity (WSI), relative contrast enhancement (RCE), edema, and presence of ulcers was internally validated as independent predictors of Crohn's disease severity. The same researchers externally validated MaRIA 3 years layer. Given the segmental predictors MaRIA uses, however, it may fail to appreciate the wide-ranging complications and total disease burden of Crohn's disease. In a 2013 prospective trial by Makanyanga et al., a magnetic resonance enterography global score (MEGS) was internally validated against fC and CRP. Used in conjunction, the measures provide an accurate measure of the activity and severity of Crohn's disease.

In-Depth [cross-sectional]: This cross-sectional assessed 50 patients with clinically active (n = 35) or inactive (n = 15) Crohn's disease based on the HBI. Ileocolonoscopy was used as the reference standard against MR. Except for a small number of patients, both assessments were performed the same day. Ileoendoscopic lesions were classified according to Crohn's Disease Endoscopic Index of Severity (CDEIS). MR imaging was performed using a 3.0 T unit after bowel preparation and after oral ingestion of a large volume of polyethylene glycol. Additionally, saline was administered rectally and IV anti peristaltic medication was given. IV gadolinium was also administered. Bowel wall thickness, ulceration, edema, pseudopolyp identification, lymph node enlargement, WSI before and after contrast, and RCE were analyzed. The chi-square test, ANOVA followed by the Bonferoni posthoc test, and Spearman rank coefficient were used for statistical analysis; results were subsequently internally validated using bootstrap bagging with 1000 samples. All paired MR evaluations were performed by two radiologists for interobserver agreement.

Complete endoscopic evaluation was completed in 36 patients (72% of total), yielding 213 colonic segments. MR and endoscopic findings were highly correlated for all parameters and interobserver agreement was very high (p < 0.001 for all). Wall thickness (p < 0.001), RCE (p = 0.013), and ulcer identification (p = 0.003) at MR were found to be independent predictors of active disease based on logistic regression analysis, with a sensitivity of 0.9 and specificity of 0.94. The MaRIA index was calculated to have a high (r = 0.81) and significant (p < 0.001) correlation with the CDEIS of each analogous colonic segment. Overall, the index has a high accuracy for detecting Crohn's disease activity (sensitivity 0.81, specificity 0.89) and for detecting ulcerative lesions (sensitivity 0.95, specificity 0.91) in the colon and terminal ileum.

Rimola J, Rodriguez S, García-Bosch O, Ordás I, Ayala E, Aceituno M, et al. Magnetic resonance for assessment of disease activity and severity in ileocolonic Crohn's disease. Gut. 2009 Aug 1;58(8):1113–20.

Additional Review:

Makanyanga JC, Pendsé D, Dikaios N, Bloom S, McCartney S, Helbren E, et al. Evaluation of Crohn's disease activity: Initial validation of a magnetic resonance enterography global score (MEGS) against faecal calprotectin. Eur Radiol. 2014 Feb 1;24(2):277–87.

Rimola J, Ordás I, Rodriguez S, García-Bosch O, Aceituno M, Llach J, et al. Magnetic resonance imaging for evaluation of Crohn's disease: validation of parameters of severity and quantitative index of activity. Inflamm Bowel Dis. 2011 Aug;17(8):1759–68.

Variable	Scoring
Deep ulceration	0 if absent, 12 if present
Superficial ulceration	0 if absent, 6 if present
Length of ulcerated mucosa	0-10, according to length in centimeters
Length of diseased mucosa	0-10, according to length in centimeters
Stenosis present	3 points if ulcerated stenosis; further 3 points if nonulcerated

Table I. Crohn's Disease Endoscopic Index of Severity (CDEIS): The first four endoscopic variables are scored for the following locations: rectum; sigmoid and left colon; transverse colon; right colon; and ileum. Total score is divided by number of locations.

Variable	Description
Bowel wall thickness	Measured in mm
Mucosal ulceration	Presence of deep depressions in mucosal surface
Mural edema	Presence of hyperintensity on T2-wedged sequences of the colon wall relative to the signal of the psoas muscle
Pseudopolyps in the lumen	Presence or absence
Enlarged regional lymph nodes	Greater than 1 cm
Wall signal intensity (WSI)	Quantitative measurement before and after IV contrast administration
Relative contrast enhancement (RCE)	RCE = (WSI postgadolinium − WSI pregadolinium) x 100 x (SD noise pregadolinium/SD noise postgadolinium)

Table II: Magnetic Resonance Index of Activity: Variables used in the statistical validation of the MaRIA index. Note that SD noise corresponds to the average of three SDs of the signal intensity measured outside the body before and after gadolinium injection. The same segmentation is used as in the CDEIS.

	0	1	2	3
Mural thickness	< 3 mm	3-5 mm	5-7 mm	> 7 mm
Mural T2 signal	Equal to normal bowel wall	Minor increase in signal	Moderate increase in signal	Marked increase in signal
Per-mural T2 signal	Equal to normal mesentery	Increase in mesenteric signal but no fluid	Small fluid rim	Large fluid rim (>2 mm)
T1 enhancement	Equal to normal bowel	Minor enhancement	Moderate enhancement	Marked enhancement
Mural enhancement pattern	N/A or homogenous	Mucosal	Layered	
Haustral loss (colon only)	None	< 1/3 segment	1/3-2/3 segment	> 2/3 segment
Multiplication factor per segment based on length of segment		0-5 cm x 1	5-15 cm x 1.5	> 15 cm x 2
	Additional extramural features that, when present, increase score by 5 points: lymph nodes, Comb sign, abscess, fistulae			

Table III. Magnetic Resonance Enterography Global Score (MEGS): A total score is calculated based the points (top row) for each given variable (left column). The same segments are evaluated as in the MaRIA index and CDEIS.

LI-RADS outlines standards for liver imaging studies assessing HCC

1. The American College of Radiology (ACR) created the Liver Imaging Reporting and Data System (LI-RADS) to standardize interpretation and reporting of liver imaging studies assessing risk for hepatocellular carcinoma (HCC).

2. Utilization of LI-RADS categories can aid in patient management decisions by suggesting diagnostic and/or treatment options.

Original Date of Publication: March 2011

Study Rundown: Chronic liver disease (CLD) and cirrhosis are risk factors for HCC, the third leading cause of cancer-related death worldwide. With these factors contributing towards development of the disease, HCC can affect a wide range of communities and counties. Early stage HCC is often asymptomatic and detection earlier is associated with better outcomes when medical treatment is offered, making screening of patients at high risk for HCC a key intervention. Screening evaluations can be completed using a variety of methods, with computed tomography (CT) or magnetic resonance imaging (MRI) being the most common.

LI-RADS, originally published in 2011 and continually updated, provides a standardized algorithmic framework for assessing HCC risk via CT or MRI. In addition to reducing variability in radiologist reporting, the framework can help clinicians by providing recommendations for how to follow-up lesions with further imaging studies, biopsies, and/or treatment. Though this system provides a standardized mechanism for lesion categorization, few prospective studies have been performed assessing how patients are differentially managed when assigned differing risk categories.

In-Depth: LI-RADS was developed by a panel of radiologists, with additional contribution from hepatologists, liver surgeons, and pathologists. The first iteration was launched in 2011 and has been updated continually since. LI-RADS provides standardized terminology for interpreting hepatic lesions and categorizing them according to their risk of HCC based on image characteristics (Table I). Categorization ranges from "Definitely Benign" (LR-1) to "Definitely HCC" (LR-5). Categorization of lesions as "Probably Benign" (LR-2),

"Intermediate Probability of HCC" (LR-3), and "Probably HCC" (LR-4) are based on 4 major image factors defined by Mitchell and colleagues including: arterial phase hyperenhancement; washout appearance following hyperenhancement; capsule appearance; and threshold growth compared with previous imaging. If there is uncertainty as to a categorization between LR-2 and LR-4, various defined ancillary image features may be used (Table 2). Additionally, there are categories for probable malignancy other than HCC (LR-M), previously treated HCC (LR5-T), and tumor within a vein (LR-5V).

Mitchell DG, Bruix J, Sherman M, Sirlin CB. LI-RADS (Liver Imaging Reporting and Data System): Summary, discussion, and consensus of the LI-RADS Management Working Group and future directions. Hepatology. 2015 Mar 1;61(3):1056–65.

Additional Review:

ACR. Archive - LI-RADS [Internet]. 2011. Available from: http://www.acr.org/Quality-Safety/Resources/LIRADS/Archive.

Purysko AS, Remer EM, Coppa CP, Leão Filho HM, Thupili CR, Veniero JC. LI-RADS: A Case-based Review of the New Categorization of Liver Findings in Patients with End-Stage Liver Disease. RadioGraphics. 2012 Nov 1;32(7):1977–95.

LI-RADS Framework

Category	Probability of HCC	Imaging Features	Management
LR-1	Definitely benign	• Diagnostic features for a benign entity OR • Lesion resolves without treatment	• Continue standard surveillance
LR-2	Probably benign	• Suggestive, but not diagnostic, features for a benign entity	• Continue standard surveillance • If >1 cm, consider accelerated follow-up, alternative imaging or multidisciplinary discussion

LR-3	Intermediate probability of HCC	• Mass HYPERenhancing in the arterial phase with NO WCT
		• Mass HYPO- or ISOenhancing in the arterial phase:
		   ○ <20 mm with ≤1 of WCT
		   ○ ≥20 mm with NO WCT
			• Variable
			• At a minimum accelerated follow-up, consider alternative imaging or multidisciplinary discussion

LR-4	Probably HCC	• Mass HYPERenhancing in the arterial phase:
		   ○ <10 mm with ≥1 of WCT
		   ○ 10-19 mm with 1 of WCT
		   ○ ≥20 mm with NO WCT
		• Mass HYPO- or ISOenhancing in the arterial phase:
		   ○ <20 mm with ≥2 of WCT
		   ○ ≥20 mm with ≥1 of WCT
			• Variable
			• Alternative imaging (if distinct advantage) and/or multidisciplinary discussion

LR-5	Definitely HCC	• Mass HYPERenhancing in the arterial phase:
		   ○ 10-19 mm with ≥2 of WCT
		   ○ ≥20 mm with ≥1 of WCT
			• Multidisciplinary discussion

LR-5V	Tumor in vein	• Definite enhancing soft tissue in vein	• Multidisciplinary discussion • Contraindication to liver transplant
LR-M	Probable malignancy, but non-specific for HCC	*Favor other malignancy* • Arterial rim HYPERenhancement • Central delayed phase enhancement • Concentric enhancement • Peripheral washout • Hepatic retraction • Biliary obstruction greater than expected for size • Targetoid on DWI or hepatobiliary phase	• Variable, may include follow-up, alternative imaging, biopsy, treatment, and/or multidisciplinary discussion
		Favor HCC • Diffuse arterial HYPERenhancement • Delayed washout • Capsule • Distinct rim • Intralesional fat • Diffuse T1 HYPERintensity • Tumor in vein • Nodule-in-nodule • Mosaic architecture • Spontaneous hemorrhage	

Table I. LI-RADS framework. WCT = Washout, Capsule, and/or Threshold Growth.
NOTE: Alternative imaging is typically considered if there is a distinct advantage to the alternative modality.
Table compiled using information from Mitchell et al. and http://www.acr.org/Quality-Safety/Resources/LIRADS

Ancillary Features: LI-RADS Framework	
Favor Benignity	**Favor Malignancy**

- Homogenous T2 HYPERintensity
- Homogenous T2 or T2* HYPOintensity
- Hepatobiliary phase ISOintensity
- No vessel distortion
- Stable or reduced diameter on follow-up scans
	- Mild-moderate T2 HYPERintensity
	- Diffusion restriction
	- Hepatobiliary/transitional phase HYPOintensity
	- Iron/fat sparing
	- Blood products
	- Diameter increase less than threshold
	- Favoring HCC specifically:
	    o Distinct rim
	    o Corona enhancement
	    o Mosaic architecture
	    o Nodule-in-nodule
	    o Intralesional fat

Table II. Ancillary Features - LI-RADS Framework. Presence of these features may be used, with caution, to downgrade or upgrade the LR category by one or more levels, up to a maximum of LR-4. Absence of one or more features should not be used to upgrade or downgrade categories. Table compiled using information from Mitchell et al. and http://www.acr.org/Quality-Safety/Resources/LIRADS.

Ovarian cancer screening does not reduce mortality

1. Randomization of patients to either yearly ovarian cancer screening with transvaginal ultrasound (TVUS) and serum CA-125 levels or usual care did not significantly reduce cancer-related mortality.

2. False-positive results among the screening cohort were associated with significant surgical morbidity, with at least one serious complication suffered by roughly one-sixth of those who underwent surgical workup.

Original Date of Publication: June 2011

Study Rundown: Ovarian cancer remains both a diagnostic and therapeutic dilemma: it is often diagnosed late in its course due to vague and nonspecific presenting symptoms, and has poor long-term survival rates once it has spread beyond a single ovary. However, surgically managed ovarian cancers that remain confined to the ovary display 5-year survival rates greater than 90%, suggesting that early recognition and treatment could lead to a substantial mortality benefit. The referenced trial, part of a series of the Prostate, Lung, Colorectal and Ovarian Cancer Screening Trial (PLCO), randomized women to either yearly screening for ovarian cancer with TVUS for 3 years and measurement of serum CA-125 levels for 5 years, or standard care with yearly bimanual examination in an effort to determine if ovarian cancer screening would yield earlier diagnoses and resultant prognostic improvements. Screening did not significantly increase the number of cases of ovarian cancer diagnosed, though the results did trend toward significance. More poignantly however, the distributions of cancer stage at diagnosis were similar between groups, with a majority diagnosed at stage III-IV, and therefore ovarian cancer-related survival remained similarly low between groups. Screening was itself not a benign intervention, with positive findings frequently requiring surgical management. Nearly 10% of women in the screening cohort had false-positive results, requiring the performance of ultimately unnecessary surgeries in which 15% of patients suffered at least one serious post-surgical complication. This trial demonstrated that annual screening with simultaneous TVUS and CA-125 does not reduce cancer-specific mortality among average risk women, but does increase the risk of harm related to the performance of invasive procedures, particularly when due to false-positive findings or overdiagnosis.

In-Depth [randomized controlled trial]: A total of 68 557 women (roughly 88.5% of non-Hispanic white ethnicity, primarily aged 55-64 years) of average risk for ovarian cancer were enrolled at 10 screening centers across the United States. Subjects were excluded from analysis if they had a pretrial history of ovarian cancer or bilateral oophorectomy. Women were randomized to either the screening arm of the trial, in which they underwent yearly TVUS for 3 years, and yearly serum CA-125 measurements for 4-6 years, or the control arm of the trial, in which they underwent only yearly bimanual examination. Due to the invasive nature of the screening tests, no blinding could be performed. The positivity threshold for TVUS included ovarian volume greater than 10 cm^3, cyst volume greater than 10 cm^3, complex ovarian cysts with solid or papillary projections into the cavity, or any mixed (solid or cystic) components within a cystic ovarian tumor. Of note, this size threshold may have been too high to effectively detect low stage ovarian tumors, which are thought to be less than 10 cm^3, but would have introduced further false-negative results. A positivity threshold of 35 U/mL was used for serum CA-125 levels. A total of 212 cases of ovarian cancer were detected in the screening arm (5.7 per 10 000 person-years) while 176 cases were detected in the control group (4.7 per 10 000 person-years; RR 1.21; 95%CI 0.99-1.48) during the mean 12.6 year follow-up period. Of the cancers detected, the majority were high grade serous cystadenocarcinomas in both groups with a similar distribution of histological subtypes and grades. No stage shift, or difference in the cancer stage at time of diagnosis, was observed between groups. The majority of tumors were diagnosed at stage III-IV, with 69% of those detected during screening being advanced stage, as compared to 78% in the control group. As a stage shift is believed to be necessary for a mortality benefit, no significant difference in cancer-related mortality was noted between the two groups (RR, 1.18; 95%CI 0.82-1.71). A total of 3285 (9.6%) women suffered false-positive screening results, 1080 of whom underwent surgical management as part of their diagnostic workup. Of these women, 163 (15%) suffered at least one major surgical complication. This trial demonstrated that screening for ovarian cancer with TVUS and serum CA-125 levels does not reduce cancer stage at the time of diagnosis or cancer-related mortality, and may in fact introduce potential harm related to the workup of false-positive results.

Buys SS, Partridge E, Black A, Johnson CC, Lamerato L, Isaacs C, et al. Effect of screening on ovarian cancer mortality: The prostate, lung, colorectal and ovarian (PLCO) cancer screening randomized controlled trial. Journal of the American Medical Association. 2011 Jun 8;305(22):2295–303.

Katayama H, Yamaguchi K, Kozuka T, Takashima T, Seez P, Matsuura K. Adverse Reactions to Ionic and Nonionic Contrast Media, A Report from the Japanese Committee on the Safety of Contrast Media. Radiology. 1990 Jun 175:621–28.

CT scans increase the risk of malignancy in children and young adults

1. In this retrospective cohort analysis of children and young adults without previous malignancy, patients exposed to multiple computed tomography (CT) scans had over 3 times the risk of developing leukemia and brain tumors.

Original Date of Publication: August 2012

Study Rundown: While the connection between radiation exposure and malignancy was previously identified, research on the subject matter drew from high-dose radiation exposure secondary to atomic bombs in Japan. At the time of its publication, this study was the first to use a cohort to examine the malignancy risk associated with low-dose radiation from CT scans. Through retrospective analysis, researchers investigated the relationship between CT-induced radiation exposure during childhood and young adulthood and development of leukemia and brain cancer, as these malignancies occur in particularly radiosensitive tissue. Children under the age of 15 who received 5-10 head CTs were exposed to around 50 milligrays (mGy) of radiation to their marrow, while 2-3 head CTs exposed these children to about 60 mGy of brain radiation. For comparison, the average chest radiograph exposes a child to 0.05 to 0.3 mGy.

Investigators reported an over 3 times increased risk of developing leukemia with exposure to ≥ 30 mGy and developing a brain tumor with ≥ 50 mGy of radiation. Limitations included using standardized CT machine settings as a proxy when assessing radiation exposure due to missing data regarding machine-specific settings. However, the use of a cohort from Great Britain's national database ensured a large study group with low risk of loss to follow-up. This was the first cohort study to investigate the potential association between lower doses of radiation than the estimated 100 mGy of radiation exposure experienced by many Japanese atomic bomb victims. While the overall incidence of these malignancies is small within the pediatric population, this study does indicate significant risks associated with over-imaging developing children. With this in mind, the Alliance for Radiation Safety in Pediatric Imaging within the United States has started the "Image Gently" campaign, a movement designed to increase awareness of healthcare practitioners and caregivers to the benefits of reducing unnecessary radiation exposure.

In-Depth [retrospective cohort]: A total of 355 191 patients seen at a Great Britain National Health Service hospital without a history of prior malignancy, but who underwent a first CT scan between 1985-2002 at ages younger than 22, were included in the study. The study group was divided such that 178 604 patients were investigated with respect to leukemia and 176 587 patients were studied with respect to brain tumors. Malignancies investigated included acute lymphoblastic leukemia, acute myeloid leukemia, myelodysplastic syndromes (MDS), leukemia excluding MDS, gliomas, meningiomas, and schwannomas. Relative risks were calculated to assess the relationship between the radiation doses expressed in mGy units and malignancy. Data were collected from a national registry and ended on December 31, 2008, at time of death, or when patients were lost to follow-up. During analysis, radiation doses were adjusted to reflect the time it typically takes to develop a malignancy. This resulted in a 2 year lag for leukemia and a 5 year lag for brain tumors.

Among the patients included in the leukemia analysis, 283 919 CT scans were completed (64% head) and 74 patients had developed leukemia on follow-up. 279 824 scans were completed for patients included in brain tumor analysis with 135 patients ultimately receiving diagnoses of brain tumors on follow-up. Significant positive associations between leukemia and CT radiation dosing ($p < 0.01$) and brain tumors and radiation ($p < 0.001$) were observed. Mean radiation dose was 51.13 mGy for patients who developed leukemia and with exposure to ≥ 30 mGy of radiation. Among those who received ≥ 30 mGy, patients were more than 3 times as likely to develop leukemia when compared to those who received < 5 mGy (RR 3.18; 95%CI 1.46-6.94). Mean radiation dose for patients who received ≥ 50 mGy and developed brain tumors was 104.16 mGy. Those who received ≥ 50 mGy of radiation were at greater than 3 times the risk of developing a brain tumor when compared to those who were exposed to < 5 mGy (RR 3.32; 95%CI 1.84-6.42).

Pearce MS, Salotti JA, Little MP, McHugh K, Lee C, Kim KP, et al. Radiation exposure from CT scans in childhood and subsequent risk of leukaemia and brain tumors: a retrospective cohort. The Lancet. 2012 Aug 4;380(9840):499–505.

Increased use of pediatric CT poses significant oncogenic risk

1. Between 1996 and 2010, the use of computed tomographic (CT) imaging increased 2- to 3-fold for children up to 14 years of age, with effective radiation doses per scan varying widely, but ranging up to 69.2 mSv/scan.

2. The highest average radiation doses were delivered by abdominal and pelvic CT scans, with up to a quarter of such scans providing over 20 mSv/scan. A corresponding lifetime attributable risk of solid oncogenesis was estimated at 1 tumor for every 300-390 scans at worst, varying by age, sex, and scan type.

Original Date of Publication: June 2013

Study Rundown: The expanding uses of pediatric imaging have dramatically improved modern diagnostic capabilities. With this expansion has come an increasing concern for the possibility of associated oncogenic risk due to the delivery of ionizing radiation from techniques such as CT. Children are thought to have increased risk of radiation-induced cancers due to their young age, reduced radiation attenuation secondary to smaller body sizes, and the potential for increased radiation doses due to a failure to appropriately alter scanning protocols from an adult to a pediatric paradigm. Previously, Mathews et al. estimated that the incidence of cancers due to childhood CT exposure was 24% higher in irradiated subjects than controls, with risk increases proportional to dose, and inversely proportional to age at exposure. The current study sought to retrospectively examine trends in CT use, including doses delivered to children during individual CT scans, and project an attributable carcinogenic risk of such scans in an effort to offer targeted dose reduction strategies. During the study period from 1996 to 2010, the authors found that CT use had sharply increased, doubling for children under age 5 and tripling for those aged 5-14 before peaking around 2007 and downtrending thereafter. Effective single scan doses were highly variable across sites and scanners, ranging from 0.03 to 69.2 mSv/scan, with up to a quarter of children receiving doses greater than 20 mSv/scan. The most frequently ordered scans were of the abdomen and pelvis, which also carried the highest average radiation dose and corresponding oncogenic risk, estimated at 25.8 to 33.9 cases per 10 000 scans for girls, and 13.1 to 14.8 cases per 10 000 for boys. Lifetime attributable solid cancer and leukemia risks were calculated based on individual organ dosimetry and were highest for girls and younger children. These data suggested that nearly 5000 future cancers could be attributed to pediatric CT use per year in the United States, and that a reduction of the highest quartile of doses could prevent over two fifths of such cancers.

In-Depth [retrospective cohort]: Between 1996 and 2010, this study retrospectively observed CT use patterns in children aged 15 or younger at six large health maintenance organizations (HMOs) within the HMO Research Network across the United States. Roughly 150 000 to 370 000 children were included in the study per year (50% female, 29% under 5 years of age.) CT use increased steadily between 1996 and 2005, peaking at a doubling of scans for children under age 5 and a tripling of scans for children aged 5 to 14. From 2007 onward, CT utilization trended down. The most commonly ordered scans were of the head, abdomen/pelvis, thorax and spine, respectively, with abdominal/pelvic scans seeing the greatest increase in use. Effective radiation doses, on a per organ basis, were calculated using age- and sex-specific computational anatomy phantoms and the abstracted study parameters of 744 randomly selected individual scans. From these data, lifetime attributable risks of cancer were projected using multiple previously published risk models based upon data from the Life Span Study of Japanese atomic bomb survivors. Solid tumor risks increased with earlier ages at exposure, increased dose, and female gender. Using abdomen/pelvis CTs as the highest risk index scenario, 1 radiation-induced tumor was predicted for every 300-390 and 670-760 scans for girls and boys, respectively.) Leukemia risks were highest for head CTs in children under age 5, at 1 case of leukemia per 5250 head CTs performed in this age group. Projection of these findings to the United States at large suggested that each year, pediatric CT imaging could conservatively be attributable to the development of 4870 future cancers. Reductions in delivered doses or scan frequency through standardized pediatric dose reduction protocols, increased use of alternative imaging modalities such as ultrasound or magnetic resonance imaging, and implementation of stricter appropriateness guidelines to reduce unnecessary scans could significantly reduce oncogenic risks. More specifically, a reduction of the highest 25% of doses delivered per scan to the median dose could prevent 43% of attributable tumors, while a 33% reduction in CTs performed would reduce cancers by an equal proportion.

Miglioretti DL, Johnson E, Williams A, Greenlee RT, Weinman S, Solberg LI, et al. The use of computed tomography in pediatrics and the associated radiation exposure and estimated cancer risk. Journal of the American Medical Association. 2013 Jun 10;167(8):700–07.

Mathews JD, Forsythe AV, Brady Z, Butler MW, Goergen SK, Byrnes GB, et al. Cancer risk in 680 000 people exposed to computed tomography scans in childhood or adolescence: data linkage study of 11 million Australians. BMJ. 2013 May 21;346:f2360.

LUNG-RADS criteria increases positive predictive value for lung cancer detection in high-risk patients

1. The American College of Radiology (ACR) developed Lung Imaging Reporting and Data System (Lung-RADS) to standardize reporting and management of CT lung cancer screenings (Table I).

2. Retrospective application of Lung-RADS criteria, notably with a higher nodule size thresholds delineating a positive screening result, showed increased positive predictive value of lung cancer diagnosis in high-risk patients receiving CT lung screenings relative to National Lung Screening Trial (NLST) nodule size thresholds.

Original Date of Publication: May 2014

Study Rundown: Early in the progression of lung cancer symptoms are rare, but persistent cough, dyspnea, chest pain, and/or weight loss may be experienced in advanced forms of the disease. Most lung cancers are caused by exposure to tobacco smoke. Because symptoms are rare in early forms of the disease it is recommended for people at increased risk for lung cancer to undergo regular screenings. Results from the National Lung Screening Trial (NLST) indicated chest CT screenings can decrease lung cancer deaths significantly relative to screenings with chest x-rays. In addition, the NLST study indicated CT screening leads to more false positives than chest x-rays, and the false positive rate is approx. 98%.

The NLST defined a positive lung CT screening result to be a nodule greater than 4 cm in diameter with no benign calcification patterns. Because increasing the threshold to diagnose a lesion as cancerous can theoretically decrease the false positive rate but also decrease the sensitivity of the screening procedure, questions have been raised about changing the thresholds for positive cancer diagnosis. Additionally, management of patients with positive screening results has not been truly standardized. Lung-RADS has sought to address these issues by increasing the thresholds for a positive screening test and providing management guidelines on how to proceed after screening. Retrospective studies by McKee and colleagues and Pinsky and colleagues indicate the positive predictive values of CT screenings of high-risk patients can be raised significantly with small or no decreases in sensitivity.

In-Depth [retrospective cohorts]: Pinsky and colleagues applied Lung-RADS criteria to published data from the NLST. Patients aged 55-74 who smoked for 30+ pack-years and still smoke or quit in the last 15 years were recruited at 33 US institutions for the study (n = 26455). Patient and nodule level information was available for analysis. To assess Lung-RADS, nodules were reclassified using categories ranging from 1 (negative screening) to 4 (suspicious), with Category 4 having various subcategories. Classification of nodules using Lung-RADS accounts for nodule size, attenuation, and nodule growth in follow-up screenings. Positive results for a new screening are 6+cm diameters for solid/part-solid nodules and 2+cm for nonsolid nodules. For follow-up screenings, 4+cm nodules and 1.5+cm of nodule growth constitutes a positive result for solid/part-solid tumors, while nonsolid nodules must still be 2+cm. The patient's screening category is based off the nodule with the highest Lung-RADS score. Lung cancer was considered present at a given screening if the diagnosis was made within 1 year of screening or before the next screening. When applying Lung-RADS criteria to baseline and follow-up screenings false-positive rates and sensitivity were significantly lower.

McKee and colleagues also retrospectively assessed application of Lung-RADS criteria to CT lung cancer screenings originally assessed using National Comprehensive Cancer Network (NCCN) criteria similar to NLST criteria. Patients were assessed at a single center and had to be at high-risk for lung cancer (as defined by NCCN), asymptomatic, have physician orders for CT lung screening, been cancer free the previous 5+ years, and not have metastatic disease (n = 2180). Reclassification of nodules to benign using Lung-RADS occurred in 17% (370/2180) of patients, decreasing positive test rates from 27.6% using NCCN criteria to 10.6%. No patients diagnosed with lung cancer following screening had their nodules reclassified to benign. PPV of baseline CT screening increased from 6.9% to 17.3%. Of 29 patients diagnosed with lung cancer on follow-up, 86.3% (25/29) were classified as Category 4.

ACR. Lung CT Screening Reporting and Data System (Lung-RADS™) - American College of Radiology [Internet]. 2014. Available from: http://www.acr.org/Quality-Safety/Resources/LungRADS.

Additional Review:

Pinsky P, Gierada D, Black W, Munden R, Nath H, Aberle D, Kazerooni E. Performance of Lung-RADS in the National Lung Screening Trial. Annals of Internal Medicine. 2015;162(7):485.

Lung-RADS Framework

Category	Descriptor	Management
0	**Incomplete**	Additional lung cancer screening CT images and/or comparison to prior chest CT examinations is needed
1	**Negative:** No nodules and definitely benign nodules	Continue annual screening with LDCT in 12 months
2	**Benign Appearance or Behavior:** Nodules with a very low likelihood of becoming a clinically active cancer due to size or lack of growth	Continue annual screening with LDCT in 12 months
3	**Probably Benign:** Probably benign finding(s) - short term follow up suggested; includes nodules with a low likelihood of becoming a clinically active cancer	6 month LDCT
4A	**Suspicious:** Findings for which additional diagnostic testing and/or tissue sampling is recommended	3 month LDCT; PET/CT may be used when there is a ≥8 mm solid component
4B	**Suspicious:** Findings for which additional diagnostic testing and/or tissue sampling is recommended	Chest CT with or without contrast, PET/CT and/or tissue sampling depending on the probability of malignancy and comorbidities. PET/CT may be used when there is a ≥8 mm solid component.
S	**Significant-other**	
C	**Prior Lung Cancer**	

Table I. Lung-RADS final assessment categories.
Table compiled using information from www.acr.org/Quality-Safety/Resources/BIRADS.

Combination mammography and breast tomosynthesis improves breast cancer screening

1. The addition of breast tomosynthesis to digital mammography in breast cancer screening improved lesion conspicuity, thereby significantly increasing the rate of cancer detection and the overall positive predictive value of screening.

2. The rate of patient recall for further workup of a positive screen was significantly reduced with the addition of tomosynthesis.

Original Date of Publication: June 2014

Study Rundown: Breast cancer screening entails yearly mammography and clinical breast exam for women aged 50-70 years, among whom it has been shown to reduce mortality. However, mammography alone suffers from a limited positive predictive value, with an excess of false-positive results believed to be due to overlapping breast tissue. Breast tomosynthesis (BT) was developed to offset this limitation. By acquiring multiple low-dose images of the breast at focal planes of varying depth and reconstructing a single image or depth stacked series of images, BT reduces the "noise" of overlapping densities within the breast to more easily highlight true abnormalities. As imaging technology has progressed with large-field, fast-reading detectors, BT has now become feasible in routine practice, and the referenced study sought to examine how large-scale combination of mammography and BT compares to mammography alone in improving upon the specificity of breast cancer screening. In a retrospective review of nearly a half million screening examinations performed before and after the introduction of combined mammography and BT in routine practice, the combination technique significantly increased the positive predictive value of a positive screening examination from 4.3% to 6.4%, and of a subsequent biopsy from 24.2% to 29.2%. This improvement was reflected in an increase in the cancer detection rate at screening from 4.2 by mammography alone to 5.4 per 1000 examinations by the combined method. Additionally, the combination of mammography and BT reduced the overall recall rate, or the proportion of patients in whom a positive screen necessitated further workup, from 107 to 91 per 1000 examinations. Together, these findings suggested that the addition of BT to routine breast cancer screening may improve screening specificity, thereby reducing unnecessary interventions due to false-positive results. However, a direct determination of sensitivity and specificity could not be calculated as the dataset did not include patient-level information on the occurrence of interval cancers. The study was additionally limited by its retrospective nature and inherent lack of randomization, introducing the potential for selection bias and differences in baseline patient characteristics to influence the results obtained.

In-Depth [retrospective cohort]: This retrospective trial was conducted at 13 separate sites over two separate periods, one prior to the introduction of BT at each institution (one year in duration), and the other following the start of standard screening with combined digital mammography and BT (average duration of 17 months). Notably, only two sites were able to replace all equipment with tomography capable devices at once, while others maintained a hybrid environment in which mammography alone was still used after the transition. A total of 454 850 screening examinations were included in the primary analysis, read by 139 radiologists across all sites, with 61.8% performed during the first period (mammography alone), and 38.2% performed during the second period (mammography + BT). Comparing those studies performed prior to the introduction of BT to mammographic screening, a specific set of metrics was tabulated to compare the efficacy of mammography with and without BT: The patient recall rate, or proportion of patients in whom a positive screen necessitated additional imaging; the cancer detection rate, or proportion of patients in whom a positive screen detected a true cancer, and the positive predictive value for both patient recall and for biopsies performed as a result of a screening examination. For mammography alone, the rate of patient recall was 107 per 1000 screens as compared to 91 per 1000 screens for mammography + BT, resulting in a decrease in the recall rate of -16 (95%CI -18 to -14; $p < 0.001$) per 1000 screens. The difference in biopsy rate between mammography without and with BT was +1.3 (95%CI 0.4-2.1; $p = 0.004$) per 1000 screens. The overall cancer detection rate (n = 815 invasive cancers, n = 392 ductal carcinoma in situ) for mammography alone was 4.2 per 1000 screens, while it increased to 5.4 per 1000 screens with the addition of tomography, resulting in an increase of 1.2 (95%CI 0.8-1.6; $p < 0.001$) per 1000 screens. When considering invasive cancers alone, the net increase in cancer detection rate was unchanged. The PPV for recall for mammography alone was 4.3% versus 6.4% with the addition of BT, for an overall increase of 2.1% (95%CI 1.7-2.5% $p < 0.001$), while for biopsy, the net increase in PPV was 5.0% (95%CI 3.0-7.0%; $p < 0.001$). A secondary analysis was performed using examinations the second period alone, comparing mammograms performed without BT to those performed with BT in an effort to address the potential for selection bias to affect the results given the hybrid nature of the transition at many sites. A statistically significant improvement in cancer detection with mammography + BT was found (p < 0.001), consistent with those findings from the primary analysis.

Friedewald SM, Rafferty EA, Rose SL, Durand MA, Plecha DM, Greenberg JS, et al. Breast Cancer Screening Using Tomosynthesis in Combination With Digital Mammography. The Journal of The American Medical Association. 2014 Jun 25;311(24):2499–2507.

Coronary CT angiography not superior to functional testing in cardiac risk management

1. Computed tomographic coronary angiography (CTCA) as the initial diagnostic test for patients at intermediate risk of coronary artery disease (CAD) was not superior to functional cardiac testing with regard to all-cause mortality or major cardiovascular events over a 2-year period.

2. Patients in the CTCA group underwent significantly more cardiac catheterizations (though with fewer procedures revealing no CAD) and subsequently had an increased rate of coronary revascularization than those in the functional testing arm.

Original Date of Publication: April 2015

Study Rundown: Patients with suspected CAD, such as those with new-onset stable angina or at least one major cardiac risk factor, require diagnostic testing to determine both their burden of disease and the appropriateness of medical or surgical intervention in cardiac risk mitigation. Noninvasive testing for CAD is indicated for such intermediate-risk, ambulatory patients and has historically involved a functional test, such as a stress electro- or echocardiogram or a nuclear stress test, any of which can reveal indirect evidence of CAD if reversible ischemia is present. However, CTCA has emerged as a viable alternative to functional testing with a theoretically increased specificity given that it provides a direct anatomical assessment. It has even been proposed that CTCA may reveal nonobstructive but prognostically significant coronary lesions. The Prospective Multicenter Imaging Study for Evaluation of Chest Pain (PROMISE) randomized outpatients with new onset, stable chest pain or with at least one major cardiac risk factor to either CTCA or functional testing for CAD in an effort to determine if noninvasive anatomical testing might improve cardiac outcomes over functional testing. Over the 2-year follow-up period from initial randomization, no significant differences were found in all-cause mortality or major cardiovascular events between the two groups, though patients in the CTCA group underwent an increased rate of cardiac catheterization and subsequent surgical or percutaneous coronary revascularization. Notably, the study was not designed or powered to assess, given its relatively short length of follow-up, if the observed increased rate of catheterization and revascularization might have affected long-term outcomes.

Within this limitation, PROMISE established that CTCA is not superior to standard functional cardiac testing in the initial workup of patients at intermediate risk of CAD. However, future trials are necessary to determine if the increased rate of revascularization observed within the CTCA group may yield a longitudinal mortality benefit.

In-Depth [randomized controlled trial]: A total of 10 003 outpatients (mean age 60±8.3 years, 52.7% women) presenting primarily with new onset, stable chest pain without a prior diagnosis of CAD were enrolled at several major medical centers across the United States. Patients were randomized to either undergo CTCA or functional cardiac testing for the non-urgent, non-invasive workup of suspected CAD, and were followed for a median period of 25 months. Functional tests utilized in the control arm of the trial included nuclear stress testing (67.5%), stress echocardiography (22.4%), and exercise electrocardiography (10.2%). The primary endpoints of the trial were all-cause mortality or major cardiovascular events (including complications from diagnostic or therapeutic cardiovascular procedures), while secondary endpoints included invasive cardiac catheterizations, particularly those that did not reveal CAD, and cumulative radiation exposure. Median cumulative radiation exposure was lower per patient in the CTCA group than the functional testing group (10.0 mSv versus 11.3 mSv; $p < 0.001$). The bulk of per patient exposure occurred secondary to nuclear stress testing, though overall exposure was greater within the CTCA group as 32.6% of patients in the functional testing group had no radiation exposure. The study was powered at 90% confidence to detect a 20% relative reduction in the primary endpoint between groups assuming an overall event rate of 8% at 2.5 years post-randomization. The true observed overall event rate was 3.1% for mortality or major cardiovascular events, with no significant difference between the CTCA group (3.3%) and the functional testing group (3.0%; adjusted hazard ratio 1.04; 95%CI 0.83-1.29; $p = 0.075$) over the median 25 month follow-up period. A similar rate of positive initial tests was observed between the two groups, with 10.7% of initial CTCAs and 11.7% of functional tests interpreted as positive. In the 90 days following randomization, 12.2% of patients in the CTCA group underwent cardiac catheterization as opposed to only 8.1% of the functional testing group, but catheterizations performed in the CTCA group significantly more likely to be positive (72.1% versus 52.5%; $p = 0.02$). Additionally, revascularization (either surgical or percutaneous) was significantly more commonly performed within the CTCA group, occurring in 6.2% of patients as compared to 3.2% in the functional testing group ($p < 0.001$). However, revascularization was not a trial end point, and the study was not adequately powered to assess the effect of this difference on long-term cardiovascular outcomes.

Douglas PS, Hoffmann U, Patel MR, Mark DB, Al-Khalidi HR, Cavanaugh B, et al. Outcomes of anatomical versus functional testing for coronary artery disease. The New England Journal of Medicine. 2015 Apr 2;372(14):1291–1300.

PI-RADS version 2: Standardized acquisition, interpretation, and reporting of prostate MRI

1. A joint steering committee have revised the original Prostate Imaging Reporting and Data System (PI-RADS) guidelines to form PI-RADS version 2 (v2), which improves the standardization of imaging acquisition and reporting in pre-therapy patients with suspected prostate cancer.

2. DWI is the predominant sequence to evaluate peripheral zone (PZ) lesions, while T2-weighted magnetic resonance imaging (MRI) is favored for evaluation of the transition zone (TZ).

3. Lesions with a PI-RADS score of ≥3 should be reported. If multiple, up to 4 should be reported with the index lesion identified.

4. The guidelines are intended to evolve as the prostate imaging community gains clinical experience in the application of PI-RADS v2.

Original Date of Publication: April 2015

Study Rundown: The European Society of Urogenital Radiology (ESUR) originally published the Prostate Imaging Reporting and Data System (PI-RADS) in 2012 to provide structured clinical guidelines for multiparametric prostate magnetic resonance imaging (mpMRI) using evidenced-based data and consensus expert opinion. This guideline was updated in 2015 by a steering committee formed by the American College of Radiology (ACR), ESUR, and AdMeTech Foundation to standardize and reduce the inter-center variability in imaging acquisition and reporting, and to improve characterization and risk stratification of patients undergoing imaging for suspected prostate cancer.

In the original version, prostatic abnormalities were scored based on individual pulse sequences on mpMRI; including T2-weighted, diffusion weighted imaging and apparent diffusion coefficient (DWI-ADC), dynamic contrast-enhanced (DCE) imaging, and (optionally) MR spectroscopy. Although the guidelines carried information regarding risk stratification, enrollment criteria for active surveillance programs, and recommendations for imaging protocols, it failed to specify how the individual sequences contributed to an overall score. This resulted in between-center variability in image acquisition and reporting.

Compared to the original version, PI-RADS v2 is more precise in its scope and purpose. It includes an overview of normal prostate anatomy, benign findings, terminology, and provides specific recommendations to assign an overall score. The following are several key differences between the original and PI-RADS v2:

- The guidelines are explicit that they only apply to pre-therapy patients being evaluated for prostate cancer, not for follow-up or post-treatment assessment.
- Only minimal technical parameters for acceptable mpMRI are given.
- MR spectroscopy is omitted and DCE is assigned a minor role.
- The overall score is based only on mpMRI, without contribution from clinical factors.

PI-RADS v2 has also defined the predominant sequence for evaluation, based on the zonal location of the abnormality; DWI for PZ lesions and T2-weighted MRI for TZ lesions. Other sequences are considered ancillary for equivocal lesions. DCE is no longer evaluated on a 5-point scale and is now either positive or negative. The 5-point scale used to evaluate DWI-ADC and T2-weighted MRI are retained from the original version. The score based on the predominant sequence is used for an overall score assignment and interpretation of cancer risk:

PI-RADS 1 – Very low (clinically significant cancer is highly unlikely to be present)

PI-RADS 2 – Low (clinically significant cancer is unlikely to be present)

PI-RADS 3 - Intermediate (the presence of clinically significant cancer is equivocal)

PI-RADS 4 – High (clinically significant cancer is likely to be present)

PI-RADS 5 - Very high (clinically significant cancer is highly likely to be present)

The following is the scoring classification for PZ and TZ lesions based on the appearance on ADC and high-b value DWI, PZ lesions based on T2-weighted MRI, and TZ lesions based on T2-weighted MRI, respectively. Please see Tables I and II for further detail:

PZ or TZ lesions based on DWI-ADC:

1. Normal on ADC maps or high-b value DWI
2. Indistinct hypointense abnormality on ADC
3. Focal mild to moderate hypointense abnormality on ADC and isointense to mild hyperintense on high-b value DWI
4. Focal markedly hypointense abnormality on ADC and markedly hyperintense on high-b value DWI; ≤1.5 cm in greatest dimension
5. Same as 4), but ≥1.5 cm in greatest dimension or definite extraprostatic extension

PZ abnormalities based on T2-weighted MRI:

1. Uniformly hyperintense (normal)
2. Linear, wedge-shaped, or diffuse mild hypointensity, usually indistinct margin
3. Noncircumscribed, rounded, moderate hypointensity
4. Circumscribed, homogenous moderately hypointense focus or mass confined to the prostate; ≤1.5 cm in greatest dimension
5. Same as 4), but ≥1.5 cm in greatest dimension or definite extraprostatic extension

TZ abnormalities based on T2-weighted MRI:

1. Homogenous intermediate signal intensity (normal)
2. Circumscribed hypointense or heterogenous encapsulated nodule(s)
3. Heterogenous signal intensity with obscured margins
4. Noncircumscribed, homogenous moderately hypointense focus or mass confined to the prostate; ≤1.5 cm in greatest dimension
5. Same as 4), but ≥1.5 cm in greatest dimension or definite extraprostatic extension

A maximum of 4 lesions with an overall score of 3, 4, or 5 are reported, with the index lesion identified. A PI-RADS score is reported for each lesion. A standardized format for reporting is recommended, though no specific model is given. The guidelines are intended to evolve with time, as radiologists gain experience in the clinical application of the PI-RADS v2 system.

ACR. PI-RADS - American College of Radiology [Internet]. 2015 [cited 2017 May 14]. Available from: https://www.acr.org/Quality-Safety/Resources/PIRADS

Additional Review:

Hamoen EHJ, de Rooij M, Witjes JA, Barentsz JO, Rovers MM. *Use of the Prostate Imaging Reporting and Data System (PI-RADS) for Prostate Cancer Detection with Multiparametric Magnetic Resonance Imaging: A Diagnostic Meta-analysis.* Eur Urol. 2015 Jun;67(6):1112–21.

PI-RADS Framework – Transition Zone Lesions			
T2W	DWI	DCE	PI-RADS
1	Any*	Any	1
2	Any	Any	2
3	≤4	Any	3
	5	Any	4
4	Any	Any	4
5	Any	Any	5

Table I. PI-RADS v2 scoring system for transitional zone lesions. *Any indicates 1-5. Table compiled with information from https://www.acr.org/Quality-Safety/Resources/BIRADS.

PI-RADS Framework – Peripheral Zone Lesions			
DWI	T2W	DCE	PI-RADS
1	Any*	Any	1
2	Any	Any	2
3	Any	–	3
		+	4
4	Any	Any	4
5	Any	Any	5

Table II. PI-RADS v2 scoring system for peripheral zone lesions. *Any indicates 1-5. Table compiled with information from https://www.acr.org/Quality-Safety/Resources/BIRADS.

The SOME trial: Screening for occult malignancy in unprovoked venous thromboembolism

1. Patients with a first unprovoked venous thromboembolism were randomized to either limited-screening for occult malignancy or limited-screening plus computed tomography (CT) of the abdomen and pelvis.

2. There were no significant differences between the two strategies in the number of occult malignancies diagnosed, and the number of occult malignancies missed by the initial screen.

Original Date of Publication: August 2015

Study Rundown: Venous thromboembolism is a common class of disease characterized by the formation of clots in the deep veins. These clots can be classified as being provoked, or unprovoked in the absence of a known risk factor (i.e., overt active cancer, current pregnancy, thrombophilia, previous clot, recent immobilization, recent major surgery). Unprovoked venous thromboembolism has been thought to be an early sign of cancer, as previous studies had demonstrated that up 10% of patients were diagnosed with malignancy in the year afterwards. Thus, an area of uncertainty for clinicians was how aggressively patients with unprovoked venous thromboembolism should be investigated for occult malignancy. The Screening for Occult Malignancy in Patients with Idiopathic Venous Thromboembolism (SOME) trial sought to address this question. In summary, the trial randomized individuals with unprovoked venous thromboembolism to either limited-screening for occult malignancy or to limited-screening plus comprehensive CT of the abdomen and pelvis. There were no significant differences between the two groups in the number of occult malignancies identified. There were also no significant differences between the two strategies in the number of malignancies initially missed on screening, but subsequently discovered. Based on these findings, a strategy of conducting limited-screening for occult malignancy may be appropriate for individuals who present with a first unprovoked venous thromboembolism.

In-Depth [randomized control trial]: A total of 854 patients from 9 participating Canadian centers were included in the intention-to-test analysis. Patients were eligible if they had a new diagnosis of first unprovoked symptomatic venous thromboembolism (i.e., proximal lower extremity deep-vein thrombosis, pulmonary embolism, or both). Exclusion criteria included age < 18 years, refusal or inability to provide informed consent, allergy to contrast media, creatinine clearance < 60 mL/minute, weight > 130 kg, ulcerative colitis, and glaucoma. Included patients were randomized in a 1:1 fashion to receive either limited occult-cancer screening (i.e., basic bloodwork, chest radiography, and recommended sex-specific screening) or limited occult-cancer screening plus comprehensive CT scan of the abdomen and pelvis. The primary outcome was newly diagnosed cancer during the 1-year follow-up period in patients with negative screen for occult malignancy. Secondary outcomes were the number of occult malignancies diagnosed, the number of early cancers diagnosed in screening and during follow-up, the incidence of recurrent venous thromboembolism, 1-year cancer-related mortality, and 1-year overall mortality.

There were no significant differences between the two groups in the number of occult cancers diagnosed. A total of 14 patients (3.2%; 95%CI 1.9 to 5.4%) in the limited-screening group and 19 patients (4.5%; 95%CI 2.9 to 6.9%) in the limited-screening plus CT group received diagnoses of occult cancers (p = 0.28). In both groups, several occult malignancies were missed by the initial screening strategies, with 4 (29%; 95%CI 8 to 58%) missed in the limited-screening group and 5 (26%; 95%CI 9 to 51%) missed in the limited-screening plus CT group (p = 1.0). Kaplan-Meier analysis showed that there was no significant difference in time to detection of missed occult cancers between the two groups (p = 0.87). There were no significant differences between the groups in the incidence of recurrent venous thromboembolism (p = 1.0), cancer-related mortality (p = 0.75), or overall mortality (p = 1.0).

Carrier M, Lazo-Langner A, Shivakumar S, Tagalakis V, Zarychanski R, Solymoss S, et al. Screening for Occult Cancer in Unprovoked Venous Thromboembolism. New England Journal of Medicine. 2015 Aug 20;373(8):697–704

Fleischner Society Guidelines, 2017 Update: Consolidated follow-up recommendations for incidental solid and subsolid pulmonary nodules

1. The revised Fleischner Society Guidelines have reduced the number of unnecessary follow-up examinations required for solid and subsolid nodules and adopted follow-up ranges to provide greater discretion in clinical decision-making.

2. In patients with low clinical risk for lung cancer, incidentally discovered nodules (solitary or multiple) smaller than 6 mm (<100 mm^3) on computed tomography (CT) do not require additional follow-up; in patients at high risk, an optional CT at 12 months is recommended.

3. No routine follow-up is recommended for ground-glass nodules (GGNs) and part-solid nodules smaller than 6 mm (<100 mm^3); follow-up until 5 years is recommended for those larger than 6 mm (>100 mm^3).

4. Risk factors for malignancy include nodule size, tobacco and other known carcinogens, family history, upper lobe location, emphysema, and pulmonary fibrosis.

Original Date of Publication: March 2017

Study Rundown: The increased use of CT in clinical practice has increased the number of incidentally discovered pulmonary nodules. These nodules can pose diagnostic dilemmas for the radiologist given the wide differential of benign and malignant etiologies. This may result in unnecessary scans and excessive ionizing radiation exposure to patients for nodules with little malignant potential. The original Fleischner Society Guidelines, published in 2005, were evidence-based recommendations regarding follow-up periods for incidentally found solid lung nodules based on size, baseline clinical risk, and nodule morphology. Complementary guidelines for subsolid nodules were issued in 2013 after it was recognized that these unique nodules carried a distinct prognosis. The updated guidelines, published in 2017, considers critical new evidence from recent, international, multi-center lung cancer screening trials in its revisions (Table 1). The new evidence is reflected in the following major changes from the original guidelines:

a. For solid nodules, the minimum size threshold that requires routine follow-up has been increased from 4 mm to 6 mm for both high and low-risk patients.
b. Solitary or multiple solid nodules smaller than 6 mm (<100 mm³) do not require additional follow-up in low risk patients; in high risk patients, an optional CT at 12 months is recommended. Stable solid pulmonary nodules between 6 mm to 8 mm require only one follow-up examination.
c. For solitary part-solid and GGN, a longer initial follow-up period is recommended, and the total duration of follow-up has been increased to 5 years.
d. Follow-up recommendations for both solid and subsolid nodules are provided as a range of time rather than specific time intervals, in order to incorporate various potential clinical risk factors as well as patient preference in determining management.
e. Volumetric thresholds have also been established corresponding to various size criteria for solid and subsolid pulmonary nodules.

Compared to the original guidelines, recent data support a less aggressive approach in the management of small solid and subsolid pulmonary nodules. The Fleischner Society constructed these guidelines based on foundational and recent literature demonstrating several key observations:

1. Patients with solid nodules smaller than 6 mm have been shown to have a cancer risk of less than 1%, even in high-risk patient population.
2. Volume doubling times for malignant solid pulmonary nodule have been well established in the 100-400-day range, while malignant subsolid nodules may present with a doubling time on the order of 3-5 years.
3. Several clinical and radiographical risk factors important in the assessment of low versus high risk must be considered in establishing follow-up periods:
    a. Size is a dominant factor in the malignant potential of nodules
    b. Nodule morphology correlates with malignant likelihood and growth rate (i.e. marginal spiculation and subsolid composition).
    c. Lung cancer occurs more often in the upper lobes, with a preference for the right lung.
    d. Emphysema and pulmonary fibrosis (especially idiopathic) are independent risk factors for malignancy.

e. Cigarette smoking portends a greater risk of lethal cancers, increasing in proportion to the degree of smoking.
f. Nodules in cigarette smokers grow faster than in nonsmokers.
g. Malignant risk of nodules increases with patient age.

Low-risk patients are defined as patients with a minimal or absent smoking history and absence of other known risk factors including a history of lung cancer in a first-degree relative, exposure to carcinogenic material (i.e., asbestos, radon, and uranium), upper lobe location, emphysema, or pulmonary fibrosis. Conversely, high-risk patients are defined as patients with a history of smoking or the aforementioned known risk factors.

The guidelines do not apply to patients with known or suspected cancers outside of the lungs, patients younger than 35 years of age, immunocompromised patients, or patients undergoing lung cancer screening. For lung cancer screening, adherence to Lung-RADS – a classification system specifically designed for the subset of patients meeting screening eligibility criteria – is recommended.

MacMahon H, Naidich DP, Goo JM, Lee KS, Leung AN, Mayo JR, Mehta AC, Ohno Y, Powell CA, Prokop M, Rubin GD. Guidelines for Management of Incidental Pulmonary Nodules Detected on CT Images: From the Fleischner Society 2017. Radiology. 2017 Feb 23:161659.

Additional Review:

Pinsky PF, Gierada DS, Black W, Munden R, Nath H, Aberle D, et al. Performance of Lung-RADS in the National Lung Screening Trial A Retrospective Assessment Performance of Lung-RADS in the NLST. Ann Intern Med. 2015 Apr 7;162(7):485–91.

	Solid Nodules		
	< 6 mm (<100 mm^3)	6-8 mm (100-250 mm^3)	> 8 mm (>250 mm^3)
Single			
Low Risk	No routine follow-up	CT at 6-12 months, then consider CT at 18-24 months	Consider CT at 3 months, PET/CT, or tissue sampling
High Risk	Optional CT at 12 months	CT at 6-12 months, then CT at 18-24 months	Consider CT at 3 months, PET/CT, or tissue sampling
Multiple			
Low Risk	No routine follow-up	CT at 3-6 months, then consider CT at 18-24 months	CT at 3-6 months, then consider CT at 18-24 months
High Risk	Optional CT at 12 months	CT at 3-6 months, then CT at 18-24 months	CT at 3-6 months, then CT at 18-24 months

Table I. 2017 Fleischner Society Guidelines for Management of Incidentally Detected Solid Pulmonary Nodules in Adults.

Subsolid Nodules		
	< 6 mm (<100 mm³)	≥6 mm (>100 mm³)
Single		
Ground Glass	No routine follow-up	CT at 6-12 months to confirm persistence, then CT every 2 years until 5 years
Part Solid	No routine follow-up	CT at 3-6 months to confirm persistence. If unchanged and solid component remains < 6 mm, annual CT should be performed for 5 years.
Multiple		
Ground Glass or Part Solid	CT at 3-6 months. If stable, consider CT at 2 and 4 years.	CT at 3-6 months. Subsequent management based on the most suspicious nodule(s).

Table II. 2017 Fleischner Society Guidelines for Management of Incidentally Detected Subsolid Pulmonary Nodules in Adults.

VII. Infectious Disease

"Research is to see what everybody else has seen, and to think what nobody else has thought."

- Albert Szent-Györgyi

Prophylactic penicillin reduces septicemia in sickle cell patients

1. This randomized, placebo-controlled, double-blinded trial demonstrated an 84% reduction in the incidence of pneumococcal septicemia among patients with sickle cell taking prophylactic penicillin when compared to those taking placebo.

2. Fifteen severe, Streptococcus pneumoniae-related infections occurred during the study with 13 occurring in patients taking placebo, 3 of which resulted in death. No patients taking prophylactic penicillin died during the study course.

Original Date of Publication: June 1986

Study Rundown: Children with sickle cell disease are at increased risk for severe, often deadly septicemia secondary to Streptococcus pneumoniae. This study investigated the use of oral penicillin prophylaxis to prevent pneumococcal sepsis. Previous research indicated the potential benefit of penicillin injections in decreasing pneumococcal septicemia in patients with compromised splenic function; however, no controlled trial of oral penicillin existed. This multicenter, randomized, double-blinded, placebo-controlled trial compared the use of twice daily penicillin to placebo vitamin C tablets using serious infection secondary to S. pneumoniae as the primary endpoint and was terminated early on account of the clear benefit of the treatment. In total, 15 cases of pneumococcal sepsis were reported, of which 13 cases occurred in patients taking placebo. Of note, 3 placebo-treated patients died from their infections. This study initiated the recommendation for all patients to undergo screening for sickle cell at birth and, for those found to be positive, to have prophylactic penicillin therapy initiated in conjunction with pneumococcal vaccination. Presently, twice daily penicillin prophylaxis from 3 months of age through 5 years old is recommended, although whether or not to stop at 5 years of age is controversial.

In-Depth [randomized controlled trial]: A total of 215 children with sickle cell disease diagnosed on hemoglobin electrophoresis and aged 3 to 36 months were recruited from 33 clinical centers and included in final analysis. Recruitment started in August 1983 and ended in February 1985. Participants needed to be asymptomatic at the time of enrollment and were randomized to receive either 125 mg of penicillin V potassium 2 times daily or a placebo of 50 mg vitamin C tablets twice daily. Patients were seen by a practitioner on study enrollment and then every 3 months. At each visit, patients were examined, had a complete blood count drawn, had their pills counted, and underwent penicillin-sensitive urine testing (to ensure compliance). Patients were nasopharyngeal swabbed for pneumococcal antibodies. While the purpose of this study was not to evaluate the efficacy of the pneumococcal vaccination, patients required vaccine administration and were given the first dose at 1 year of age and then at 2 years of age. The primary endpoint of the study was a severe infection such as bacteremia, meningitis, or pneumonia resulting in hospitalization secondary to S. pneumoniae with a severe infection due to any other organism considered a secondary endpoint.

The study was concluded 8 months earlier than planned after 15 episodes of pneumococcal septicemia were reported, with 13 cases among patients taking placebo and 2 among those taking penicillin. These were the only S. pneumoniae-related infections and amounted for an 84% reduction in pneumococcal septicemia with significantly less penicillin-treated patients experiencing S. pneumoniae infections compared to those on placebo ($p < 0.005$). Three of the placebo-treated patients died as a result of their pneumococcal infection, despite all having been vaccinated according to the recommended regimen. No children receiving prophylactic penicillin died from infectious causes during the trial. No adverse effects of the treatment were noted.

Gaston MH, Verter JI, Woods G, Pegelow C, Kelleher J, Presbury G, et al. Prophylaxis with Oral Penicillin in Children with Sickle Cell Anemia. New England Journal of Medicine. 1986 Jun 19;314(25):1593–9.

Albumin in cirrhotic patients with spontaneous bacterial peritonitis

1. In cirrhotic patients with spontaneous bacterial peritonitis (SBP), albumin infusion on days 1 and 3 of treatment, in addition to antibiotics, significantly reduced the risk of developing renal impairment and mortality when compared with antibiotics alone.

Original Date of Publication: August 1999

Study Rundown: Renal impairment during SBP is a known risk factor for in-hospital mortality and is thought to be due to low effective circulating volume (ECV). This reduction in ECV is likely due to third-spacing, as well as excessive vasodilation resulting from systemic inflammatory response. Albumin is able to increase the ECV by providing higher oncotic pressures in the vasculature. This randomized, controlled study sought to determine the benefits of albumin in patients treated for SBP. A total of 126 patients with SBP were randomized to receive antibiotics with albumin infusions, or albumin alone. The study found that patients treated with both antibiotics and albumin had significantly lower rates of renal impairment and mortality when compared to those receiving antibiotics alone.

In-Depth [randomized controlled trial]: This study involved 126 patients with cirrhosis who were diagnosed with SBP and randomized them to receive 1) antibiotics with albumin infusion or 2) antibiotics alone. Patients were recruited from 7 university hospitals in Spain. Patients in the albumin group received a 1.5 mg/kg dose of albumin on day 1 within 6 hours of enrollment in the study, and this was followed by a 1 mg/kg dose on day 3 of the study. All patients were treated with intravenous cefotaxime (dose-adjusted based on serum creatinine). After the resolution of infection, all patients were started on norfloxacin 400 mg daily prophylaxis. All investigators were blinded to treatment group assignment. Patients were included in the study if they had a polymorphonuclear cell count in the ascitic fluid > $250/mm^3$, were between 18-80 years of age, had no antibiotic treatment within 1 week before the diagnosis of SBP (except for norfloxacin prophylaxis), did not have other infections/shock/gastrointestinal bleeding/ileus/grade 3 or 4 hepatic encephalopathy/organic nephropathy (i.e., proteinuria, hematuria, abnormal renal ultrasound), did not have human immunodeficiency virus infection, and had serum creatinine ≤265 µmol/L. Primary endpoints of the study were development of renal impairment (i.e., non-reversible deterioration of renal function during hospitalization) and mortality.

Patients receiving both antibiotics and albumin experienced significantly lower rates of renal impairment, when compared with patients being treated with antibiotics alone (10% vs. 33%, p = 0.002). Moreover, patients in the antibiotics and albumin group experienced significantly lower mortality both in-hospital (10% vs. 29%, p = 0.01) and at 3 months (22% vs. 41%, p = 0.03), when compared with patients receiving antibiotics alone.

Sort P, Navasa M, Arroyo V, Aldeguer X, Planas R, Ruiz-del-Arbol L, et al. Effect of Intravenous Albumin on Renal Impairment and Mortality in Patients with Cirrhosis and Spontaneous Bacterial Peritonitis. New England Journal of Medicine. 1999 Aug 5;341(6):403–9.

Adjuvant dexamethasone improves outcomes in adult bacterial meningitis

1. Treatment with dexamethasone significantly reduced morbidity and mortality in adults with bacterial meningitis.

2. There was no significant difference in risk of adverse events with corticosteroid treatment.

Original Date of Publication: November 2002

Study Rundown: Bacterial meningitis is a neurological emergency with high fatality rates and results in neurologic deficits in nearly a third of survivors. Streptococcus pneumoniae and Neisseria meningitidis are the most common causes of bacterial meningitis, accounting for 80% of adult cases. Pneumococcal meningitis refers to infection caused by S. pneumoniae while meningococcal meningitis refers to infection by N. meningitidis. Bacterial meningitis is suspected in patients presenting with the classic triad of fever, neck stiffness and altered mental status. The triad has a low sensitivity but almost all patients present with at least two of four symptoms: headache, fever, neck stiffness and altered mental status. Culture and stain of a cerebrospinal fluid (CSF) obtained by lumbar puncture is the definitive method of diagnosis and identification of the etiologic agent. However, there is a significant risk of brain herniation with the lumbar puncture due to high cranial pressure. Thus neuroimaging, typically by cranial computed tomography (CT), is recommended before lumbar puncture to detect brain shift. Antibiotic therapy is initiated as soon as possible.

This study found that early adjuvant dexamethasone (10 mg every 6 hours for four days) reduced morbidity and mortality in adults with acute bacterial meningitis. The beneficial effect of dexamethasone was clear in patients with pneumococcal meningitis but a significant benefit was not shown in patients with meningococcal meningitis, possibly due to the limited number of patients in this subgroup. There was some concern regarding delay in treatment initiation due to informed-consent procedures and the time required for cranial CT and lumbar puncture when it was indicated for patients. Previous studies suggested that 2- and 4-day regimens of dexamethasone therapy are equally effective. This study used and recommended a 4-day regimen, initiated before or with the first dose of antibiotics. Although the reduction in mortality in this study was not associated with a higher rate of neurologic sequelae, corticosteroids may be associated with ischemic injury to neurons and so further research should investigate cognitive impairment in adults treated with and without dexamethasone.

In-Depth [randomized controlled trial]: A total of 301 patients with suspected meningitis were randomly assigned to receive dexamethasone 10 mg intravenously Q6H or placebo for four days along with usual antibiotic therapy. Patients were eligible for the trial if they were ≥17 years of age, had suspected meningitis in combination with a cloudy CSF, bacteria in CSF on Gram staining, or CSF leukocyte count > 1000/mm³. Exclusion criteria included hypersensitivity to beta-lactam antibiotics or corticosteroids, pregnancy, cerebrospinal shunt, treatment with antibiotics in the previous 48 hours, and a history of active tuberculosis or fungal infection. The primary outcome was the score on the Glasgow Outcome Scale, where a score of 5 indicates a favorable outcome and a score from 1-4 indicates an unfavorable outcome, eight weeks after undergoing randomization.

Patients in the dexamethasone group were less likely to experience an unfavorable outcome than patients in the placebo group at eight weeks after enrollment (RR 0.59; 95%CI 0.37-0.94). The absolute risk reduction for an unfavorable outcome was 10% in patients treated with dexamethasone. Mortality was also lower in the dexamethasone group than the placebo group (RR 0.48; 95%CI 0.24-0.96). Dexamethasone did not significantly improve or worsen neurologic sequelae (e.g., hearing loss) in survivors. Patients receiving dexamethasone were less likely to develop impaired consciousness (11% vs. 25%, p = 0.002) and were less likely to have seizures (5% vs. 12%, p = 0.04) or cardiorespiratory failure (10% vs. 20%, p = 0.02).

De Gans J, van de Beek D. Dexamethasone in Adults with Bacterial Meningitis. New England Journal of Medicine. 2002 Nov 14;347(20):1549–56.

The CURB-65 score: Risk stratifying patients with community-acquired pneumonia

1. Patients with community-acquired pneumonia (CAP) were stratified into mortality risk groups using a 5-point score.

2. One point was awarded for each of the following on initial presentation: confusion, urea > 7 mmol/L, respiratory rate > 30/min, low systolic (<90 mm Hg) or diastolic (<60 mm Hg) blood pressure, age > 65 years.

3. Patients who received a score of ≥3 were found to be at a high-risk of mortality (>19%) and require admission.

Original Date of Publication: May 2003

Study Rundown: The CURB-65 score was developed as a simple 5-point clinical tool for risk stratifying patients presenting with community-acquired pneumonia. Patients with a score of 0-1 may suitable for home management (i.e., low-risk). Patients with a score of 2 may require a short inpatient stay (i.e., intermediate-risk), while those with scores ≥3 should be managed in hospital (i.e., high-risk). Compared to the 20-variable Pneumonia Severity Index (PSI), the CURB-65 score is much easier to remember and apply clinically. In the CURB-65 score, one point is awarded for each of the following: confusion, urea > 7mmol/L, respiratory rate > 30/min, low systolic (<90 mmHg) or diastolic (<60 mm Hg) blood pressure, and age > 65 years on initial assessment. This prospective cohort study describes how the score was derived and validated. In summary, the CURB-65 score is a simple tool to aid clinical decision-making in stratifying patients presenting with community-acquired pneumonia into low-, intermediate-, and high-risk groups in terms of mortality, thereby assisting in management decisions.

In-Depth [prospective cohort]: Data from 1068 adult patients admitted with CAP in three prospective studies (conducted in the UK, New Zealand, and the Netherlands) were amalgamated. The main outcome measure was 30-day mortality. The dataset was divided into an 80% derivation cohort and a 20% validation cohort. Based on the modified British Thoracic Society (mBTS) assessment tool, the association between the "CURB" score and 30 day-mortality was examined, and prognostic variables were elucidated, including newly identified independent factors separate from CURB. Prognostic features not readily available during an initial hospital assessment were excluded from the clinical prediction rule for practical relevance. The CURB-65 (a six-point score from 0 to 5, one point for each variable present) enabled patients to be stratified according to mortality risk. The score (Figure) involved one point for each of **C**onfusion, **U**rea > 7 mmol/L, **R**espiratory rate > 30/min, low systolic (<90 mm Hg) or diastolic (<60 mm Hg) **B**lood pressure, and age > **65** years on initial patient assessment. All results were tested against the aforementioned validation cohort, which confirmed the increasing mortality pattern.

CURB-65 score	Mortality risk
0	0.7%
1	3.2%
2	3%
3	17%
4	41.5%
5	57%

Table I. CURB-65 score and associated patient mortality risk

Lim WS, Eerden MM van der, Laing R, Boersma WG, Karalus N, Town GI, et al. Defining community acquired pneumonia severity on presentation to hospital: an international derivation and validation study. Thorax. 2003 May 1;58(5):377–82.

Quadrivalent HPV vaccine in young women

1. Prophylactic use of a quadrivalent vaccine against human papillomavirus (HPV) strains 6, 11, 16, and 18 significantly reduced the incidence of HPV infection and HPV-associated genital disease 30 months after vaccination.

2. No significant adverse effects were observed secondary to the vaccinations.

Original Date of Publication: April 2005

Study Rundown: HPV infection causes cervical cancer in women worldwide, and while routine screening with Pap smears and close follow up of pre-cancerous lesions have reduced the risk of cervical cancer, it has not eliminated it. This study examined the efficacy of a quadrivalent vaccine in reducing the incidence of HPV infection due to the four most common strains: 6, 11, 16, and 18. These 4 strains have been linked with 70% of cervical cancers and 90% of genital warts. The vaccine is comprised of 3 injections months apart from each other and the participants were followed over the course of 36 months. In summary, the incidence of HPV infection and HPV-associated diseases were significantly lower in the vaccinated group when compared with the unvaccinated group 3 years post-vaccination. These results indicated that the vaccine may prevent infection and consequently reduce the prevalence of HPV-associated diseases. However, the study only followed the women for 3 years post-vaccination and could not demonstrate the vaccine's long-term efficacy.

In-Depth [randomized controlled trial]: This phase II randomized, multicenter, double-blind placebo-controlled study that randomized 552 women to either receive the quadrivalent HPV vaccine or a placebo injection in 3 doses, with the second and third doses administered at 2 and 6 months, respectively, after the first dose. All participants were between the ages of 16-23 years of age, not pregnant, had no history of abnormal Pap smears, and had 4 or fewer male sex partners in their lifetime. Women with history of cleared HPV infection were included in the study. Patients were followed for 36 months and had gynecological exams that included a Papanicolau test and HPV cervical swab testing on day 1, and at 7, 12, 24, and 36 months from the initiation of the study. The primary endpoint was the difference in incidence of HPV infection and/or HPV-associated genital disease.

Under the modified intention-to-treat analysis, the incidence of HPV infection and associated disease was significantly lower in the vaccinated group (6 vs. 48 participants, 89% efficacy difference, 95%CI 73-94%, p < 0.0001). Notably, the incidence of HPV infections, HPV-associated disease (e.g., condylomata acuminata, vulvar intraepithelial neoplasia, vaginal intraepithelial neoplasia), and cervical intraepithelial neoplasia were all significantly lower in vaccinated patients compared to those receiving placebo. All women who completed the vaccination regimen mounted an antibody response following the last dose of the vaccine, and a majority (76-100%) maintained seropositivity at 36 months (percentages differ for each HPV type). Adverse effects of the vaccination were of mild and moderate severity, with the most common being pain at the site of injection and a headache following the injection.

Villa LL, Costa RLR, Petta CA, Andrade RP, Ault KA, Giuliano AR, et al. Prophylactic quadrivalent human papillomavirus (types 6, 11, 16, and 18) L1 virus-like particle vaccine in young women: a randomised double-blind placebo-controlled multicentre phase II efficacy trial. Lancet Oncol. 2005 May;6(5):271–8.

Tenofovir-emtricitabine more effective and safer than zidovudine-lamivudine in HIV treatment

1. A significantly higher percentage of patients receiving tenofovir, emtricitabine, and efavirenz had human immunodeficiency virus (HIV) viral load < 50 copies/mL, when compared to those taking zidovudine, lamivudine, and efavirenz.

2. Significantly more patients discontinued medication in the zidovudine-lamivudine group due to adverse events than in the tenofovir-emtricitabine group.

Original Date of Publication: January 2006

Study Rundown: Highly-active antiretroviral therapy (HAART) has significantly changed the clinical management and outcomes of HIV patients across the world. Prior to this study, zidovudine or tenofovir coupled with either lamivudine or emtricitabine, and efavirenz were the recommended HAART regimens. This 2006 paper took ART-naive and otherwise healthy HIV patients and randomly assigned them to either the tenofovir-emtricitabine regimen or the zidovudine-lamivudine regimen for 48 weeks and recorded the effects on viral load as well as adverse effects. Results revealed a significantly higher proportion of patients in the tenofovir-emtricitabine group achieved a viral load < 50 copes/mL than their counterparts in the zidovudine-lamivudine group. More patients in the zidovudine-lamivudine group discontinued therapy due adverse effects, the most common being marked anemia. While the study was open-label, their primary and secondary objectives were objective data, which reduces the impact of potential observer bias.

In-Depth [randomized controlled trial]: This 2006 study was a multicenter, open-label, randomized controlled trial that assigned 500 patients with HIV to either the standard ART regimen of zidovudine, lamivudine, and efavirenz or to the newer drugs tenofovir, emtricitabine, and efavirenz for 48 weeks. All patients were previously diagnosed with HIV and had never taken anti-viral therapy in the past. None of the participants had any other significant lab abnormalities. There was no cutoff CD4 count. Patients were followed for 48 weeks and viral load, CD4 count, standard labs, and adverse events were recorded. The primary outcome was reaching a viral load of equal or fewer than 400 copies/mL. The secondary outcomes included HIV RNA levels of less than 50 copies/mL, a positive trend in CD4 count, and the prevalence of adverse events.

The tenofovir-emtricitabine group surpassed the zidovudine-lamivudine group in the primary and all secondary outcomes. The group also had a significantly higher percentage of patients who achieved HIV RNA levels of less than 400 copies per milliliters (84% vs. 73%, 95%CI 4.0-19.0%, p = 0.002) as well as less than 50 copies per milliliters (80% vs. 70%, 95%CI 2.0-17.0%, p = 0.02) than those in the zidovudine-lamivudine group. Those patients also had a significant increase in their CD4 cell counts (190 vs. 158 cells; 95%CI 9-55; p = 0.002) and fewer significant adverse effects from the drugs. There was also lower incidence of resistance development in the tenofovir-emtricitabine group compared to the zidovudine-lamivudine group.

Gallant JE, DeJesus E, Arribas JR, Pozniak AL, Gazzard B, Campo RE, et al. Tenofovir DF, Emtricitabine, and Efavirenz vs. Zidovudine, Lamivudine, and Efavirenz for HIV. New England Journal of Medicine. 2006 Jan 19;354(3):251–60.

Vancomycin superior to metronidazole for severe C. difficile diarrhea

1. Metronidazole and vancomycin were similarly effective in treating mild cases of Clostridium difficile (C. difficile)-associated diarrhea (CDAD).

2. Vancomycin was superior to metronidazole in treating severe cases of CDAD.

Original Date of Publication: August 1, 2007

Study Rundown: C. difficile is a leading cause of antibiotic associated diarrhea and nosocomial infection. This study was the first randomized, controlled trial of metronidazole versus vancomycin treatment for CDAD that stratified cases according to disease severity. No significant difference in efficacy was found in treating mild disease. However, vancomycin was superior to metronidazole in treating severe cases of CDAD. The findings are significant to treatment guidelines, as vancomycin is a more expensive drug and its use comes with the risk of selecting for vancomycin-resistant enterococci. Strengths of the study included its large sample size and the study design to reduce bias. In summary, the study suggests that severe cases of CDAD may benefit from treatment with vancomycin rather than metronidazole, given the higher cure rates demonstrated with vancomycin therapy.

In-Depth [randomized controlled trial]: Published in Clinical Infectious Diseases in 2007, this was the first randomized, controlled study to compare vancomycin and metronidazole treatment of C. difficile-associated diarrhea based on disease severity. Patients were classified as having severe disease if they had endoscopic evidence of pseudomembranous colitis, were treated in the intensive care unit or had two or more of the following characteristics: 1) age > 60 years, 2) temperature > 38.3°C, 3) albumin level < 2.5 mg/dL, or 4) peripheral WBC count > 15,000 cells/mm^3 within 48 hours of study entry. The investigators assessed cure as resolution of diarrhea by day 6 of treatment and negative result of C. difficile-toxin A at days 6 and 10 of treatment. In mild cases of disease, metronidazole treatment resulted in cure in 90% of patients and vancomycin treatment resulted in cure in 98% of patients ($p = 0.36$). In severe cases of disease, metronidazole cured 76% of patients while vancomycin cured 97% of patients ($p = 0.02$).

Zar FA, Bakkanagari SR, Moorthi KMLST, Davis MB. *A Comparison of Vancomycin and Metronidazole for the Treatment of Clostridium difficile–Associated Diarrhea, Stratified by Disease Severity.* Clin Infect Dis. 2007 Aug 1;45(3):302–7.

Early initiation of antiretroviral therapy significantly improves HIV survival

1. **The relative risk of death was significantly higher in patients who deferred antiretroviral therapy compared to those who initiated treatment early on,**

2. **This finding remained significant after adjustment for independent risk factors of age, history of injection drug use and HCV infection.**

Original Date of Publication: April 2009

Study Rundown: Published in NEJM in 2009, this study analyzed data collected by the North American AIDS Cohort Collaboration on Research and Design (NA-ACCORD). Results revealed that all-cause mortality was significantly higher in patients who deferred antiretroviral therapy until CD4+ counts fell below 2 thresholds of 350 and 500 cells/mm^3. This effect remained significant after adjustment for independent risk factors of age, history of injection drug use and HCV infection. The improvement in survival associated with early treatment initiation may have been the result of earlier control of viral replication or protection of immune function. Strengths of the study included the large sample size and measurement of survival as a primary outcome. Limitations of the study included those inherent to an observational study design. It remains unclear at what point an asymptomatic HIV-infected patient should initiate antiretroviral therapy to balance the benefit of treatment with toxicity, but this study contributes to the body of evidence supporting earlier treatment.

In-Depth [prospective cohort]: Two analyses were conducted on separate patients groups. The first analysis included 8362 patients who had a baseline CD4+ count of 351 to 500 cells/mm^3. The rate of death from any cause was compared in those who initiated antiretroviral therapy within 6 months of this count (early-therapy group) with those who deferred treatment until CD4+ count fell below this range (deferred-therapy group). The second analysis included 9155 patients who had a CD4+ count higher than 500 cells/mm^3 and made the same comparison between those who initiated therapy early with those who deferred treatment. The relative risk of death was markedly higher in the deferred-therapy group in both analyses.

Kitahata MM, Gange SJ, Abraham AG, Merriman B, Saag MS, Justice AC, et al. Effect of Early versus Deferred Antiretroviral Therapy for HIV on Survival. New England Journal of Medicine. 2009 Apr 30;360(18):1815–26.

Fidaxomicin vs. vancomycin in C. difficile infection

1. Fidaxomicin was non-inferior to vancomycin in achieving clinical cure of Clostridium difficile (C. difficile) infection.

2. Fidaxomicin therapy significantly reduced the rate of recurrence and significantly increased the rate of global cure of C. difficile infection when compared with vancomycin therapy.

Original Date of Publication: February 2011

Study Rundown: C. difficile infection is a common complication affecting patients treated with antibiotics. The incidence of C. difficile infection is increasing rapidly and mortality from C. difficile is steadily rising. Infections manifest with a range of symptoms, from diarrhea to inflammation of the entire colon, potentially necessitating surgical management. Recent data have been concerning, as numerous studies have shown poorer response to treatments and higher rates of recurrence compared with previous decades. Currently, the commonly used antibiotics for treating C. difficile are metronidazole and vancomycin. Fidaxomicin is a newer macrocyclic antibiotic that was designed to selectively eradicate C. difficile. It is more active than vancomycin in vitro and is minimally absorbed into the bloodstream, thereby remaining in feces in high concentrations.

This phase 3, non-inferiority trial was performed to compare the effects of fidaxomicin and vancomycin in treating C. difficile infection. Results demonstrated that fidaxomicin was non-inferior to vancomycin in achieving clinical cure of C. difficile infection. Rates of recurrence were significantly lower in the fidaxomicin group when compared with the vancomycin group. The rates of global cure (i.e., cure without recurrence) were significantly higher in the fidaxomicin group. In 2011, fidaxomicin received full U.S. Food and Drug Administration approval for treating C. difficile infection. The cost of a 10-day course of fidaxomicin is typically many times more expensive than a course of oral vancomycin. Thus, the cost of fidaxomicin has been a major barrier to wider use.

In-Depth [randomized controlled trial]: This phase 3, non-inferiority trial compared fidaxomicin with vancomycin in treating C. difficile infection. A total of 629 patients were recruited from 67 sites across Canada and the United States and randomized to receive a 10-day course of fidaxomicin 200 mg orally every 12 hours or vancomycin 125 mg orally every 6 hours. Patients were eligible if they were 16 years of age or older, had a diagnosis of C. difficile infection (i.e., change in bowel habits, ≥3 unformed bowel movements in 24 hours prior to randomization), and a stool specimen positive for C. difficile toxin A, B, or both in the 48 hours prior to randomization. Patients were excluded if they had life-threatening or fulminant C. difficile infection, toxic megacolon, a history of inflammatory bowel disease (i.e., ulcerative colitis, Crohn's), or more than one occurrence of C. difficile infection in the 3 months before the study. The primary endpoint was the rate of clinical cure (i.e., resolution of diarrhea with no need for antimicrobials on the second day after treatment finished). The secondary endpoints were recurrence of C. difficile infection in the 4-week period after finishing therapy and global cure rates (i.e., resolution of diarrhea without recurrence).

In the modified intention-to-treat, 88.2% of patients treated with fidaxomicin and 85.8% of those treated with vancomycin met criteria for clinical cure. In the per-protocol analysis, the proportions experiencing clinical cure were 92.1% and 89.8% in the fidaxomicin and vancomycin groups, respectively. In both instances, criteria for non-inferiority were met. The rates of recurrence were significantly lower in the fidaxomicin group compared to the vancomycin group in both the modified intention-to-treat (15.4% vs. 25.3%, p = 0.005) and per-protocol analyses (13.3% vs. 24.0%, p = 0.004). The rates of global cure were also significantly higher in patients treated with fidaxomicin as compared with vancomycin (74.6% vs. 64.1%, p = 0.006 for modified intention-to-treat; 77.7% vs. 67.1%, p = 0.006 for per-protocol). There were no significant differences between the groups in the rates of adverse events.

Louie TJ, Miller MA, Mullane KM, Weiss K, Lentnek A, Golan Y, et al. Fidaxomicin versus Vancomycin for Clostridium difficile Infection. New England Journal of Medicine. 2011 Feb 3;364(5):422–31.

Early antiretroviral therapy reduces HIV-1 transmission in couples

1. Human immunodeficiency virus (HIV-1) transmission rates were significantly lower in the early-therapy group compared to the delayed-therapy group.

2. Patients in the early-therapy group had lower incidence of HIV-related clinical events with a lower viral load and higher CD4 cell count than those whose therapy was delayed.

Original Date of Publication: August 2011

Study Rundown: Previous studies had demonstrated that combination therapy significantly reduced the rate of HIV-1 replication and the viral load in genital secretions. Since HIV transmission is highly linked with viral concentrations in blood and genital secretions, it was hypothesized that initiating early treatment of HIV-positive individuals would reduce the likelihood of sexual transmission. This study revealed that treatment of HIV with antiretroviral therapy (ART) reduced HIV-1 transmission between serodiscordant couples. The participants who started ART early also showed a reduction in the viral load and an increase in CD4 count while those in the delayed-therapy group on average had a modest decline in CD4 counts over the course of the study. ART also proved beneficial to reducing the incidence of HIV-related clinical events. The participants in both groups did not differ with regards to gender, location, marital status, education level, self-reported sexual activity, condom use, and baseline CD4 count and viral load. The partners of HIV-infected individuals who eventually tested positive for the HIV virus were tested to ascertain whether the patient was infected heir partner. In summary, the delayed-therapy group had a significantly higher incidence of linked transmission between couples than those in the early-therapy group.

In-Depth [randomized controlled trial]: This 2011 study randomized 1763 serodiscordant couples to either early or delayed retroviral therapy for the HIV-infected partner and looked at the rate of seroconversion in the non-infected partner over a five-year period. Participants all had CD4 cell counts between 350-550 cells per cubic millimeter and had not received antiretroviral therapy in the past. The delayed therapy group was started on antiretroviral medication once their cell counts dropped below 250 or they developed an AIDS-defining infection. Antiretroviral medications varied between the sites. All participants had sexual intercourse with one monogamous partner, as per self-reported measures.

The primary outcome was the seroconversion of the non-infected partner. Secondary outcomes included incidence of HIV-1 related clinical events and adverse events from ART. The study demonstrated that the rate of seroconversion in the early-therapy group was significantly lower than in the delayed-therapy group (HR 0.11; 95%CI 0.04-0.32). Moreover, there was significantly lower incidence of linked transmission between couples in the early-therapy group, as compared to the delayed-therapy group (HR 0.04; 95%CI 0.01-0.27). The early therapy group also had a lower incidence of HIV-related clinical events (HR 0.59; 95%CI 0.4-0.88). Most of the difference in HIV-related clinical events was driven by the higher incidence of extrapulmonary tuberculosis in the delayed-therapy group.

Cohen MS, Chen YQ, McCauley M, Gamble T, Hosseinipour MC, Kumarasamy N, et al. Prevention of HIV-1 Infection with Early Antiretroviral Therapy. New England Journal of Medicine. 2011 Aug 11;365(6):493–505.

Fecal transplantation in recurrent C. difficile infection

1. Treating recurrent Clostridium difficile (C. difficile) infection with an infusion of donor feces resulted in significantly higher cure rates than treating with vancomycin-alone or vancomycin with bowel lavage.

2. Adverse events after feces infusion included diarrhea, cramping, and belching.

Original Date of Publication: January 2013

Study Rundown: Previous studies demonstrated that vancomycin was superior to metronidazole in treating severe C. difficile-associated diarrhea. Additional studies also revealed that fidaxomicin was non-inferior to vancomycin in achieving clinical cure of C. difficile infection. In many patients, however, antibiotic treatment does not lead to sustained response, and these patients often require repeated or long tapering courses of vancomycin in attempts to achieve cure. While many factors have been suggested for C. difficile recurrence, one commonly cited reason is the destruction of the normal intestinal flora from repeated bouts of antibiotic therapy. Early non-randomized trials had explored the efficacy of gastrointestinal infusions of feces from healthy donors to treat recurrent C. difficile infection, and the results were promising. The purpose of this small randomized, controlled trial was to explore the efficacy of donor feces infusion in treating recurrent C. difficile infection. In summary, the study revealed that patients receiving donor feces infusion were significantly more likely to achieve cure without relapse in the 10 weeks after starting therapy. While these results are promising, larger, multicenter trials are needed to study the generalizability of these findings. Moreover, trials with longer follow-up are necessary to assess the duration of the effect.

In-Depth [randomized controlled trial]: This open-label, randomized, controlled trial was originally published in NEJM in 2013. Participants in the trial were randomized to three treatment groups: 1) infusion of donor feces (preceded by a short course of vancomycin and bowel lavage), 2) a standard vancomycin regimen, and 3) a standard vancomycin regimen with bowel lavage. Patients were eligible for the trial if they were > 18 years old, had a life expectancy > 3 months, and had a relapse of C. difficile after an adequate course of antibiotics ($\geq$10 days of vancomycin or metronidazole). Exclusion criteria included recent chemotherapy, HIV infection with CD4 < 240, prolonged use of prednisolone

≥60 mg daily, pregnancy, use of antibiotics for other infections, and admission to intensive care or requiring vasopressors. Patients who experienced recurrence after the first infusion were given a second infusion from a different donor. The primary endpoint was cure without relapse in the 10 weeks after starting therapy, or 10 weeks after the second infusion. A total of 43 patients underwent randomization. In the feces infusion group, 81% of patients were cured after the first infusion, and 94% were cured overall. Cure rates were 31% and 23% for the vancomycin-alone and vancomycin with lavage groups, respectively. Patients in the feces infusion group had significantly higher rates of cure ($p < 0.01$ for both comparisons after one infusion, $p < 0.001$ for overall cure rate). Most patients (94%) had diarrhea immediately after receiving donor feces, while cramping (31%) and belching (19%) were also common. These symptoms resolved within 3 hours in all patients.

Van Nood E, Vrieze A, Nieuwdorp M, Fuentes S, Zoetendal EG, de Vos WM, et al. Duodenal Infusion of Donor Feces for Recurrent Clostridium difficile. New England Journal of Medicine. 2013 Jan 31;368(5):407–15.

The iPrEx trial: Preexposure prophylaxis reduces HIV transmission in men and transgender women who have sex with men

1. In human immunodeficiency virus (HIV)-seronegative men and transgender women who have sex with men, preexposure prophylaxis with antiretrovirals significantly reduced the risk of HIV infection when compared with placebo.

2. There were similar rates of serious adverse events in both groups, though patients taking antiretroviral preexposure prophylaxis were significantly more likely to experience nausea and unintentional weight loss.

Original Date of Publication: December 2010

Study Rundown: Despite advances in treatment and measures to reduce the risk of transmission, HIV continues to be spread at high rates with approximately 2.7 million new infections occurring annually worldwide. Postexposure prophylaxis is recommended after exposure to HIV-infected fluids, though this requires recognition of exposure and for therapy to start within 72 hours. Preexposure prophylaxis, that is taking antiretroviral medications to prevent infection, has been proposed as a means of further reducing HIV transmission. The Preexposure Prophylaxis Initiative (iPrEx) trial explored the effects of preexposure prophylaxis with a combination of emtricitabine (FTC) and tenofovir (TDF) in men and transgender women who have sex with men at high-risk of HIV infection as compared with placebo.

In summary, individuals who were randomized to receive FTC-TDF experienced significantly lower risk of new HIV infection than those were treated with placebo. Of the people randomized to the FTC-TDF group, it was found that those with detectable levels of the study drug had an even larger reduction in the risk of HIV infection when compared with those who did not have detectable levels of the study drug. This was the first randomized trial to explore the effects of preexposure prophylaxis with FTC-TDF. Since its publication, several other randomized trials have been published to support the utility of preexposure prophylaxis in other populations, including heterosexuals, serodiscordant couples, and injection drug users. Preexposure is now commonly recommended in individuals at high-risk of HIV infection, alongside other preventive methods.

In-Depth [randomized controlled trial]: A total of 2499 participants were enrolled from 11 sites in 6 countries (i.e., Peru, Ecuador, South Africa, Brazil, Thailand, United States). Individuals were included if they were male at birth and had sex with men, ≥18 years of age, HIV-seronegative, and at high-risk for acquisition of HIV (e.g., high number of sexual partners, unprotected receptive anal intercourse, transactional sex, known partner with HIV). At each follow-up visit, participants received HIV testing, testing and treatment for other sexually transmitted infections, and counseling regarding safe sexual practices. Participants were randomized to treatment with daily emtricitabine (FTC) and tenofovir (TDF) combination therapy or placebo.

Study participants were followed for 3324 person-years, with the median duration of observation being 1.2 years. HIV seroconversion was noted in 110 patents, though 10 had HIV RNA present in their baseline samples. Of the 100 individuals with emergent HIV infection, 36 were in the FTC-TDF group and 64 were in the placebo group, which represented a relative reduction in incidence of 44% (95%CI 15 to 63%, $p = 0.005$). In the FTC-TDF group, those with detectable levels of the study drug experienced a relative reduction in HIV risk of 92% (95%CI 40 to 99%, $p < 0.001$) when compared to those without detectable levels. There were no significant differences between the 2 groups in the rates of serious adverse events ($p = 0.57$). Those in the FTC-TDF group had significantly higher rates of nausea and unintentional weight loss ($p = 0.04$).

Grant RM, Lama JR, Anderson PL, McMahan V, Liu AY, Vargas L, et al. Preexposure chemoprophylaxis for HIV prevention in men who have sex with men. The New England Journal of Medicine. 2010;363(27):2587-2599.

The VALENCE Trial: Sofosbuvir–ribavirin for hepatitis C

1. This trial demonstrated that in patients with hepatitis C virus (HCV) rates of virologic response were high in those who received sofosbuvir–ribavirin (93%) as compared to placebo (85%) 12 weeks post-treatment.

2. Virologic response rates in HCV genotype 3 infection were increased in participants without liver cirrhosis (91%) as compared to those who had a liver cirrhosis diagnosis (68%).

Original Date of Publication: May 2014

Study Rundown: The VALENCE trial assessed the impact of the combination nucleotide polymerase inhibitor and antiviral agent sofosbuvir–ribavirin on sustained virologic response in patients with HCV genotypes 2 and 3. Patients with HCV genotype 2 in the sofosbuvir-ribavirin group had significant improvements in virologic response as compared to placebo, sustained 12 weeks after a 12-week treatment period. Similarly, patients who received sofosbuvir-ribavirin in the HCV genotype 3 group had significantly improved virologic response as compared to placebo at 12 weeks after an extended treatment time (24 weeks). In patients with HCV genotype 3, presence of liver cirrhosis was associated with reduced efficacy of sofosbuvir-ribavirin. In summary, the VALENCE trial demonstrated that sofosbuvir-ribavirin improves viral response in patients with HCV genotypes 2 and 3 as compared to placebo.

In-Depth [randomized control trial]: In the VALENCE trial, patients diagnosed with chronic infection with HCV genotypes 2 or 3 were randomized into receiving either sofosbuvir-ribavirin (n = 334) or a placebo (n = 85). After 12 weeks, the study was unblinded and placebo participation was discontinued. Patients with HCV genotype 2 had significant improvements in viral response as compared to placebo 12 weeks after a 12-week treatment regimen (93%; 95%CI 85-98). Patients with HCV genotype 3 also demonstrated significant improvement in viral response 12 weeks following an extended 24-week treatment period (85%; 95%CI 80-89). Response rate did not differ across HCV genotype 2 subgroups, although in HCV genotype 3 patients with liver cirrhosis treatment response in the study group was blunted (87% versus 62% viral response). No significant difference in adverse events was seen across study groups.

Zeuzem S, Dusheiko GM, Salupere R, Mangia A, Flisiak R, Hyland RH, et al. Sofosbuvir and Ribavirin in HCV Genotypes 2 and 3. New England Journal of Medicine. 2014 May 22;370(21):1993–2001.

STOP-IT Trial: Short-course antimicrobial therapy in the treatment of intraabdominal infection

1. This study determined that amongst patients with complicated intraabdominal infections who had undergone appropriate source-control procedures, similar outcomes were achieved after shorter fixed-duration antibiotic therapy (4 days) compared to a longer course of antibiotics (8 days).

2. There was no significant difference in rates of subsequent infections between the two study groups.

Original Date of Publication: May 2015

Study Rundown:

Complicated intraabdominal infections are common across the world. Despite varying presentations and etiologies, the basic management is similar, involving source control procedures, rescuscitation if patients develop systemic inflammatory syndrome, and antibiotic therapy. However, the appropriate duration of antibiotic therapy remains unclear. The objective of this randomized controlled trial was to compare two different strategies in duration of antibiotic therapy for the management of patients with intraabdominal infection. Results of this study found that amongst patients with intrabdominal infection who had already been treated with source control procedures, a fixed course of antibiotic therapy (median 4-day duration) had similar outcomes to patients treated with a longer course of antibiotics (median 8-day duration). Limitations of this study include its rigid inclusion criteria (patients with inadequate source control were excluded, and only a few immunosuppressed patients were included). Furthermore, the rate of noncompliance was rather high at 18% amongst patients in the experimental group. Finally, the study was underpowered and thus proof of equivalence could not be claimed. Nonetheless, this study was significant in suggesting outcomes in patients with intraabdominal infections who received a fixed 4-day antibiotic treatment duration were similar to outcomes in patients treated with a longer duration of antibiotics after source control procedures.

In-Depth [randomized controlled trial]: 518 patients who presented with complicated intraabdominal infections and had been adequately treated with source control procedures underwent 1:1 randomization in the Study to Optimize Peritoneal Infection Therapy (STOP-IT) multicenter trial. Patients were either randomized to receive a fixed 4 full days of antimicrobial therapy (n = 258, experimental group) or antimicrobial therapy until 2 days after resolution of physiological abnormalities related to systemic inflammatory syndrome (n = 260, control group). Results demonstrated that the composite primary outcome (recurrent intraabdominal infection, death, surgical-site infection) occurred in 56/257 patients in the experimental group compared to 58/260 patients in the control group (absolute difference, −0.5 percentage point; 95%CI −7.0-8.0; p = 0.92). Furthermore, there was a significant difference in duration of therapy between the experimental group (median duration = 4 days) and the control group (median duration = 8 days) (absolute difference, −4.0 days; 95%CI −4.7 to −3.3; p < 0.001). Altogether, the results of this study support the use of short-course antimicrobial therapy for patients with complicated intraabdominal infections who had already undergone intervention for source control.

Sawyer RG, Claridge JA, Nathens AB, Rotstein OD, Duane TM, Evans HL, et al. Trial of Short-Course Antimicrobial Therapy for Intraabdominal Infection. Massachusetts Medical Society; 2015.

On-demand preexposure prophylaxis decreases HIV infection in high-risk men

1. HIV-1 acquisition rates were significantly lower in men who used tenofovir-disoprovil fumarate (TDF) and emtricitabine (FTC) preexposure prophylaxis (PrEP).

2. TDF-FTC was associated with significantly higher rates of gastrointestinal (GI) complaints and elevated serum creatinine levels.

Original Date of Publication: December 2015

Study Rundown: Studies have shown potential for effective PrEP of HIV infections with antivirals such as TDF or FTC. However, these studies examined daily oral regimens, which may underestimate efficacy due to issues with daily adherence. An on-demand program of PrEP may be more efficacious as issues with adherence could be lower, especially in high-risk populations such as men who have sex with men (MSM). This double-blind randomized controlled trial examined the efficacy and safety of sexual activity-dependent PrEP with TDF-FTC in MSM. The acquisition rates of HIV-1 were significantly decreased in men who used TDF-FTC before and after sexual activity as compared to placebo: a relative risk reduction of 86%. There were no significant differences in serious adverse events and no deaths in the study. The TDF-FTC group had higher rates of GI adverse events (nausea, vomiting, diarrhea, abdominal pain) and renal adverse events (elevations in serum creatinine). Strengths of this study include examining a novel manner of drug administration in a HIV high-risk group. Limitations include a relatively short follow-up, which does not provide information on long-term adherence.

In-Depth [randomized control trial]: This double-blind, modified intention-to-treat, randomized controlled trial was conducted at six study sites in France and one in Canada from February 2012 to October 2014. Inclusion criteria were HIV-negative status men or transgendered female sex adults who have sex with men. Those with hepatitis B or C infection, chronic kidney disease or specific transaminase abnormalities were excluded. Men were randomized to either TDF-FTC or placebo. All participants received risk-reduction counselling and condoms and regularly tested for HIV and other sexually transmitted infections. The primary endpoint was the diagnosis of HIV-1 infection defined as the first evidence of HIV antibodies or p24 antigen in serum as determined by an ELISA assay.

A total of 400 participants who did not have HIV infection were enrolled: 199 in the TDF-FTC and 201 in the placebo group. The median follow-up was 9.3 months (interquartile range [IQR] 4.9 to 20.6). Participants in both the TDF-FTC and placebo group took a median of 15 pills per month (p = 0.57). Of the 16 HIV-1 infections that occurred during follow-up, 2 occurred in the TDF-FTC group (incidence 0.91 per 100 person-years) and 14 in the placebo group (incidence 6.60 per 100 person-years), a relative reduction of 86% (95%CI 40-98, p = 0.002). There were no significant differences between groups in the frequency of serious adverse events, including zero deaths in the study period. The TDF-FTC group did have significantly higher rates of gastrointestinal events (14% vs. 5%, p = 0.002) and significant increases in serum creatinine (18% vs. 10%, p = 0.03).

Molina J-M, Capitant C, Spire B, Pialoux G, Cotte L, Charreau I, et al. On-Demand Preexposure Prophylaxis in Men at High Risk for HIV-1 Infection. New England Journal of Medicine. 2015 Dec 3;373(23):2237–46.

Bezlotoxumab associated with lower recurrence of C. difficile infection: The MODIFY I and II trials

1. Bezlotoxumab therapy associated with significantly lower rate of recurrent *C. difficile* infection compared to placebo.

2. Actoxumab not efficacious when administered aloine or in combination with bezlotoxumab in reducing rates of recurrent *C. difficile* infection.

Original Date of Publication: January 2017

Study Rundown: In hospitalized patients, *C. difficile* is a widespread cause of infectious diarrhea. An emerging approach in preventing the recurrence of *C. difficile* infection involves co-administering toxin-neutralizing monoclonal antibodies along with standard of care of antibiotics. Actoxumab and bezlotoxumab are human monoclonal antibodies that target *C. difficile* toxins A and B, respectively. In the Monocolona antibodies for C. Difficile Therapy (MODIFY I and II) Trials, researchers aimed to determine the efficacy of administering both antibodies (with antibiotics) together, separately and against placebo in reducing rates of symptomatic *C. difficile* recurrence. They found that bezlotuxumab was associated with a significantly lower rate of recurrent infection compared to placebo, with both having a similar safety profile. Additionally, in subgroup analysis, researchers also demonstrated that for participants categorized as high risk for recurrent infection (i.e. patients > 65 years of age, immunocompromised), bezlotuxumab was similarly efficacious compared to placebo in preventing recurrent infection. In contrast, actoxumab failed to provide benefit in prevention *C. difficile* recurrence. Limitations of the study include lack of standardization of standard-of-care antibiotics and potential underestimation of severe baseline *C. difficile* infection, given many initial assessments were performed on patients already receiving antibiotics. Overall, this is a well-powered study with optimal follow-up that suggests neutralization of toxin B via bezlotuxumab may reduce disease recurrence.

In-Depth [randomized control trial]: In these nearly identical double-blind, randomized, placebo controlled trials conducted between 2011 and 2015, 2655 adults receiving standard-of-care antibiotics to prevent *C. difficile* infection were randomized to receive either bezlotuxumab (n = 781), bezlotuxumab and actoxumab (n = 773), actoxumab (n = 232) and placebo (n = 773). Of note, only the MODIFY I trial included a single-therapy actoxumab group – the second trial excluded it due to it's demonstrated lack of efficacy. The primary end point was recurrent infection, defined as a new episode after initial clinical cure within 12 weeks after treatment infusion. In the MODIFY I trial, for the bezlotoxumab-only and placebo groups, recurrence rates were 17% (67 of 386) and 28% (109 of 395), respectively (95%CI 15.9 to -4.3; $p < 0.001$). Similarly, in the MODIFY II trial, for the bezlotoxumab-only and placebo groups, recurrence rates were 16% (62 of 395) and 26% (97 or 378), respectively (95%CI 17.4 to -5.9; $p < 0.001$). The bezlotoxumab and actoxumab combination groups were also more efficacious in reducing recurrence compared to placebo. Rates of adverse events were similar between groups, with the most common events being abdominal pain, diarrhea and nausea.

Wilcox MH, Gerding DN, Poxton IR, Kelly C, Nathan R, Birch T, et al. Bezlotoxumab for Prevention of Recurrent Clostridium difficile Infection. New England Journal of Medicine. 2017 Jan 26;376(4):305–17.

VIII. Nephrology

"There are two possible outcomes: if the result confirms the hypothesis, then you've made a measurement. If the result is contrary to the hypothesis, then you've made a discovery."

- Enrico Fermi

The MDRD trial: Protein intake and blood pressure control in renal insufficiency

1. Reducing protein intake and lowering blood pressure targets did not significantly delay the rate of decline of glomerular filtration rate (GFR) in patients with renal insufficiency.

2. In patients with renal insufficiency and elevated baseline proteinuria (≥1 g/day in moderate insufficiency, ≥3 g/day in severe insufficiency), lower blood pressure targets significantly delayed the progression of renal disease.

Original Date of Publication: March 1994

Study Rundown: At the time of the Modification of Diet in Renal Disease (MDRD) trial in 1994, studies had shown that dietary protein restriction and blood pressure control delayed the progression of renal disease in animal models. The MDRD trial sought to assess whether dietary and blood pressure changes can similarly delay worsening renal insufficiency in humans. The study involved both patients with moderate (GFR between 25-55 mL/min/1.73m^2) and severe renal insufficiency (GFR 13-24 mL/min/1.73m^2), and randomized patients to different levels of protein intake and blood pressure control. At the 3-year mark, the rate of decline in GFR did not significantly differ between different degrees of protein consumption or blood pressure control. In subsets of patient with elevated baseline proteinuria (≥1 g/day in moderate insufficiency, ≥3 g/day in severe insufficiency), lower blood pressure control significantly slowed the progression of renal disease. A major limitation of the study was its low recruitment of minority patients, as 85% of study participants were white. The authors remarked that the study's 53 black patients had a significantly more rapid rate of GFR decline than the rest of the participants, suggesting that renal disease progression may differ for different patient populations. In summary, the MDRD trial demonstrated that reducing protein intake and stricter blood pressure control did not significantly alter the rate of decline in GFR in patients with moderate or severe renal insufficiency.

In-Depth [randomized controlled trial]: Originally published in 1994 in NEJM, this randomized trial was comprised of 2 studies involving 840 patients. The first study examined individuals with moderate renal insufficiency (GFR 25-55 mL/min/1.73m^2), while the second involved those with severe insufficiency (GFR 13-24 mL/min/1.73m^2). Eligible patients were between 18-70 years old, had creatinine concentrations within defined limits (1.2-7.0 mg/dL or 106-619 μmol/L for women, 1.4-7.0 mg/dL or 124-619 μmol/L for men) or a creatinine clearance rate < 70 mL/min/1.73m^2 of body surface area, and a mean arterial pressure ≤125 mmHg. The exclusion criteria included pregnancy, being excessively under- or overweight (i.e., < 80% or > 160% of standard body weight), having diabetes mellitus and requiring insulin therapy, urinary protein excretion rate > 10 g/day, and a history of renal transplantation or other chronic medical conditions.

Patients with moderate renal insufficiency (GFR of 25-55 ml/min/1.73m^2) were randomized to a usual- (1.3 g/kg/day) or low-protein diet (0.58 g/kg/day), and usual- (<140/90 mmHg) or low-blood pressure control (<130/80 mmHg). Patients with severe renal insufficiency (GFR of 13-24 ml/min/1.73m^2) were randomized to receive low- (0.58 g/kg/day) or very low-protein diet (0.28 g/kg/day), and usual- (<140/90) or low-blood pressure control (<130/80). GFR was measured at 2 and 4 months, and every 4 months thereafter as an indicator of renal disease progression. The primary endpoint was the rate of change in GFR. In patients with moderate renal insufficiency, there was no significant difference in the rate of decline in GFR between the diet or blood pressure groups at the 3-year mark. In patients with severe renal insufficiency, the rate of GFR decline also did not differ significantly between the diet and blood pressure groups at 3 years. Subgroup analyses were performed based on baseline proteinuria. Patients with moderate insufficiency and ≥1 g/day of proteinuria were found to have significantly slower rates of decline in GFR when they were managed to lower blood pressure targets. The rate of decline in GFR was also significantly slower in patients with severe insufficiency and baseline proteinuria ≥3 g/day when they lower blood pressure was targeted.

Klahr S, Levey AS, Beck GJ, Caggiula AW, Hunsicker L, Kusek JW, et al. The Effects of Dietary Protein Restriction and Blood-Pressure Control on the Progression of Chronic Renal Disease. New England Journal of Medicine. 1994 Mar 31;330(13):877–84.

Non-contrast CT sensitive and specific for kidney stones

1. Among patients with acute flank pain, non-contrast computed tomography (CT) of the abdomen and pelvis demonstrated a sensitivity of 97% and a specificity of 96% for the diagnosis of kidney stones.

2. Non-contrast CT was associated with a low false negative rate and was able to suggest alternative diagnoses in a significant number of patients without evidence of kidney stones, thus increasing the overall diagnostic yield.

Original Date of Publication: January 1996

Study Rundown: Kidney stones, or nephrolithiasis, are a common cause of pain among patients presenting to the emergency department. Historically, the evaluation of patients with suspected nephrolithiasis consisted of plain radiographs together with clinical history, physical examination, and laboratory data. However, this combination was associated with a high false negative rate. The diagnostic yield was improved with the widespread adoption of intravenous pyelography (IP), a fluoroscopic technique in which dye is introduced into the urinary tract and imaged by x-rays in real-time. The use of IP improved stone detection but was associated with higher radiation exposure and the need for contrast administration, and the false negative rate remained high. There remained a significant need for a fast, accurate diagnostic technique among patients with suspected stone disease. With the introduction of CT into standard practice, there was a strong push towards its adoption as the standard for evaluation of nephrolithiasis given its high spatial and contrast resolution.

In the present study, patients with symptoms concerning for nephrolithiasis were imaged with non-contrast CT of the abdomen and pelvis to determine the presence or absence of stones within the urinary tract. These patients then underwent a combination of repeat imaging, surgery, or close clinical follow-up to determine the final diagnosis. The results suggested that non-contrast CT was highly sensitive and specific for the nephrolithiasis, as well as associated with few false negative findings. Moreover, because of the ability to imaging other structures within the abdomen and pelvis in high resolution, CT was able to identify possible alternative diagnosis, such as appendicitis or infection, in nearly 33% of patients without evidence of stones. The study was limited by the use of a composite reference standard and the lack of outcome data. Today, non-contrast CT in conjunction with ultrasonography remains the diagnostic gold standard among patients with suspected kidney stones.

In-Depth [prospective cohort]: A total of 292 consecutive patients referred for evaluation of possible nephrolithiasis at a single center underwent non-contrast CT of the abdomen and pelvis by standard protocol. Images were blindly reviewed by 2 radiologists with expertise in CT interpretation, and imaging diagnoses were made by consensus. Findings considered positive for nephrolithiasis included direct visualization of a stone within the ureters or bladder, or unilateral collecting system dilation and perinephric stranding without direct stone visualization. Of the original cohort that underwent imaging, 210 patients (98 male, 112 female; age range 18-85 years) went on to have diagnostic confirmation in the form of surgery, repeat imaging, or clinical follow-up. The results of the study suggested a sensitivity and negative predictive value of 97%, and a specificity and positive predictive value of 96%. The overall diagnostic accuracy of non-contrast CT in the evaluation of patients with suspected nephrolithiasis was 97%. Thirty-one patients without evidence of stone disease on CT (27.6%) were found to have unsuspected extra-renal abnormalities, the most common of which was symptomatic adnexal masses.

Smith RC, Verga M, McCarthy S, Rosenfield AT. Diagnosis of acute flank pain: value of unenhanced helical CT. American Journal of Roentgenology. 1996 Jan 1;166(1):97–101.

The IDNT: Irbesartan protects from renal deterioration in diabetic nephropathy

1. Irbesartan significantly reduced the risk of doubling of serum creatinine concentration, developing end-stage renal disease, or death from all causes.

2. Serum creatinine concentration increased at a slower rate in patients receiving irbesartan compared to amlodipine and placebo groups.

Original Date of Publication: September 2001

Study Rundown: The Irbesartan Diabetic Nephropathy Trial (IDNT) assessed the ability of an angiotensin-II-receptor blocker (ARB), irbesartan and a calcium channel blocker (CCB), amlodipine to protect against renal deterioration in patients with nephropathy due to type 2 diabetes mellitus (T2DM). At the time of this publication, inhibitors of the renin-angiotensin-aldosterone system were known to be effective in patients with nephropathy due to type 1 diabetes but no major trial had investigated these agents in patients with nephropathy due to T2DM. While no significant differences were observed between the amlodipine and placebo treatment groups, irbesartan was associated with a significantly lower relative risk of a composite end point that included doubling of serum creatinine concentration, onset of end-stage renal disease, and death from any cause. Irbesartan was also associated with a slower rate of increase in serum creatinine concentration. These protective effects were found to be independent of the drug's benefit in lowering blood pressure. In summary, the ARB irbesartan carries renoprotective effects in addition to lowering blood pressure in patients with nephropathy due to T2DM.

In-Depth [randomized controlled trial]: This trial randomly assigned 1715 patients with a documented diagnosis of T2DM and hypertension to 1 of 3 treatment arms: 1) the ARB, irbesartan, 2) the CCB, amlodipine, or 3) placebo. The target blood pressure for all patients was the same (135/85 mmHg or less) and blood pressure was managed as needed with antihypertensive agents other than ACE inhibitors, ARBs, and CCBs. The primary endpoint was a composite of doubling of baseline serum creatinine concentration, development of end-stage renal disease, or death from any cause. A composite cardiovascular end point was measured as a secondary outcome. The relative risk of the primary end point was not significantly different between the placebo and amlodipine groups. Patients receiving irbesartan had a 20% lower relative risk of the primary end point than patients in the placebo group (p = 0.02) and a 23% lower risk that those in the amlodipine group (p = 0.006). There was no significant difference in the occurrence of the composite cardiovascular outcome among the three groups. Serum creatinine concentration increased at significantly slower rates in the irbesartan group than in the placebo and amlodipine groups. Hyperkalemia requiring discontinuation of trial medication occurred more frequently in the irbesartan group than in the placebo and amlodipine groups.

Lewis EJ, Hunsicker LG, Clarke WR, Berl T, Pohl MA, Lewis JB, et al. Renoprotective Effect of the Angiotensin-Receptor Antagonist Irbesartan in Patients with Nephropathy Due to Type 2 Diabetes. New England Journal of Medicine. 2001 Sep 20;345(12):851–60.

The RENAAL trial: Losartan in diabetic nephropathy

1. In patients with type II diabetes mellitus (T2DM) and nephropathy, losartan at a dose of 50-100 mg daily significantly reduced the risk of developing end-stage renal disease (ESRD) compared to placebo.

2. While losartan was linked to a significant reduction in the degree of proteinuria in these patients, it did not have a related reduction in mortality when compared with placebo.

Original Date of Publication: September 2001

Study Rundown: Diabetic nephropathy is a leading cause of ESRD. Previous studies had shown that blockade of the renin-angiotensin system slowed the progression of renal disease in patients with type I diabetes. The Reduction of Endpoints in NIDDM with the Angiotensin II Antagonist Losartan (RENAAL) study was the one of the first to assess the effect of disrupting the renin-angiotensin system in patients with T2DM. The study demonstrated that in T2DM patients already receiving conventional anti-hypertensive therapy, the use of the angiotensin-II-receptor antagonist losartan significantly decreased the risk of ESRD. Losartan therapy also was associated with a significant decrease in the degree of proteinuria. There was no significant difference between the groups in mortality rates. One limitation of this study was the high rate at which patients discontinued the study drug. About 53.5% of patients in the placebo group and 46.5% of patients in the losartan group stopped taking their study medication early. In summary, the findings of this study support the use of losartan in delaying the progression of renal disease in patients with T2DM and nephropathy.

In-Depth [randomized controlled trial]: This trial included 1513 patients from 250 centers in 28 countries. Eligible patients were between 31-70 years of age with diagnoses of type 2 diabetes and nephropathy (i.e., urinary protein ≥ 0.5 g/24 hours and serum creatinine between 115-254 µmol/L). Patients who had type 1 diabetes, non-diabetic renal disease, or a history of heart failure were excluded. Moreover, patients who had recent myocardial infarction (MI), percutaneous coronary intervention (PCI), coronary artery bypass grafting (CABG), or cerebrovascular event were excluded. Patients received conventional anti-hypertensive therapy as needed, in addition to either losartan or placebo. Permitted anti-hypertensive therapy included calcium channel blockers, diuretics, alpha-blockers, and beta-blockers, but not angiotensin converting enzyme (ACE) inhibitors or angiotensin-II-receptor antagonists other than losartan. Treatment was administered for a mean of 3.4 years. The primary outcome measure was time to the composite endpoint comprised of ESRD (i.e., need for dialysis or renal transplantation), doubling of serum creatinine level, and death. The secondary endpoints were morbidity and mortality from cardiovascular causes, progression of renal disease, and changes in the degree of proteinuria.

The daily dose of losartan ranged from 50-100 mg daily with 71% of patients receiving 100 mg. Losartan treatment significantly reduced the incidence of the primary endpoint when compared to placebo (43.5% vs. 47.1%, 16% risk reduction, p = 0.02). This difference was driven by significant reductions in the risk of doubling serum creatinine (21.6% vs. 26.0%, 25% risk reduction, p = 0.006) and the risk of end-stage renal disease (19.6% vs. 25.5%, 28% risk reduction, p = 0.002) in the losartan group. There was no significant difference between the two groups in mortality (21.0% vs. 20.3%, p = 0.88). Moreover, there was no difference between the groups in the secondary endpoint of morbidity and mortality from cardiovascular causes. Patients in the losartan group, however, did experience significant reductions in the amount of proteinuria when compared with those receiving placebo (p < 0.001).

Brenner BM, Cooper ME, de Zeeuw D, Keane WF, Mitch WE, Parving H-H, et al. Effects of Losartan on Renal and Cardiovascular Outcomes in Patients with Type 2 Diabetes and Nephropathy. New England Journal of Medicine. 2001 Sep 20;345(12):861–9.

Percutaneous radiofrequency ablation effective in small, exophytic renal cell carcinoma

1. Percutaneous radiofrequency ablation (RFA) demonstrated high efficacy and safety in patients with exophytic renal cell carcinoma (RCC) tumors up to 5 cm.

2. Large RCC tumors with central renal sinus involvement were associated with increased treatment failure.

Original Date of Publication: February 2003

Study Rundown: RCC is the most common primary kidney malignancy and results in approximately 14 000 deaths annually in the United States. Historically, definitive management of RCC consisted of invasive surgery with radical or partial nephrectomy. Non-invasive management options, including RFA, are alternative modalities for treatment of RCC for patients ineligible for surgical intervention or with the need for nephron-sparing therapy. The purpose of this landmark prospective trial was to report the effectiveness of and to delineate the tumor characteristic most amenable to RFA.

The prospective trial reported the results of 34 patients that underwent RFA for treatment of RCC. The primary outcome was evidence of technical success, which was demonstrated by lack of active disease on follow-up imaging. At the conclusion of the study, all exophytic RCC tumors were successfully treated, regardless of size. The majority of tumors that underwent successful treatment required only one RFA session; large tumors (>3 cm) were associated with multiple ablation sessions. Additionally, large tumors that demonstrated involvement of the central renal sinus were associated with an increased incidence of treatment failure. There were no cases of locally recurrent disease or development of metastatic disease in patients with successful RFA treatment. Complications occurred in a small number of patients, with no cases of death or dialysis requirement due to RFA. The trial was limited by a small sample size and did not include any data for small (<3 cm) tumors with renal sinus involvement. However, this prospective trial demonstrated the effectiveness of using RFA in RCC up to 5 cm in size and not involving the renal pelvis.

In-Depth [prospective cohort]: This was a prospective, single center trial analyzed the results of 34 consecutive patients with biopsy-confirmed RCC that underwent RFA in the United States. Inclusion criteria included ineligibility for surgery due to medical comorbidities, life expectancy > 1 year, and presence of solitary kidney. Patients were excluded if there was a lack of a safe percutaneous path for tumor access on imaging. The primary outcome was overall treatment success, which was defined as the absence of enhancement in the area of the tumor on 1 month follow-up imaging. Each RCC tumor was characterized with contrast-enhanced CT scan to determine size and location within the kidney. Tumors with extension into the peri-renal fat space with no involvement of the renal sinus were categorized as exophytic. Additionally, tumors greater than 3 cm in cross-sectional diameter were categorized as large. Overall, 42 tumors from 34 patients underwent RFA. All exophytic RCC tumors (n = 29) had a technically successful ablation, regardless of size. Successful ablation was achieved for size as large as 5 cm in diameter. The majority of small (89%) and large (70%) exophytic tumors only required a single session ablation therapy. Only 5 out of 12 large RCC tumors with central renal sinus involvement demonstrated successful ablation. There were no small tumors involving the central renal sinus. In univariate analysis, large tumors with involvement of the central renal sinus were a significant negative predictor of treatment success (p = 0.01). After a median follow-up of 9.9 months, there was no evidence of imaging recurrence or development of metastatic disease in patients that underwent successful RFA treatment. Four complications occurred in a total of 54 ablation sessions. These included one minor hemorrhage, two major hemorrhages, and one ureteral stricture. No patients required dialysis post-RFA treatment.

Gervais DA, McGovern FJ, Arellano RS, McDougal WS, Mueller PR. Renal Cell Carcinoma: Clinical Experience and Technical Success with Radio-frequency Ablation of 42 Tumors. Radiology. 2003 Feb 1;226(2):417–24.

The CHOIR trial: Targeting lower hemoglobin levels in patients with anemia and chronic kidney disease

1. In patients with anemia and chronic kidney disease, treatment with epoetin α to a lower hemoglobin target significantly reduced the incidence of death, myocardial infarction (MI), hospitalization for congestive heart failure (CHF), and stroke.

2. Achieving the lower hemoglobin target required significantly lower doses of epoetin α.

Original Date of Publication: November 2006

Study Rundown: This study found that in patients with anemia and chronic kidney disease, treating with epoetin α to a higher hemoglobin target was linked with a significantly higher risk of negative events, including death, MI, hospitalization for CHF, and stroke when compared to a lower target. Moreover, achieving the higher target required about double the dose of epoetin α, a costly medication. While this study was a multicenter, randomized trial, it was criticized for its relatively small size, high rates of withdrawal from the study, and the fact that it was not double-blinded. In summary, treating anemia in patients with chronic kidney disease using epoetin α to a lower hemoglobin target (i.e., ≥11.3 g/dL) significantly reduced the risk of composite events compared to a high target (i.e., ≥13.5 g/dL). Significantly lower doses of epoetin α were required to achieve the lower hemoglobin target.

In-Depth [randomized controlled trial]: The Correction of Hemoglobin and Outcomes in Renal Insufficiency (CHOIR) trial was an open-label, randomized study exploring the use of epoetin α in treating anemia associated with chronic kidney disease. The trial sought to determine if treating with epoetin α to target a higher hemoglobin level (i.e., ≥13.5 g/dL) would improve outcomes when compared to a lower target (i.e., ≥11.3 g/dL). The targets were adjusted partway through the trial, as the initial targets were 13.0-13.5 g/dL for the high-hemoglobin group and 10.5-11.0 g/dL for the low-hemoglobin group. Patients were included if they were at least 18 years of age, had a hemoglobin < 11.0 g/dL, and had chronic kidney disease (i.e., GFR 15-50 ml/min/1.73m^2 using MDRD). The primary endpoint was the time to a composite of death, MI, hospitalization for CHF, or stroke.

The study was terminated early in May 2005 at the second interim analysis on the recommendation of the data and safety monitoring board. At that time, 1432 participants had been enrolled from 130 states from across the United States, with 715 in the high-hemoglobin group and 717 in the low-hemoglobin group. Analyses were based on intention-to-treat, though 549 (38.3%) patients withdrew from the study prematurely. There was a significantly increased risk of composite event in the high-group compared to the low-group (HR 1.34; 95%CI 1.03-1.74). Of note, death (29.3%) and hospitalization for CHF (45.5%) accounted for 74.8% of the composite events. It was also noted that patients in the high-group required almost double the dose of epoetin α to achieve the target when compared to the dose required to achieve the low-target.

Singh AK, Szczech L, Tang KL, Barnhart H, Sapp S, Wolfson M, et al. Correction of Anemia with Epoetin Alfa in Chronic Kidney Disease. New England Journal of Medicine. 2006 Nov 16;355(20):2085–98.

The ADVANCE trial: Intensive glycemic control reduces the risk of nephropathy in diabetes

1. In diabetic patients, intensive glycemic control significantly reduced the risk of new or worsened nephropathy when compared to conventional glycemic control.

2. There was no significant reduction in major macrovascular events associated with intensive blood sugar control.

Original Date of Publication: June 2008

Study Rundown: Glycated hemoglobin (HbA1c) levels are used as a marker of glycemic control in diabetic patients. Previous studies, such as the ACCORD and UKPDS trials, demonstrated that tighter glycemic control reduced the risk of microvascular complications (i.e., nephropathy, retinopathy, and neuropathy). The ACCORD trial, however, also noted that there was significantly higher risk of mortality in patients who underwent tight glycemic control (i.e., target HbA1c < 6.0%). Moreover, there was no strong evidence demonstrating that better glycemic control significantly improved rates of macrovascular complications (i.e., myocardial infarction, stroke). The Action in Diabetes and Vascular Disease: Preterax and Diamicron Modified Release Controlled Evaluation (ADVANCE) trial sought to assess the effects of intensive glycemic control (i.e., target HbA1c ≤6.5%) on vascular outcomes. The findings demonstrated that patients in the intensive group had significantly lower risk of new/worsening nephropathy and new-onset microalbuminuria when compared with standard therapy. There were no significant differences between the groups in the rates of macrovascular complications or all-cause mortality. Importantly, the risk of severe hypoglycemia was significantly higher in patients undergoing intensive therapy.

In-Depth [randomized controlled trial]: The study included 11 140 participants from 215 centers in 20 countries. Patients were eligible if they were ≥55 years of age, were diagnosed with type 2 diabetes mellitus at ≥30 years of age, and had a history of micro- or macrovascular disease. Exclusion criteria included a definite indication for or contraindication to any of the study drugs, or a definite indication for long-term insulin therapy at study entry. Included patients were randomized to either intensive glucose control (i.e., target HbA1c ≤6.5%) or standard glucose control (i.e., based on local guidelines). The intensive control group received gliclazide and other adjuvants to achieve target HbA1c, while the control group received treatment as per local guidelines. The primary outcome was a composite of macrovascular (i.e., myocardial infarction, stroke, or death from cardiovascular event) and microvascular events (nephropathy or retinopathy). Median follow-up time was 5 years. At the end of the follow-up period, the mean HbA1c levels were 6.5% and 7.3% in the intensive and standard groups, respectively. There were no significant differences between the 2 groups with regards to the incidence of major macrovascular events (HR 0.94; 95%CI 0.84-1.06) and death from any cause (HR 0.93; 95%CI 0.83-1.06). The intensive group had a significantly lower rate of major microvascular events (HR 0.86; 95%CI 0.77-0.97), which was driven by a significantly lower risk of new or worsening nephropathy (HR 0.79; 95%CI 0.66-0.93) and new-onset microalbuminuria (HR 0.91; 95%CI 0.85-0.98). There was no significant difference between the 2 groups in terms of the risk of new or worsening retinopathy. The risk of severe hypoglycaemia, however, was significantly higher in the intensive group (HR 1.86; 95%CI 1.42-2.40).

ADVANCE Collaborative Group, Patel A, MacMahon S, Chalmers J, Neal B, Billot L, et al. Intensive blood glucose control and vascular outcomes in patients with type 2 diabetes. New England Journal of Medicine. 2008 Jun 12;358(24):2560–72.

The Symplicity HTN-2 trial: Renal denervation effective for treatment-resistant hypertension

1. Renal denervation significantly reduced blood pressure in patients suffering from treatment-resistant hypertension.

2. Renal denervation was not associated with a significantly higher rate of adverse events in comparison to control.

Original Date of Publication: December 2010

Study Rundown: Approximately half of hypertensive patients do not experience a reduction in blood pressure despite treatment with pharmaceutical agents and/or lifestyle changes. Efferent sympathetic outflow from kidneys can stimulate renin release and increased tubular sodium reabsorption, thereby increasing blood pressure. Afferent sympathetic outflow from kidneys can influence central sympathetic signals and contribute to neurogenic hypertension. Previous non-randomized trials suggest that renal denervation can successfully ameliorate treatment-refractory hypertension.

The Symplicity HTN-2 trial was the first study to randomize patients with treatment-resistant hypertension (i.e., persistent hypertension despite compliance with three or more antihypertensive drugs) to receive renal denervation or not. Results revealed that renal denervation significantly reduced blood pressure in treatment-refractory patients. Treatment with renal denervation was not linked with significantly higher rates of adverse events. There was no major injury to the renal arteries or evidence of worsening renal function associated with the denervation procedure. Limitations of the study include the low percentage of patients (17%) in both experimental groups that reported having used an aldosterone antagonist prior to the study. This raises the concern that the participants' hypertension may not have been resistant to all available effective drug therapies. Additionally, study participants were only monitored for 6 months, thus the long-term effects of renal denervation were not assessed. It should be noted that more recent studies have shown similar results extended to 24 months. In summary, the results of the Symplicity HTN-2 trial suggest that catheter-based renal denervation can be safely and effectively used to reduce blood pressure in treatment-refractory hypertensive patients.

In-Depth [randomized controlled trial]: The Symplicity HTN-2 trial was a randomized, controlled trial involving 106 participants from Europe, Australia, and New Zealand. Eligible patients were between the ages of 18 and 85 with a systolic blood pressure (BP) of at least 160 mmHg, despite compliance with at least three hypertensive drugs. Exclusion criteria included a glomerular filtration rate (GFR) of less than 45 mL/min/1.73 m^2, type 1 diabetes mellitus, valvular heart disease, and pregnancy. Renal denervation was performed using the Symplicity catheter to apply radiofrequency treatments along both renal arteries. Changes in the baseline doses of anti-hypertensive drugs were not permitted during the trial. Patients' BP was measured at 1, 3, and 6 months using office-based and home-based blood pressure machines. Adverse effects were assessed by measuring serum creatinine concentration, cystatin C concentration, and urine albumin-to-creatinine ratio. Kidneys in the denervation group were also imaged by ultrasound. Results based on office-based BP measurements showed that renal denervation resulted in a significant BP decrease of 32/12 mmHg ($p < 0.0001$), while the control group experienced no significant change. At 6 months, office-based BP of patients in the denervation group was significantly lower than the control group (between-group difference of 33/11 mmHg, $p < 0.0001$). Home-based BP was also significantly lower in the denervation group (between-group difference of 22/12 mmHg, $p < 0.001$). There was no difference in estimated GFR, serum creatinine, and cystatin C levels between the two groups.

Symplicity HTN-2 Investigators, Esler MD, Krum H, Sobotka PA, Schlaich MP, Schmieder RE, et al. Renal sympathetic denervation in patients with treatment-resistant hypertension (The Symplicity HTN-2 Trial): a randomised controlled trial. Lancet. 2010 Dec 4;376(9756):1903–9.

Gadolinium-containing contrast associated with nephrogenic fibrosing dermopathy and systemic fibrosis

1. Among patients with end-stage renal disease (ESRD), gadolinium (Gd) containing MRI contrast agents were found to trigger nephrogenic fibrosing dermopathy (NFD) or nephrogenic systemic fibrosis (NSF) within 1 month of administration.

2. The half-life of gadolinium is dramatically prolonged in ESRD and when combined with metabolic acidosis, may contribute to dissociation of the Gd-ligand complex, allowing tissue precipitation of Gd salts.

Original Date of Publication: June 2006

Study Rundown: Gadolinium-containing contrast agents are used in MRI examinations to reduce the T1 relaxation time of water molecules as they intermittently bind to the paramagnetic metal center, providing increased MR signal. They are typically considered very safe agents even among those with renal insufficiency, with a low rate of adverse reactions and a half-life of roughly 2 hours in those without kidney disease. However, among patients with impaired renal function, that half-life may extend to as long as 120 hours, and it has been proposed that this prolonged exposure may lead to Gd-salt deposition within body tissues and subsequent complications, such as NFD or NSF. NFD is an acquired, idiopathic disease of those with renal failure characterized by painful thickening and induration of the skin, particularly in the distal extremities. NSF is a variant of the same disease in which there is systemic involvement beyond the skin, affecting the joints, lungs, heart or liver.

The present study described a case-control series in which patients with ESRD underwent Gd-enhanced MR angiography (MRA) and developed symptoms of either NFD or NSF, and was among the first publications to describe the association between Gd and these diseases. Of the 9 patients who underwent Gd-enhanced MRA over 2 years, 5 developed skin symptoms suggestive of NFD with characteristic histopathological changes. The most significant differences between those who developed symptoms and those who did not were the presence of a significant metabolic acidosis and a prolonged history of dialysis among those affected versus those unaffected. Despite the inherent limitations of a case-control series study examining a rare disease entity with limited sampling, this study introduced a now common association between Gd-contrast agents and NFD or NSF among ESRD patients.

In-Depth [case-control study]: This series identified 9 dialysis-dependent patients (mean age 58±10.3 years) over a 2-year period who underwent Gd-enhanced MRA with gadopentetic acid, 5 of whom developed skin symptoms suggestive of NFD with characteristic histopathological changes. Baseline characteristics of those affected were compared to those unaffected in an effort to identify potential risk factors for the development of NFD or NSF. In each index case, skin changes occurred 2-4 weeks following the initial administration of gadopentetic acid, and clinical courses were uneventful. Only two major differences were identified between the two patient groups: their mean time on dialysis and their pH values. Those affected had a mean time on dialysis of 36±16.5 months versus 23.75±12.5 months for those unaffected. Additionally, those affected uniformly displayed a metabolic acidosis with an average pH of 7.29±0.04 and serum bicarbonate of 19.5±1.7 mmol/L versus 7.39±0.01 and 22.95±0.58 mmol/L respectively, for those unaffected. A laboratory review including antinuclear antibodies, antineutrophil cytoplasmic antibodies, antiphospholipid antibodies, immune complexes, anti-glomerular basement membrane antibodies and complement factors were unremarkable among both those affected and unaffected. A single affected patient displayed decreased levels of protein C and increased levels of Factor VIII. No medications were identified in common between any of the nine patients.

In those with ESRD, the half-life of Gd-containing compounds is significantly prolonged, and multiple metabolic derangements are often present including metabolic acidosis. This may predispose to dissociation of the Gd ion from its contrast complex, allowing formation of Gd-salts with free anions such as phosphate, which is often increased in concentration in dialysis patients. It was proposed, though without direct evidence, that these salts may precipitate into tissues and trigger the symptoms of NFD or NSF in susceptible patients.

Grobner T. Gadolinium – a specific trigger for the development of nephrogenic fibrosing dermopathy and nephrogenic systemic fibrosis? Nephrology Dialysis Transplantation. 2006 Jan 21:1104–08.

The DOSE trial: Loop diuretic strategies in acute decompensated heart failure

1. This study found that mode of administration (bolus vs. continuous infusion) and dosage (low vs. high) of loop diuretics had no significant effect on the primary endpoints of overall effectiveness or safety of therapy.

2. Higher doses of loop diuretics led to significantly greater diuresis, improved dyspnea, and fewer adverse events than lower doses.

Original Date of Publication: March 2011

Study Rundown: Loop diuretics were first approved by the U.S. Food and Drug Administration (FDA) in 1966 and had become widely prescribed for patients with congestive heart failure. However, in the intervening decades, scant prospective data was generated to guide the optimal administration of these drugs. There remained concern that higher doses of loop diuretics, while generating greater diuresis, could worsen renal function and activate the sympathetic nervous system, thereby leading to worse outcomes. Additionally, limited pharmacokinetic data suggested that continuous infusions of intravenous (IV) loop diuretics were superior to boluses. In this setting of clinical uncertainty, the Diuretic Optimization Strategies Evaluation (DOSE) trial was conducted in 2008 to gauge the safety and effectiveness of different dosing strategies of loop diuretics for patients with acute decompensated heart failure.

This study compared bolus doses vs. infusions and also compared low vs. high doses of loop diuretics. There were no differences in the primary effectiveness endpoint (72-hour qualitative symptom improvement) or the primary safety endpoint (72-hour increase in serum creatinine) when comparing bolus or continuous infusion administration of loop diuretic. While there were also no differences in the primary endpoints between patients receiving low doses or high doses of loop diuretics, higher doses were associated with greater total diuresis, greater relief of dyspnea, and fewer adverse events overall. Additionally, there were no differences between the low or high dose regimens when it came to 60-day mortality or rehospitalization.

In summary, among patients with acute decompensated heart failure, the mode of administration (bolus vs. infusion) and dosage of IV loop diuretics had no significant effect on the overall effectiveness or safety of therapy, though higher doses may be preferable to lower doses with regards to various secondary endpoints.

In-Depth [randomized controlled trial]: This prospective, double-blind, randomized trial was conducted at 26 institutions in the United States and Canada. A total of 308 patients meeting the inclusion criteria (history of congestive heart failure on an oral daily dose of furosemide between 80-240 mg or equivalent, admission to hospital for an acute decompensation within the previous 24 hours) were randomized to bolus vs. continuous infusion and low vs. high dose IV administration of loop diuretics in a 2×2 factorial design. Low doses were equivalent to each patient's baseline oral loop diuretic dose prior to hospitalization, while high doses were set at 2.5 times the level of baseline oral dosages. Dosage of the loop diuretic could be adjusted based on clinical factors at 48 hours, and at 72 hours all patients were made open-label for continued management. Co-primary endpoints of effectiveness (qualitative symptom assessment improvement) and safety (change in serum creatinine) were quantified in serial assessments over the first 72 hours. Because of its dual nature, for both primary endpoints a p-value of < 0.025 was considered significant. Several secondary endpoints were also measured at 72 hours, and a composite clinical outcome of mortality and rehospitalization was assessed at 60 days.

There were no differences between the continuous dosing and bolus dosing when it came to the primary measures of overall symptom improvement ($p = 0.47$) and creatinine change ($p = 0.45$). Though there was a non-significant trend towards improvement of overall symptoms with higher loop diuretic doses, there were also no significant differences between low and high dosing strategies with regards to the co-primary endpoints ($p = 0.06$ and $p = 0.21$). With regards to secondary endpoints, the higher dosing strategy was associated with improvement in qualitative dyspnea ($p = 0.04$), greater total diuresis ($p = 0.001$), and fewer adverse events ($p = 0.03$). There was additionally no difference in the length of hospital stay or the number of days patients remained alive and out of the hospital between the different administrations and dosages.

Felker GM, Lee KL, Bull DA, Redfield MM, Stevenson LW, Goldsmith SR, et al. Diuretic strategies in patients with acute decompensated heart failure. The New England Journal of Medicine. 2011;364(9):797-805.

The CREDENCE trial: The effect of canagliflozin on renal function

1. In this study, a composite of end-stage kidney disease, double of serum creatinine, and renal or cardiovascular death was significantly lower in diabetic patients taking canagliflozin (43.2%) as compared to a placebo (61.2%).

2. Cardiovascular death, myocardial infarction, stroke, and heart failure hospitalization rates were also lower in the canagliflozin group.

Original Date of Publication: June 2019

Study Rundown: The Canagliflozin and Renal Events in Diabetes with Established Nephropathy Clinical Evaluation (CREDENCE) trial demonstrated that canagliflozin, a sodium–glucose cotransporter 2 (SGLT2) inhibitor, is superior to placebo in patients with type 2 diabetes in preventing renal dysfunction. The canagliflozin group had significantly lower rates of the primary composite outcome of end-stage kidney disease, double of serum creatinine, and renal or cardiovascular death as well as each outcome individually when compared to controls. Cardiovascular outcomes including cardiovascular death, myocardial infarction, and stroke were also significantly lower in the study group. Amputation and fracture rates did not differ between groups. The trial was limited in that it was stopped at interim analysis at recommendation of the safety monitoring committee. Although, previous large trials of SGLT2 inhibitors suggest that effect size was likely not overestimated due to trial interruption. In summary, the CREDENCE trial is a novel demonstration of the renal-protective effects of canagliflozin in patients with type 2 diabetes.

In-Depth [randomized control trial]: In the CADENCE trial, patients with type 2 diabetes and chronic kidney disease were randomized to either treatment with canagliflozin (n = 2,202) or treatment or placebo (n = 2,199). The trial was double blinded to reduce risk of bias and outcomes were adjudicated by blinded independent adjudication committees. In patients in the canagliflozin group, the primary composite end point of end-stage kidney disease, a doubling of serum creatinine level, and renal or cardiovascular death was significantly lower than in controls (HR 0.70; 95%CI 0.59-0.82). Cardiovascular death, myocardial infarction, stroke, and hospitalization (HR 0.68; 95%CI 0.54-0.86) as well as hospitalization for heart failure (HR 0.61; 95%CI 0.47-0.80) were also significantly lower in the study group. Although, risk of amputation or fracture did not differ between groups.

Perkovic V, Jardine MJ, Neal B, Bompoint S, Heerspink HJL, Charytan DM, et al. Canagliflozin and Renal Outcomes in Type 2 Diabetes and Nephropathy. New England Journal of Medicine. 2019 Jun 13;380(24):2295–306.

IX. Neurology

> "Nature uses only the longest threads to weave her patterns, so that each small piece of her fabric reveals the organization of the entire tapestry"
>
> - Richard P. Feynman

The NASCET: Carotid endarterectomy in symptomatic stenosis

1. **Carotid endarterectomy, in addition to medical therapy, significantly reduced the risk of major and fatal stroke in patients with symptomatic, high-grade (70-99%) carotid stenosis.**

Original Date of Publication: August 1991

Study Rundown: The North American Symptomatic Carotid Endarterectomy Trial (NASCET) was one of the first trials to provide strong evidence in favor of carotid endarterectomy, in addition to medical therapy, in treating symptomatic carotid artery stenosis. The trial was originally conceived in response to the rising rates of carotid endarterectomy without strong evidence to support its use in prophylaxis against cerebrovascular events. Results demonstrated significant benefits for patients suffering from high-grade carotid stenosis (70-99%), who had recently experienced transient ischemic attack, monocular blindness, or non-disabling stroke. These findings were consistent with findings from the European Carotid Stenosis Trial. At the time, questions remained regarding the benefits of carotid endarterectomy in patients with asymptomatic carotid stenosis, and this has been explored in subsequent trials. In summary, carotid endarterectomy in addition to medical therapy significantly reduced the absolute risk of ipsilateral stroke and major or fatal ipsilateral stroke in patients with high-grade, symptomatic, carotid artery stenosis.

In-Depth [randomized controlled trial]: Patients were recruited from 50 centers across Canada and the United States and randomized to either medical therapy alone (i.e., antiplatelet, antihypertensive, antilipid, antidiabetic therapy, as needed), or medical therapy with carotid endarterectomy. Patients were eligible for the trial if they provided informed consent, were < 80 years old, and had a cerebrovascular event (i.e., transient ischemic attack, monocular blindness, non-disabling stroke) in the previous 120 days with ipsilateral carotid stenosis of 30-99% (as per carotid ultrasonography). Patients were assessed at 30 days, every three months for the first year, and every four months subsequently for death or stroke. The trial was stopped prematurely by the monitoring and executive committees according to a pre-planned rule because of evidence demonstrating treatment efficacy in patients with high-grade stenosis (70-99%) undergoing endarterectomy. The trial involving medium-grade stenosis (30-69%) continued.

A total of 659 patients with high-grade stenosis were part of the final analyses. At two years, there was a significant reduction in the absolute risk of ipsilateral stroke by 17% (±3.5%, $p < 0.001$) and major or fatal ipsilateral stroke by 10.6% (±2.6%, $p < 0.001$).

North American Symptomatic Carotid Endarterectomy Trial Collaborators. Beneficial effect of carotid endarterectomy in symptomatic patients with high-grade carotid stenosis. New England Journal of Medicine. 1991 Aug 15;325(7):445–53.

The SPAF trial: Warfarin and aspirin reduce the risk of stroke in atrial fibrillation

1. Patients with atrial fibrillation are at higher risk of ischemic stroke and systemic embolism.

2. Compared to placebo, warfarin and aspirin significantly reduced the risk of ischemic stroke and systemic embolism in patients with atrial fibrillation.

3. Today, antithrombotic therapy remains a vital consideration in managing patients with atrial fibrillation, though many more agents are available.

Original Date of Publication: August 1991

Study Rundown: Patients with atrial fibrillation have a higher risk of ischemic stroke. It is suspected that atrial fibrillation increases the risk of left atrial thrombi, which subsequently increases the risk of cardioembolic stroke. Thus, many patients with atrial fibrillation are treated with antithrombotic therapy to reduce the risk of stroke and systemic embolism. The Stroke Prevention in Atrial Fibrillation (SPAF) trial was conducted to determine the effects of warfarin and aspirin on ischemic stroke and systemic embolism as compared to placebo. While preliminary results had been published previously, this paper described the final results of the trial.

In summary, it was found that both warfarin and aspirin significantly reduced the risk of ischemic stroke and systemic embolism when compared with placebo. Patients on warfarin experienced a 67% reduction in this risk, while those on aspirin experienced a 42% reduction compared to patients taking placebo. Both warfarin and aspirin were compared directly to placebo, but not to one another. This study was one of the first randomized trials demonstrating that antithrombotic therapy reduced the risk of ischemic stroke and systemic embolism in patients with atrial fibrillation, and antithrombotic therapy remains a key consideration in managing these patients today.

In-Depth [randomized controlled trial]: This randomized trial was conducted at 15 centers. Inclusion criteria were electrocardiographically documented atrial fibrillation in the 12 months prior to enrollment, no prosthetic heart valves, no echocardiographic evidence of mitral stenosis, and no other requirements for or contraindications to aspirin or warfarin. Patients who had experienced a stroke or transient ischemic attack > 2 years before enrollment were also eligible. Exclusion criteria included transient, self-limited atrial fibrillation episodes, prosthetic heart valves, stroke or TIA within the preceding 2 years, life expectancy < 2 years due to another medical condition (e.g., metastatic cancer), and chronic renal failure. Included patients were randomized to treatment with warfarin (dose-adjusted to international normalized ratio between 2.0 and 4.5), aspirin 325 mg daily, or placebo. The primary outcome was ischemic stroke or systemic embolism, while secondary outcomes were myocardial infarction, TIA, unstable angina requiring hospitalization, and death.

A total of 1330 patients were randomized. When compared to placebo, patients in the warfarin group experienced significantly lower rates of ischemic stroke and systemic embolism (2.3% vs. 7.4% per year; risk reduction 67%, 95%CI 27 to 85%, $p = 0.01$). Patients taking aspirin also experienced significantly lower rates of ischemic stroke and systemic embolism when compared with those on placebo (3.6% vs. 6.3% per year; risk reduction 42%, 95%CI 9 to 63%, $p = 0.02$). The rate of major bleeding was between 1 to 2% per year in the warfarin and aspirin groups.

Stroke Prevention in Atrial Fibrillation Investigators. Stroke prevention in atrial fibrillation study: Final results. Circulation. 1991;84(2):527-539.

Interferon beta-1b reduces exacerbations in relapsing-remitting multiple sclerosis

1. In patients with relapsing-remitting multiple sclerosis (MS), treatment with interferon beta-1b (IFNB) significantly reduced the rate of MS exacerbations in a dose-dependent fashion.

2. Serial magnetic resonance imaging (MRI) revealed less MS activity in patients with increasing doses of IFNB.

3. There was no difference in disability caused by IFNB treatment.

Original Date of Publication: April 1993

Study Rundown: This landmark trial, conducted by the IFNB Multiple Sclerosis Study Group, randomized patients with relapsing-remitting MS to low-dose IFNB, high-dose IFNB, or placebo. Patients on IFNB experienced lower rates of disease exacerbation and were found to have less activity on serial MRI compared to placebo. Moreover, patients taking the higher dose of IFNB experienced significantly lower rates of relapse and MRI activity as compared to those on the lower dose, thereby demonstrating dose-dependent effect. Over a 3 year period, however, there was no significant difference in overall disability between the 3 groups. In summary, this study was vital in establishing the efficacy of IFNB as a treatment for relapsing-remitting MS and it remains a commonly used medication for this disease.

In-Depth [randomized controlled trial]: This trial enrolled patients with relapsing-remitting MS from 11 medical centers across the U.S. and Canada. In order to be enrolled, patients must have been suffering from the illness for at least 1 year and must not have received any treatment for 30 days prior to enrollment. Patients were randomized to receive placebo, 1.6 million international units (MIU) IFNB, or 8 MIU IFNB. The primary endpoint was the annual exacerbation rate and proportion of patients free of exacerbations. Exacerbations were defined as the appearance of a new symptom or the worsening of an old symptom that could be clinically attributed to MS. In addition, each patient had a brain MRI at baseline and on a yearly basis afterwards. At 3 years of follow-up, the exacerbation rates were 1.21 for the placebo group, 1.05 for the 1.6 MIU group, and 0.84 for the 8 MIU group ($p = 0.0004$). Furthermore, MRIs at the 3-year mark demonstrated a

17.1% increase in mean lesion area for patients in the placebo group and a 1.1% increase for the 1.6 MIU group, while the 8 MIU group experienced a 6.2% decrease compared to baseline MRIs. Over the 3-year period, there was no statistically significant difference between the groups with regards to total disability, as measured by the Kurtzke EDSS score.

Paty DW, Li DKB et al. Interferon beta-1b is effective in relapsing-remitting multiple sclerosis II. MRI analysis results of a multicenter, randomized, double-blind, placebo-controlled trial. Neurology. 1993 Apr 1;43(4):662–662.

The WARSS: Warfarin vs. aspirin in preventing recurrent ischemic stroke

1. Warfarin was not superior to aspirin in preventing recurrent ischemic stroke in patients with a prior noncardioembolic ischemic stroke.

2. There was no significant difference in the rate of major hemorrhage when comparing warfarin to aspirin.

Original Date of Publication: November 2001

Study Rundown: Previous studies demonstrated that warfarin was associated with lower rates of embolic stroke in patients with atrial fibrillation when compared to aspirin. Additionally, while aspirin was the treatment of choice for the prevention of recurrent events in noncardioembolic ischemic strokes, a substantial rate of recurrence was observed clinically. The Warfarin-Aspirin Recurrent Stroke Study (WARSS) therefore sought to investigate whether warfarin may be superior to aspirin in the prevention of recurrent ischemic stroke in patients with prior noncardioembolic strokes. The study showed no significant difference between warfarin and aspirin in the prevention of recurrent ischemic strokes. In other words, warfarin did not decrease the rate of recurrent stroke in patients with a prior noncardioembolic stroke, as it did for patients with atrial fibrillation. Because the WARSS study was only powered to detect a 30% relative reduction in primary outcome, it is possible that the study was underpowered to detect more modest treatment effects. Additionally, while there was no difference in rates of major hemorrhage (e.g., intracranial, intraspinal, dural/epidural bleeding) between aspirin and warfarin use, patients on warfarin had significantly more minor hemorrhages (e.g., gastrointestinal bleeding, ecchymoses). In summary, the results of the WARSS suggest that aspirin is a reasonable choice for prophylaxis against recurrent noncardioembolic ischemic stroke, given that warfarin requires closer monitoring, without being more effective.

In-Depth [randomized controlled trial]: This randomized, double-blinded clinical trial was conducted in 48 academic centers in the U.S. A total of 2206 patients aged 30-85 with a noncardioembolic ischemic stroke within the previous 30 days and scores of 3 or more on the Glasgow Outcome Scale were randomized to receive warfarin (dosed to a target INR of 1.4-2.8) or aspirin 325 mg daily. The primary endpoint was death from any cause or recurrent ischemic stroke. Rates of major hemorrhage (e.g., intracranial, intraspinal) and minor hemorrhage (e.g., gastrointestinal, ecchymoses) were also recorded. There was no significant difference between the warfarin and aspirin groups in the time to the primary endpoint (HR 1.13; 95%CI 0.92-1.38). There was also no difference in the rates of major hemorrhage (p = 0.10), though rates of minor hemorrhage were significantly higher in the warfarin group (p < 0.001). Finally, there was no significant difference in time to the primary endpoint due to patient differences in gender, ethnicity, or subtype of prior stroke.

Mohr JP, Thompson JLP, Lazar RM, Levin B, Sacco RL, Furie KL, et al. A Comparison of Warfarin and Aspirin for the Prevention of Recurrent Ischemic Stroke. New England Journal of Medicine. 2001 Nov 15;345(20):1444–51.

Aspirin vs. warfarin in atherosclerotic intracranial stenosis

1. There was no significant difference between warfarin and aspirin in preventing recurrent stroke in patients with significant atherosclerotic intracranial stenosis.

2. Warfarin therapy significantly increased the risk of major hemorrhage compared to aspirin.

Original Date of Publication: March 2005

Study Rundown: This trial randomized patients who were recently diagnosed with a stroke due to intracranial atherosclerotic stenosis to prophylactic treatment with either high-dose aspirin or warfarin. The trial was stopped early because the warfarin treatment group had a much higher incidence of major hemorrhages compared to the aspirin treatment group. There was no significant difference in the rate of stroke recurrence between the two groups. In summary, this study demonstrated that aspirin should be used for secondary prophylaxis in patients who suffered an ischemic stroke due to significant atherosclerotic intracranial stenosis. Warfarin was associated with increased risk of major hemorrhage and did not provide added benefit over aspirin in preventing a second stroke.

In-Depth [randomized controlled trial]: This trial involved enrollment of 569 patients with intracranial stenosis from 59 sites in North America. In order to participate, patients had to have experienced a transient ischemic attack (TIA) or non-disabling stroke within 90 days prior to enrollment that was attributed to 50-90% stenosis of a major intracranial artery. Patients were excluded if they had any evidence of 50-90% stenosis of the extracranial carotid artery, evidence or history of atrial fibrillation, or other non-atherosclerotic causes of intracranial artery stenosis. Patients were randomized to receive 5 mg of warfarin daily or 650 mg of aspirin twice daily. A non-blinded investigator made dosage changes based on side effects and INR value. The rest of the investigating team and the patients were blinded to the treatment arms. The primary endpoint was occurrence of ischemic or hemorrhagic stroke or death from any vascular cause. Study follow-up was expected to be 36 months, however the trial was stopped early due to a significant increase of adverse events in the warfarin group. The warfarin group experienced significantly more major hemorrhages than the aspirin group (HR 0.39 95%CI 0.18-0.84) after a mean of 1.8 years of follow-up. There was no significant difference in primary endpoint outcomes between the two groups (HR 1.04, 95%CI 0.73-1.48).

Chimowitz MI, Lynn MJ, Howlett-Smith H, Stern BJ, Hertzberg VS, Frankel MR, et al. Comparison of Warfarin and Aspirin for Symptomatic Intracranial Arterial Stenosis. New England Journal of Medicine. 2005 Mar 31;352(13):1305–16.

The CARESS trial: Dual antiplatelet therapy superior to monotherapy in symptomatic carotid stenosis

1. **Dual antiplatelet therapy with clopidogrel and aspirin significantly reduced the risk of microembolic events in patients with symptomatic carotid stenosis compared to aspirin alone.**

2. **There was no significant difference between the two groups in the risk of bleeding.**

Original Date of Publication: May 2005

Study Rundown: The Clopidogrel and Aspirin for Reduction of Emboli in Symptomatic Carotid Stenosis (CARESS) trial evaluated combination antiplatelet therapy (i.e., clopidogrel and aspirin) compared to aspirin alone to prevent embolic events in patients with symptomatic carotid stenosis. The study used microembolic signals (MES) detected by transcranial Doppler (TCD) ultrasound as a surrogate marker for antiplatelet efficacy and risk of TIA or stroke. In summary, dual antiplatelet therapy was associated with a significant 39.8% relative risk reduction in the proportion of patients who were positive for MES after one week of treatment. Further, the frequency of MES was significantly reduced in the dual therapy group compared to the monotherapy group. There was no increased risk of bleeding associated with combination therapy. Although the trial did not assess a clinical end point, it demonstrated that MES detected by TCD is a feasible outcome measure.

In-Depth [randomized controlled trial]: This randomized, double-blind, multicenter study involved 11 centers located in France, Germany, Switzerland, and the United Kingdom. Eligible patients were > 18 years old, had ≥50% stenosis, and had TIA or stroke in the past 3 months. These patients were evaluated for MES using TCD ultrasound. Exclusion criteria included having clinical/imaging evidence of hemorrhagic transformation, carotid endarterectomy scheduled within the next 2 weeks, acoustic window that did not allow TCD recording, atrial fibrillation or other major cardiac source of embolism, thrombolysis within the last 2 weeks, and anticoagulation within the past 3 days, amongst other factors. Patients in whom MES were detected were randomized to receive clopidogrel plus aspirin or aspirin monotherapy. Those in the dual therapy group received a loading dose of 300 mg of clopidogrel on day 1, followed by 75 mg once daily up to day 7. Both groups received 75 mg of aspirin once daily for the duration of the study. The primary endpoint was the proportion of patients who were MES positive on day 7. Secondary endpoints included the proportion of patients who were MES positive on day 2 and the rate of embolization (in number of MES per hour) on days 2 and 7. After screening for MES with TCD, 107 patients were randomized to receive either dual therapy or monotherapy.

On intention-to-treat analysis, dual therapy was associated with a significant reduction in the proportion of patients who were MES positive on day 7 (RRR 39.8%; 95%CI 13.8% to 58.0%; p = 0.0046). MES frequency per hour was reduced in the dual therapy group compared to the monotherapy group at both day 7 (embolization rate reduction 61.4%; 95%CI 31.6% to 78.2%; p = 0.001) and day 2 (embolization rate reduction 61.6%; 95%CI 34.9% to 77.4%; p < 0.001). There was no significant difference in bleeding between the two treatment groups

Markus HS, Droste DW, Kaps M, Larrue V, Lees KR, Siebler M, et al. Dual Antiplatelet Therapy With Clopidogrel and Aspirin in Symptomatic Carotid Stenosis Evaluated Using Doppler Embolic Signal Detection The Clopidogrel and Aspirin for Reduction of Emboli in Symptomatic Carotid Stenosis (CARESS) Trial. Circulation. 2005 May 3;111(17):2233–40.

Donepezil and vitamin E in Alzheimer's disease

1. **High-dose vitamin E supplementation did not significantly slow progression in Alzheimer's disease (AD).**

2. **Donepezil, a cholinesterase inhibitor, significantly reduced the risk of progression to AD early in treatment.**

Original Date of Publication: June 2005

Study Rundown: Around 80% of people who meet criteria for amnestic mild cognitive impairment develop AD within the next 6 years. There has been significant research focused on ways of slowing down the process of cognitive impairment, including medications such as donepezil and supplements such as vitamin E. This study compared donepezil (a cholinesterase inhibitor), high-dose vitamin E supplementation, and placebo concerning their effect at slowing down the progression to AD. The study found that while donepezil had a modest, but significant, effect early on in treatment, vitamin E was not superior to placebo. In summary, this study showed the modest effects of donepezil at reducing the progression to AD and that vitamin E was not effective in slowing down the progression of mild cognitive impairment. As shown in previous studies, this study also demonstrated that being a carrier of the APO-E e4 allele is the most significant risk factor in developing AD. Given the allele's propensity for AD, it was included as a covariate when running statistical analysis of data. However, the paper did not show any data concerning the covariate.

In-Depth [randomized controlled trial]: This multicenter, randomized, double-blind, placebo-controlled trial took 769 subjects with mild cognitive impairment from across the United States and Canada and randomized them to receive either 2000 IU of vitamin E with a placebo, 10 mg of donepezil with a placebo, or placebos for both. All patients also took a daily multivitamin. Subjects were screened for mild cognitive impairment by several independent measures and were all between 55-90 years of age. The primary end point was time to the development of possible or probable Alzheimer's disease, which was defined according to clinical criteria by multiple independent national neurological and Alzheimer's disease organizations. Secondary outcomes included scores on a variety of assessment scales testing different aspects of cognition. Patients were followed for 3 years. Results showed that there was no significant difference in progression to AD between the vitamin E group and the placebo group at any time during the 3 year trial (numerical data not provided in paper). Donepezil, on the other hand, did show modest reduction in risk of progression to AD compared to placebo, for the first 12 months of the trial (p = 0.004 at 6 months and p = 0.04 at 12 months). During years 2 and 3, the hazard ratios were lower, but still significant (p = 0.03 for both years). However, by 36 months, the three groups did not differ significantly in the number of subjects who had progressed to AD (63 in donepezil group vs. 73 in placebo group, p = 0.21). Secondary outcomes showed minor improvements in some of the assessments in the donepezil group compared to the placebo group but the differences were confined to the first 18 months of the study. The one marker that stood out was the APO-E e4 allele, with 76% of AD cases in the study occurring among carriers of the allele (p < 0.001).

Petersen RC, Thomas RG, Grundman M, Bennett D, Doody R, Ferris S, et al. Vitamin E and Donepezil for the Treatment of Mild Cognitive Impairment. New England Journal of Medicine. 2005 Jun 9;352(23):2379–88.

The ESPRIT trial: Aspirin with dipyridamole after cerebral ischemia

1. The combination of aspirin and dipyridamole was superior to aspirin alone in the secondary prevention of major vascular events.

2. Patients on combination therapy were more likely to discontinue the trial medication due to adverse effects.

Original Date of Publication: May 2006

Study Rundown: Daily aspirin as a secondary preventive measure was previously shown to reduce the risk of vascular events in patients with a history of transient ischemic attack. There was, however, uncertainty as to whether dipyridamole in combination with aspirin added any additional benefits. The European/Australasian Stroke Prevention in Reversible Ischemia (ESPRIT) trial was a large, multicenter randomized controlled trial of aspirin with dipyridamole versus aspirin alone following cerebral ischemia of arterial origin. When the results of this trial were included in a meta-analysis of combination therapy versus aspirin alone, a clear benefit was demonstrated in the prevention of vascular death, stroke, or myocardial infarction (MI). A potential limitation of the study is its non-blinded design; however, outcomes were verified by an auditing committee that was unaware of treatment assignment. In summary, the findings of the ESPRIT trial suggest that patients should be prescribed both aspirin and dipyridamole following cerebral ischemia of arterial origin.

In-Depth [randomized controlled trial]: Published in the Lancet in 2006, this randomized controlled trial assigned 2739 patients with a history of a transient ischemic attack within the past 6 months to receive a combination of aspirin and dipyridamole or aspirin alone. The primary outcome was a composite of death from all vascular causes, non-fatal stroke, non-fatal MI or major bleeding complication. Of the patients assigned to the combination treatment, 470 (34%) discontinued the trial medication largely due to adverse effects, while 184 (13%) of the patients assigned to aspirin alone discontinued their medication. The primary outcome occurred in 173 (13%) patients assigned to combination therapy versus 216 (16%) of those assigned to aspirin alone (HR 0.80; 95%CI 0.66-0.98). The investigators updated a previously conducted meta-analysis with the addition of these results and found an overall risk ratio of 0.82 (95%CI 0.74-0.91) for the composite outcome of vascular death, non-fatal stroke or non-fatal MI.

ESPRIT Study Group, Halkes PHA, van Gijn J, Kappelle LJ, Koudstaal PJ, Algra A. Aspirin plus dipyridamole versus aspirin alone after cerebral ischaemia of arterial origin (ESPRIT): randomised controlled trial. Lancet. 2006 May 20;367(9523):1665–73.

The SPARCL trial: Atorvastatin reduces the risk of stroke in patients with recent stroke or transient ischemic attack

1. In patients with recent stroke or transient ischemic attack (TIA), high-dose atorvastatin significantly reduced the risk of fatal stroke compared to placebo.

2. Atorvastatin also significantly reduced the risk of cardiovascular events.

Original Date of Publication: August 2006

Study Rundown: While this trial demonstrated that atorvastatin after stroke or TIA significantly reduced the risk of fatal stroke, there were several criticisms of this trial. One of the main criticisms of the study was the use of industry funding. Moreover, many of the contributors received consulting fees and grant support from various pharmaceutical companies. Lastly, the study was not powered to examine the effect on mortality. Nevertheless, the Stroke Prevention by Aggressive Reduction in Cholesterol Levels (SPARCL) trial has been influential, and has informed the AHA/ASA recommendation for statin therapy in patients with prior stroke and TIA. In summary, statins should be considered in patients soon after a stroke or transient ischemic attack to reduce the risk of subsequent stroke and cardiovascular events.

In-Depth [randomized controlled trial]: Published in NEJM in 2006, the SPARCL trial sought to determine whether atorvastatin would reduce the incidence of stroke or cardiovascular events in patients with recent stroke or TIA. A total of 4731 patients were randomized to either the treatment group receiving 80 mg of atorvastatin per day or to the placebo group. The primary endpoint was the incidence of fatal or nonfatal stroke. A number of cardiovascular events were also measured as secondary outcomes. Patients were eligible for inclusion if they were 18 years of age and had an ischemic or hemorrhagic stroke or TIA in the 1-6 month period prior to randomization. Patients were recruited from 205 different centers, and patients were followed for a mean of 4.9 years. Low-density lipoprotein (LDL) cholesterol levels were similar between the two groups at baseline and decreased by 53% in the atorvastatin group while remaining unchanged in the placebo group at one month after randomization. Atorvastatin was associated with a relative risk reduction of 16% for the primary end point of fatal or nonfatal stroke, which was significant according to the prespecified adjusted model (adjusted HR 0.84; 95%CI 0.71-0.99; p = 0.03). The statin was also associated with a significant reduction in risk of cardiovascular events, including nonfatal myocardial infarctions, acute coronary events, and revascularization (HR 0.80; 95%CI 0.69-0.92; p = 0.002). Overall mortality rates were the same in the two groups (p = 0.98).

Amarenco P, Bogousslavsky J, Callahan A, Goldstein LB, Hennerici M, Rudolph AE, et al. High-dose atorvastatin after stroke or transient ischemic attack. New England Journal of Medicine. 2006 Aug 10;355(6):549–59.

The ABCD2 score: Risk of stroke after transient ischemic attack

1. The ABCD2 score is a validated, seven-point, risk-stratification tool to identify patients at high risk of stroke following a transient ischemic attack (TIA).

2. Patients with scores ≥4 were found to be at considerably higher risk of stroke in the 2-day period following a TIA. These patients may require urgent intervention as inpatients.

Original Date of Publication: January 2007

Study Rundown: The ABCD2 score is a 7-point score for identifying patients who have suffered a TIA at the highest risk of stroke in the following 2-day period. The score was created by merging 2 previously validated clinical decision rules - the ABCD and the California scores. The ABCD score was created to estimate the 7-day risk of stroke following a TIA, while the California score predicted the 90-day risk. The 2 scores shared many features, and were combined in hopes of developing a more widely validated model to identify patients at the highest risk of stroke 2 days after a TIA, thereby allowing clinicians to determine if patients required urgent management.

Since its publication, the ABCD2 score has become widely used by front-line healthcare providers to risk stratify patients with TIA and determine how urgently these patients should be seen for subsequent assessment and treatment. While its c statistic was similar to those of the ABCD and California scores, the ABCD2 score has been more widely validated and has been shown to accurately predict the risk of stroke at 2, 7, and 90 days following a TIA. Some have criticized the ABCD2 score for only taking into account clinical features and not giving consideration to investigations. Moreover, the score has been shown to be predictive of carotid embolic sources, but less useful for cardiac sources of emboli.

In-Depth [randomized controlled trial]: Study cohorts were drawn from the Kaiser-Permanente Medical Care Plan in Northern California, United States and from Oxfordshire, United Kingdom. The c statistic was calculated to measure predictive ability. All combinations of factors from the ABCD and California scores were tested for their c statistic, and the combination with the highest statistic for 2-day risk of stroke was selected and validated. In total, the two derivation groups and four validation groups included 4809 individuals with TIA. The new composite score was named the ABCD2 score (Figure), because it took into account age, blood pressure, clinical features, duration, and diabetes mellitus diagnoses.

Risk factor	Points
Age ≥60 years	1
Blood pressure elevation (systolic > 140 mmHg and/or diastolic ≥90 mmHg)	1
Clinical features	
Unilateral weakness	2
Speech disturbance without weakness	1
Duration of symptoms	
≥60 minutes	2
10-59 minutes	1
Diabetes mellitus	1

Table I. The ABCD2 score: Risk factors and point scores for patients who have suffered a transient ischemic attack

ABCD2 scores were grouped into low-, moderate-, and high-risk categories. The rate of strokes are considerably higher with ABCD2 scores ≥4, and patients who are classified as moderate- and high-risk may require more urgent specialist assessment, investigation, and treatment to prevent stroke (Figure).

ABCD2score	Patients	2-day risk (%)	7-day risk (%)	90-day risk (%)
Low (0-3)	1,628	1.0	1.2	3.1
Moderate (4-5)	2,169	4.1	5.9	9.8
High (6-7)	1,012	8.1	11.7	17.8

Table II. ABCD2 scores and associated 2 day, 7 day and 90 day risk.

Johnston SC, Rothwell PM, Nguyen-Huynh MN, Giles MF, Elkins JS, Bernstein AL, et al. Validation and refinement of scores to predict very early stroke risk after transient ischaemic attack. Lancet. 2007 Jan 27;369(9558):283–92.

CT not sufficient to rule out early subarachnoid hemorrhage

1. In a retrospective review of 119 patients presenting with sudden headache, computed tomography (CT) scan within 12 hours of symptom onset failed to identify all patients with proven subarachnoid hemorrhage (SAH).

2. Lumbar puncture 12 hours after symptom onset definitively diagnosed all patients with SAH.

Original Date of Publication: March 1995

Study Rundown: SAH is most commonly due to a ruptured saccular aneurysm and is associated with high rates of mortality and significant neurologic morbidity. Although non-contrast CT scans provide high sensitivity in detection of SAH within 24 hours, given the significant morbidity associated with a missed diagnosis, definitive diagnosis by lumbar puncture is generally recommended when a CT scan is negative. The purpose of this landmark retrospective trial was to determine whether a non-contrast CT scan earlier in the presentation (within 12 hours) can improve the accuracy for SAH detection and remove the need for lumbar puncture.

Of 175 retrospectively reviewed patients presenting with acute headache, 119 consecutive patients with lumbar puncture-confirmed SAH received a CT scan within 12 hours of presentation. At the conclusion of the trial, there was evidence of subarachnoid blood on CT in 117 cases. Two cases of SAH were reported normal with no evidence of blood or other abnormalities on repeat interpretation. Both cases underwent angiography which demonstrated aneurysmal bleed in the PICA and posterior communicating artery, respectively. The results of this study demonstrated that CT scan cannot definitively rule out SAH in patients who present within 12 hours after onset of symptoms. Therefore, further diagnostic testing for xanthochromia via lumbar puncture is recommended in patients with normal head CT scans. This trial was one of the first studies to demonstrate the diagnostic accuracy of CT for SAH detection in patients who present early after symptom onset. Although a recent study by Cortnum et al. suggests that improved detection with modern CT scanners may obviate the need for lumbar puncture in this setting, the results of the study by Van Der Wee et al. have still been used to inform recent guidelines from the American Stroke Association which continue to recommend the use of lumbar puncture in patients suspected of having SAH with a normal CT head examination.

In-Depth [retrospective cohort]: This study retrospectively reviewed patient outcomes of 175 patients who presented to two hospitals in the Netherlands with acute headache between 1989 and 1993. Patients were excluded if they had any focal neurological deficits or if their CT scan was performed 12 hours after the onset of symptoms. The CT scans were assessed by a neuroradiologist and two neurologists. The primary outcome was the accuracy of CT scans in detecting the presence of SAH. At the conclusion of the trial, 117 (67%) patients demonstrated evidence of SAH on CT. However, lumbar puncture identified two patients (2%) with confirmed SAH that had normal CT scans. The two patients without CT evidence of SAH were found to have a PICA aneurysm and PCA aneurysm, respectively. Of the 117 patients with CT evidence of SAH, the distribution of etiologies consisted of ruptured aneurysms from the anterior cerebral artery (n = 29), carotid artery (n = 26), middle cerebral artery (n = 17), and posterior circulation (n = 5).

van der Wee N, Rinkel GJ, Hasan D, van Gijn J. Detection of subarachnoid haemorrhage on early CT: is lumbar puncture still needed after a negative scan? J Neurol Neurosurg Psychiatry. 1995 Mar;58(3):357–9.

Additional Review:

Cortnum S, Sørensen P, Jørgensen J. Determining the sensitivity of computed tomography scanning in early detection of subarachnoid hemorrhage. Neurosurgery. 2010 May;66(5):900–2.

Connolly ES, Rabinstein AA, Carhuapoma JR, Derdeyn CP, Dion J, Higashida RT, et al. Guidelines for the Management of Aneurysmal Subarachnoid Hemorrhage A Guideline for Healthcare Professionals From the American Heart Association/American Stroke Association. Stroke. 2012 Jun 1;43(6):1711–37.

Thrombolysis harmful in acute ischemic strokes with large area of parenchymal hypoattenuation

1. Parenchymal hypoattenuation of greater than 33% of the middle cerebral artery (MCA) territory on computed tomographic (CT) imaging within 6 hours of onset of an acute stroke was predictive of poor neurologic outcomes with intravenous thrombolytic therapy (tPA) and an increased risk of hemorrhagic conversion.

2. Like those with a large area of focal hypoattenuation, patients without parenchymal abnormalities on CT showed a significantly increased risk of cerebral hemorrhage and no significant change in neurologic outcomes at 90-days post-tPA; however, those with small (<33% of MCA territory) regions of hypoattenuation showed a significant improvement in long-term function.

Original Date of Publication: November 1997

Study Rundown: Acute ischemic stroke occurs when blood supply to a region of the brain is disrupted, leading to characteristic symptomatology related to the location of the lesion. After clinical examination, the mainstay of stroke diagnostics depends upon neuroimaging to aid in lesion localization and characterization of its type, size, and the extent of irreversible ischemia to guide therapeutic intervention. While recent trials have established mechanical thrombectomy as the optimal therapeutic strategy in large-vessel occlusions, the initial management of ischemic strokes presenting within 3-6 hours of onset was previously established by the ECASS and NINDS trials, which revealed that early tPA administration may achieve chemical recanalization and improve neurologic recovery. Both modern directed intra-arterial therapies and standard intravenous tPA administration are predicated on the concept that the affected tissue has not progressed to complete infarction, or that there is a region of hypoperfused or "penumbral" tissue within the affected vascular territory that may be rescued by the restoration of blood flow. The referenced study sought to determine if a large area of hypoattenuation on initial CT, indicative of terminal ischemic edema, may portend poorer outcomes with standard tPA treatment. Patients presenting with acute ischemic stroke within 6 hours of symptom onset underwent baseline head CT and were randomized to receive either tPA or placebo. Patients were then prospectively subcategorized into one of three groups according to the extent of visible MCA territorial hypoattenuation: no visible defects, 33% or less, or more than 33% of the region affected, and neurologic outcomes were recorded at 90 days post-treatment. The authors found that those with greater than 33% of the MCA territory visibly hypoattenuated and those with no visible hypoattenuation on initial CT imaging did not have a statistically significant improvement in long-term neurologic recovery, but did suffer a significantly increased risk of fatal cerebral hemorrhage secondary to tPA therapy. Those with hypoattenuation visible in less than 33% of the MCA territory were not at significantly increased risk of hemorrhagic conversion and demonstrated an improvement in long-term neurologic recovery, as observed in the previously referenced trials. This analysis was instrumental in demonstrating that the extent of completed ischemia visible on CT could predict outcomes after stroke therapy.

In-Depth [randomized controlled trial]: A total of 620 patients presenting with acute, ischemic hemispheric stroke within 6 hours of symptom onset were randomized to either receive intravenous tPA or placebo in a double-blinded fashion across multiple European medical centers. All patients underwent baseline head CT, and were prospectively categorized into one of three groups according to the extent of hypoattenuation visible within the affected MCA territory: no hypoattenuation visible, less than 33% (small territory), or greater than 33% (large territory.) Of those enrolled, 336 patients had no visible parenchymal hypoattenuation, while 215 displayed a small region, and only 52 displayed a large region of hypoattenuation, and no significant differences in baseline characteristics were noted between the subcategories except for their presenting clinical stroke scores (progressively worsened for those with larger areas of infarction; $p < 0.0001$.) The degree of presenting hypoattenuation was significantly associated with an increased baseline risk of poor neurologic outcomes as assessed within the placebo-treated groups ($p < 0.0001$). Among patients treated with intravenous tPA, no statistically significant effect on long-term neurologic recovery was noted for patients with either no initial parenchymal hypoattenuation or those with a large area of parenchymal hypoattenuation. However, 14 of 198 patients (7%) in these two groups died secondary to cerebral hemorrhage, while only 2 of 190 patients (1%) in the corresponding placebo-treated groups suffered the same complication. Patients who presented with a small area of hypoattenuation displayed an OR for good neurologic recovery of 3.43 following tPA treatment, while those with a large or no area of hypoattenuation did not show a significant difference in their odds of recovery (OR 0.41, 95%CI 0.06-2.70; OR 1.27, 95%CI 0.82-1.95, respectively.) This study established the lack of benefit and subsequent risks of utilizing intravenous thrombolytic therapy in patients with greater than one-third of the MCA territory visibly infarcted.

Von Kummer R, Allen KL, Holle R, Bozzao L, Bastianello S, Manelfe C, et al. Acute stroke: Usefulness of early CT findings before thrombolytic therapy. Radiology. 1997 Nov 1;205(2):327–33.

Hacke W, Kaste M, Fieschi C, Toni D, Lesaffre E, Kummer R von, et al. Intravenous Thrombolysis With Recombinant Tissue Plasminogen Activator for Acute Hemispheric Stroke: The European Cooperative Acute Stroke Study (ECASS). JAMA. 1995 Oct 4;274(13):1017–25.

The National Institute of Neurological Disorders and Stroke rt-PA Stroke Study Group. Tissue plasminogen activator for acute ischemic stroke. The New England Journal of Medicine. 1995 Dec 14;333(24):1581–87.

Diffusion-weighted MRI highly sensitive for acute stroke

1. Among patients with acute neurologic deficits presenting within 6 hours of symptom onset, diffusion-weighted magnetic resonance imaging (DWI) was significantly more sensitive and specific for the diagnosis of ischemic stroke compared non-contrast computed tomography (NCCT).

Original Date of Publication: September 2002

Study Rundown: Thrombolysis is a widely accepted method for the management of acute ischemic stroke, with the goal of opening blocked vessels to restore blood flow to at-risk brain tissue. One of the primary requirements for the administration of intravenous thrombolytic drugs is the exclusion of intracranial hemorrhage as an explanation for a patient's acute neurologic symptoms. NCCT is the method of choice for fast and accurate detection of intracranial bleeding. Its performance in the detection of early acute ischemic stroke, however, is generally poor, with a reported sensitivity of approximately 40-60% within the first 6 hours from symptom onset. DWI is an attractive alternative imaging technique that allows for the high-resolution depiction of areas of reduced blood flow in the brain much earlier than is generally possible with NCCT.

In this comparative trial, patients presenting to the emergency department with symptoms concerning for acute ischemic stroke were assigned to undergo both NCCT and DWI in a randomized order. For each patient and for each imaging study, the presence or absence of stroke was determined alongside other parameters to determine the diagnostic utility of both methods. The results suggested that DWI is significantly more sensitive and specific than NCCT for the diagnosis of acute ischemic stroke. Additionally, researchers found that inter-reader reliability differed greatly between the two imaging modalities, with almost perfect agreement when using DWI and only modest agreement when using NCCT, suggesting that DWI is less susceptible to interpretive errors than NCCT. This was the first trial to provide a head-to-head comparison of the two diagnostic imaging methods for stroke, and it served to significantly strengthen the evidence base in support of DWI that had been built in prior trials.

In-Depth [prospective cohort]: In this study, 54 consecutive patients presenting to a single academic medical center emergency department with symptoms concerning for acute ischemic stroke were prospectively enrolled to undergo both

NCCT and DWI in a randomized order. Primary inclusion criteria included presentation for evaluation within six hours of symptom onset and a National Institute of Health Stroke Scale (NIHSS) greater than 3, with higher values indicating greater stroke severity. All images were read by expert neuroradiologists and stroke neurologists and categorized according to the presence or absence of ischemic stroke, the vascular distribution of the stroke, the stroke subtype (none, lacunar, territorial, or hemodynamic), and other parameters. Readers were blinded to the specific details of each case.

Overall, NCCT demonstrated a sensitivity and specificity of 61% and 65%, respectively, for the diagnosis of acute ischemic stroke, and inter-reader reliability was moderate. DWI significantly outperformed NCCT, with a sensitivity and specificity of 91% and 95%, respectively, and almost perfect inter-reader reliability. Notably, no acute lacunar infarcts were visible on NCCT while four were diagnosed using DWI, suggesting that DWI may also be superior for the identification of specific stroke subtypes. All infarcts in this study were within the middle cerebral artery distribution, and the mean NIHSS of enrolled patients was 11 (range 3-27). The mean time from initial evaluation to the receipt of diagnostic imaging was comparable for both modalities (NCCT = 180 minutes, DWI = 189 minutes).

Fiebach JB, Schellinger PD, Jansen O, Meyer M, Wilde P, Bender J, et al. CT and Diffusion-Weighted MR Imaging in Randomized Order Diffusion-Weighted Imaging Results in Higher Accuracy and Lower Interrater Variability in the Diagnosis of Hyperacute Ischemic. Stroke. 2002 Sep 1;33(9):2206–10.

The ISAT trial: endovascular coiling superior to neurosurgical clipping in selected patients with aneurysmal subarachnoid hemorrhage

1. In patients with aneurysmal subarachnoid hemorrhage (SAH), endovascular coiling demonstrated significantly better survival compared to neurosurgical clipping.

2. Patients with ruptured posterior and middle cerebral artery were underrepresented in the cohort due to expert consensus for preferential endovascular coiling and neurosurgical clipping, respectively.

Original Date of Publication: October 2002

Study Rundown: Ruptured intracranial aneurysms are the most common cause of spontaneous SAH and are associated with significant morbidity and mortality. Historically, management options have included open neurosurgical clipping and endovascular therapy with detachable coiling. Choice of treatment was previously based on a combination of clinical judgement and the availability of technical expertise in endovascular therapy at referral centers. The purpose of the landmark International Subarachnoid Aneurysm Trial (ISAT) was to compare the safety and efficacy of endovascular coiling to neurosurgical clipping in patients deemed suitable for either treatment.

The ISAT trial randomized over 2000 patients with aneurysmal SAH to either neurosurgical clipping or endovascular coiling. At the conclusion of the trial, endovascular coiling demonstrated a 23% relative risk and 7% absolute risk reduction in significant disability or death compared to surgical clipping. The results of the ISAT trial thus favored endovascular clipping over surgical clipping in the treatment of ruptured intracranial aneurysm. However, extrapolation of these findings to all patients and aneurysm types was limited by the narrow scope of the ISAT population. During the enrollment phase of the trial, 80% of patients screened were excluded for not meeting the requirement for their aneurysm to be judged as equally amenable to neurosurgical or endovascular therapy. Over 80% of the included patients had aneurysms in the anterior cerebral or internal carotid artery. Posterior circulation and middle cerebral artery aneurysms were underrepresented due to expert consensus for preferential endovascular coiling and neurosurgical clipping, respectively; thus the results of ISAT were not applicable to these patient populations.

In-Depth [randomized controlled trial]: The ISAT trial was an open-labeled, multicenter randomized controlled trial that compared the efficacy and safety of endovascular coiling to neurosurgical clipping in patients with SAH secondary to a ruptured intracranial aneurysm. Patients were screened in all participating centers if they had imaging-confirmed SAH and intracranial aneurysm. Patients were evaluated by both a neurosurgeon and an interventional radiologist and were included if the target lesion was felt to equally amenable to either endovascular coiling or neurosurgical clipping. The primary end-point was overall disability or survival at 2 months and 1 year, as measured by the modified Rankin scale. Secondary outcomes included rates of hospital admission or episodes of re-bleeding. The trial was stopped after the planned interim analysis at 1 year.

Overall, 2143 patients out of 9559 screened met the inclusion/exclusion criteria and were randomized. There were no significant differences in baseline characteristics between the group randomized to endovascular treatment (n = 1073) and neurosurgery (n = 1070). However, 83% of patients had aneurysms in the anterior cerebral or internal carotid arteries. Patients with posterior circulation and middle cerebral artery aneurysms represented only 2.7% and 14.1% of patients, respectively. At the conclusion of the trial, patients randomized to endovascular coiling demonstrated significantly lower rates of disability or death at 1 year compared to surgical clipping (23.7% versus 30.6%; p = 0.019). Patients in the endovascular group had a relative- and absolute risk reduction of disability or death of 22.6% (95%CI 8.9% to 34.2%) and 6.9% (2.5% to 11.3%), respectively. The risk of re-bleeding after 1-year was 2 per 1276 patients in the endovascular group and 0 per 1081 patients in the neurosurgery group.

Molyneux A. International Subarachnoid Aneurysm Trial (ISAT) of neurosurgical clipping versus endovascular coiling in 2143 patients with ruptured intracranial aneurysms: a randomised trial. The Lancet. 2002 Oct 26;360(9342):1267–74.

The ECASS III trial: Administering alteplase up to 4.5 hours after onset of acute ischemic stroke improves neurological outcomes

1. Alteplase administered between 3 to 4.5 hours after the onset of acute ischemic stroke was associated with improved functional outcomes at 90 days, compared to placebo.

Original Date of Publication: September 2008

Study Rundown: Previously, the National Institute of Neurological Disorders and Stroke (NINDS) trial demonstrated that, compared to placebo, treatment of acute ischemic stroke with tissue plasminogen activator (t-PA) within 3 hours of symptom onset significantly improved functional outcomes 3 months after the incident. However, there remained uncertainty regarding the efficacy and safety of administering t-PA more than 3 hours after the onset of acute ischemic stroke. Two previous European trials (i.e., ECASS I and II) had investigated the use of alteplase up to 6 hours after the onset of stroke, but these studies did not demonstrate any benefits. The ECASS III trial was a randomized, controlled trial designed to explore the efficacy and safety of utilizing alteplase, a recombinant t-PA, 3 to 4.5 hours after the onset of stroke.

Treating acute ischemic stroke patients with intravenous alteplase 3 to 4.5 hours after the onset of symptoms significantly improved neurological outcomes at 3 months compared to placebo. While patients in the alteplase group experienced a significantly higher risk of intracranial hemorrhage, mortality was not significantly different between the groups. Some clinicians criticized the trial for excluding patients with severe stroke signs and for a change of protocol during the trial. Regardless, its findings have informed practice as current recommendations suggest administering recombinant t-PA up to 4.5 hours after the onset of acute ischemic stroke.

In-Depth [randomized controlled trial]: This double-blind, placebo-controlled trial examined the use of alteplase at a dose of 0.9 mg/kg. Patients were eligible for the trial if they had a stroke with a clearly defined time of onset, a measurable deficit, and a computed tomographic scan of the brain that demonstrated no evidence of intracranial hemorrhage at baseline. Exclusion criteria included stroke or serious head trauma in the preceding 3 months, major surgery in the past 14 days, history of intracranial hemorrhage, rapidly improving or minor symptoms, and seizure at the onset of stroke. The study involved 821 patients and had a primary outcome measure of disability at 90 days, as assessed using the modified Rankin Scale. The secondary outcome measure was a global measure at 90 days as determined using the modified Rankin Scale, Barthel Index, NIHSS, and Glasgow Outcome Scale. Safety outcomes included mortality at 90 days, intracranial hemorrhage (any, symptomatic), symptomatic edema, or other events. Patients in the alteplase group were significantly more likely to have favorable outcomes of both the primary and secondary outcomes when compared to the placebo group. Patients in the alteplase group, however, experienced a significantly higher risk of intracranial hemorrhage, including symptomatic intracranial hemorrhage, in the first 36 hours after treatment ($p < 0.001$). There were no significant differences between the groups in terms of mortality.

Hacke W, Kaste M, Bluhmki E, Brozman M, Dávalos A, Guidetti D, et al. Thrombolysis with Alteplase 3 to 4.5 Hours after Acute Ischemic Stroke. The New England Journal of Medicine. 2008 Sep 25;359(13):1317–29.

MR CLEAN: Intraarterial Treatment for Acute Ischemic Stroke

1. In this phase 3 randomized, controlled trial, intraarterial treatment for acute ischemic stroke with usual care was associated with a significant improvement in functional independence versus usual care alone.

2. Use of intraarterial treatment was not associated with an improvement in mortality or occurrence of symptomatic intracerebral hemorrhage.

Original Date of Publication: January 2015

Study Rundown: The Multicenter Randomized Clinical Trial of Endovascular Treatment for Acute Ischemic Stroke in the Netherlands (MR CLEAN) was designed to assess whether the addition of intraarterial treatment to usual care of acute ischemic stroke improved efficacy versus usual care alone. Overall, the absolute difference in functional independence via modified Rankin score was 13.5 percentage points in favor of intraarterial treatment (32.6%) versus only usual care (19.1%). This treatment effect persisted in the study's various subgroups, including subgroups based on age or National Institutes of Health Stroke Scale (NIHSS). There was no significant difference between groups for serious adverse events during 90-day follow-up (p = 0.31). Strengths of this study included its comprehensive inclusion of all intraarterial treatments at stroke centers in the Netherlands during the trial period. Major limitations, however, included the asymmetric group sizes (233 in intervention *vs.* 267 in control). Furthermore, these results should be interpreted with some caution, as, although intraarterial treatment proved to be beneficial, nearly 9% of patients in the intervention group had embolization into another vascular territory when assessed on digital-subtraction angiography.

In-Depth [randomized, controlled trial]: The MR CLEAN study was conducted at 16 stroke centers across the Netherlands between December 2010 and March 2014, with a total of 502 participants with acute occlusion in the anterior circulation artery. Addition of intraarterial treatment comprised either delivery of a thrombolytic agent or mechanical thrombectomy at the discretion of the attending physician. Overall, the intervention group saw a significant improvement in functional outcome as measured by the modified Rankin score at 90 days (13.5 percentage points in favor of intervention), with an adjusted odds ratio of 2.16. Although there was no significant difference between groups for serious adverse events, 5.6% of patients in the intervention group had clinical signs of new ischemic stroke in a new vascular territory within 90 days, versus 0.4% in the control group. Complications related to the intraarterial intervention included embolization into new vascular territory (8.6% of patients), vessel dissection (1.7%) and vessel perforation (0.9%). The improved treatment effect in the intervention group persisted within subgroups stratified by age, NIHSS score, or Alberta Stroke Program Early Computed Tomography Score.

Berkhemer OA, Fransen PSS, Beumer D, van den Berg LA, Lingsma HF, Yoo AJ, et al. A Randomized Trial of Intraarterial Treatment for Acute Ischemic Stroke. New England Journal of Medicine. 2015 Jan 1;372(1):11–20.

Intraarterial therapy and t-PA increase reperfusion and functional independence after acute ischemic stroke

1. Across several randomized controlled trials (Table I), patients treated with intraarterial therapy and intravenous (IV) tissue plasminogen activator (t-PA) had consistently improved functional outcomes compared to patients that received IV t-PA alone.

2. Patients were more likely to achieve successful reperfusion after receiving both intraarterial and medical therapy.

3. The addition of intraarterial therapy to usual care did not increase rates of mortality or serious adverse events.

Original Dates of Publication: Multiple 2015 Trials

Study Rundowns: The intravenous (IV) administration of alteplase, a tissue plasminogen activator (t-PA) involved in the breakdown of blood clots, has long been the mainstay in treating acute ischemic stroke. However, a narrow therapeutic time window and various contraindications (i.e. recent surgery, coagulation abnormalities, history of intracranial hemorrhage) have limited the number of patients who qualify for t-PA therapy. IV alteplase is also less effective in penetrating through proximal occlusions of major intracranial arteries, which account for over a third of acute anterior-circulation strokes. Intraarterial therapy includes the chemical dissolution of clots with locally delivered thrombolytic agents and/or clot retrieval through thrombectomy with mechanical devices. While a number of trials have been conducted to evaluate the efficacy of intraarterial therapy compared to more conventional treatment, concerns surrounding the design and execution of these studies left uncertainty on the role of intraarterial therapy in managing acute ischemic stroke in conjunction with alteplase.

As part of the Multicenter Randomized Clinical Trial of Endovascular Treatment for Acute Ischemic Stroke in the Netherlands (MR CLEAN), patients with proximal arterial occlusion in the anterior cerebral circulation received intraarterial treatment with usual care or usual care alone. Berkhemer and colleagues found that at 90 days of follow-up, patients that received intraarterial therapy in addition to usual care had significantly improved functional outcomes. The results of computed tomography angiography (CTA) also showed that after 24 hours, patients assigned to the intervention group were significantly less likely to have residual occlusion. There were no significant differences in the occurrence of serious adverse events; however, a higher proportion of patients from the interventional group demonstrated clinical signs of a new ischemic stroke in a different vascular territory. Given the invasive nature of intraarterial therapy, these patients were also subject to procedure-related complications not seen in the control group.

Campbell and colleagues subsequently conducted the Emergency Neurological Deficits – Intra-Arterial (EXTEND-IA) trial to evaluate whether the use of computed tomographic (CT) perfusion imaging could be used in maximizing the therapeutic potential of intraarterial interventions. Specifically, CT perfusion imaging was used to identify patients with a dual target of vessel occlusion and evidence of salvageable tissue; patients with large ischemic cores and without evidence of clinically significant salvageable ischemic brain tissue were not included in the study. Unlike the MR CLEAN trial where various forms of intraarterial therapy were employed, patients in this study received intraarterial therapy using a stent retriever and IV alteplase, or alteplase alone within 6 hours of stroke onset. As the results of an interim analysis strongly favored the intervention, this trial was stopped early, demonstrating that CT perfusion imaging can be effectively used to identify patients with the greatest potential to benefit from endovascular therapy. Specifically, early combination endovascular therapy and IV alteplase was associated with significantly earlier neurologic improvement when compared to the receipt of IV alteplase alone. Patients in the intervention group also achieved greater overall reperfusion after 24 hours, corresponding to improved functional outcomes measured at 90 days. The use of CT perfusion imaging also shortened the time to treatment initiation. The results of this study were echoed in the Endovascular Treatment for Small Core and Anterior Circulation Proximal Occlusion with Emphasis on Minimizing CT to Recanalization Times (ESCAPE) trial published in the same issue of The New England Journal of Medicine (NEJM).

Like the EXTEND-IA trial, patients in the ESCAPE trial were initially evaluated using CT and CTA, and considered eligible if they had a small infarct core, an occluded proximal artery in the anterior circulation, and moderate-to-good collateral circulation. Unlike the ESCAPE trial, however, enrollment up to 12 hours after the onset of stroke symptoms was permitted, and intraarterial therapy was not restricted to the use of retrievable stents. As this study was also terminated early, results reflected that of an interim analysis, where the intervention was significantly favored with respect to improved functional outcomes. The mortality rate among patients that received both intraarterial therapy and IV alteplase was also significantly decreased when compared to patients that received alteplase alone, and rates of symptomatic intracerebral hemorrhage did not significantly differ. The median time from initial imaging to groin puncture and median time to first visualization of reflow in the middle cerebral artery in the intervention group were also considerably reduced compared to previous studies, including the EXTEND-IA trial.

Less than six months after the release of the EXTEND-IA and ESCAPE trials, the results of the Solitaire with the Intention for Thrombectomy as Primary Endovascular Treatment (SWIFT PRIME) emerged. Using similar methodology to the EXTEND-IA and ESCAPE studies, namely strict imaging eligibility requirements, Saver and colleagues further confirmed that patients receiving IV t-PA and thrombectomy using a stent retriever had significantly better functional outcomes at 90 days, with the proportion of patients achieving functional independence far exceeding that observed in patients that received t-PA alone. The proportion of patients with successful reperfusion in the intervention group was also twice as high as that seen in the control group, without significantly increasing the risk of serious adverse events or 90-day mortality. This study also noted that patients who received IV t-PA at another hospital before being transferred to a study site for thrombectomy had less favorable outcomes, where levels of functional independence in these patients did not significantly from that observed in patients receiving t-PA alone.

The REVASCAT study also reiterated the value of administering combination intraarterial and medical therapy. Like the prior studies, following visualization of an occlusion in the proximal anterior circulation without a large core, patients were randomized to receive thrombectomy using a stent retriever and medical therapy or medical therapy alone. Consistent with the aforementioned studies, patients in the intervention group had significantly improved functional outcomes compared to those that received medical therapy alone. Patients that received intraarterial therapy were also significantly more likely to exhibit dramatic neurologic improvements at 24 hours, without an increase in the risk experiencing serious adverse events or death.

Berkhemer OA, Fransen PSS, Beumer D, van den Berg LA, Lingsma HF, Yoo AJ, et al. A Randomized Trial of Intraarterial Treatment for Acute Ischemic Stroke. The New England Journal of Medicine. 2015 Jan;372(1):11-20.

Campbell BCV, Mitchell PJ, Kleinig TJ, Dewey HM, Churilov L, Yassi N, et al. Endovascular Therapy for Ischemic Stroke with Perfusion-Imaging Selection. The New England Journal of Medicine. 2015 Mar;372(11):1009-18.

Goyal M, Demchuk AM, Menon BK, Eesa M, Rempel JL, Thornton J, et al. Randomized Assessment of Rapid Endovascular Treatment of Ischemic Stroke. The New England Journal of Medicine. 2015 Mar;372(11):1019-30.

Saver JL, Goyal M, Bonafe A, Diener H-C, Levy EI, Pereira VM, et al. Stent-Retriever Thrombectomy after Intravenous t-PA versus t-PA Alone in Stroke. The New England Journal of Medicine. 2015 Jun;372(24):2285-95.

Jovin TG, Chamorro A, Cobo E, de Miquel MA, Molina CA, Rovira A, et al. Thrombectomy within 8 Hours after Symptom Onset in Ischemic Stroke. The New England Journal of Medicine. 2015 Jun;372(24):2296-306.

	Study population	Methodology	Results	Key findings
MR CLEAN (2015)	- Patients ≥18 years of age with proximal arterial occlusion in the anterior circulation established with CTA, magnetic resonance angiography (MRA) or digital-subtraction angiography (DSA) - Patients must have been within 6 hours of symptom onset	- RCT (n=500) - Endovascular therapy (intra-arterial thrombolysis and/or mechanical thrombectomy) and IV t-PA vs. IV t-PA alone - Primary outcome: functional outcome by modified Rankin scale (MRS) at 90 days	- Improved functional outcomes by MRS at 90 days in endovascular group (OR 1.67, 95% CI 1.21-2.30) - 75.4% of intervention group had no intracranial occlusion on follow-up CTA (OR 6.88, 95%CI 4.34-10.94) - No difference in occurrence of serious adverse events (p = 0.31) between groups	- Endovascular therapy was associated with improved function outcome compared to IV t-PA alone - No increase in serious adverse events with endovascular therapy
EXTEND-IA (2015)	- Patients with anterior circulation ischemic stroke established with CTA - Patients must have had a dual target of vessel occlusion and evidence of salvageable tissue on perfusion imaging and received IV t-PA within 4.5 hours of symptom onset	- RCT (n=70) - Mechanical thrombectomy and IV t-PA vs. IV t-PA alone - Primary outcome(s): reperfusion (% reduction in perfusion-lesion volume at 24 hours) and early neurologic improvement by NIH stroke scale	- Median % reperfusion at 24 hours in the endovascular group was 100% compared to 37% in IV t-PA only group (OR 4.7, 95% CI 2.5-9.0) - Higher proportion of patients from intervention group achieved early neurologic improvement (OR 6.0, 95% CI 2.0-18.0) - Improved functional outcomes by MRS at 90 days in thrombectomy group (OR 2.0, 95% CI 1.2-3.8)	- Mechanical thrombectomy improved reperfusion, early neurologic recovery and functional outcomes compared to IV t-PA alone - CT perfusion imaging can be used to identify patients with the greatest potential to benefit from endovascular therapy, and shorten time to treatment initiation

ESCAPE (2015)	- Patients ≥18 years of age with a small infarct core, proximal intracranial occlusion in the anterior circulation, and moderate-good collateral circulation by CTA - Patients were enrolled up to 12 hours after symptom onset and must have received IV t-PA within 4.5 hours of symptom onset	- RCT (n=316) - Mechanical thrombectomy and IV t-PA vs. IV t-PA alone - Primary outcome: function outcome by MRS at 90 days	- Improved functional outcomes by MRS at 90 days in thrombectomy group (OR 2.6, 95% CI 1.7-3.8) - Intervention associated with reduced mortality (RR 0.5, 95% CI 0.3-1.0)	- Mechanical thrombectomy was associated with improved functional outcomes and reduced mortality compared to IV t-PA alone
SWIFT PRIME (2015)	- Patients with confirmed occlusions in the proximal anterior intracranial circulation without large ischemic-core lesions detected through imaging - Patients must have been within 6 hours of symptom onset and must have IV t-PA within 4.5 hours of symptom onset	- RCT (n=196) - Mechanical thrombectomy with stent retriever and IV t-PA vs. IV t-PA alone - Primary outcome: functional outcome by MRS at 90 days	- Improved functional outcomes by MRS at 90 days in thrombectomy group (p<0.001) - Successful reperfusion (≥90%) at 27 hours was more frequent in the intervention group (p<0.001) - No difference in occurrence of serious adverse events (p = 0.54)	- Mechanical thrombectomy was associated with improved functional outcomes compared to IV t-PA alone

Trial	Inclusion criteria	Design	Results	Conclusion
REVASCAT (2015)	- Patients age 18-85 years with anterior circulation ischemic stroke without evidence of a large ischemic core on imaging - Patients must have been within 8 hours of symptom onset and must have received IV t-PA within 4.5 hours of stroke onset without evidence of revascularization within 30 minutes of t-PA	- RCT (n=206) - Thrombectomy with stent retriever and IV t-PA vs. IV t-PA - Primary outcome: functional outcome by MRS at 90 days	- Improved functional outcomes by MRS at 90 days in thrombectomy group (OR 1.7, 95%CI 1.05-2.8) and dramatic neurologic improvement at 24 hours (OR 5.5, 95% CI 2.9-10.3) - Mortality (p = 0.60) and rates of intracranial hemorrhage (p = 1.00) did not significantly differ at 90 days	- Mechanical thrombectomy was associated with improved function outcomes, without an increased risk of mortality or intracranial hemorrhage compared to IV t-PA alone

Table I. Key stroke trials.

Thrombectomy between 6 and 24 hours after acute stroke reduces disability: The DAWN trial

1. Thrombectomy performed between 6 and 24 hours after onset of acute stroke in patients with a mismatch between stroke symptoms and infarct volume results in better disability outcomes compared to standard care alone.

2. Adverse events of intracranial hemorrhage and 90-day mortality do not differ significantly between thrombectomy and standard care-treated patients.

Original Date of Publication: January 2018

Study Rundown: Acute stroke management with thrombectomy aims to increase cerebral perfusion in order to minimize ischemic damage. Prior studies have indicated a clinical advantage to performing thrombectomy within 6 hours of stroke onset, with decreasing clinical benefit as time to thrombectomy increases. After 6 hours from stroke onset relatively fewer studies are available to aid in determining optimal stroke management with thrombectomy. In this study, the DAWN (DWI or CTP Assessment with Clinical Mismatch in the Triage of Wake-Up and Late Presenting Strokes Undergoing Neurointervention with Trevo) trial compares stroke patients with a mismatch between their clinical deficits and infarct volume treated 6 to 24 hours after symptom onset with thrombectomy plus standard care compared to standard care alone. Primary endpoints of disability and functional independence were both improved in the thrombectomy group compared to the standard treatment group at 90 days post treatment. Rates of internal hemorrhage and 90-day mortality did not significantly differ between the two groups. This study provides significant evidence supporting thrombectomy treatment between 6 and 24 hours after stroke onset. Study strengths include participation of numerous multinational treatment centers and extensive subgroup analysis, and a notable weakness is exclusion of patients with large volume infarcts.

In-Depth [randomized control trial]: This prospective, multicenter trial conducted between 2014 and 2017 randomized 206 patients to thrombectomy plus standard care (n = 107) and standard care (n = 99) groups. Eligible patients had occlusion of either the intracranial internal carotid artery, proximal middle cerebral artery, or both with a last known well time between 6 and 24 hours prior to treatment. Included patients also had a mismatch between their clinical symptom severity and infarct volume as defined by the National Institutes of Health Stroke Scale (NIHSS). Concomitant stenting was not performed in the thrombectomy group. The modified Rankin scale was used to assess co-primary endpoints of disability and functional independence. Patients in the thrombectomy group were less disabled at 90 days post-treatment compared to the standard care group (5.5 vs 3.4 Rankin score, respectively; 95% confidence interval 1.1 to 3.0). Rates of functional independence at 90 days were 49% in the thrombectomy group and 13% in the control group (adjusted difference 33%; 95% credible interval 22 to 40). Subgroup analysis indicated significantly improved disability scores for thrombectomy-treated patients for almost all assessments (except for unwitnessed stroke). Rates of intracerebral hemorrhage (6% vs 3%, p = 0.50) and 90-day mortality (19% vs 18%, p = 1.00) did not differ between the thrombectomy and standard care groups, respectively.

Nogueira RG, Jadhav AP, Haussen DC, Bonafe A, Budzik RF, Bhuva P, et al. Thrombectomy 6 to 24 Hours after Stroke with a Mismatch between Deficit and Infarct. New England Journal of Medicine. 2018 Jan 4;378(1):11–21

POINT trial: Clopidogrel and Aspirin for Acute Ischemic Stroke

1. In this randomized, controlled trial, combination therapy with aspirin and clopidogrel resulted in a lower risk of major ischemic events at 90 days versus aspirin alone for patients with acute ischemic stroke or high-risk transient ischemic attack.

2. Combination therapy with aspirin and clopidogrel resulted in a higher risk of major hemorrhage event at 90 days than aspirin alone.

Original Date of Publication: July 2018

Study Rundown: The Platelet-Oriented Inhibition in New TIA and Minor Ischemic Stroke (POINT) trial evaluated the use of dual antiplatelet therapy (clopidogrel with aspirin) versus aspirin alone to reduce the risk of recurrent stroke in patients with acute ischemic stroke or high-risk transient ischemic attack (TIA). Although the trial showed improved efficacy for dual antiplatelet therapy versus aspirin alone ($P = 0.02$), it was ultimately halted before completion due to a clear risk of increased major hemorrhage for participants in the treatment arm. Notably, although risk of recurrent ischemic stroke was reduced for the dual antiplatelet group, there was no significant difference in efficacy for reducing myocardial infarction events ($P = 0.46$) or death from ischemic vascular causes ($P = 0.52$). Based on these results, the authors estimate that, per 1000 patients treated with dual antiplatelet therapy, 15 ischemic events would be prevented, and 5 major hemorrhages would be precipitated by 90 days. The main strength of this study was its relatively large sample size and strong trial design, taking place at numerous centers internationally. Limitations, however, include the exclusion of certain patient groups, such as those with moderate, severe or cardioembolic strokes, limiting the generalizability of this study.

In-Depth [randomized, controlled trial]: The POINT trial randomized a total of 4881 patients at 269 centers across the world between May 2010 and December 2017. Eligible patients had had either an acute ischemic stroke scored as less than 3 on the National Institutes of Health Stroke Scale (NIHSS) or a TIA with a score of greater than 4 on the ABCD^2 scale within 12 hours. Those in the clopidogrel group received a 600mg loading dose on day 1, followed by 75mg per day. Aspirin dose ranged from 50-325mg per day in both groups. Overall, those receiving aspirin with clopidogrel had a significantly improved primary efficacy outcome (a composite of ischemic stroke, myocardial infarction or death from ischemic vascular event) versus aspirin alone (P = 0.02). However, these significant differences did not persist in secondary efficacy outcomes for myocardial infarction or death from ischemic event in isolation. Major hemorrhage, the primary safety outcome, occurred in 0.9% of the dual antiplatelet group and 0.4% of the aspirin group (P = 0. 02). This exceeded the prespecified boundary for safety signal, thus resulting in trial discontinuation in August 2017.

Johnston SC, Easton JD, Farrant M, Barsan W, Conwit RA, Elm JJ, et al. Clopidogrel and Aspirin in Acute Ischemic Stroke and High-Risk TIA. New England Journal of Medicine. 2018 Jul 19;379(3):215–25.

OVIVA trial: Oral versus Intravenous Antibiotics for Bone and Joint Infection

1. This randomized, controlled trial found that oral antibiotics were noninferior to intravenous antibiotics for treatment failure at 1 year when started within 6 weeks of complex orthopedic infections.

2. There was no significant difference in the rate of major adverse events between the two groups.

Original Date of Publication: January 2019

Study Rundown: The Oral Versus Intravenous Antibiotics for Bone and Joint Infection (OVIVA) trial was a multicenter, randomized controlled trial assessing noninferiority for risk of treatment failure at 1 year for oral versus intravenous antibiotics. Overall, oral antibiotics were shown to be noninferior to intravenous antibiotics when initiated within 6 weeks of surgery (risk difference = -1.4). Likewise, there were no significant differences in the percentage of participants with at least one serious adverse event (p = 0.58). Notably, median hospital stay was significantly longer in the intravenous (14 days) versus oral (11 days) groups (p < 0.001). Based on these results, the authors support the use of oral antibiotics in the early treatment of complex orthopedic infections, however they acknowledge this may not be appropriate for all patient groups. Some strengths of this trial were its diverse patient population, with good generalizability, and high trial retention. Limitations, however, included its open-label nature. The trial did not actually assess or compare specific antibiotic agents versus others, relying on local expertise to decide. Finally, given that the trial's selection criteria were so inclusive and heterogenous, this makes drawing more nuanced conclusions about its population difficult.

In-Depth [randomized, controlled trial]: The OVIVA trial was conducted at 26 sites in the United Kingdom, including a per-protocol analysis of 909 participants with complex bone or joint infection. The majority (60.6%) were treated with surgical intervention, and antibiotic treatment was initiated within 6 weeks of presentation in all cases. The difference in the risk of treatment failure between oral and intravenous antibiotics at 1 year was -1.4 percentage points, meeting the prespecified noninferiority criteria. The number of participants experiencing at least one serious adverse events did not differ between groups, and adverse events were most common related to operative site or antibiotic-related. Episodes of *C. difficile* diarrhea also did not significantly differ between groups. Median hospital stay was significantly longer for the intravenous group (14 days) versus the oral group (11 days) (p < 0.001). Patient-reported outcome measures did not significantly differ.

Li H-K, Rombach I, Zambellas R, Walker AS, McNally MA, Atkins BL, et al. Oral versus Intravenous Antibiotics for Bone and Joint Infection. New England Journal of Medicine. 2019 Jan 31;380(5):425–36.

X. Obstetrics and Gynecology

"No amount of experimentation can ever prove me right; a single experiment can prove me wrong."

- Albert Einstein

Antenatal steroids promote fetal lung maturity

1. In a randomized trial, preterm infants whose mothers received steroids were less likely to experience respiratory distress syndrome (RDS) and perinatal mortality.

Original Date of Publication: October 1972

Study Rundown: Respiratory complications of preterm birth are an important and common cause of preterm morbidity and mortality. Prior to 34 weeks gestational age, fetal lungs are considered immature due to the lack of surfactant present in pulmonary alveoli. As the fetal lungs develop, they begin to produce greater quantities of surfactant. Specifically, lecithin production and the ratio of lecithin to sphingomyelin (L/S ratio) in fetal amniotic fluid increase. The L/S ratio is a marker of fetal lung maturity with an L/S ratio < 1.5 is associated with an increased risk of RDS while an L/S ratio > 2 is associated with fetal lung maturity and a decreased risk of RDS. As of the late 1969s, no interventions existed to reduce the respiratory morbidity associated with preterm birth. In the late 1960s, animal studies in lambs and rabbits demonstrated that fetal lung maturity was accelerated in fetuses whose mothers received glucocorticoids prior to preterm delivery. These studies stimulated obstetricians and scientists to examine whether fetal lung maturity could be similarly improved in humans. Unlike some other animals (e.g. cows), the human placenta is relatively permeable to glucocorticoids such that maternal administration of steroids permits transfer of these medicines to the preterm fetus.

This classic trial from the 1970s demonstrated that maternal antenatal steroids confer a significant reduction in risk of perinatal death and RDS in preterm infants. Subsequent investigations would go on to support these findings and establish additional fetal benefits of steroid administration, including decreased risk for intraventricular hemorrhage. This landmark trial changed practice such that women at risk for imminent preterm delivery are now recommended to receive a course of antenatal steroids, which consists of 2 doses of intramuscular betamethasone administered 24 hours apart. Strengths included randomized, double-blinded design and standardized, objective assessment of RDS. Limitations included a small sample size of women who delivered at the same institution in New Zealand.

In-Depth [randomized controlled trial]: A total of 213 women with threatened preterm labor were randomized to receive betamethasone (n = 117) or placebo (n = 96) and received tocolysis with ethanol or salbutamol in attempts to delay delivery for 48-72 hours after the first betamethasone injection. Pharmacists randomized patients to allow healthcare providers to remain blinded to group assignments. Primary outcomes investigated were perinatal mortality and RDS, assessed via the Silverman Score, a system that incorporates respiratory rate, grunting, and chest retractions. Secondary outcomes included intraventricular hemorrhage.

Perinatal death was less common in the infants of mothers who received antenatal betamethasone compared to placebo (6 vs. 18%, p = 0.02). RDS was 66% less likely to occur among infants whose mothers received betamethasone compared to infants whose mothers were randomized to placebo (9 vs. 26%, p < 0.01). No infants in the treatment group experienced hyaline membrane disease or intraventricular hemorrhage compared to incidences of 7% and 5%, respectfully, in the control group.

Liggins GC, Howie RN. A controlled trial of antepartum glucocorticoid treatment for prevention of the respiratory distress syndrome in premature infants. Pediatrics. 1972;50(4):515-25.

A standard for fetal growth in pregnancy

1. After an initial rapid period of curvilinear growth, fetal weight was found to increase at a more linear rate through term.

Original Date of Publication: November 1976

Study Rundown: As of the 1970s, there was not a standard for fetal growth in pregnancy. As such, it was not possible to adequately or reliably monitor growth, preventing optimal fetal monitoring and precluding insight into how numerous obstetric and medical conditions could affect the developing fetus. For example, the effects of maternal or obstetric pathology (e.g., chronic hypertension, preeclampsia, diabetes) on intrauterine growth could not be evaluated in the absence of a fetal growth standard. Additionally, diagnostic measurements of fetal growth, which can be used to estimate gestational age when a mother is not aware of her last menstrual period or the date of conception, were not possible. Previous investigations on the subject were limited by unreliable weight measurements of deceased neonates due to weighing of formalin-fixed fetuses. The largest prior study included 5000 Caucasian infants born to women of low socioeconomic status living at a high altitude such that results were not readily applicable to other populations. In the present work, authors compared fetal weight and growth measurements of tens of thousands of fetuses and newborns to determine a standard for intrauterine fetal growth.

This landmark study plotted the weights and gestational ages from more than 31 000 pregnancies to create the first standard for fetal growth in pregnancy appropriate for widespread use in the U.S. This was the first investigation to systematically evaluate growth standards by gestational age in a large and diverse population of American women. Strengths included the largest and most comprehensive assessment of fetal growth to date and use of information from 2 centers. Lack of accounting for biological sex, race, or maternal parity in fetal growth rate models may confound results. Though future investigations could improve upon this model, this classic initial investigation effectively demonstrated that after an initially rapid period of curvilinear growth, fetal weight increases in a more linear fashion through term.

In-Depth [retrospective cohort]: A total of over 31 268 fetuses and infants were assessed to characterize fetal growth rate, or weight gain per week of pregnancy.

Data was obtained from 430 medical terminations performed at 8 to 21 weeks gestation in Chapel Hill and from 30 772 liveborn singleton infants delivered from 21 through 44 weeks estimated gestational age in Cleveland. All participants had reliable dating, defined as dating by last menstrual period consistent with clinician-measured fundal height. Percentiles of fetal weight gain by gestational age were plotted with 2-pointed weighted means. Simple linear regression was used to model crown-rump length by gestational age. Fetal growth rate is denoted by median fetal weight (grams, g) by estimated week of gestation.

The relationship between fetal growth and gestational age was initially curvilinear during a period of rapid growth in early pregnancy and then noted to become linear as fetal growth rate stabilizes. In contrast, weekly fetal weight gain increased throughout pregnancy to a maximum of just over 200 g/week from 34-36 weeks. At term, 37 weeks gestation, fetal weights were 2580 g at the 25th percentile, 2870 g at the 50th percentile, 3160 g at the 75th percentile, and 3470 g at the 90th percentile. The majority (>50%) of infants at the premature gestational age of 30 weeks were low birthweight and weighed < 1500 g.

Brenner WE, Edelman DA, Hendricks CH. A standard of fetal growth for the United States of America. American journal of obstetrics and gynecology. 1976;126(5):555-64.

HELLP syndrome is variant of preeclampsia

1. The syndrome of hemolysis, elevated liver enzymes and low platelets (HELLP) was defined as a destructive, consumptive coagulopathy on the spectrum of preeclampsia.

Original Date of Publication: January 1982

Study Rundown: The syndrome of HELLP is a high-risk obstetrical condition that is characterized by thrombocytopenia, hemolysis (microangiopathic hemolytic anemia), and elevated liver enzymes. HELLP syndrome is thought to be first described in a small case series in the 1950s, but remained poorly understood for decades thereafter. Previously, small case series identified a number of laboratory abnormalities in pregnant women with elevated blood pressures, including thrombocytopenia, hemolysis, and transaminitis. However, these investigations attributed transaminitis to nonobstetric etiologies, such as hepatitis. Then, a small case series described 5 severely ill pregnant patients with transaminitis and biopsy-proven liver damage in the absence of severely elevated blood pressures. This report highlight our lack of understanding of whether newly elevated blood pressures in pregnancy was a highly reproducible or requisite feature of new liver dysfunction in pregnancy. The present study was the first to define a unifying diagnosis of HELLP syndrome as elevated blood pressures, thrombocytopenia, hemolysis, and liver dysfunction in pregnancy.

This landmark case series was the first to characterize the classical features of HELLP syndrome, as well as the remarkably high maternal morbidity, and characterized the disease as a consumptive process on the spectrum of preeclampsia. Investigators demonstrated that both normotensive and hypertensive women can experience HELLP, making serial laboratory testing in preeclamptic patients, and high indices of suspicion advisable. Findings contributed to improved early recognition, timely diagnosis and treatment of this highly morbid condition in pregnancy. Strengths included comprehensive review of clinical presentation, disease course, and maternal and neonatal outcomes as well as thorough assessment and discussion of findings, existing literature and possible pathophysiologic mechanisms of disease. Limitations included a descriptive study and small sample size of 29 patients at a single institution.

In-Depth [case series]: All pregnant women diagnosed with HELLP syndrome at a single institution in Arizona (n = 29) were followed over a 30 month period. Outcomes included obstetric and neonatal morbidity and mortality including eclampsia, severe-range blood pressures (blood pressures ≥160/110), proteinuria (2+ or greater on urine dip), thrombocytopenia (platelets < 100,000), and microangiopathic hemolytic anemia (MAHA). Once the diagnosis of HELLP syndrome was made, women were delivered expediently via induction of labor in the setting of a favorable cervix or cesarean section in the instance of an unfavorable cervix.

Nausea, right upper quadrant pain, transaminitis, proteinuria and thrombocytopenia were present in 100% of women with HELLP syndrome and 97% had MAHA on peripheral blood smear. Severe-range blood pressures occurred in 30% of primigravid and 78% of multiparous women with HELLP, while eclampsia occurred in 15% of primigravid and 11% of multiparous women. Numerous women developed HELLP syndrome within 2 weeks of hospitalization for preeclampsia. Adverse maternal and fetal outcomes included 1 maternal death (3%) and 3 neonatal deaths (9%). Twin gestation (11%), chronic hypertension (10%), and diabetes mellitus (7%) pre-existent to pregnancy were prevalent in women diagnosed with HELLP.

Weinstein L. Syndrome of hemolysis, elevated liver enzymes, and low platelet count: a severe consequence of hypertension in pregnancy. American journal of obstetrics and gynecology. 1982;142(2):159-67.

Low maternal serum α-fetoprotein associated with fetal aneuploidy

1. Compared to healthy controls, women whose pregnancies were complicated by fetal aneuploidy had lower levels of maternal serum α-fetoprotein (AFP).

2. This study supported use of maternal serum AFP as a serum screening test for aneuploidy.

Original Date of Publication: April 1984

Study Rundown: Serum screening for aneuploidy is a relatively modern concept in the United States. As of the 1980s, no screening tests existed for fetal aneuploidy, an abnormal number of chromosomes. The only available antenatal testing for chromosomal disorders was diagnostic, invasive, and associated with an increased risk of pregnancy loss. Invasive prenatal diagnostic testing via amniocentesis or amniotic fluid cell culture and was primarily reserved for women of advanced maternal age (AMA, ≥35 years) while low-risk pregnant women were not recommended to undergo testing. Development of a noninvasive screening test for aneuploidy would permit risk assessment in young women and decrease morbidity associated with invasive testing. Previous investigations identified a relationship with elevated maternal serum AFP, a protein produced primarily in the fetal liver, and an increased risk for neural tube defects. Follow-up investigations demonstrated that low levels of maternal serum AFP were associated with pregnancy loss. Authors of the present work then encountered a healthy 28-year-old pregnant woman who was incidentally noted to have an undetectable (very low) serum AFP level in the second trimester and went on to deliver an infant with trisomy 18. This index case motivated a case-control study comparing maternal serum AFP levels in women who delivered infants with aneuploidy to maternal serum AFP levels in women who delivered healthy infants.

This landmark study characterized the relationship between low maternal serum AFP and an increased risk of fetal aneuploidy, making it the first study to identify a serum marker associated with aneuploidy and initiating the development of routine noninvasive screening tests for aneuploidy. Further investigations would go on to define gestational-age-dependent cutoffs for maternal serum AFP levels, below which women are now counseled regarding an increased risk for aneuploidy and can be referred for invasive diagnostic testing. Strengths included gestational age matching and investigation at 2 sites. Limitations included retrospective design, a small number of cases (n = 53), and missing maternal age data, which is an established confounder for fetal aneuploidy.

In-Depth [case-control study]: From a series of over 3800 amniocenteses performed at Albert Einstein in New York and Case Western in Ohio, a total of 41 cases of fetal autosomal trisomy were identified. Levels of corresponding maternal serum AFP were obtained from cases and compared to levels in > 40 000 gestational-age-matched controls. The primary outcome of interest was difference in serum α-fetoprotein between cases and controls. Results are presented as multiples of the mean (MOM).

Compared to gestational-age matched controls, 88% of pregnancies affected by fetal autosomal trisomy had corresponding maternal serum AFP levels below the median (p < 0.01). Maternal serum AFP levels were below 0.4 MOM in 25% of aneuploidy cases compared to 11.2% of healthy controls. Similarly, serum AFP levels below 0.25 MOM occurred in 14% of cases compared with 5.3% of controls.

Merkatz IR, Nitowsky HM, Macri JN, Johnson WE. An association between low maternal serum alpha-fetoprotein and fetal chromosomal abnormalities. American journal of obstetrics and gynecology. 1984;148(7):886-94.

Atypia predicts progression to endometrial cancer

1. **Among women with endometrial hyperplasia, cytologic atypia was the most important predictor of progression to carcinoma.**

Original Date of Publication: July 1985

Study Rundown: Endometrial cancer is the most common gynecologic malignancy and affects 3% of all American women in their lifetime. Further, the incidence of endometrial cancer is increasing in concert with the rising obesity epidemic in the United States. Risk factors for endometrial adenocarcinoma include obesity, anovulation and advanced age. Fortunately, the majority of these cancers are diagnosed early due to the common presenting symptom of postmenopausal bleeding. Evaluation of postmenopausal bleeding in women at increased risk for endometrial cancer typically includes endometrial sampling via endometrial biopsy or dilation and curettage. Pathology might reveal benign findings, malignancy, or a premalignant lesion: endometrial hyperplasia. Endometrial hyperplasia encompasses a group of heterogenous noninvasive endometrial proliferations that are histological precursors to cancer. Prior to the 1980s, physicians and scientists knew little about which histologic characteristics conveyed the highest risk for cancer progression. Previous investigations identified an increased risk of progression with complex atypical hyperplasia but did not parse out whether cytologic (typical or atypical) or architectural (simple or complex) characteristics were more predictive of progression to cancer. In the present work, researchers followed women with hyperplasia for an average of 13 years to determine the risk of progression by cytologic and architectural characteristics.

This landmark study demonstrated that cytologic atypia is the most important risk factor for progression of endometrial hyperplasia to cancer. Strengths included central pathology review and complete access to the clinical record. Limitations included observational design whereby women with the most strikingly abnormal histology and symptomatology might have undergone hysterectomy earlier and biased results toward the null. Findings of this investigation changed clinical practice such that women with hyperplasia with atypia who have completed childbearing are now recommended to undergo hysterectomy. Later studies would demonstrate that up to 43% of women with complex atypical hyperplasia on endometrial sampling are found to have endometrial cancer on hysterectomy.

In-Depth [retrospective cohort]: A total of 170 women underwent dilation and curettage that demonstrated some degree of hyperplasia from 1940-1970 and did not undergo hysterectomy for at least 1 year. The mean time between curettage and hysterectomy was 13.4 years. Simple hyperplasia was defined as an increased number of endometrial glands; complex hyperplasia was denoted by glands with irregular outlines with marked structural complexity and back-to-back crowding; atypical hyperplasia was defined as proliferation of cells demonstrating nuclear atypia and loss of polarity. The primary outcome assessed was progression of hyperplasia to carcinoma as evidenced on subsequent curettage or hysterectomy. The frequency of regression and persistence of hyperplasia were also assessed.

Among women with endometrial hyperplasia, progression to carcinoma occurred in 1% of patients with simple, typical hyperplasia, 3% of women with complex, typical hyperplasia, 8% of women with simple, atypical hyperplasia and 29% of women with complex, atypical hyperplasia. Only 1.6% of women with typical hyperplasia progressed to carcinoma compared with 23% of women with atypical hyperplasia ($p = 0.001$).

Kurman RJ, Kaminski PF, Norris HJ. The behavior of endometrial hyperplasia. A long-term study of "untreated" hyperplasia in 170 patients. Cancer. 1985;56(2):403-12.

Nurses' Health Study: Postmenopausal estrogen associated with cardiovascular risk

1. Healthy postmenopausal women on estrogen were less likely to develop major cardiovascular disease or experience cardiovascular mortality.

2. Results were not reproduced in follow-up randomized controlled trials.

Original Date of Publication: September 1991

Study Rundown: The impact of exogenous estrogen use on cardiovascular disease risk has been a topic of debate for decades. In the mid 1980s, conflicting results were published from 2 prospective investigations assessing the impact of estrogen use on cardiovascular disease risk. In 1985, initial findings from four years of follow-up from the Nurses' Health Study (NHS), a large prospective observational study of healthy nurses, identified a decreased risk for cardiovascular disease among women on supplemental estrogen therapy. In the same issue of the The New England Journal of Medicine, findings from the Framingham Heart study, a large prospective cohort study, demonstrated a 50% increased risk for cardiovascular morbidity among women over 50 years old on estrogen. These contradictory findings led to significant confusion in clinical practice and popular media.

The NHS presents data from 10 years of follow-up comparing the risk of major coronary disease between postmenopausal women taking estrogen and those not taking estrogen. While results demonstrated reduction in cardiovascular morbidity in women on estrogen, subsequent investigations would disprove this finding. Randomized controlled trials from the Women's Health Initiative (WHI) demonstrated no benefit to estrogen-only therapy and an increased cardiovascular risk associated with combined estrogen-progestin hormone replacement therapy (HRT), such that HRT is no longer recommended for primary prevention of cardiovascular morbidity. These 2 studies differed in patient age (NHS 30-63 years of age, WHI 50-79 years of age) and in study design (NHS was a cohort study, while WHI was a randomized trial). The NHS is one of the most famous and well-studied examples of how bias can impact epidemiologic investigation. In this study, healthy user bias, compliance bias (or adherer effect), and confounding by socioeconomic status contributed to an incorrect conclusion.

In-Depth [prospective cohort]: A total of 48 470 healthy, postmenopausal nurses aged 30-63 years in the NHS were followed for 10 years to compare the incidence of cardiovascular morbidity and mortality in women on exogenous estrogen and those not on HRT. Participants completed follow-up questionnaires every 2 years. Cardiovascular disease outcomes assessed included nonfatal myocardial infarction, fatal coronary heart disease, coronary artery bypass graft procedure, stroke, and total cardiovascular mortality. Established and potential risk factors, smoking, diabetes, hyperlipidemia and hypertension, were accounted for in multivariate analysis.

Postmenopausal women who elected to take estrogen HRT experienced a 44% reduced risk of major coronary disease compared to women who did not take HRT (RR 0.56; 95%CI 0.40-0.80). This risk reduction was similar when analysis was restricted to healthy nonsmokers without diabetes, hypertension, or hyperlipidemia (RR 0.53; 95%CI 0.31-0.91). Age-adjusted relative risk of cardiovascular mortality in women on estrogen was 0.72 (95%CI 0.55-0.95, p = 0.02).

Stampfer MJ, Colditz GA, Willett WC, Manson JE, Rosner B, Speizer FE, et al. Postmenopausal estrogen therapy and cardiovascular disease. Ten-year follow-up from the nurses' health study. The New England Journal of Medicine. 1991;325(11):756-62.

Human papillomavirus infection is associated with adenocarcinoma of the cervix

1. Human papillomavirus (HPV) types 16 and 18 were present in a high proportion of cervical disease and termed oncogenic subtypes.

2. Infection with HPV subtypes 16 or 18 conferred at least a 60-fold increased risk of developing cervical cancer.

Original Date of Publication: March 1992

Study Rundown: HPV was first linked to cervical cancer in the early 1980s. Since that time, molecular biologists worked to better understand the relationship between HPV exposure, infection and cervical cancer. Regarding exposure and infection, studies demonstrated variable association with exposure and subsequent persistent HPV infection. With respect to cervical cancer, a large investigation demonstrated that HPV strains 16 and 18 were present in 70% of all cervical cancer specimens, suggesting these 2 strains were associated with development of dysplasia and cancer. Other HPV serotypes were detected in low-risk cervical pathology but were much less frequent. Thus, the proportion of women exposed to HPV who would develop persistent infection and of those, the proportion who would develop cervical cancer, remained unclear.

In this landmark work, authors assessed the incidence of HPV in healthy controls, the clinicopathologic relationship of 15 common HPV strains, and condylomatous, premalignant, and malignant cervical disease. Authors determined that the HPV subtypes 16, 18, 45 and 56 were the most commonly found subtypes in cervical dysplasia and neoplasia. Additional novel findings included a frequency (6%) of HPV infection in the normal population, which was remarkably low considering the frequency with which women are exposed. Strengths included a large sample size with over 2500 subjects and blinding of scientists performing HPV probes to the clinical cervical diagnoses. Limitations included secondary analysis, case-control study design, and use of a convenience sample which may subject findings to selection or recall bias.

In-Depth [case-control study]: A total of 2627 women previously recruited into the studies performed at Life Technologies on HPV infection and cervical neoplasia study submitted to retesting of previously-collected 731 biopsy specimens and 1896 cervical swabs for HPV testing for the most common 15 subtypes. Controls were defined as healthy (normal) and cases were defined as condyloma, premalignant, or invasive/malignant cervical disease by final surgical pathology. The primary exposure of interest was infection with each of the most common 15 HPV subtypes and cervical disease. The incidence of HPV infection in each patient group was assessed and outcomes included continued healthy status, borderline atypia, low-grade squamous intraepithelial lesion (LSIL), high-grade squamous intraepithelial lesion (HSIL), and cancer. Data were presented as relative risk values, which were estimated from odds ratios.

HPV infection was detected in 79% of women with cervical dysplasia or neoplasia, 24% of women with borderline atypia, and 6% of normal subjects. Multiple HPV risk categories were identified: high-risk, or oncogenic, subtypes 16 (present in 47% of HSIL and 47% of cancers) and subtypes 18 (in 7% of HSIL and 27% of cancers), intermediate-risk types 31, 33, 35, 51, 52, 58 (in 24% of HSIL and 11% of cancers), and low-risk subtypes 6, 11, 42, 43, 44 (in 0% of cancers and 20% of LSIL). The relative risk of cervical disease associated with oncogenic HPV subtypes ranged from 65-236 for cervical cancer and 31-296 for high-grade dysplasia.

Lorincz AT, Reid R, Jenson AB, Greenberg MD, Lancaster W, Kurman RJ. Human papillomavirus infection of the cervix: relative risk associations of 15 common anogenital types. Obstetrics and gynecology. 1992;79(3):328-37.

Folic acid for prevention of neural tube defects

1. In women seeking pregnancy, periconceptional folic acid was associated with decreased likelihood of having a fetus with a neural tube defect (NTD).

Original Date of Publication: December 1992

Study Rundown: In the late 1980s, neural tube defects complicated between 2 and 3 out of every 1000 pregnancies, at which time it was established that folic acid was associated with a reduced incidence of recurrent NTDs in women with a prior pregnancy complicated by an NTD. However, the overwhelming majority (>90%) of neural tube defects occurred in women without a history of pregnancy complicated by NTD. Therefore, whether or not periconceptional (prior to pregnancy and throughout the period of organogenesis or 8 completed weeks of gestation) folic acid supplementation conferred a decreased incidence of the first occurrence of NTD was unknown. Folic acid, also known as vitamin B9, is necessary to complete numerous cellular processes including DNA synthesis and repair, cell division, and growth. While the exact mechanism by which folate deficiency contributes to neural tube defects is unknown, multiple theories exist. Differential methylation of the insulin-like growth factor 2 gene contributes to normal intrauterine fetal development and occurs in the presence of adequate folate such that folate deficiency might impair development and lead to NTDs. Folate deficiency might also contribute to the development of neural tube defects by disallowing post-translational methylation of the cytoskeleton, which is requisite for differentiation of neural structures.

This landmark study was the first to demonstrate that periconceptional folate supplementation was associated with reduction in the first incidence of NTDs. Strengths included randomized, double-blinded design. Lack of blinding may bias adherence to treatment or results and inclusion of a Hungarian-only population may limit generalizability. These findings stimulated further investigations that would go on to confirm these results in ethnically diverse populations and contribute to the current recommendation for daily, periconceptional intake of 400-600 mcg (0.4-0.6 mg) in healthy women and 4 mg of folic acid supplementation in women with a history of fetal NTD or who are taking anti-epileptic medications.

In-Depth [prospective cohort]: A total of 7540 women planning pregnancy, of which 4753 went on to achieve pregnancy, were randomized to receive 1 tablet of a multivitamin supplement containing 800 mcg of folic acid (n = 2104) or a placebo trace element (n = 2052). Participants began taking their supplement at least 1 month prior to conception and continued through the date of their second missed menses, which corresponds to 8 completed weeks of gestation or the completion of organogenesis. The primary outcome was development of a fetus or infant with a neural-tube defect or congenital malformation.

Compared to women randomized to placebo, women randomized to folic acid supplement were less likely to conceive a child with a neural tube defect (0 vs. 6 cases, 0.0% vs. 0.3%, p = 0.03) or a congenital malformation (1.33% vs. 2.29%, p = 0.02). The incidence of cleft lip or cleft palate did not differ between groups.

Czeizel AE, Dudas I. Prevention of the first occurrence of neural-tube defects by periconceptional vitamin supplementation. The The New England Journal of Medicine. 1992;327(26):1832-5.

Preterm infants benefit from delayed cord clamping

1. Preterm infants randomized to delayed umbilical cord clamping for 30 seconds after birth required less cardiorespiratory intervention, less supplemental oxygen, and fewer blood transfusions compared to controls.

Original Date of Publication: January 1993

Study Rundown: Prematurity is a major contributor to neonatal morbidity, mortality, and healthcare costs in the United States. As of 2015, more than 11% of all births in the United States were preterm. Preterm infants experience increased risk for multiple complications, but are most in danger of compromise secondary to delivery prior to fetal lung maturation. Due to this risk of respiratory failure at delivery, preterm infants have traditionally been handed off to awaiting neonatal intensive care unit staff as soon as possible following birth. The urgency of this hand-off prompted immediate cord clamping by obstetricians. While there was an abundance of research detailing the adverse neonatal events associated with delayed cord clamping (e.g., volume overload, polycythemia, hyperbilirubinemia) and a dearth of literature on adverse events associated with immediate cord clamping (e.g., hypovolemia), there were numerous and repeated hypotheses that delayed cord clamping was particularly beneficial for preterm infants who are at increased risk for hypovolemia, anemia and respiratory failure. In this classic study, authors conducted the first randomized investigation to assess whether delaying cord clamping for 30 seconds of additional placental transfusion was associated with fetal benefit in preterm infants.

Researchers demonstrated that preterm infants randomized to delayed umbilical cord clamping experienced less respiratory compromise and required fewer blood transfusions. Strengths included randomized design and assessment of numerous markers of respiratory, cardiac, and hematologic function. Limitations included single-site investigation and small sample size of 36 infants. Findings stimulated additional investigations further characterizing these benefits and contributed to the determination that delayed cord clamping is associated with health benefits for the preterm neonate.

In-Depth [randomized controlled trial]: A total of 36 women pregnant from 27 to 33 weeks gestation were randomized to delayed cord clamping for 30 seconds (n = 17, "delayed cord clamping") or conventional management with immediate cord clamping (n = 19, "controls"). Primary outcomes were markers of neonatal circulation and oxygenation and included initial red blood cell volume, peak serum bilirubin, need for blood transfusion, and markers of respiratory impairment. Minimum arterial-alveolar oxygen tension ratios were used as a surrogate marker of cardiopulmonary function. Secondary outcomes included need for supplemental oxygen and mechanical ventilation.

Preterm infants randomized to delayed cord clamping had superior cardiopulmonary function from day 1 of life ($p = 0.02$), required fewer days of supplemental oxygen (3 vs. 10 days, $p < 0.01$) and required less supplemental oxygen ($p < 0.01$) compared to controls. Preterm infants in the delayed cord clamping group required a lower median volume of transfused red blood cells compared to infants in the control group (0 mL vs. 23 mL, $p = 0.03$). The majority of both groups of infants (n = 13 for both) required mechanical ventilation.

Kinmond S, Aitchison TC, Holland BM, Jones JG, Turner TL, Wardrop CA. Umbilical cord clamping and preterm infants: a randomised trial. BMJ. 1993 Jan 16;306(6871):172–5.

Anal sphincter disruption common with forceps-assisted vaginal delivery

1. The anal sphincter was disrupted in 80% of forceps-assisted vaginal deliveries and 35% of spontaneous vaginal deliveries.

2. Sphincter injury occurred only in the setting of an episiotomy or perineal laceration.

Original Date of Publication: December 1993

Study Rundown: Vaginal delivery and operative vaginal delivery are associated with lower overall morbidity and mortality compared to cesarean delivery. However, vaginal delivery is associated with a higher risk of pelvic floor dysfunction, including morbidities such as anal incontinence that can greatly impair quality of life. As of the 1990s, existing research on anal sphincter dysfunction after vaginal delivery was limited by retrospective design that precluded assessment of chronology and causality. As such, whether anal incontinence following vaginal delivery occurred as the result of obstetrical trauma or was caused by a progressive denervation of the anal sphincter muscles following occult pudendal nerve injury in labor remained unknown. The development of anal endosonography, which assesses both anal sphincter integrity and neurophysiologic function, permitted diagnosis of anal sphincter injuries in real time. Authors of the present work used this new technology to assess the integrity of the external anal sphincter before and after delivery to determine the incidence of mechanical and neurological trauma affecting the anal sphincter.

This cohort study was the first to prospectively evaluate the integrity and function of the anal sphincter before and after vaginal delivery. Findings identified a moderately common incidence of sphincter disruption with spontaneous vaginal delivery and a high incidence of disruption with forceps-assisted vaginal delivery. Further, results demonstrated that the majority of anal sphincter trauma occurred with the first vaginal delivery. Strengths of the investigation included assessment of structural integrity and neurophysiologic function by various modalities (anal endosonography, manometry and perineometry), stratification of outcomes by parity, and a similar proportion of black and white women enrolled. Future investigations would go on to confirm that forceps-assisted vaginal delivery and episiotomy are strong risk factors for high-order perineal lacerations and anal sphincter disruption.

In-Depth [prospective cohort]: A total of 202 consecutive pregnant women including both nulliparous (n = 135) and parous (n = 67) women were examined during the last 6 weeks of pregnancy and reevaluated 6 to 8 weeks after delivery. Anal sphincter structural integrity and neurophysiologic function were assessed with anal endosonography, manometry, perineometry, and pudendal nerve motor latency. Primary outcome was a defect in the internal or external anal sphincter. Secondary outcomes included symptomatology, such as stool, and flatal incontinence.

The incidence of anal sphincter defect at 6 weeks postpartum was 35% in primiparous women. In parous pregnant women, 40% had a pre-existing anal sphincter defect and the incidence increased only 4% after delivery, implying that the majority of sphincter damage occurs with the first delivery. Among women who underwent forceps-assisted vaginal delivery (n = 10), 8 women (80%) experienced anal sphincter injury compared to 0 out of 5 sphincter injury after vacuum-assisted deliveries. All external anal sphincter injuries occurred in the setting of episiotomy or laceration. Sphincter defects were strongly associated with bowel symptoms (p < 0.001).

Sultan AH, Kamm MA, Hudson CN, Thomas JM, Bartram CI. Anal-sphincter disruption during vaginal delivery. The The New England Journal of Medicine. 1993;329(26):1905-11.

The ACTG 076 Trial: Zidovudine for reduction of maternal-infant HIV transmission

1. Among pregnant women with human immunodeficiency virus (HIV), those randomized to zidovudine experienced a significant reduction in maternal-infant HIV transmission.

Original Date of Publication: November 1994 | 3942 Citations

Study Rundown: The primary cause of HIV infection in young children is maternal-infant transmission. In the 1990s, a staggering 15-45% of infants delivered to women with HIV were infected, mostly during the process of labor and delivery. Despite medicine's best treatments, pediatric HIV infection remained a fatal disease, underscoring the importance of preventing transmission. Prior research demonstrated that zidovudine (also known as AZT) reduced maternal transmission of HIV in animal models. Promising Phase I studies in pregnant women suggested that zidovudine was safe for use. In the present work, researchers hypothesized that zidovudine administered in the antepartum, intrapartum, and neonatal periods would be associated with a reduction in maternal-infant transmission of HIV. After the first interim analysis demonstrated benefit to zidovudine therapy for reduction of maternal-infant HIV transmission, the Data Safety Monitoring Board altered the study protocol to recommend zidovudine to all women.

Findings from the landmark, AIDS Clinical Trials Group 076 (ACTG 076) trial demonstrated that a regimen of zidovudine administered in the antepartum, intrapartum and neonatal periods was associated with a significant reduction in maternal-neonatal HIV transmission. Findings supported the universal administration of antiretroviral therapy in the antepartum period, zidovudine intravenously in labor, and zidovudine syrup for neonates of pregnant women with HIV. Incorporation of study findings into practice affected a meaningful risk reduction in maternal-infant HIV transmission. Subsequently, in resource-rich settings, the risk of maternal-infant HIV transmission rate dropped from 20-45% with no treatment to < 1% with zidovudine regimen, abstinence from breastfeeding, and cesarean delivery at 37 weeks for maternal HIV viral load > 1000. Study strengths included the multicenter, international trial with parsimonious randomized design and outcome ascertainment at multiple times.

Results may not apply to women with a high viral load and assessment of teratogenicity was limited due to enrollment of women only after the first trimester.

In-Depth [randomized controlled trial]: A total of 363 HIV-positive pregnant women with CD4 counts > 200 not previously on antiretroviral therapy were randomized to receive zidovudine (n = 180) or placebo (n = 183) in this multicenter, international (United States and France) clinical trial by the AIDS Clinical Trials Group (ACTG 076). Women randomized to zidovudine received antepartum zidovudine orally 5 times daily, intrapartum intravenous zidovudine and zidovudine for the newborn for the first 6 weeks of life. Primary outcome was the incidence of HIV infection in newborns at 18 months of life as detected by enzyme immunoassay and confirmed by Western blot and serial HIV cultures.

Pregnant, HIV-positive women randomized to a regimen of zidovudine in the antepartum, intrapartum and neonatal periods experienced a 67.5% risk reduction in maternal-fetal HIV transmission (95%CI 0.4-0.8, $p < 0.0001$). The proportion of HIV-infected infants was 8% in the zidovudine group compared with 26% among women in the placebo group.

Connor EM, Sperling RS, Gelber R, Kiselev P, Scott G, O'Sullivan MJ, et al. Reduction of maternal-infant transmission of human immunodeficiency virus type 1 with zidovudine treatment. Pediatric AIDS Clinical Trials Group Protocol 076 Study Group. The The New England Journal of Medicine. 1994;331(18):1173-80.

Cervical length indicates risk of preterm delivery

1. Transvaginal cervical length was inversely associated with risk of spontaneous preterm delivery (PTD) in a dose-dependent manner.

Original Date of Publication: February 1996

Study Rundown: Spontaneous PTD is a vexing problem encountered in clinical obstetrics. Over 11% of all deliveries in the United States are complicated by PTD. Currently, PTD remains the leading cause of neonatal morbidity and mortality and causes complicated and hard to treat cardiorespiratory, neurologic, ophthalmologic, and gastrointestinal problems. Although a history of prior spontaneous PTD is an established risk factor strongly associated with PTD, risk factors for the first spontaneous PTD remained poorly characterized. For years, clinicians suspected that shorter cervical lengths were associated with preterm parturition, or the premature, inappropriate softening and shortening of the gravid cervix. However, assessment of the relationship between cervical length and PTD has been complicated by lack of a reliable measure of cervical length. The long-time standard for cervical length measurement, the digital cervical exam, was an imprecise measurement with high intra and inter-observer variability. As transvaginal ultrasound evolved in the late half of the 20th century to become part of standard prenatal care, sonographic cervical length measurement emerged as a standardized, reliable and reproducible method of measuring cervical length. The present work represents the largest and most well designed multi-center prospective investigation of the association of cervical length and incidence of spontaneous preterm delivery.

This landmark, multi-center prospective study demonstrated that cervical length is an indicator of cervical competency and is inversely proportional to the incidence of spontaneous PTD. Strengths of this investigation included large, population-based sample and enrollment of women with ultrasound-confirmed, nonanomalous singleton pregnancies. A program of ultrasound operator training and quality control minimized variability in measurements to the greatest extent possible. Inclusion of women with a history of prior PTD, who comprised 16% of the sample, introduced the opportunity for nonrandom misclassification and confounding since women with a history of PTD are more likely to have a short cervix and to experience PTD. Future investigations would go on to reproduce these findings in both primigravid populations and women with a history of prior spontaneous PTD. Future investigations have reproduced the findings presented herein and highlight an inverse association with second trimester cervical length and risk of preterm delivery.

In-Depth [prospective cohort]: A total of 2915 women with singleton pregnancies were enrolled across 10 university-affiliated clinics in this study conducted by the Maternal Fetal Medicine (MFM-U) Network from 1992 through 1994. Cervical length was measured by transvaginal ultrasound at 24 and 28 weeks gestation and the incidence of spontaneous preterm delivery was assessed. Spontaneous PTD was defined as delivery at a gestational age less than 35 weeks. Women with cervical lengths > 75%ile were considered the referent group.

At 28 weeks gestation, women with cervical lengths ≤75th percentile were more than twice as likely to experience PTD (RR 2.80; $p < 0.003$) and those with cervical lengths ≤50th percentile experienced an even higher risk of PTD (RR 3.52; $p < 0.001$). At 24 weeks gestation, women with cervical lengths ≤75th percentile were also more likely to experience PTD (RR 1.98; $p < 0.01$) compared to the referent group. The incidence of PTD increased with shorter cervical length (RR 5.4 if ≤25th percentile, RR 9.6 if ≤10th percentile, RR 13.9 if ≤5th percentile, RR 24.9 if ≤1st percentile).

Iams JD, Goldenberg RL, Meis PJ, Mercer BM, Moawad A, Das A, et al. The length of the cervix and the risk of spontaneous premature delivery. National Institute of Child Health and Human Development Maternal Fetal Medicine Unit Ne2rk. The New England Journal of Medicine. 1996;334(9):567-72.

Adverse pregnancy outcomes linked to thrombophilias

1. The incidence of genetic thrombophilias was higher in women with adverse pregnancy outcomes.

Original Date of Publication: January 1999

Study Rundown: Inadequate placental perfusion is associated with numerous adverse pregnancy outcomes including placental abruption, growth restriction, and stillbirth. Certain thrombophilic mutations, including mutations of Factor V Leiden, prothrombin, and methylenetetrahydrofolate reductase (MTHFR) are associated with an increased risk of thromboembolic complications. Other thrombophilias including deficiencies of Protein C, Protein S, and antithrombin III also increase a woman's clot risk. In pregnancy and the postpartum period, thrombosis risk is increased due to hepatic effects of elevated serum estrogen and progesterone-mediated venous stasis. In the setting of thrombophilias, researchers proposed that thrombosis of the maternal vessels supplying the placenta (e.g. intervillous and spiral artery thrombosis) may contribute to inadequate perfusion of the fetal-placental unit and contribute to an increased risk for adverse pregnancy outcomes. To address this question, researchers investigated whether adverse obstetric outcomes of severe pre-eclampsia, placental abruption, fetal growth retardation and stillbirth were related to thrombophilias by comparing the incidence of thrombophilias among women who experienced adverse obstetric outcomes to the incidence in women with uncomplicated deliveries.

This investigation was the first to identify a high prevalence of thrombogenic mutations in women who experienced severe obstetric complications. Findings imply that women with genetic thrombophilias are at increased risk for adverse pregnancy outcomes including severe preeclampsia, placental abruption or stillbirth. Notably, however, recent investigations failed to substantiate this association. Diagnosis of pre-eclampsia has changed over the years and may contribute to mixed results, but would be unlikely to contribute to systemic directional bias. Following this landmark study, additional investigations have explored the benefit of prophylactic anticoagulation in pregnancy for high-risk thrombophilias.

In-Depth [case-control study]: A total of 220 women were tested for genetic thrombophilias in the postpartum period and the incidence of thrombophilias was compared among women who experienced uncomplicated pregnancies (n = 110) and those who experienced obstetric complications including placental abruption, severe preeclampsia, fetal growth restriction and stillbirth (n = 110). Exposures of interest were the Factor V Leiden mutation, MTHFR mutation, prothrombin mutation, Protein C deficiency, Protein S deficiency, Antithrombin III deficiency, and the presence of anticardiolipin antibodies.

Women who experienced adverse pregnancy outcomes were more likely to have a thrombogenic mutation (52% vs. 17%, p < 0.001). Specifically, more women with adverse pregnancy outcomes were found to be carriers of the Factor V Leiden mutation (20 vs. 6 %, p = 0.003), MTHFR mutation (22 vs. 8%, p = 0.005), prothrombin mutation (10 vs. 3%, p = 0.03) or have a deficiency in protein C, S, or antithrombin III or anticardiolipin antibodies (13 vs. 1%, p < 0.001).

Kupferminc MJ, Eldor A, Steinman N, Many A, Bar-Am A, Jaffa A, et al. Increased frequency of genetic thrombophilia in women with complications of pregnancy. The New England Journal of Medicine. 1999;340(1):9-13.

Uterine artery embolization effective for uterine fibroids

1. Bilateral uterine artery embolization (UAE) was associated with high clinical efficacy in patients with uterine fibroids.

2. Major complications were rare but included endometria ischemia, endometritis, and permanent amenorrhea.

Original Date of Publication: October 1999

Study Rundown: Uterine fibroids are the most common benign pelvic tumor in women, affecting up to 40% of females over the age of 35 in the United States. Historically, definitive management of patients with symptomatic uterine fibroids consisted of surgical intervention with hysterectomy. UAE, which employs an endovascular approach, was developed to provide a uterus-sparing option for patients who either prefer a less invasive approach or are not eligible for surgery. The purpose of this early retrospective study was to evaluate the effectiveness of UAE in the treatment of uterine fibroids.

The retrospective review included 60 consecutive patients that were referred for UAE with polyvinyl alcohol (PVA) particles for treatment of symptomatic fibroids. The primary outcome of interest was clinical and symptomatic improvement post-UAE. Secondary outcomes included post-procedural complications and sonographic evaluation of residual fibroid volume at follow-up. At the conclusion of the trial, 59 of 60 patients underwent successful bilateral UAE. The majority of patients reported either moderate or marked clinical improvement of their previous symptoms by 2 years follow-up. Furthermore, there was an approximately 50% reduction of dominant fibroid volume in this cohort on ultrasound follow-up. There were two cases of treatment failure resulting in hysterectomy. One case demonstrated permanent amenorrhea post UAE. The results of this trial provided evidence for the use of UAE as an effective, minimally invasive treatment modality for symptomatic fibroids. However, the study is limited by a small sample size and lack of a comparison group to myomectomy or hysterectomy. Additional randomized trials have since demonstrated similar efficacy compared to surgical intervention.

In-Depth [retrospective cohort]: This was a retrospective review of 60 consecutive patients (mean age: 43.5; range 27-66) that underwent UAE for symptomatic fibroids at a single institution in the United States. No patients were excluded from the study. With the exception of one patient, all underwent bilateral UAE with permanent PVA. Each patient underwent routine clinical and ultrasound follow-up at regular intervals at 6 weeks, then at 2, 6, 12, 18, and 24 months. The primary outcome of interest was symptomatic improvement as determined by patient-reported abnormal bleeding and pain Likert scale. Secondary outcomes of interest included rates of complications as well as dominant fibroid volume post-procedure. After a mean follow up of 10.2 months, 47 of 54 (87%) patients and 41 of 45 (91%) patients reported either moderate or marked improvement in abnormal bleeding and pain, respectively. Additionally, 92% of patients demonstrated reduction in the dominant fibroid volume with an average volume reduction of 48.8% (range: -522% to 100%). Two patients required an additional embolization procedure due to recanalization; treatment failure occurred in one patient that required hysterectomy. Common post-procedure complications were abdominal pain (100%), fever (34%), and post-embolization syndrome (10%). Significant complications were rare but included moderate groin hematoma (n = 1), permanent amenorrhea (n = 1), and delayed infection resulting in hysterectomy (n = 1). There was no specific report of patient disposition post-procedure, but 22 patients (37%) required same-day hospital admission for pain management. Univariable analysis demonstrated that patients with large fibroid volume reduction on ultrasound ($p < 0.001$) or with a previous history of myomectomy ($p < 0.02$) were less likely to undergo hysterectomy post-UAE. Additionally, younger patients were more likely to experience treatment failure ($p < 0.02$).

Goodwin SC, McLucas B, Lee M, Chen G, Perrella R, Vedantham S, et al. Uterine Artery Embolization for the Treatment of Uterine Leiomyomata Midterm Results. J Vasc Interv Radiol. 1999 Oct;10(9):1159–65.

Doppler velocimetry predicts fetal anemia

1. Among fetuses at risk for maternal red cell alloimmunization, peak systolic velocity in the middle cerebral artery was a sensitive predictor of moderate or severe fetal anemia.

Original Date of Publication: January 2000

Study Rundown: Maternal red cell alloimmunization is a morbid, immunogenic phenomenon associated with a high risk of fetal anemia that complicates less than 1% of pregnancies. Maternal alloimmunization results when a pregnant woman previously sensitized to a paternally-derived red cell antigen is re-exposed by a fetus that carries the same paternally-derived antigen. In response, maternal antibodies are produced, cross the placenta, bind to antigens on fetal red blood cells, and cause hemolysis. In severe cases, hemolysis can progress to severe fetal anemia, hydrops fetalis, and fetal death. As of the late 1990s, women at risk for alloimmunization underwent invasive testing via serial cordocentesis, the standard of care, or amniocenteses to diagnose fetal anemia. Cordocentesis permitted direct measurement of fetal hemoglobin, but exposed women to a 1-2% risk of fetal loss and a 50% risk of fetal-maternal hemorrhage, which worsens alloimmunization. Amniocentesis carried less risk, but was unreliable at diagnosis anemia due to the wide variation in bilirubin levels in amniotic fluid. Researchers hypothesized that measuring peak systolic velocity in a fetal cerebral artery might permit reliable yet noninvasive anemia diagnosis. A prior study demonstrated that peak systolic velocity through the fetal MCA, as measured by ultrasound, was increased in anemic infants. In this study, researchers compared measurement of peak systolic middle cerebral artery velocimetry to the current standard of care, invasive cordocentesis, for diagnosis of fetal anemia among infants at risk for maternal alloimmunization.

This landmark research demonstrated that increased peak systolic velocity through the fetal middle cerebral artery is a sensitive predictor of moderate or severe fetal anemia. Findings allowed for noninvasive diagnosis of fetal anemia and prevent fetuses with mild anemia from exposure to the morbidity and mortality associated with invasive testing. Authors calculated that institution of doppler velocimetry for screening and diagnosis of fetal anemia would prevent an estimated 140 pregnancy losses associated with cordocentesis each year. Strengths included multicenter study, concomitant measurement of hemoglobin by both direct (cordocentesis) and indirect (doppler velocimetry) methods, and use of a control population. Limitations included small sample size to evaluate variation in velocity associated with diagnosis of the rare, fatal outcome of fetal hydrops (n = 11).

In-Depth [cross-sectional study]: A total of 111 fetuses at risk for anemia due to maternal red cell alloimmunization underwent measurement of hemoglobin concentration via invasive cordocentesis and via noninvasive measurement of MCA peak systolic velocity using doppler velocimetry. Hemoglobin values in at-risk infants were compared to the hemoglobin values of 265 normal fetuses in this comparative cross-sectional study. The outcome of interest was moderate fetal anemia, defined as hemoglobin < 0.65 times the median hemoglobin concentration in normal fetuses and severe anemia, defined as < 0.55 times the median.

Peak MCA systolic velocity values greater than 1.5 times the median conferred 100% sensitivity and a 100% negative predictive value for the diagnosis of moderate or severe fetal anemia. The relationship between multiples of the median of peak systolic velocity with moderate to severe fetal anemia was significant (p < 0.001). Among infants at risk for anemia related to maternal alloimmunization, 32% had mild anemia, 4% had moderate anemia and 28% had severe anemia.

Mari G, Deter RL, Carpenter RL, Rahman F, Zimmerman R, Moise KJ, Jr., et al. Noninvasive diagnosis by Doppler ultrasonography of fetal anemia due to maternal red-cell alloimmunization. Collaborative Group for Doppler Assessment of the Blood Velocity in Anemic Fetuses. The New England Journal of Medicine. 2000;342(1):9-14.

The Term Breech Trial: Cesarean delivery improves perinatal outcome

1. Among women with term fetuses in breech malpresentation, cesarean delivery was associated with reduction in perinatal and neonatal mortality and morbidity.

Original Date of Publication: October 2000

Study Rundown: While the majority of fetuses in breech malpresentation spontaneously convert to cephalic presentation by term (37 weeks gestation), a minority remain in footling, complete, or frank breech malpresentation. If these 3-4% of women fail or decline to undergo external cephalic version, these women with persistent breech malpresentation have historically been recommended to undergo a planned cesarean section. This recommendation was based on findings from earlier studies that may have been biased by lack of randomization, delivery attendants inexperienced in vaginal breech extraction and broad eligibility criteria that included poor candidates for vaginal breech delivery (e.g., anomalous, compromised or footling breech-presenting fetuses). Accordingly, clinicians continued to question whether vaginal breech delivery represented a safe mode of delivery in the appropriate clinical setting, such as a multiparous patient in active labor. Because vaginal delivery is a nearly universally safer procedure for the mother, further rigorous assessment of the neonatal outcomes associated with a vaginal breech delivery was merited.

Term Breech Trial demonstrated that serious perinatal and neonatal complications were less common when women with fetuses in breech malpresentation were delivered by planned cesarean section. The absolute difference in neonatal complications during delivery and throughout the first 6 weeks of life was small but clinically significant. As a result of these findings, nulliparous women with persistent breech malpresentation at term are typically counseled toward cesarean delivery. Strengths included randomized design, strict eligibility criteria and intention-to-treat analysis. Limitations included lack of randomization stratification by study site and dichotomization of parity (nulliparous or not), which introduced bias if clinician skill varied by center or if successful vaginal delivery varied between primiparous and multiparous women, respectively. Additional investigation restricting to parous women presenting in spontaneous active labor would provide insight into whether cesarean section confers significant fetal benefit in women with the highest likelihood of successful vaginal breech delivery.

In-Depth [randomized controlled trial]: Across more than 120 sites, a total of 2083 women with a term singleton pregnancy in persistent frank or complete breech malpresentation were randomized to undergo planned cesarean delivery (n = 1041) or planned vaginal birth (n = 1042) in this multicenter, randomized controlled trial. Primary outcomes included neonatal mortality or serious neonatal morbidity. Secondary outcomes assessed were maternal mortality or serious maternal morbidity. Outcomes were assessed from delivery through 6 weeks postpartum via intention-to-treat analysis.

For delivery of term fetuses in breech malpresentation, neonatal mortality and serious morbidity were less common in women randomized to cesarean compared to trial of vaginal birth (1.6% vs. 5.0%, RR 0.33; 95%CI 0.2-0.6, p < 0.0001). Among women randomized to planned cesarean delivery, 90% delivered by cesarean whereas only 57% of those randomized to planned vaginal birth delivered vaginally. Maternal mortality and serious maternal morbidity did not differ between groups (p = 0.35).

Hannah ME, Hannah WJ, Hewson SA, Hodnett ED, Saigal S, Willan AR. Planned caesarean section versus planned vaginal birth for breech presentation at term: a randomised multicentre trial. Term Breech Trial Collaborative Group. Lancet. 2000;356(9239):1375-83.

The TARGET trial: Anastrazole superior to tamoxifen for breast cancer

1. Postmenopausal women with advanced breast cancer randomized to anastrazole experienced an increase in time to progression and a more favorable side effect profile compared to women randomized to tamoxifen.

Original Date of Publication: November 2000

Study Rundown: Postmenopausal breast cancer is classically a hormone-responsive disease whereby the majority of tumors require estrogen stimulation to grow. Tamoxifen is a selective estrogen receptor modulator (SERM) that antagonizes estrogen receptors in the breast and uterus and acts as an agonist, or activator, of estrogen receptors in bone. In the treatment of postmenopausal breast cancer, chemotherapy and endocrine treatment in the form of tamoxifen therapy have been shown to be beneficial. While tamoxifen is associated with increased survival and reduced incidence of contralateral breast cancer, tamoxifen has also been associated with a 2-3 fold increased risk of endometrial cancer. Further, while tamoxifen is an estrogen receptor antagonist in breast tissue, it can also act as a partial agonist such that it may not maximally suppress the effects of estrogen systemically. In the late 1990s, researchers hypothesized that aromatase inhibitors, which inhibit the enzyme aromatase and thus block the peripheral conversion of androgens to estrogens in adipose tissue, would permit more complete estrogen suppression. Anastrazole, also known as arimidex, is an aromatase inhibitor that demonstrated promise in prolonging survival in women with advanced stage breast cancer. In the present work, researchers conducted a large international randomized trial comparing the efficacy and tolerability of anastrazole and tamoxifen among women with advanced postmenopausal breast cancer.

Results from the North American arm of the Tamoxifen or Arimidex Randomized Group Efficacy and Tolerability (TARGET) trial demonstrated that anastrazole is at least equivalent to tamoxifen as first-line therapy for postmenopausal breast cancer. Further, anastrazole was associated with a longer time to progression (or death) interval and a decreased risk of thromboembolic events and vaginal bleeding compared to tamoxifen. Findings changed practice recommendations whereby the standard of care for postmenopausal women with a new diagnosis of breast cancer now includes an aromatase inhibitor. Women with breast cancer who undergo prophylactic, risk-reducing bilateral salpingo-oophorectomy (e.g., for BRCA1 or BRCA2 mutation carriers) are also recommended to start anastrazole for breast cancer therapy following surgical menopause.

In-Depth [randomized controlled trial]: A total of 353 postmenopausal women with advanced breast cancer were enrolled across 97 study sites in the United States and Canada to daily treatment with anastrazole 1 mg (n = 171) or tamoxifen 20 mg (n = 182) in this randomized, double-blind multicenter study comparing the efficacy and tolerability of these 2 drugs as first-line treatment of advanced breast cancer in postmenopausal women. Primary outcome assessed was time to progression (TTP), defined as the time to objective disease progression or death, whichever occurred first. Other outcomes assessed included tolerability, objective response, time to treatment failure, response duration, duration of benefit and side effects. Equivalence was defined as a hazards ratio comparing tamoxifen to anastrazole with a lower 95% confidence limit of $\geq$ 0.80 (i.e., a 20% or greater advantage to tamoxifen must be ruled out with at least 95% certainty).

Women randomized to tamoxifen were 44% more likely to experience disease progression and a shorter TTP interval compared to women randomized to anastrazole (HR 1.44; 6 vs. 11 months, $p < 0.01$). Anastrazole met criteria for equivalence to tamoxifen for first-line treatment of postmenopausal breast cancer (lower one-sided 95%CI 1.16). A higher proportion of women in the anastrazole group demonstrated clinical benefit to therapy compared to women in the tamoxifen group (59 vs. 46%, $p = < 0.01$). Rates of thromboembolic events and vaginal bleeding were higher in women on tamoxifen.

Nabholtz JM, Buzdar A, Pollak M, Harwin W, Burton G, Mangalik A, et al. Anastrozole is superior to tamoxifen as first-line therapy for advanced breast cancer in postmenopausal women: results of a North American multicenter randomized trial. Arimidex Study Group. Journal of clinical oncology : official journal of the American Society of Clinical Oncology. 2000;18(22):3758-67.

The ORACLE trial: Antibiotics improve preterm outcomes

1. Among infants born to women with preterm premature rupture of membranes (PPROM), women randomized to erythromycin experienced a lower incidence of adverse neonatal outcomes.

2. Women randomized to antibiotics experienced prolongation of pregnancy compared to the placebo group.

Original Date of Publication: March 2001

Study Rundown: PPROM is a common cause of preterm birth. Following PPROM, approximately 50% of women will deliver within 1 week. As such, the majority of infants born to women with PPROM are exposed to risks associated with prematurity including respiratory distress syndrome, necrotizing enterocolitis, intraventricular hemorrhage, and retinopathy of prematurity as well as risks of cerebral palsy, blindness, and deafness. Further, leakage of amniotic fluid in PPROM can expose the fetus to oligohydramnios and associated Potter sequence complications such as pulmonary hypoplasia, pneumothorax, and skeletal deformities. Because PPROM involves a breech in the integrity of the amniotic membrane, fetuses exposed to PPROM also experience an increased risk of complications associated with intrauterine infection, including chorioamnionitis, neonatal sepsis, and hypoxemic ischemic encephalopathy. Previous research demonstrated that subclinical chorioamnionitis plays a role in degrading the amniotic membrane such that most experts agree that the etiology of PPROM is infectious. Researchers theorized that administering antibiotics to women who experience PPROM would improve overall neonatal health. As of the late 1990s, trials of antibiotics in the setting of PPROM demonstrated an association with prolongation of pregnancy but not with reduced risks of adverse neonatal outcomes.

In this large randomized controlled trial, researchers investigated the impact of 3 different antibiotic regimens for use in PPROM (erythromycin, amoxicillin-clavulanic acid, or both) compared to placebo on neonatal outcomes and demonstrated that, compared to placebo, the use of antibiotics following PPROM, specifically erythromycin, was associated with reduction in adverse neonatal outcomes. Results also confirmed findings of previous investigations that antibiotics were associated with pregnancy prolongation. In contrast, amoxicillin-clavulanic acid was associated with an increased incidence of necrotizing enterocolitis. Strengths included large sample size and multicenter study with 4 treatment arms to distinguish the impact of various treatments compared with placebo. The study was conducted in the United Kingdom and results may not apply to populations with differing demographic compositions.

In-Depth [prospective cohort]: A total of 4826 women with PPROM in a singleton pregnancy were randomized to receive erythromycin (n = 1197), amoxicillin-clavulanic acid (n = 1212), both (n = 1192), or placebo (n = 1225) 4 times daily for 10 days or until delivery, whichever came first. Intention-to-treat analysis was applied to evaluate the composite primary outcome of neonatal death, chronic lung disease or major cerebral abnormality between treatment groups. Secondary outcomes included prolongation of pregnancy, maternal outcomes and specific neonatal outcomes including necrotizing enterocolitis.

Among women with PPROM, the neonates of women randomized to erythromycin experienced a lower incidence of the composite primary outcome of severe adverse neonatal events compared to controls (11.2% vs. 14.4%, p = 0.02). Maternal erythromycin use was also associated with prolongation of pregnancy and reduced need for surfactant. Use of either antibiotic regimen containing amoxicillin-clavulanic acid was associated with a higher incidence of neonatal necrotizing enterocolitis (p = 0.0005).

Kenyon SL, Taylor DJ, Tarnow-Mordi W, Group OC. Broad-spectrum antibiotics for preterm, prelabour rupture of fetal membranes: the ORACLE I randomised trial. ORACLE Collaborative Group. Lancet. 2001;357(9261):979-88.

The MAGPIE trial: Magnesium lowers eclampsia risk

1. Women with pre-eclampsia randomized to receive magnesium treatment were less than 50% as likely to seize compared to controls.

Original Date of Publication: June 2002

Study Rundown: Pre-eclampsia is a multi-system hypertensive disorder of pregnancy associated with significant maternal morbidity and mortality. Worldwide, approximately 50 000-60 000 women die from manifestations of pre-eclampsia each year. Eclampsia, defined as convulsions or seizures superimposed on pre-eclampsia (hypertensive disease of pregnancy with laboratory evidence of organ dysfunction), affects 1 in 2000 deliveries and is associated with a high maternal mortality rate. One difficult decision for providers is how and when to administer medications to prevent the development of seizures in women with pre-eclampsia. In the 1990s, various anticonvulsants including benzodiazepines, phenytoin and barbiturates were used to prevent eclamptic seizures. Around this time, a systematic review of 4 trials comparing anticonvulsants to placebo for eclampsia prophylaxis identified magnesium as the drug with the most potential to reduce the risk of eclampsia. Theories for how magnesium sulfate might reduce the risk of eclampsia include relaxation of vascular smooth muscle, improvement in endothelial function, and blockage of central N-methyl-D-aspartate receptors to decrease neuronal excitability. The magnitude of eclampsia risk reduction attributable to magnesium, however, and the tolerability and fetal impacts of magnesium therapy were unknown. In the Magnesium Sulphate for the Prevention of Eclampsia (MAGPIE) trial, researchers randomized pre-eclamptic women in labor with to receive magnesium sulfate or placebo and assessed rates of eclampsia.

This trial demonstrated that magnesium meaningfully reduced the risk of eclamptic seizures among women with pre-eclampsia. Findings provided reliable evidence that intrapartum magnesium was an intervention that reduced maternal morbidity and mortality associated with pre-eclampsia. This international investigation was 12 times larger than the previous largest trial on the topic and took over 3.5 years to complete. Strengths included elegant, blinded study design with central randomization and sensitivity analyses. Drawbacks included variability in the route of administration by site (intramuscular or intravenous) and inconsistent loading dosing (4 mg or 5 mg).

In-Depth [randomized controlled trial]: A total of 10 141 pregnant women with pre-eclampsia, defined as persistently elevated blood pressures greater than 140/90 and proteinuria, were enrolled in this blinded, placebo-controlled international trial across 33 countries. Women were randomized on the basis of gestational age, severity of pre-eclampsia and proximity to delivery. Primary outcomes included eclampsia and fetal or infant death. Analysis was performed via intention-to-treat and effect estimates are presented as RR and number needed to treat (NNT).

Women randomized to magnesium experienced a 58% lower risk of eclampsia (95%CI 40-71% reduced risk) compared to women allocated to placebo (RR 0.32; $p < 0.0001$). The overall NNT to prevent 1 seizure was 91 women; the NNT to prevent 1 seizure in severe pre-eclamptics was 63 women and the NNT to prevent 1 seizure in women with pre-eclampsia without severe features was 109. Women on magnesium were more likely to report side effects, most commonly flushing, compared to controls (24% vs. 5%). There were no differences in risk of fetal or neonatal death between groups.

Altman D, Carroli G, Duley L, Farrell B, Moodley J, Neilson J, et al. Do women with pre-eclampsia, and their babies, benefit from magnesium sulphate? The Magpie Trial: a randomised placebo-controlled trial. Lancet. 2002;359(9321):1877-90.

The WHI trial: Risks outweigh benefits of combination hormone replacement therapy

1. Combination estrogen and progestin hormone replacement therapy (HRT) following menopause was associated with an increased risk of cardiovascular disease, venous thromboembolism, and invasive breast cancer.

2. Among 10 000 women taking combination HRT for 1 year, there would be 7 more cardiovascular events, 8 more strokes, 8 more pulmonary emboli, 8 more cases of invasive breast cancer, 6 fewer colorectal cancers, and 5 fewer hip fractures.

Original Date of Publication: November 2002

Study Rundown: Whether post-menopausal HRT impacts cardiovascular disease, breast and colorectal cancers, or osteoporotic fractures was a topic of great interest in medicine in the late 20th century. Previous investigations produced conflicting results, and the majority of studies demonstrated a reduced risk of cardiovascular disease associated with estrogen-only HRT. In 1991, observational research from the Nurse's Health study demonstrated a reduced risk of major coronary disease in women on postmenopausal estrogen replacement therapy. However, many worried that this observational data was subject to numerous forms of bias, including healthy user and compliance bias. As of the early 1990s, there were no randomized trials evaluating how hormone replacement therapy impacted overall health. The Women's Health Initiative (WHI) clinical trial was designed to assess the impact of HRT in healthy women.

This landmark study demonstrated that combined HRT was associated with an increased risk of venous thromboembolism, stroke, and breast cancer. Results provided solid evidence that HRT should not be used for the primary prevention of cardiovascular morbidity and showed that overall, risks outweighed benefits to combination HRT. Strengths included randomized, controlled design, low rate of loss to follow-up, and an ethnically diverse study population. Results may not apply to women undergoing the menopausal transition, the time when most women seek therapy for vasomotor symptoms, due to an average age in the study of 63 years (compared to an average age of menopause of 51 years in the United

States). Future analyses might restrict investigation to short-courses of HRT in symptomatic women undergoing the climacteric (menopausal) transition.

In-Depth [randomized controlled trial]: A total of 16 608 healthy, postmenopausal women aged 50-79 years were randomized to receive daily combined estrogen and progestin HRT (0.625 mg conjugated equine estrogen and 2.5 mg medroxyprogesterone acetate; n = 8 506) or placebo (n = 8 102). Clinical outcomes were assessed via telephone questionnaire conducted by certified study staff. Outcomes included cardiovascular disease (cardiovascular death, nonfatal MI, stroke), venous thromboembolic event (deep vein thrombosis, pulmonary embolism), breast cancer, endometrial cancer, colorectal cancer, fractures (hip, vertebral, other osteoporotic), and death due to other causes. The study was prematurely terminated by the data safety and monitoring board for evidence of breast cancer harm with combination HRT such that the average follow-up time was 5.2 years instead of the planned 8.5 years.

Compared to placebo, women randomized to combination HRT were more likely to experience venous thromboembolism (aHR 2.11; 95%CI 1.26-3.55). In unadjusted models, women on combination HRT experienced a 29% increased risk of cardiovascular event (95%CI 1.02-1.63), a 41% increased risk of stroke (95%CI 1.07-1.85) and a 26% increased risk of invasive breast cancer (95%CI 1.00-1.59) compared to controls. Women on HRT were less likely to experience colorectal cancer (HR 0.63; unadjusted 95%CI 0.43-0.92) and osteoporotic fracture (aHR 0.76; 95%CI 0.63-0.92) compared to women randomized to placebo.

Rossouw JE, Anderson GL, Prentice RL, LaCroix AZ, Kooperberg C, Stefanick ML, et al. Risks and benefits of estrogen plus progestin in healthy postmenopausal women: principal results From the Women's Health Initiative randomized controlled trial. Jama. 2002;288(3):321-33.

Progesterone injections for recurrent preterm birth

1. In women with a history of preterm birth, those randomized to weekly progesterone injections were less likely to experience repeat preterm delivery.

2. Number needed to treat to prevent 1 preterm birth was 6 women.

Original Date of Publication: June 2003

Study Rundown: Preterm birth is common, morbid, and the major contributor to the relatively high infant mortality rate in the United States. Currently, preterm delivery complicates 11.2% of pregnancies in the United States. The strongest predictor of spontaneous preterm birth is a history of prior preterm birth whereby women with this history experience a 2.5 fold increased risk for recurrent preterm birth. The etiology of spontaneous preterm birth involves impairment of normal cervical physiology in pregnancy. Despite much study, the mechanisms responsible for impaired cervical physiology remain poorly characterized. Trials of interventions to decrease the risk of recurrent preterm birth, including strict bed rest, tocolytics, and antibiotics, have failed to identify effective preventive management. Early, small studies investigating the impact of a metabolite of progesterone, 17 alpha-hydroxyprogesterone caproate (17OHPc) for reduction of preterm delivery showed promise, although others identified no benefit. There is biologic plausibility for progesterone supplementation preventing onset or propagation of preterm parturition through prevention of gap junction formation in cervical stroma or antagonism of oxytocin.

The results of this landmark trial in women with prior spontaneous preterm birth demonstrated a reduced incidence of preterm delivery before 37 weeks among women randomized to progesterone injections. Treatment also associated with pregnancy prolongation and a significant reduction in neonatal morbidities. These findings changed clinical practice such that it is now recommended that women with a history of prior preterm birth receive weekly progesterone injections from 16 through 36 weeks gestation. Strengths included randomized double-blinded design and use of an inert, injectable placebo. As most preterm deliveries occur in women with no history of preterm delivery, the findings of this investigation will not affect primary prevention.

In-Depth [randomized controlled trial]: Women were enrolled at 19 different clinical centers and randomized in a 2:1 ratio to receive weekly injections of 250 mg 17-OHPc (n = 310) or inert oil placebo (n = 153) from the time of enrollment through 36 weeks gestation in this double-blinded trial. Pregnant women with a history of prior preterm delivery between 20 weeks and 36 weeks 6 days, a current pregnancy between 15 and 20 weeks gestation, and a documented ultrasound between 14 and 21 weeks gestation were eligible. A 2:1 intervention-to-placebo randomization ratio was used to minimize the number of women receiving painful placebo injections of no direct benefit. Women with multifetal gestations, fetal anomalies, planned cerclage, and other high-risk maternal fetal conditions that increase risk for preterm delivery not related to cervical insufficiency were excluded. Primary outcome was preterm delivery prior to 37 weeks gestation. Secondary outcomes included birth weight and neonatal morbidities.

Among women with a history of prior spontaneous preterm birth, those randomized to weekly progesterone injections were less likely to experience preterm delivery before 37 weeks (36 vs. 55%, $p < 0.01$), before 35 weeks (21 vs. 31%, $p = 0.02$) and before 32 weeks gestation (11 vs. 20%, $p = 0.02$) compared to controls. NNT to prevent 1 preterm birth was 6 (95%CI 3.6-11.1). Survival analysis demonstrated significant prolongation of pregnancy with progesterone injections compared to placebo ($p = 0.01$). Infants of women randomized to progesterone injections experienced lower incidences of necrotizing enterocolitis, intraventricular hemorrhage, and need for supplemental oxygen.

Meis PJ, Klebanoff M, Thom E, Dombrowski MP, Sibai B, Moawad AH, et al. Prevention of recurrent preterm delivery by 17 alpha-hydroxyprogesterone caproate. The New England Journal of Medicine. 2003;348(24):2379-85.

The TOLAC study: Risks of labor after Cesarean delivery

1. Very few women undergoing a trial of labor after Cesarean delivery (TOLAC) experienced uterine rupture.

2. The absolute risk of permanent neurological impairment in infants born to women undergoing TOLAC is similarly very low.

Original Date of Publication: December 2004

Study Rundown: Cesarean delivery is associated with higher maternal morbidity and mortality than vaginal delivery. Each additional cesarean section further increases a woman's risk for abnormal placentation and other complications of pregnancy and childbirth. In 1990, the United States Public Health Service set a goal cesarean delivery rate of 15% and a goal vaginal birth after cesarean (VBAC) rate of 35% in efforts to reduce the incidence of cesarean delivery. Accordingly, the incidence of cesarean section dropped and the incidence of TOLAC increased. Subsequently, however, preliminary reports emerged citing an increased incidence of adverse, highly undesirable complications associated with TOLAC including uterine rupture, intrapartum fetal demise, and perinatal morbidity. These studies discouraged providers from recommending TOLAC and in turn, the VBAC rate dropped. Thus, over the course of 20 years, the rate of VBAC in the United States fluctuated from a nadir of 3% in 1981 to a peak of 28% in 1996 then down to 13% in 2002. Yet, throughout this time, no prospective studies existed to guide practice recommendations, such that these drastic fluctuations in VBAC incidence were largely attributable to shifts in popular opinion.

Findings of this landmark trail demonstrate an acceptably low rate of uterine rupture associated with TOLAC and highlight an increased risk of rupture associated with prostaglandin use. This study is one of the largest observational trials performed assessing maternal and perinatal complication rates associated with TOLAC. Limitations included selection bias where women willing to undergo TOLAC may have been more likely to achieve vaginal delivery (e.g. more favorable cervix), biasing results toward the null. Future investigations might assess the incidence of uterine rupture by specific prostaglandin agent to evaluate if all prostaglandins, as opposed or one specific type, are associated with increase in rupture risk.

In-Depth [prospective cohort]: Trained research personnel at 19 academic medical centers across the United States enrolled > 30 000 women with a prior cesarean delivery and a current singleton pregnancy at ≥ 20 weeks gestation from 1999 through 2002. Clinical data from these 19 centers was collected and pooled to create the Cesarean registry. All study sites were centers in the National Institute of Child Health and Human Development Maternal-Fetal Medicine Units (MFM-U) Ne2rk. Outcomes of interest included uncommon and rare maternal and fetal complications, including uterine rupture and infants with hypoxic-ischemic encephalopathy. The study was planned to take 3 years but an appreciable decline in the rate of trial of labor after Cesarean during the study period necessitated extending data collection for an additional year.

Uterine rupture occurred in < 1% of women (124 out of 17 898) undergoing TOLAC. Compared to those in spontaneous labor, women whose labor was induced (OR 2.86, 95%CI 1.75-4.67) or augmented (OR 2.42, 95%CI 1.49-3.93) were more likely to experience rupture. In the incidence of rupture, permanent and severe neurological impairment occurred in 5.6% of infants (7 out of 124). Among all women undergoing TOLAC, the absolute risk of permanent neonatal neurological impairment was < 1% (0.46 per 1000 women). Rate of intrapartum fetal demise was similar between groups (p > 0.4 for all).

Landon MB, Hauth JC, Leveno KJ, Spong CY, Leindecker S, Varner MW, et al. Maternal and perinatal outcomes associated with a trial of labor after prior cesarean delivery. The New England Journal of Medicine. 2004;351(25):2581-9.

Head cooling improves outcome in neonatal encephalopathy

1. Among term infants with neonatal encephalopathy associated with mild electroencephalography (EEG) changes, those randomized to head cooling had lower likelihood of death and severe neurodevelopmental disability.

Original Date of Publication: January 2005

Study Rundown: Hypoxic-ischemic encephalopathy (HIE) is a highly morbid cause of acute neurological injury at birth and occurs in 1-2 babies per 1000 term livebirths. HIE occurs as a result of total brain anoxia, or the deprivation of oxygen affecting the entire brain, and has been implicated in over 20% of neonatal deaths. In severe HIE, neonates demonstrate marked EEG changes, are stuporous or flaccid and may demonstrate generalized hypotonia, absent neonatal reflexes, fixed or dilated pupils, and cardiorespiratory failure. It is a deeply upsetting diagnosis for parents and healthcare providers both due to the upsetting presenting signs and because no specific clinical intervention has been shown to improve outcome. Prior studies demonstrating improved neurological recovery in adult cardiac arrest patients treated with moderate hypothermia motivated neonatologists to apply the same principle to neonates with HIE. Numerous small research studies demonstrated improved electrophysiological and functional neurologic outcomes following reduction in brain temperature of 2-5°C but treatment protocols varied widely. In the present work, researchers investigated whether 72 hours of selective head cooling started within 6 hours of birth improves neurodevelopmental outcome at 18 months in infants with moderate or severe HIE.

This landmark study demonstrated that head cooling for encephalopathic infants with mild to moderate EEG changes resulted in improved survival without severe neurologic disability at 18 months. Infants with more severe EEG changes were less likely to benefit from head cooling. Findings support the use of selective head cooling among those infants with HIE and less than severe EEG changes. Strengths included multicenter, randomized trial with an ethnically and geographically diverse population. A higher proportion of severely abnormal EEG findings and Apgar scores in the cooling group may bias results toward the null. The vast majority of subjects initiated cooling 4 hours after birth such that the relatively late onset of treatment may have also reduced the benefit of treatment.

In-Depth [randomized controlled trial]: A total of 234 term infants with moderate to severe neonatal encephalopathy and EEG changes were randomized to receive head cooling (n = 116) or conventional care (n = 118). Infants requiring high-dose anticonvulsants, those with major congenital anomalies, severe growth restriction, or otherwise considered critically ill were excluded. Primary outcome was death or severe neurodevelopmental disability at age 18 months.

Among infants with HIE and mild-moderate EEG changes, those randomized to selective head cooling experienced improved survival and a lower risk of death or severe neurodevelopmental disability at 18 months (OR 0.47, 95%CI 0.26-0.87). The number needed to treat was 6 (95%CI 3-27). Infants with the most severe EEG changes did not derive benefit from head cooling (p = 0.51).

Gluckman PD, Wyatt JS, Azzopardi D, Ballard R, Edwards AD, Ferriero DM, et al. Selective head cooling with mild systemic hypothermia after neonatal encephalopathy: multicentre randomised trial. Lancet. 2005;365(9460):663-70.

Intraperitoneal chemotherapy improves advanced ovarian cancer survival

1. Women with advanced-stage (≥Stage III) ovarian cancer randomized to intraperitoneal chemotherapy achieved an increase in overall survival compared to controls.

Original Date of Publication: January 2006

Study Rundown: Ovarian cancer is the most deadly gynecologic malignancy. Due to nonspecific presenting symptoms and disease predilection for early intraabdominal spread via peritoneal lymphatics, the majority of patients present with advanced-stage disease. As of the early 2000s, the standard of care for women with advanced disease involved optimal tumor reductive surgery, defined as resection of all disease > 1 cm, followed by adjuvant intravenous chemotherapy. The most common chemotherapy regimen involved 6 cycles of paclitaxel and a platinum analogue, such as cisplatin. The peritoneal cavity is the primary site of disease in ovarian cancer, which triggered researchers to postulate that applying chemotherapy locally to the peritoneal cavity might improve disease response and decrease toxicities associated with intravenous chemotherapy. Previous trials comparing intravenous only (IV) versus intravenous plus intraperitoneal (IV/IP) chemotherapy produced mixed results: one demonstrated a significant survival advantage in the IV/IP group while another showed an improvement in the progression-free interval but not survival.

This landmark Phase 3 clinical trial compared the standard of care, IV cisplatin/paclitaxel, to IV paclitaxel with IP cisplatin/paclitaxel and found that the IV/IP regimen was associated with increase in both progression-free survival and overall survival. However, the minority (<50%) of patients in the IV/IP group completed 6 cycles of treatment due to toxicities including fatigue, pain and neurologic side effects. Findings changed clinical practice such that patients with advanced-stage ovarian cancer who seek to maximize survival at the cost of an increased risk of treatment-associated toxicities are now offered IP chemotherapy. Strengths included parsimonious, multicenter, randomized controlled trial through the Gynecologic Oncology Group (GOG). Central review of the complete medical record by GOG physician-scientists permitted adherence to strict inclusion and exclusion criteria. Findings are limited by a low completion rate of IV/IP regimen due to toxicities, which may bias results toward the null.

In-Depth [randomized controlled trial]: A total of 415 women with Stage III ovarian carcinoma or primary peritoneal carcinoma who underwent optimal tumor reductive surgery (no residual mass greater than 1.0cm) were randomized to receive intravenous cisplatin/paclitaxel ("IV," n = 210) or intravenous paclitaxel followed by intraperitoneal cisplatin/paclitaxel ("IV/IP," n = 205) for 6 cycles of chemotherapy occurring every three weeks at one of the Gynecologic Oncology Group (GOG) clinical centers across the United States (Columbus, New York, Irvine, Philadelphia, Oklahoma, Baltimore). Primary outcome was duration of overall survival. Secondary outcomes included progression-free survival, quality of life and treatment-associated toxicities.

Among women with Stage III ovarian cancer who underwent optimal tumor reductive surgery, those randomized to IV/IP chemotherapy experienced an increased duration of overall survival (67 vs. 50 months, p = 0.03) and a longer progression-free survival (24 vs. 18 months, p = 0.05) compared to those randomized to IV chemotherapy. Compared to women receiving standard IV chemotherapy alone, women in the IV/IP group were more likely to report toxicities including fatigue, pain and neurologic side effects but experienced a similar quality of life 1 year after treatment.

Armstrong DK, Bundy B, Wenzel L, Huang HQ, Baergen R, Lele S, et al. Intraperitoneal cisplatin and paclitaxel in ovarian cancer. The New England Journal of Medicine. 2006;354(1):34-43.

The HAPO trial: Hyperglycemia and adverse pregnancy outcomes

1. Impaired glucose tolerance on the 2-hour glucose tolerance test was associated with increased odds of primary cesarean delivery, large for gestational age (LGA) infants, cord-blood serum C-peptide > 90th percentile and neonatal hypoglycemia.

2. Impaired glucose tolerance was also associated with increased risk of preterm delivery, shoulder dystocia and preeclampsia.

Original Date of Publication: May 2008

Study Rundown: The Pedersen hypothesis, postulated by Jorgen Pedersen in 1952, states that maternal hyperglycemia leads to fetal hyperglycemia, invoking an exaggerated production of insulin in the neonate. This increased insulin production acts as a fetal growth factor and contributes to metabolic derangements after delivery. Considering the numerous and meaningful risks of adverse pregnancy outcomes associated with maternal diabetes pre-existent to pregnancy, researchers questioned whether women with gestational diabetes, who have a lesser degree of glucose intolerance, also experience increased risk for adverse pregnancy outcomes. However, assessment of whether gestational diabetes is associated with adverse outcomes is complex. Diagnostic criteria for gestational diabetes were originally designed to identify women at risk for developing diabetes later in life, not to predict the degree of maternal hyperglycemia in pregnancy. Historically, there has been a lack of consensus guidelines on diagnosis such that the 1-hour, 2-hour and 3-hour oral glucose tolerance tests (OGTT) have all been used to diagnose gestational diabetes. Confounders like obesity and co-existent medical morbidities that track closely with glucose intolerance and adverse neonatal outcomes further complicate assessment. In the present work, researchers used a large international cohort to prospectively assess the incidence of adverse outcomes including fetal macrosomia, primary cesarean delivery, and elevated cord-blood serum C-peptide levels between women with normal and those with impaired glucose tolerance testing.

This landmark study demonstrated that impaired carbohydrate tolerance in pregnancy, even less severe than overt diabetes, is associated with an increased risk of adverse pregnancy outcomes. Findings of an elevated umbilical cord blood serum C-peptide level are consistent with the Pedersen hypothesis of neonatal insulin production and underscore the need for uniform diagnostic and therapeutic thresholds. Results from this investigation contributed to the recommendations for universal screening for gestational diabetes between in pregnancy. Limitations included lack of adjustment for maternal BMI, gestational weight gain, and history of a prior macrosomic infant.

In-Depth [randomized controlled trial]: Across 15 centers in 9 countries, a total of 25 505 women with ongoing pregnancies underwent a 75-gram oral glucose tolerance test from 24 to 32 weeks gestation. Results remained blinded if fasting blood glucose was 105 mg/dL or less and 2-hour blood glucose was 200 mg/dL or less. Women with overt diabetes diagnosed on testing were unblinded and excluded from analysis. Primary outcomes were delivery via primary cesarean section, large for gestational age (LGA) infant, neonatal hypoglycemia and cord-blood serum C-peptide > 90th percentile. Additional outcomes assessed included delivery before 37 weeks gestation, shoulder dystocia, and preeclampsia.

Impaired glucose tolerance in the fasting, 1 hour and 2 hour glucose levels was associated with an increased odds of an LGA infant (ORs 1.38, 1.46, 1.38, respectively), cord-blood serum C-peptide level > 90th percentile (ORs 1.55, 1.46, 1.37), neonatal hypoglycemia (ORs 1.08, 1.08, 1.13) and primary cesarean delivery (ORs 1.11, 1.10, 1.08) as well as increased odds of preterm delivery (ORs 1.05, 1.18, 1.16), shoulder dystocia (ORs 1.18, 1.23, 1.22) and preeclampsia (ORs 1.21, 1.28, 1.28).

Group HSCR, Metzger BE, Lowe LP, Dyer AR, Trimble ER, Chaovarindr U, et al. Hyperglycemia and adverse pregnancy outcomes. The New England Journal of Medicine. 2008;358(19):1991-2002.

Magnesium for the prevention of cerebral palsy

1. Among women with imminent preterm delivery, babies of women randomized to magnesium were less likely to be diagnosed with moderate or severe cerebral palsy.

Original Date of Publication: August 2008

Study Rundown: Cerebral palsy, the leading cause of childhood disability, is a group of syndromes characterized by motor and postural dysfunction. A strong risk factor for cerebral palsy is preterm birth, which is associated with as many as a third of cerebral palsy cases. In the early-mid 2000s, research identified an increased prevalence of cerebral palsy among very preterm infants (28-32 weeks gestation). The survival of preterm (<37 weeks gestation) and very preterm infants born in the United States drastically improved in recent decades such that more premature infants survive to childhood. In the setting of improved survival, researchers have been working to prevent, mitigate and treat morbidities associated with prematurity, including cerebral palsy. A retrospective investigation identified a lower odds ratio of cerebral palsy among premature infants whose mothers received magnesium. However, previous studies enrolled women in preterm labor, who are often recommended to receive magnesium for its purposes as a uterine tocolytic. The present study achieves greater parsimony by enrolling women without other indications for magnesium therapy to specifically evaluate the benefit of intrapartum magnesium for fetal neuroprotection in premature infants born between 24 and 31 weeks.

This randomized, placebo-controlled trial evaluated the benefit of intrapartum administration of magnesium sulfate for fetal neuroprotection in women at risk for imminent preterm delivery between 24 and 31 weeks gestation. Follow-up exams at 2 years of age showed a decrease of almost 50% in the diagnosis of moderate or severe cerebral palsy in infants whose mothers received magnesium. Along with other studies, this landmark investigation indicated that magnesium could significantly reduce the risk of cerebral palsy in the group of infants at highest risk for developing this disabling condition. Strengths included elegant study design and high follow-up rate of 96%. Inclusion of women with both singleton and twin gestations receiving care at 20 delivery centers across the United States allows for widely applicable results. Limitations included potential selection bias, with 40% of eligible participants (1602/3843) declining to participate.

In-Depth [randomized controlled trial]: Multicenter trial of 2241 women at risk for imminent delivery between 24 and 31 weeks of gestation were randomly assigned to receive magnesium sulfate (6 g loading dose followed by 2 g/hour infusion) or placebo. Women with hypertension, pre-eclampsia, or those requiring magnesium for tocolysis were excluded. Outcomes assessed included the primary composite outcome of stillbirth or infant death within 1 year. Secondary outcomes assessed were moderate or severe cerebral palsy beyond 2 years of age. The diagnosis of cerebral palsy was rigorously determined by an annually certified pediatrician or pediatric neurologist. Diagnosis was made if children met 2 or more strictly defined criteria, including motor delay, abnormal muscle tone or reflexes, persistence of primitive reflexes, and movement abnormality.

Among women with imminent delivery between 24 and 31 weeks gestation, those randomized to receive magnesium sulfate were 45% less likely to be diagnosed with moderate or severe cerebral palsy at 2 years of life (1.9% vs. 3.5%, RR 0.55; $p = 0.03$). Risk of fetal death did not differ between groups (9.5 vs. 8.5%, $p = 0.4$). Obstetrical outcomes and a range of other neonatal outcomes, including respiratory distress, intraventricular hemorrhage, necrotizing enterocolitis and retinopathy of prematurity were similar between groups (all $p > 0.5$).

Rouse DJ, Hirtz DG, Thom E, Varner MW, Spong CY, Mercer BM, et al. A randomized, controlled trial of magnesium sulfate for the prevention of cerebral palsy. The New England Journal of Medicine. 2008;359(9):895-905.

XI. Ophthalmology

"Somewhere, something incredible is waiting to be known."

- Carl Sagan

The ONTT: Intravenous steroids lead to faster visual recovery in optic neuritis

1. In patients with first presentation of optic neuritis, treatment with intravenous methylprednisolone followed by oral prednisone resulted in faster visual recovery when compared to placebo, though only a small benefit persisted by 6 months.

2. The use of oral prednisone alone demonstrated no benefit in terms of visual recovery and appeared to increase the risk of recurrent episodes of optic neuritis compared to placebo.

Original Date of Publication: February 1992

Study Rundown: Optic neuritis is an inflammatory condition affecting the optic nerve and is most commonly associated with multiple sclerosis (MS). Clinically, it can present with a wide range of impairment in visual acuity, color vision, contrast sensitivity, and/or visual fields. In the 1990s, both ophthalmologists and neurologists were commonly using oral steroids to treat optic neuritis, though oral and intravenous steroid regimens had not yet been evaluated in a randomized controlled trial.

The Optic Neuritis Treatment Trial (ONTT) compared the effectiveness and safety of different steroid regimens in treating optic neuritis. The study found that intravenous methylprednisolone followed by oral prednisone hastened the rate of visual recovery in optic neuritis compared to placebo, with some improvement in vision noted at 6 months after treatment. Use of oral prednisone alone was shown to have no benefit compared to placebo, though it did lead to significantly higher rates of recurrent optic neuritis. Since the publication of the ONTT, subsequent studies have found that intravenous steroids do accelerate visual recovery in optic neuritis, though there were no differences in long-term visual outcomes.

In-Depth [randomized controlled trial]: This open-label, randomized trial recruited patients between 18-46 years of age with acute unilateral optic neuritis with visual symptoms lasting ≤8 days, a relative afferent pupillary defect (RAPD), and visual field defect in the affected eye. Exclusion criteria included previous optic neuritis in the same eye or evidence of a systemic disease, other than MS, that could cause optic neuritis. A total of 457 patients were randomized to either i) intravenous methylprednisolone 250 mg q6h for 3 days followed by oral prednisone 1 mg/kg for 11 days, ii) oral prednisone 1 mg/kg for 14 days, or 3) placebo. Steroid treatment was followed by a short oral taper. Patients were followed for 24 months. The primary outcomes were visual fields and contrast sensitivity measured at 6 months.

Patients treated with methylprednisolone had a higher rate of return to normal vision in visual fields ($p = 0.0001$) and contrast sensitivity ($p = 0.02$), with a trend towards improved visual acuity ($p = 0.09$) compared to placebo. At 6 months, patients in the methylprednisolone group experienced better contrast sensitivity ($p = 0.026$) and color vision ($p = 0.033$), with no differences noted in visual acuity ($p = 0.664$). There were no significant differences in the rates of recovery for oral prednisone patients compared to placebo in all measures of vision ($p > 0.05$). By 24 months, 20 (13%) patients in the methylprednisolone group, 42 (27%) patients in the oral prednisone group, and 24 (15%) patients in the placebo group had experienced ≥1 new episode of optic neuritis. The oral prednisone group had a higher rate of new episodes of optic neuritis compared with placebo (RR 1.79, 95%CI 1.08-2.95).

Beck RW, Cleary PA, Anderson MM, Keltner JL, Shults WT, Kaufman DI, et al. A randomized, controlled trial of corticosteroids in the treatment of acute optic neuritis. The Optic Neuritis Study Group. N Engl J Med. 1992 Feb 27;326(9):581–8.

The EVS: Vitrectomy results in better visual outcomes for light-perception patients

1. In patients with endophthalmitis after recent lens implantation, immediate vitrectomy significantly improved visual outcomes for patients presenting with light-perception visual acuity compared to vitreous tap. In patients with better than light-perception vision at the time of presentation, there was no benefit with vitrectomy.

2. Systemic antibiotics do not provide any further benefit when added to intraocular antibiotics in either vitrectomy or vitreous tap.

Original Date of Publication: December 1995

Study Rundown: Endophthalmitis is a condition characterized by inflammation of all intraocular structures, usually secondary to bacterial infection, and is one of the most challenging complications of ocular surgery. Vitrectomy, a procedure to remove vitreous humor from the eye, was thought to be advantageous in managing endophthalmitis, though prior studies were inconclusive and often suffered from selection bias. Furthermore, while intraocular antibiotic injections were considered standard of care, the role of systemic antibiotics remained unclear.
The Endophthalmitis Vitrectomy Study (EVS) was a randomized controlled trial that sought to establish the role of pars plana vitrectomy and systemic intravenous antibiotics in the treatment of endophthalmitis. The study found that, in patients with light-perception (LP) visual acuity at presentation, immediate vitrectomy tripled the frequency of achieving 20/40 vision, doubled the frequency of achieving 20/100 vision, and reduced the frequency of severe vision loss by half. In patients with better than LP visual acuity at presentation, vitrectomy was not shown to be beneficial compared to vitreous tap/biopsy. Systemic antibiotics were found to have no benefit and were not recommended as part of routine endophthalmitis treatment to reduce side effects, cost, and hospital length of stay.

In-Depth [randomized controlled trial]: This multicenter, randomized controlled trial recruited patients with clinical signs and symptoms of bacterial endophthalmitis after having cataract or lens implantation in the preceding 6 weeks, with obscured second order arterioles either due to hypopyon or cloudy media (but clear enough to view the iris and perform pars plana vitrectomy), and a visual acuity between 20/50 and light-perception (LP). Exclusion criteria included pre-existing eye disease limiting best corrected visual acuity beyond 20/100, previous intraocular surgery apart from simple cataract surgery or lens implantation, and previous treatment for endophthalmitis. A total of 420 patients were randomized using a 2×2 factorial design to i) vitrectomy (VIT) or b) vitreous tap/biopsy (TAP) and i) intravenous antibiotics (amikacin and vancomycin) or ii) no intravenous antibiotics. Patients were followed for 9-12 months. The primary outcomes were visual acuity and ocular media clarity at final visit.

At 3 months, patients treated with VIT experienced higher rates of clear media than patients receiving TAP (86% vs. 75%, p = 0.004). This difference was not seen at the final study visit, except in patients with initial LP vision (VIT 78% vs. TAP 52%, p = 0.007). Comparing patients who received systemic antibiotics with those who did not, there was no significant difference in media clarity noted at any time. There were no differences between the VIT and TAP groups in terms of achieving 20/40 or 20/100 visual acuity, though VIT therapy did significantly reduce the risk of severe visual loss (5/200 or worse) compared to TAP (8% vs. 15%, p = 0.03). Again, systemic antibiotic treatment did not influence the likelihood of visual improvement. In the subgroup of patients with LP vision initially, VIT resulted in significantly greater chances of achieving 20/40 vision (33% vs. 11%) and 20/100 vision (56% vs. 30%), and a lower chance of severe visual loss (20% vs. 47%) when compared to TAP (p < 0.001 for all comparisons).

Endophthalmitis Vitrectomy Study Group. Results of the Endophthalmitis Vitrectomy Study. A randomized trial of immediate vitrectomy and of intravenous antibiotics for the treatment of postoperative bacterial endophthalmitis. Endophthalmitis Vitrectomy Study Group. Arch Ophthalmol. 1995 Dec;113(12):1479–96.

The CNTG trial: Intra-ocular pressure reduction slows progression of normal-tension glaucoma

1. Reduction of intra-ocular pressure (IOP) with topical medications in normal-tension glaucoma significantly reduced risk of progression to visual field impairment and/or optic disc damage.

Original Date of Publication: July 1998

Study Rundown: Increased intraocular pressure (IOP) is known to be a significant risk factor for glaucoma. However, some patients with glaucoma demonstrate normal IOP, known as normal tension glaucoma (NTG). Prior to the Collaborative Normal Tension Glaucoma (CNTG) study, it was unclear whether reducing IOP would be beneficial in this subset of patients as well. The CNTG trial randomized approximately 140 patients with NTG to observation or IOP-lower treatments. After an average of eight years of follow-up, the study found that lowering IOP significantly reduced the incidence of visual field impairment and/or optic disc damage compared to control. Cataracts occurred at a substantially higher rate in the treatment group, potentially cofounding the result; however, the significant benefit of reducing IOP in NTG patients remained after statistical correction. Limitations include that providers were not blinded to randomization, although the outcome assessors were masked. In addition, not all patients in the observation arm were randomized, and the time required to reach the goal of 30% IOP decrease was prolonged. Sample size was also quite limited compared to other randomized controlled trials in ophthalmology. Nonetheless, this study demonstrates that IOP reduction even in NTG patients may be beneficial.

In-Depth [randomized controlled trial]: Approximately 140 patients diagnosed with NTG (normal IOP with optic disc abnormalities) were randomized to the observation arm or treatment arm involving the use of topical ocular antihypertensive drops and/or filtration surgery to decrease IOP by 30%. Patients were evaluated every 3-6 months with optic disc imaging and visual field testing. If the patient were thought to have glaucomatous progression, images were forwarded to a masked review committee, which would confirm the findings. Kaplan-Meier survival analysis showed that after correction, mean survival time was 2,049 ± 129 days and 1,427 ± 139 days in the treatment and observation arms, respectively (p = 0.005). A significantly higher rate of cataract was found in the treatment arm (38% vs. 14%, p = 0.0011), which affected visual field testing. When the data was corrected for this confounder, the significance of IOP lowering treatment still remained (p = 0.0034). IOP lowering therefore may be beneficial in delaying the progression of glaucoma even in NTG patients.

Collaborative Normal-Tension Glaucoma Study Group. Comparison of glaucomatous progression between untreated patients with normal-tension glaucoma and patients with therapeutically reduced intraocular pressures. Collaborative Normal-Tension Glaucoma Study Group. Am J Ophthalmol. 1998 Oct;126(4):487–97.

Collaborative Normal-Tension Glaucoma Study Group. The effectiveness of intraocular pressure reduction in the treatment of normal-tension glaucoma. Collaborative Normal-Tension Glaucoma Study Group. Am J Ophthalmol. 1998 Oct;126(4):498–505.

The AREDS1: Zinc and antioxidant supplementation reduce progression of age-related macular degeneration in high-risk patients

1. In patients with advanced age-related macular degeneration (AMD) in one eye only or intermediate AMD in either eye, zinc and antioxidant supplementation reduced the risk of progression to advanced AMD and reduced the risk of moderate vision loss.

2. In patients with early stage AMD, supplementation did not reduce the risk of progressing to advanced AMD. No supplementation is recommended in early stage AMD, as the baseline risk of progression is low.

Original Date of Publication: October 2001

Study Rundown: AMD is the leading cause of irreversible vision loss in the world in individuals 65 years of age and older. Until the Age-Related Eye Disease Study 1 (AREDS1), no therapies were available to prevent the progression of AMD. Epidemiologic and animal studies had suggested that zinc and antioxidant vitamins could potentially be beneficial in treating AMD by targeting and reducing oxidative stress.

The AREDS1 was a randomized controlled trial that sought primarily to evaluate the effects of high-dose zinc and antioxidants on the progression of AMD and vision loss. The study found that, in those at high-risk of developing advanced AMD, a combination of zinc and antioxidants reduced the risk by 25% and reduced the risk of moderate vision loss by 19%. In patients with no AMD or early AMD, there was no benefit observed with supplementation, though the risk of progression was low with placebo.

In-Depth [randomized controlled trial]: This multicenter, randomized, controlled trial recruited patients between 55-80 years of age with a best-corrected visual acuity of ≥20/32 in the study eye and a range of AMD abnormalities (i.e., from no abnormalities to one eye with features of advanced AMD). Exclusion criteria included obscured ocular media preventing macular photographs, any eye disease that could complicate assessment of AMD, and previous ocular non-cataract surgery. A total of 3640 patients were assigned to 4 ordinal categories of AMD (1-4) based on the extent of their macular findings, and subsequently randomized 1:1:1:1 to treatment with 1) zinc alone, 2) antioxidants alone, 3) zinc and antioxidants, and 4) placebo. The antioxidant formulation was a combination of vitamin C, E, and beta carotene, while the zinc formulation consisted of zinc and cupric acid. Patients were followed for 5 years or longer. The primary outcomes were disease progression, treatment for advanced AMD, and visual acuity loss of ≥15 letters. A p-value ≤0.01 was considered statistically significant.

Category 2 (early AMD), 3 (intermediate AMD), and 4 (advanced AMD in one eye) patients had a 1.3%, 18%, and 43% probability of progression to advanced AMD, respectively, in the placebo group by 5 years. Compared with placebo, zinc and antioxidant therapy led to significantly lower risk of progression to advanced AMD (OR 0.72; 99%CI 0.52-0.98, p = 0.007); the risk of progression was further reduced when category 1 and 2 patients were excluded from analysis (OR 0.66; 99%CI 0.47-0.91, p = 0.001). After excluding category 1 and 2 patients, zinc and antioxidant treatment also significantly reduced the risk of moderate vision loss compared to placebo (OR 0.73; 99%CI 0.54-0.99, p = 0.008).

Age-Related Eye Disease Study Research Group. A randomized, placebo-controlled, clinical trial of high-dose supplementation with vitamins C and E, beta carotene, and zinc for age-related macular degeneration and vision loss: AREDS report no. 8. Arch Ophthalmol. 2001 Oct;119(10):1417–36.

The OHTS trial: Topical ocular hypotensive medication reduces risk of open-angle glaucoma

1. At 5 years, the probability of developing open-angle glaucoma was significantly lower in the group that received topical ocular hypotensive medication compared to the observed group.

2. Older age, male gender, African-American ethnicity, larger cup-to-disc ratios, higher IOP, greater visual field deficits, heart disease, and reduced cornea thickness were predictors of the development of glaucoma.

Original Date of Publication: June 2002

Study Rundown: Glaucoma is the leading cause of irreversible blindness worldwide, and is thought to result from increased intraocular pressure (IOP). Prior to the Ocular Hypertension Treatment Study (OHTS), the efficacy of topical ocular hypotensive medications was unclear. In this study, over 1,500 patients were randomized to receive treatment or simply be observed. After 5 years, the probability of developing glaucoma was 60% lower in the group that received ocular hypotensive medication compared to the observed group. Treatment was not associated with an increase in side effects compared to the observation arm. Older age, male gender, African-American ethnicity, larger cup-to-disc ratios, higher IOP, greater visual field deficits, heart disease, and thinner corneas were found to be predictive of open-angle glaucoma. Limitations to the study include the fact that neither patients nor physicians were blinded to the randomization, although the endpoint evaluators were masked. The OHTS trial demonstrates that ocular anti-hypertensive treatment significantly reduces the incidence of primary open-angle glaucoma, and that patients identified as high-risk could benefit from earlier treatment.

In-Depth [randomized controlled study]: Approximately 1,636 patients who had no prior glaucomatous damage but elevated IOP in both eyes were randomized into treatment or observation arms. The treatment arm involved reducing IOP by 20% to at least 24 mm Hg using various topical hypotensive medications. Patients were evaluated semi-annually, including visual field testing and optic disc imaging. Masked reviewers assessed for signs of glaucomatous damage from these studies. After 5 years, the probability of developing primary open-angle glaucoma (POAG) was 4.4% and 9.5% in the treatment and observation groups, respectively (HR 0.40; 95%CI 0.27-0.59). In univariate analysis, age, sex, ethnicity, cup-to-disc ratios, elevated IOP, and thinner central corneal thickness (CCT) were found to increase the risk of developing glaucoma. Patients with significantly thin corneas (<555 μm) were found to have a hazard ratio of 3.4, reflecting how CCT can be an essential metric in risk assessment. Ultimately, the OHTS trial demonstrated that topical ocular antihypertensive therapy is essential to reducing progression to glaucoma, and identifying criteria to risk stratify patients.

Gordon MO, Beiser JA, Brandt JD, Heuer DK, Higginbotham EJ, Johnson CA, et al. The Ocular Hypertension Treatment Study: baseline factors that predict the onset of primary open-angle glaucoma. Arch Ophthalmol. 2002 Jun;120(6):714-720; discussion 829-830.

Kass MA, Heuer DK, Higginbotham EJ, Johnson CA, Keltner JL, Miller JP, et al. The Ocular Hypertension Treatment Study: a randomized trial determines that topical ocular hypotensive medication delays or prevents the onset of primary open-angle glaucoma. Arch Ophthalmol. 2002 Jun;120(6):701-713; discussion 829-830.

The EMGT: Reducing intraocular pressure slows progression of glaucoma

1. Treatment using laser trabeculoplasty and topical betaxolol hydrochloride to reduce intraocular pressure (IOP) is associated with delayed progression of glaucoma.

2. Treatment to decrease IOP was associated with an increase in nuclear lens opacity grading indicative of cataract formation.

Original Date of Publication: October 2002

Study Rundown: Previous epidemiological studies had suggested that few patients with elevated IOP developed glaucoma when left untreated. This challenged two assumptions at the time: firstly, the belief that glaucoma was caused by elevated IOP, and secondly, the thought that reducing IOP was a means of treating glaucoma. The Early Manifest Glaucoma Trial (EMGT), which commenced in 1992, was the first adequately powered, randomized trial that assessed the effectiveness of reducing IOP in the treatment of patients with previously untreated glaucoma. Its results showed that reduction of IOP through laser trabeculoplasty and topical betaxolol significantly delayed the onset of disease progression by a median of 18 months compared to the untreated control group. The benefits of treatment remained when participants were stratified according to IOP level, degree of visual damage, age, and presence of exfoliative glaucoma. However, IOP reduction was also associated with a significant increase in cataract formation based on nuclear opacity measurements.

Limitations of the trial include the study's homogeneous patient population, consisting predominantly of white patients. Study participants were also required to have an IOP ≤30 mm Hg, which precluded the study from assessing the effect of IOP reduction in patients with higher initial IOP levels. Also, for ethical reasons, participants in the control group were monitored only until the onset of disease progression, at which point participants were then given appropriate treatment at the time. This design prevented the study from observing the natural history of glaucoma for an extended period of time. In summary, while the results of the EMGT do not conclusively show that elevated IOP causes glaucoma, it does confirm that elevated IOP is an important component of glaucoma's pathophysiology, and that reducing IOP can help slow the progression of glaucoma in patients of various age, IOP level, and other characteristics. This finding supports efforts to improve early-detection of elevated IOP in patients.

In-Depth [randomized controlled trial]: The EMGT was a randomized trial that enrolled 255 patients from two Swedish cities. Eligible patients had to have had a diagnosis of newly detected, previously untreated open-angle glaucoma, reproducible visual deficits, and be between 50 and 80 years of age. Exclusion criteria included having severe visual field defects, a mean IOP > 30 mm Hg, and significant cataractous lens changes. A total of 129 participants were randomized to receive treatment to reduce IOP through laser trabeculoplasty and topical betaxolol, while 126 participants were randomized to receive no treatment. All patients were monitored until the moment of disease progression, whereupon appropriate treatment was administered for all patients. Progression of glaucoma was assessed via measurements of visual field defects and optic disc cupping. All graders for these measurements were blinded.

Median follow-up was 6 years (range 51-102 months). The study demonstrated that treatment to reduce IOP was associated with a significantly lower frequency of glaucoma progression when compared with no treatment (45% vs. 62%, $p = 0.007$). This benefit of reducing IOP remained when patients were stratified according IOP level, degree of visual damage, age, and presence of exfoliation. The median time to progression for the treatment group was 18 months longer than for the control group. The study also found that treatment to reduce IOP levels was associated with a significant increase in nuclear opacities, when compared with no treatment ($p = 0.002$).

Heijl A, Leske MC, Bengtsson B, Hyman L, Bengtsson B, Hussein M, et al. Reduction of intraocular pressure and glaucoma progression: results from the Early Manifest Glaucoma Trial. Arch Ophthalmol. 2002 Oct;120(10):1268–79.

The AREDS2: No benefit from additional carotenoid and omega-3-fatty acid supplementation to original AREDS formulation

1. There was no added benefit observed with adding lutein and zeaxanthin, omega-3-fatty acids (DHA and EPA), or the combination to the original AREDS formulation in reducing progression to advanced age-related macular degeneration (AMD) in high-risk patients.

2. Because of the suspected association between beta-carotene and increased lung cancer risk in smokers, beta-carotene can be replaced by lutein and zeaxanthin in recent and current smokers requiring AREDS supplementation.

Original Date of Publication: May 2013

Study Rundown: The Age-Related Eye Disease Study 1 (AREDS1) demonstrated lower progression to advanced AMD and risk of moderate vision loss in high-risk patients with the supplementation of high-dose zinc and antioxidants, which became known as the AREDS1 formulation. Since the original trial, new evidence suggested that other carotenoids (lutein and zeaxanthin) and omega-3-fatty acids (DHA and EPA) could potentially further reduce the risk of progression. In smokers, it was also noted that beta-carotene may be associated with a higher risk of incident lung neoplasm.

The AREDS2 was a randomized controlled trial that sought primarily to evaluate the effects adding these carotenoids and omega-3-fatty acids to the original AREDS1 formulation on the risk of progression to advanced AMD. The investigators also explored the effects of eliminating beta-carotene from and lowering the dose of zinc in the original formulation. The study found that there was no added benefit of these new supplements in any combination on the progression of AMD or in preventing vision loss. Similarly, eliminating beta-carotene and lowering zinc showed no statistically significant effect. In patients with low lutein and zeaxanthin intake at baseline, supplementing these carotenoids may offer some benefit, as demonstrated in the study subgroup analyses. Given the potential link between beta-carotene and lung cancer in recent and current smokers, it was suggested that substituting lutein and zeaxanthin may be a reasonable option in this patient population.

In-Depth [randomized controlled trial]: This multicenter, randomized, controlled trial recruited patients between 55-80 years of age, at high-risk for developing advanced AMD (i.e., bilateral large drusen or large drusen in 1 eye and advanced AMD in the other eye), who had agreed to stop pre-existing supplements containing study therapies (lutein, zeaxanthin, DHA, EPA, vitamin C/E, beta carotene, zinc, copper), and demonstrated reasonable adherence (i.e., took at least 75% of supplements during run-in phase). Exclusion criteria included obscured ocular media preventing macular photographs, any eye disease that could complicate assessment of AMD, previous ocular non-cataract surgery, and systemic disease with poor 5-year survival (e.g., oxalate kidney stones, Wilson disease, hemochromatosis, lung cancer). A total of 4203 patients were randomized to either i) lutein and zeaxanthin, ii) DHA and EPA, iii) lutein, zeaxanthin, DHA ,and EPA, or iv) placebo. These supplements were taken in addition to the original AREDS formulation, which consisted of vitamin C/E, beta carotene, zinc, and copper. Consenting patients underwent a secondary randomization to evaluate variations of the AREDS formulation, specifically regimens with i) no beta-carotene, ii) low dose zinc, iii) no beta carotene and low dose zinc, or iv) the original AREDS formula. Patients were followed for 5 years. The primary outcome was progression/treatment for advanced AMD at 5 years.

Unfortunately, none of the additional supplement combinations significantly delayed progression to advanced AMD when compared to placebo: i) lutein and zeaxanthin (HR 0.90, 98.7%CI 0.76-1.07, p = 0.12), ii) DHA and EPA (HR 0.97, 98.7%CI 0.82-1.16, p = 0.70), iii) lutein, zeaxanthin, DHA, and EPA (HR 0.89, 98.7%CI 0.75-1.06, p = 0.10). With regards to adjusting the original AREDS formula, lowering zinc (HR 1.06, 95%CI 0.95-1.19, p = 0.32) and eliminating beta-carotene (HR 1.07, 95%CI 0.94-1.20, p = 0.31) also did not significantly reduce progression rate compared to placebo. A subgroup analysis demonstrated that patients in the lowest quintile of baseline lutein and zeaxanthin dietary intake may benefit from lutein and zeaxanthin supplementation (HR 0.74, 95%CI 0.59-0.94, p = 0.01). There were no statistically significant differences between the groups in terms of the risk of serious adverse events.

Age-Related Eye Disease Study 2 Research Group. Lutein + zeaxanthin and omega-3 fatty acids for age-related macular degeneration: the Age-Related Eye Disease Study 2 (AREDS2) randomized clinical trial. JAMA. 2013 May 15;309(19):2005–15.

XII. Pediatrics

> ""The important thing is not to stop questioning. Curiosity has its own reason for existing. One cannot help but be in awe when one contemplates the mysteries of eternity, of life, of the marvellous structure of reality. It is enough if one tries to comprehend only a little of this mystery every day.""
>
> - Albert Einstein

Childhood febrile seizure characteristics associated with epilepsy diagnosis

1. Children with febrile seizures, complex febrile seizures, and febrile seizures of early onset (before 6 months of age) had a variably increased risk of developing epilepsy when compared to individuals without febrile seizures.

2. Abnormal performance on neurologic testing was linked to increased epilepsy risk.

Original Date of Publication: November 1976

Study Rundown: Previous research indicated an increase in unprovoked seizures following childhood febrile seizures. The researchers in this study were the first to try to define the risk factors associated with progression from childhood febrile seizure to epilepsy. As a part of the Collaborative Perinatal Project of the National Institute of Neurological and Communicative Disorders and Stroke, researchers developed this multi-center, large prospective cohort study. Children were followed from birth to age 7, during which time febrile and afebrile seizure activity as well as overall development were examined. Results demonstrated that individuals who experienced febrile seizures with and without complex features, those who tested abnormally on developmental screening prior to their first febrile seizure, and children with early febrile seizures were significantly more likely to be diagnosed with epilepsy by the age of 7.

This study was limited by its lack of consideration of potential covariates, including whether or not a child was started on anticonvulsant therapy. Other studies have found that early first febrile seizures (before 5 years of age), repeated febrile seizures, prolonged febrile seizure length, and a family history of cerebral palsy were potential contributors to childhood epilepsy.

In-Depth [prospective cohort]: Conducted in 12 teaching hospitals, 54 000 children born to mothers enrolled in the Collaborative Perinatal Project were recruited for study inclusion. Children were followed from birth to 7 years of age. Parents were interviewed regarding the occurrence of seizures, convulsions, and changes in consciousness at 4, 8, 12, 18, and 24 months with annual follow-up continuing from 2 to 7 years of age. Interviews were completed by trained individuals. Medical records were obtained for each medically managed seizure episode. Neurologic and developmental assessments were completed throughout the study with standard physical examination at 4 months of age, psychological assessment at 8 months of age, and pediatric and neurologic assessment at 1 year of age. "Febrile seizures" were defined as any seizure occurring with fever in a child 1 month to 7 years of age. "Afebrile seizures" were defined as recurrent seizure without fever before 4 years of age or 1, isolated afebrile seizure episode after 2 years of age. "Epilepsy" was defined as recurrent afebrile seizures with at least 1 occurring after 2 years of age. No associated known acute neurologic illness could be present in order for these diagnoses to be made. Complex features of seizures were defined as seizure duration longer than 15 minutes, more than 1 seizure in 24 hours, and focal seizure activity.

Of the children included, 1706 experienced at least one febrile seizure and were followed to study completion at 7 years of age. Among these children, 550 (32%) had at least 1 more febrile seizure, but no afebrile seizure, while 52 children (3%) had at least 1 afebrile seizure during the study, and 34 (2%) met criteria for a diagnosis of epilepsy. Of the 39 179 children who did not have a febrile seizure and were followed for 7 years, 199 were diagnosed with epilepsy. Significantly more individuals were diagnosed with epilepsy following a first febrile seizure with complex features when compared to those with only afebrile seizures (41 vs. 5 per 1000, $X^2 = 70$, $p < 0.001$). Children with complex febrile seizures had significantly greater rates of epilepsy than those who had febrile seizures without complex features (41 vs. 15 per 1000, $X^2 = 7.8$, $p < 0.01$). Children with febrile seizures without complex features were diagnosed at higher rates than those who had afebrile seizures (15 vs. 5 per 1000, $p < 0.001$). Children with any abnormal findings on assessments prior to first seizure were significantly more likely to meet criteria for epilepsy when compared to those with normal screenings (39 v. 12 per 1000, $X^2 = 11$, $p < 0.001$). An 18-fold increase in risk of epilepsy was noted among children who had both complex first febrile seizure and abnormal screening performance compared to those with no febrile seizure (92 vs. 5 per 1000, $X^2 = 79$, $p < 0.001$). Previously normal children without complex seizures had significantly higher rates of epilepsy than those with afebrile seizures (11 vs. 5 per 1000, $X^2 = 4.0$, $p < 0.05$). There was a significant increase in epilepsy by 7 years of age among children who had febrile seizures during their first 6 months of life when compared to those who had them beyond the first year (57 vs. 15 per 1000, $X^2 = 7.6$, $p < 0.01$).

Nelson KB, Ellenberg JH. Predictors of Epilepsy in Children Who Have Experienced Febrile Seizures. New England Journal of Medicine. 1976 Nov 4;295(19):1029–33.

Initial guidelines for prolonged fever in children

1. Among 100 children presenting to one children's hospital for prolonged febrile illnesses, the majority of cases were of an infectious etiology (52 cases).

2. Febrile illness due to infectious causes were significantly more likely to occur in younger children, while those due to inflammatory conditions were significantly more likely to occur in older children.

Original Date of Publication: April 1975

Study Rundown: The issue of prolonged febrile illness in children presents a diagnostic challenge to pediatric practitioners. At the time of this study's publication, there were no guidelines for diagnosis and management of children with fevers of unknown origin (FUO), a term still without a clear definition today. It is often defined as temperature > 38.3°C for at least 8 days without any obvious cause following initial outpatient or hospital evaluation. This study investigated prolonged fever in 100 children in order to better define guidelines for the care of those with FUO, defined in this study as a temperature > 38.5°C, $\geq$ 5 times during a 2-week period.

Of the 100 records included, the most common fever etiology was infection (52 cases). Findings indicated that significantly more young children had fevers of infectious etiologies, while significantly more older children had collagen-inflammatory fever etiologies. Based on the findings that 62% of children had stories and presentations consistent with etiology, researchers recognized the importance of a thorough history and physical in diagnosis. With 80% of children receiving antibiotics prior to official diagnosis and no resolution in their symptoms, the use of antibiotic therapy prior to hospitalization was discouraged and use of diagnostic cultures encouraged. In addition, erythrocyte sedimentation rate (ESR) testing and protein analysis were deemed more useful than complete blood count (CBC) and urinalysis (UA). Other procedures and imaging techniques were helpful when indicated by the history and physical.

This study was limited by its small sample size, lack of patient racial/ethnic diversity, and use of a single institution as a source of patient reports. Decades and multiple studies and reports on FUO later, many of the conclusions drawn from this landmark study still stand. Infection remains the most common cause of prolonged febrile illness. The importance of history and physical in diagnosing children with FUO continues to be emphasized; however specific recommendations for initial testing now include CBC, ESR, C-reactive protein, blood cultures, UA and culture, chest radiograph, tuberculosis testing, electrolytes, and blood urea nitrogen, creatinine, liver panel, and HIV serology.

In-Depth [retrospective cohort]: A total of 100 patient records of children (65% male and 91 white) seen at a tertiary children's hospital for prolonged fever during 1966 to 1973 were included in analysis. Prolonged fever defined as a temperature of $> 38.5\,°C$ on ≥ 5 times during a 2-week period without final diagnosis from a referring physician. Temperatures were taken either rectally or by an equivalent method. Results were analyzed using X^2 testing with final diagnoses as determined by laboratory testing when appropriate and then categorized as "infectious-presumed viral," "infectious-nonviral," "collagen-inflammatory," "malignancy," "miscellaneous," or "undiagnosed." In addition, fever patterns, use of antipyretics, symptoms, physical findings, laboratory results, and radiologic findings were recorded.

Of 100 patients, most were diagnosed with infectious causes of their fevers (52 cases), with 17 secondary to presumed viral illness, 20 due to collagen-inflammatory disorders, 6 secondary to malignancy, and 10 from miscellaneous causes. When cases were divided by age into either younger than 6 years of age (52 cases) or older than 6 years of age (48 cases), it was found that significantly more younger patients were diagnosed with infection than older patients (34 vs. 18, $p < 0.05$), while significantly more of those diagnosed with collagen-inflammatory diseases were older than 6 years (16 vs. 4, $p < 0.05$). The most common presenting symptoms of febrile patients were head, ear, eye, nose, and throat symptoms (72 cases). Only 27 patients had physical signs directly related to their final diagnoses. White blood cell count and low hematocrit from CBC did not significantly relate to fever etiology. ESR was significantly related to non-serious fever etiology in the 20 children with ESR < 10 mm/hr. Thirty-four of 74 children tested had reversed albumin-globulin ratios. Of these, significantly more patients with collagen-inflammatory disease had reversal compared to those with viral diagnoses (75% vs. 20%, $p < 0.05$). In addition, electrophoresis patterns differed significantly among patients with viral disorders showing a uniform decrease in albumin and increase in globulin.

Pizzo PA, Lovejoy FH, Smith DH. Prolonged Fever in Children: Review of 100 Cases. Pediatrics. 1975 Apr 1;55(4):468–73.

Artificial surfactant improves respiratory distress syndrome in infants

1. In 10 infants treated for respiratory distress syndrome (RDS) with artificial surfactant, significant improvements in blood pressure, acid-base status, arterial oxygenation, and radiologic findings were observed.

2. Infants also required significantly less oxygen therapy and ventilator pressure following surfactant administration.

Original Date of Publication: January 1980

Study Rundown: Hyaline membrane disease (HMD), now known as infant RDS, is a pulmonary disease of young infants most often linked to fetal immaturity. After the landmark 1959 discovery by Avery et al. connecting insufficient surfactant with RDS, methods of treating the disease were investigated. As surfactant was known to reduce lung surface tension, making it easier to maintain patent alveoli, this study built upon work in animals as the first trial of artificial surfactant treatment for RDS in human infants.

Using a mixture of natural and synthetic lipids including dipalmitoyl lecithin (the primary component of surfactant) and phosphatidyl glycerol, researchers administered artificial surfactant to 10 infants diagnosed with RDS and examined their laboratory, clinical examination, and radiologic changes. Significant reductions in systolic blood pressure (SBP), along with improvements in arterial oxygenation, arterial-alveolar oxygen concentration differences, acid-base balance, and radiologic findings were observed. Infants also required significantly less inspired oxygen and ventilator pressure after surfactant administration. This study was limited by a lack of randomization, comparison to control infants, and its small sample size. Despite these factors, this study led to future, large, randomized, clinical trials that further solidified the benefits of artificial surfactant use among infants with RDS. Antenatal corticosteroids coupled with post-delivery surfactant and ventilation are now commonplace treatments for infants in neonatal intensive care as they significantly improve clinical outcomes among infants suffering from poor lung development.

In-Depth [prospective cohort]: Ten infants with diagnosed RDS (mean gestational age = 30.2 weeks, mean birthweight = 1552 g) were included in the study. Prior to surfactant administration, ventilator settings were noted and not changed. Arterial oxygen tension (P_aO_2), carbon dioxide tension (P_aCO_2), and pH were recorded 30-90 minutes before and again 10-20 minutes before surfactant administration to provide a snapshot of each infant's physiologic state. No significant differences were noted between these 2 time periods. About 10 mL of artificial surfactant (150 μmol lipid phosphorus/kg) was suspended in normal saline and put into the infants' endotracheal tubes. Infants were then moved into different positions to ensure the solution was distributed to each lung segment and the infant was ventilated with a respirator. Up to 3 hours post-administration P_aO_2, $PaCO_2$, acid-base balance, and radiographic findings were assessed without alteration in ventilator settings. Following this assessment, ability to reduce inspired oxygen concentration (F_iO_2) and respiratory pressure were noted.

On clinical examination, significant increases in SBP post-administration was observed in the 6 infants who had continuous blood pressure monitoring (37 ± 5 mmHg pre vs. 59 ± 4 mmHg post, $p < 0.02$). PO_2 increased significantly (45 ± 7 mmHg pre vs. 212 ± 46 mmHg post, $p < 0.005$), PCO_2 decreased significantly (50 ± 4 mmHg pre vs. 33 ± 2 mm Hg post, $p < 0.005$), and pH increased significantly (7.13 ± 0.05 pre vs. 7.31 ± 0.04, $p < 0.05$). Three hours post-administration, F_iO_2 were able to decrease significantly from $81\pm7\%$ to $38\pm5\%$ ($p < 0.01$) and, within 6 hours of administration, inspiratory pressure could be reduced from 30 ± 2 cm H_2O to 22 ± 2 cm H_2O ($p < 0.02$). The difference in alveolar and arterial O_2 concentration decreased significantly as well 474 ± 49 mmHg to 189 ± 29 ($p < 0.005$) 3 hours post-administration and to 120 ± 18 mmHg ($p < 0.001$) 30 hours post-administration. At an average of 6 hours post-administration complete radiologic resolution of RDS was observed. Two of the 10 infants studied died due to causes unrelated to RDS or surfactant administration. No serious adverse events were linked to surfactant use.

Fujiwara T, Maeta H, Chida S, Morita T, Watabe Y, Abe T. Artificial surfactant therapy in hyaline-membrane disease. Lancet. 1980 Jan 12;1(8159):55–9.

Avery M, Mead J. Surface properties in relation to atelectasis and hyaline membrane disease. AMA Am J Dis Child. 1959 May 1;97(5I):517–23.

IVIg with aspirin reduces coronary aneurysms in Kawasaki disease

1. Children with Kawasaki disease treated with a combined regimen of aspirin and intravenous gamma globulin (IVIg) experienced significantly lower rates of coronary artery aneurysms when compared to those receiving aspirin only.

2. Children treated with the combined regimen had significantly shorter fevers and a greater decrease in inflammatory markers when compared to those treated with aspirin alone.

Original Date of Publication: August 1986

Study Rundown: Kawasaki disease, also known as Kawasaki syndrome, is an inflammatory vascular condition characterized by persistent fever, oral erythema, conjunctivitis, lymphadenopathy, and rash with risk of lasting coronary artery aneurysm or ectasia. At the time of the current study, standard care for Kawasaki disease included aspirin, which was thought to aid in reducing inflammation without reducing the disease's cardiovascular complications. This study was the first to expand upon the proposed efficacy of high-dose IVIg in preventing Kawasaki-related cardiac problems when compared to aspirin. Prior studies used low-dose (100mg) IVIg and had poor study design.

In this study, researchers found that children receiving combined therapy had a significantly lower incidence of aneurysms, fever duration, and inflammatory markers by day 5 of treatment when compared to those receiving aspirin only. This study was limited in its lack of blinding among practitioners administering the treatment regimen and differences in hospitalization status (all patients undergoing IVIg required hospitalization, whereas those receiving aspirin only were not). This was the first study to provide evidence of the efficacy of high-dose IVIg in managing the cardiac and inflammatory outcomes of Kawasaki disease.

In-Depth [randomized controlled trial]: From February 1984 to September 1985, 168 children with diagnosed Kawasaki disease were recruited from 6 care centers throughout the United States. Kawasaki disease was diagnosed in individuals with 5 of 6 clinical features (fever, nonexudative conjunctivitis, oral changes, extremity changes, rash, and cervical lymphadenopathy). Participants were randomized into 1 of 2 treatment groups: 1) 100mg/kg of aspirin every 16 hours for 14 days (n = 84) or 2) 400mg (high-dose) IVIg for the first 4 days of treatment along with the aspirin regimen described previously (n = 84). Demographics, baseline laboratory testing, and follow-up salicylate levels of the groups did not differ significantly. Coronary artery pathology was assessed using echocardiography at enrollment as well as 2 and 7 weeks after enrollment. Secondary outcomes included fever duration and reduction in inflammatory markers (white-cell count, absolute granulocyte count, α_1-antitrypsin level, absolute neutrophil count, and platelet count). Imaging was read by 2 pediatric echocardiographers blinded to the study. T-tests to compare means and Mantel-Haenszel methods along with logistic regression were completed to assess the effect of IVIg on the treatment regimen.

A total of 311 follow-up echocardiograms were completed. At 2-week follow-up, significantly fewer children in the combined treatment group had coronary artery abnormalities when compared to those treated only with aspirin (8% vs. 23.1%, p < 0.01). This difference was also observed at 7-week follow-up (3.8% vs. 17.7%, p = 0.005). Using Mantel-Haeszel methods and logistic regression, it was determined that at 2 weeks, children who had the combined treatment regimen were one third as likely to have coronary aneurysms and, at 7 weeks, one fifth as likely when compared to children treated with only aspirin (95%CI). Children treated with a combined regimen experienced a significantly greater drop in body temperature during the first 2 days of treatment than with aspirin ($1.30 \pm 0.16°C$ drop vs. $0.42 \pm 0.11°C$, p = 0.001). By day 5 of treatment, those with treated with combined therapy had a significant greater decrease in white cell count (p < 0.0001), absolute granulocytes (p = 0.0001), and alpha$_1$ anti-trypsin levels (p = 0.05). Absolute neutrophil count and platelet count did not differ by treatment group. No serious adverse effects of IVIg were experienced.

Newburger JW, Takahashi M, Burns JC, Beiser AS, Chung KJ, Duffy CE, et al. The Treatment of Kawasaki Syndrome with Intravenous Gamma Globulin. New England Journal of Medicine. 1986 Aug 7;315(6):341–7.

Prone sleeping position and heavy bedding associated with sudden infant death syndrome

1. A significant increase in sudden infant death syndrome (SIDS) was observed among infants who slept prone as opposed to sleeping on their side or supine.

2. A significant increase in SIDS risk was observed among infants who were wrapped in more blankets, wore heavier clothing to bed, or were in a home that was heated overnight when compared to control infants.

Original Date of Publication: July 1990

Study Rundown: This study aimed to further elucidate the role of sleeping position, bedding, and environmental temperature in SIDS. Researchers found that prone position during sleep, heavy bedding/bed clothing, and overnight heating in homes significantly increased the risk of infants dying from SIDS. The study was limited in its generalizability through use of a study population from a single geographic location. Despite this, the study further supported the theories that SIDS deaths commonly resulted from prone infant position and increased infant heat exposure. Following this study and multiple other publications supporting findings regarding sleep positioning, the United States and many other countries initiated "Back to Sleep" campaigns now known as "Safe to Sleep," encouraging caretakers to place infants in the supine position to reduce SIDS incidence. Significant reductions in SIDS were seen following these campaigns. While side sleeping has not been identified as a SIDS risk factor, it is discouraged by pediatricians as infants can roll over from their sides onto their abdomens. In addition, further work has identified other SIDS-associated risk factors including loose bedding, soft sleeping surfaces, and bed-sharing.

In-Depth [case-control study]: All sudden infantile deaths in 2 counties of England were reported and, for each infant, 2 control infants living in the same neighborhood were identified. Researchers visited bereaved families soon after death and on several other occasions during the following months in order to gather a full social and medical history at the time of death. This included discussing sleeping position, sleep timing, clothing and blankets in the crib, and heating conditions in the room. To assess the heaviness of infant bedding and blankets, the thermal resistance of these materials was calculated and expressed in units of tog, where higher tog indicates heavier materials. Comparable histories were taken for control infants with attention paid to the 24 hours before the research visit. X^2 testing along with Mantel-Haenszel tests, and multiple logistic regression models were used to assess the difference between groups and risks associated with sudden death.

A total of 72 infants died suddenly during the study period (mean age = 94.4 days) and 144 control infants (mean age = 97.0 days) were included for comparison. Among the 72 infants who died, 5 were found to have pathologic causes contributing to their deaths, while the remaining 67 had no known cause and their deaths were therefore deemed secondary to SIDS. Among the 67 SIDS cases, 62 infants had been put to sleep in the prone position, while 76 of the 134 control infants slept prone. Prone positioning was associated with an 8.8 times increased risk of SIDS when compared to control infants (relative risk [RR] 8.8, 95%CI 7.0-11.0, $p < 0.001$). Infants who died of SIDS were wrapped in significantly heavier bedding than control infants (9.1 tog vs. 8.0 tog, $p < 0.05$). After controlling for sleep position, a significant increased risk with heavier bedding/heavier bed clothing was observed (RR 1.14 for each 1 tog increase above 8 tog, 95%CI 1.03-1.28, $p < 0.05$). Overnight home heating was seen in significantly more homes of infants who died than controls and was associated with a significantly increased risk of SIDS death (28 of 67 vs. 34 of 134, RR 2.7, 95%CI 1.4-5.2, $p < 0.01$).

Fleming PJ, Gilbert R, Azaz Y, Berry PJ, Rudd PT, Stewart A, et al. Interaction between bedding and sleeping position in the sudden infant death syndrome: a population based case-control study. BMJ. 1990 Jul 14;301(6743):85–9.

Lead exposure in childhood associated with worse cognitive performance

1. Among children exposed to lead early in life, serum lead levels at 24 months of age were significantly associated with decreased cognitive performance on measures of intelligence and educational achievement at 10 years old.

2. Each 0.48 μmol/L (10 μg/dL) increase in serum lead at 24 months of age was associated with a 5.8 point decline in a measure of intelligence quotient (IQ) and an 8.9 point decline in educational achievement score during cognitive testing at 10 years of age.

Original Date of Publication: December 1992

Study Rundown: At the time of this publication, prior studies investigating early, low-level lead exposure and cognition later in life had mixed findings. Previous reports assessed the potential connection between lead levels and cognitive performance into preschool years. This was the first study to investigate the effects of early low-level lead exposure on cognitive performance into school age. One hundred forty-eight children were assessed from birth to 10 years of age for serum lead levels and cognitive development through IQ testing via the Wechsler Intelligence Scale for Children-Revised (WISC-R) and the Kaufman Test of Educational Achievement Brief Form (K-TEA). Findings indicated that high serum lead levels at 24 months of age were significantly associated with lower IQ and neuropsychiatric performance at 10 years old, a finding which was upheld after controlling for covariates.

This study was limited by the potential role of bias towards children available for follow-up as multiple participants were lost from 5 years of age to 10 years old. In addition, this cohort was of higher socioeconomic status (SES) and intelligence than the average citizen, which may have allowed for an enhanced view of the cognitive effects of lead, but makes the findings less generalizable compared to previous study cohorts of lower SES. This study demonstrated that even at low levels, early lead exposure can lead to poor cognitive development through school age. Combined with previous work, these findings encouraged the Centers for Disease Control to lower the benchmark for toxic lead levels to the current level of 0.24 μmol/L (5 μg/dL).

In-Depth [prospective cohort]: Two hundred forty-nine infants born between August 1979 and August 1981 were recruited from Brigham and Women's Hospital in Boston, Massachusetts with umbilical blood lead levels in the ranges required for eligibility. Infants were considered for study inclusion if their umbilical cord blood lead levels were below the 10%ile at the time of the study (<0.15 μmol/L or 3μg/dL), around the 50%ile (0.31 μmol/L or 6.5 μg/dL), or above the 90%ile (≥0.48 μmol/L or 10 μg/dL) indicating, respectively, "low," "medium," or "high" prenatal lead exposure. Infants' lead levels and development were evaluated at 6, 12, 18, 24, and 57 months of age and then again at 10 years old. Primary cognitive outcomes were assessed through the use of the WISC-R and K-TEA.

Of the initial cohort, 148 children were included in the final analysis as they completed the entire study course. Of those, 116 had serum lead measurements at all 7 time points, including birth (mean 0.14 μmol/L or 2.9 μg/dL). Multiple regression analysis was completed with appropriate adjustment for confounders. Overall, participants had cognitive scores about 1 SD above the national average. After controlling for covariates, only the lead levels of children at 24 months of age (mean lead level < 0.34 μmol/L or < 7 μg/dL) were significantly associated with cognitive performance including the full-scale WISC-R IQ and K-TEA battery composite. Each 0.48 μmol/L (10 μg/dL) increase in serum lead was associated with a 5.8 point decline in the IQ measure and 8.9 point decline in the K-TEA composite ($p < 0.01$, $p < 0.001$, respectively). No significant association between lead levels and cognitive scores was seen at any other age.

Bellinger DC, Stiles KM, Needleman HL. Low-Level Lead Exposure, Intelligence and Academic Achievement: A Long-term Follow-up Study. Pediatrics. 1992 Dec 1;90(6):855–61.

PROS network study examines pubertal onset by race/ethnic groups

1. In a study population of girls 3-12 years of age, African American females developed secondary sexual characteristics significantly earlier than white females.

2. African American females had earlier menarche at 12.16 years of age, compared to 12.88 years of age among white females.

Original Date of Publication: April 1997

Study Rundown: The onset of female pubertal changes varies greatly by race/ethnicity. As the start of secondary characteristics marks a significant physiologic and psychological change in an individual's life, being able to anticipate onset is essential to providing proper medical care. Prior to the initiation of this work, no nationally representative, racially diverse data was available to assess female pubertal status in the United States. This cross-sectional study stood as the first to investigate secondary sexual characteristics and menses onset among girls 3-12 years of age that could provide evidence representative of national norms.

This study included children form the American Academy of Pediatrics Practice-based Research in the Office Settings (PROS) Network. Researchers found that African American girls developed secondary sexual characteristics, including breast development, axillary hair, and pubic hair significantly earlier than white females. All girls started puberty 6 months to a year earlier than reported in prior studies. The average age of menarche in African American females was 12.16 years of age compared to 12.88 years in white females. This study was limited by potential selection bias with non-random sample selection, the lack of hormone testing to provide a potential endocrinologic etiology for these developmental differences, and participants being heavier and taller, on average, than girls in the nationally-representative height and weight values provided by the Health and Nutrition Examination Surveys. Findings from this study indicated that the initiation of sex education and physician counseling should be tailored accordingly to earlier pubertal changes among girls. Follow-up work to this initial paper was completed and published as documented below to dispel confusion regarding studies investigating this subject matter after 1997. Another, more recent publication supported these findings, indicating that thelarche onset differed by race/ethnicity and started earlier in those with higher BMI.

In-Depth [cross-sectional study]: A total of 17 077 female patients (90.4% white, 9.6% African American) aged 3-12 years from the PROS Network were included in the study. Sexual maturity was staged by physicians trained and assessed in their ability to use Tanner staging criteria. In addition, a survey with questions regarding demographics, medical history, presence or absence of menses, and development of breast, pubic, and axillary hair was completed. Axillary hair was designated according to an original scale with stage 1 as no hair, stage 2 as sparse hair, and stage 3 as adult, mature hair. With and without controlling for height and weight, African American girls were found to develop secondary sexual characters significantly earlier than white girls (8.87 years vs. 9.96 years for breast development, 8.78 years vs. 10.51 years for pubic hair, and 10.01 vs. 11.80 stage 2 axillary hair development; p < 0.001 for all findings). The average age of menses onset was 12.16 years for African American girls and 12.88 years for white girls. Significantly more African American females had menses at the age of 12 when compared to white girls (62.1% vs. 35.2%, p < 0.001).

Herman-Giddens ME, Slora EJ, Wasserman RC, Bourdony CJ, Bhapkar MV, Koch GG, et al. Secondary Sexual Characteristics and Menses in Young Girls Seen in Office Practice: A Study from the Pediatric Research in Office Settings Network. Pediatrics. 1997 Apr 1;99(4):505–12.

Biro FM, Greenspan LC, Galvez MP, Pinney SM, Teitelbaum S, Windham GC, et al. Onset of Breast Development in a Longitudinal Cohort. Pediatrics. 2013 Nov 4;132(6):1019-27.

Transcutaneous bilirubinometry linked to decreased serum testing and cost in infants

1. In a 2-year study period, researchers observed a significant decrease in the number of infants undergoing bilirubin serum testing after introduction of a transcutaneous bilirubinometer (TcB) in a single hospital's newborn nursery.

2. The use of the transcutaneous instrument decreased hospital costs by $1625 each year when compared to serum bilirubin measurements.

Original Date of Publication: April 1997

Study Rundown: At the time of this study, one of the most commonly completed laboratory tests in the newborn nursery was the serum bilirubin level, second only to other routine genetic and metabolic screening tests. Researchers proposed that the use of a transcutaneous instrument for bilirubin measurements would be an effective way to decrease unnecessary serum bilirubin testing as well as reduce costs in the nursery setting.

As the use of a TcB was integrated into the nursery work environment, researchers observed a significant decrease in the number of serum bilirubin measurements completed. In addition, significantly fewer low serum bilirubin (< 10 mg/dL) measurements were obtained over the course of the study, indicating a potential decrease in unnecessary serum tests secondary to TcB use. TcB monitor use was also associated with an estimated decrease in annual hospital expenses secondary to bilirubin monitoring of about $1625. This study was limited in its lack of a control group, lack of generalizability due to the study population coming from a single nursery, and complications with the practicality of the TcB device. However, the results suggested that TcB use could reduce the need for unnecessary invasive testing in addition to lowering overall costs. Today, this device is commonly used as its validity and reliability has been reaffirmed in numerous studies.

In-Depth [prospective cohort]: On November 1, 1990, the TcB meter was introduced for regular use in the William Beaumont Hospital Department of Pediatrics newborn nursery. The number of serum bilirubin measurements along with the estimated total costs for performing the tests was calculated for newborns in the nursery from July 1990 to December 1992. Costs included salary for laboratory staff, supply costs, and time required for the procedure. Information from 12 625 infant admissions were included in the analysis. Data from July 1990 to December 1990 admissions were considered "pre-jaundice meter" as hospital staff adjusted to TcB use. A 40% decrease in infants requiring at least 1 serum bilirubin test and a 56% decrease in those requiring at least 2 were seen by study completion ($p < 0.0001$). Over the course of the study, bilirubin levels less than 10 mg/dL decreased significantly, starting at 46% of readings progressing to 27% of readings at the study conclusion ($p < 0.0001$). When the costs related to serum and transcutaneous bilirubin measurements were calculated, it was found that nearly $1625 per year for a cohort of 12 625 infants would be saved through regular TcB use.

Maisels MJ, Kring E. Transcutaneous Bilirubinometry Decreases the Need for Serum Bilirubin Measurements and Saves Money. Pediatrics. 1997 Apr 1;99(4):599–600.

The ACE trial: Adverse childhood exposures associated with poor health in adulthood

1. A significant dose-response relationship was observed between childhood exposures, adult health risk behaviors and adult disease states.

Original Date of Publication: May 1998

Study Rundown: At the time of this study, researchers had just begun investigating the role of childhood trauma on the development of adult medical conditions. Through a retrospective approach, the Adverse Childhood Experiences (ACE) trial investigated the influence of childhood abuse on adult disease risk factors, disease incidence, quality of life, use of healthcare resources, and death. Overall, 8056 adults completed a standardized questionnaire addressing their exposure to various forms of adverse events including abuse and household dysfunction. Researchers found individuals who experienced adverse childhood exposures to be at increased risk of having both health-related risk factors such as smoking and obesity as well as illnesses such as ischemic heart disease and malignancy in adulthood. These risk increases were largely present in a dose-response fashion. While this study was limited by its retrospective design and reliance on self-reporting for both adverse exposures and health status, the prevalence of adverse exposures was consistent with national averages. These findings emphasized the importance of preventative measures in childhood and extending into adulthood to reduce childhood adverse exposure, the development of health risk factors, and ultimately disease development and mortality.

In-Depth [retrospective cohort]: A total of 8056 adults (mean age = 56.1 years, 52.1% female, 79.4% white) who underwent standardized medical evaluation at a large United States adult healthcare clinic from August-November of 1995 and January-March of 1996 were included. Following examination, patients received a mailed copy of the study questionnaire, which inquired about childhood psychological, physical, and sexual abuse along with household dysfunction metrics. Responses were then related to self-reported present health risk factors, adult disease conditions with high mortality rates, and overall health status. Risk factors investigated included physical inactivity (defined as no physical activity participation in the past month), severe obesity (defined as body mass index > 35 kg/m^2), current smoking, attempted suicide, depressed mood (defined as 2 or more weeks of depressed mood over the past year), alcohol abuse, illicit drug use, intravenous drug use, history of sexually transmitted infections, and high numbers of total sexual partners (defined as > 50 partners). Logistic regression analysis was completed with adjustment for potential confounders to investigate the relationship between the number of childhood exposures to risk factors and adult medical conditions.

Overall, 52% of respondents experienced > 1 adverse childhood exposure and 6.2% reported exposure to > 4 adverse events. Substance abuse was the most common adverse exposure (25.6%) with a housemate being imprisoned as the least common (3.4%). Individuals who experienced 1 adverse exposure had a median probability of exposure to at least 1 more adverse exposure of 80%. Increases in number of exposures were associated with increased odds of developing health risk factors and adult disease conditions. Linear regression accounting for age, gender, race, and educational level as covariates, revealed a significant dose-response relationship between the number of adverse childhood exposures and each of the risk factors ($p < 0.001$) as well as the development of ischemic heart disease, cancer, emphysema, hepatitis or jaundice, fractures, and poor health on self-report ($p < 0.05$).

Felitti VJ, Anda RF, Nordenberg D, Williamson DF, Spitz AM, Edwards V, et al. Relationship of Childhood Abuse and Household Dysfunction to Many of the Leading Causes of Death in Adults. American Journal of Preventive Medicine. 1998 May 1;14(4):245–58.

Sleep-disordered breathing associated with poor academics and surgical improvement

1. Sleep-associated gas exchange abnormalities were highly prevalent among a first-grade study cohort with poor academic performance. About 18% of participants had oxygenation abnormalities assessed during overnight observation.

2. School performance improved significantly among children who received surgical intervention for abnormal breathing patterns during sleep.

3. Symptoms of disordered sleep were significantly worse among children who did not undergo surgical tonsillectomy and adenoidectomy.

Original Date of Publication: September 1998

Study Rundown: Previous studies indicated that a substantial portion of children suffered from obstructive sleep apnea (OSA) and primary snoring (PS), disorders linked to pulmonary hypertension, failure to thrive, systematic hypertension, and behavioral disturbances. To prevent these negative outcomes, children with sleep disorders often underwent tonsillectomy and adenoidectomy. Despite prior research, no prospective, controlled trial had investigated the potential cognitive outcomes of individuals with OSA. Researchers in this study aimed to determine whether or not sleep-associated gas exchange abnormalities (SAGEA) among children performing poorly in school was related to academic difficulties and whether or not surgical intervention aided in resolution of cognitive and disordered sleep symptoms.

Results demonstrated that a large number of cohort participants had PS (22.2%) and SAGEA (18.1%) and that both school performance and symptoms could improve through surgical intervention. This study was limited in the use of SpO_2 as a measure of oxygenation, which does not indicate whether obstruction or a lower respiratory process is responsible for desaturation and in the use of academic performance as the sole measure of cognition. Despite these limitations, this study added evidence obtained in a prospective, controlled manner to mostly case study-based findings. Current recommendations encourage adenotonsillectomy to prevent the physical, behavioral, and cognitive complications discussed here, with particular attention paid to assessing for potential residual disease requiring further intervention.

In-Depth [prospective cohort]: Two hundred ninety-seven first-grade students in the lowest 10%ile of their class were recruited for study participation in an overnight study. To assess sleep-disordered breathing symptoms, parents completed an OSA Syndrome (OSAS) questionnaire regarding childhood sleep behavior and respiratory compromise. Subsequently, the children underwent overnight respiratory analysis including pulse oximetry (SpO_2) and transcutaneous carbon dioxide tension (T_{CCO2}). SAGEA was diagnosed based upon a high score on the questionnaire along with 2 desaturations (periods of > 5% reductions in baseline SpO_2 or SpO_2 < 90%) per hour and/or an elevated T_{CCO2} > 8 mmHg compared with normal, waking values during an overnight study. Children without changes in SpO_2 or T_{CCO2}, but an elevated questionnaire score were diagnosed with PS. Children testing positive for SAGEA were followed 3 months and then 1 year after diagnosis date to assess if patients underwent surgical intervention. Cognitive outcomes were assessed through school records both 1 year before and 1 year after completion of the overnight study. For analysis, children were grouped into those who had no abnormalities on overnight study (CO), those with PS, those with SAGEA who went untreated (NT), and those who were treated surgically (TR). Two-way analyses of variance, Newman-Keuls tests, and paired *t* tests were completed.

Of the 297 children tested, 66 met criteria for PS (22.2%) and 54 for SAGEA (18.1%). Twenty-four had surgical treatment for their disorder (TR), while 30 went untreated (NT). In comparing academic scores between groups, mean grades among the TR group increased significantly from first to second grade (2.43 ± 0.17 in first grade vs. 2.87 ± 0.19, $p < 0.001$). Only 2 of the 24 children in the TR group remained in the lowest 10%ile following intervention. Those in the NT group had no significant improvement in grades. Upon follow-up questionnaire administration to parents of NT and TR children, untreated children scored significantly higher, indicating worse symptoms, compared to surgically treated children (10.4 ± 2.6 in NT vs. 1.7 ± 2.4 in TR, $p < 0.001$).

Gozal D. Sleep-Disordered Breathing and School Performance in Children. Pediatrics. 1998 Sep 1;102(3):616–20.

The Bogalusa Heart Study: Childhood weight status and cardiovascular risk factors

1. In children, a higher body mass index (BMI) was associated with increased frequencies of cardiac risks factors

2. Among the cardiovascular risk factors assessed, overweight youth had the highest odds of having elevated insulin levels.

Original Date of Publication: June 1999

Study Rundown: The Bogalusa Heart Study was initiated in 1972 in Bogalusa, Louisiana, and stands as the longest running biracial study of children. Although an abnormal BMI was an established risk factor for multiple adverse health outcomes at the time of the investigation, this study added insight into the connection between early weight risk and cardiovascular health. It was also one of the first trials to factor sex, race/ethnicity, and age into analysis. Eleven percent of the 9167 children included in the study were overweight. Cardiac risk factors increased in prevalence as BMI increased beyond the 85%ile, with considerable risk elevations as BMI increased from the 95%ile to 97%ile and beyond. Among the risk factors, overweight youth were found to have the highest odds of having elevated insulin levels. Being overweight was considered an effective screening tool for cardiovascular risk with over 50% of overweight participants having at least 1 risk factor (positive predictive value [PPV] > 50%). Differences between African Americans and whites were noted when examining diastolic blood pressure (DBP) and insulin levels. Low density lipoprotein cholesterol (LDLC), DBP, and systolic blood pressure (SBP) differed significantly between age groups. While BMI is a useful surrogate for assessing weight status, it has limited accuracy among certain populations including those with very high or low levels of muscle mass. Despite this limitation, this study produced results agreeing with previous findings and strengthened the evidence to support prevention and early intervention for overweight youth.

In-Depth [cross-sectional study]: Nine thousand one hundred sixty-seven children, 5-17 years of age (mean age = 11.9 years; 48% female; 36% black) were drawn from 7 cross-sectional studies completed during 1973-1994 within the larger Bogalusa Heart Study. Age, race/ethnicity, weight, height, triceps and subscapular skinfolds measurements, total cholesterol (TC), triglycerides (TG),

LDLC, high-density lipoprotein cholesterol (HDLC), SBP, DBP, and fasting insulin levels were all included in analysis. Logistic regression analyses were completed to assess the association between risk factors and BMI. Eleven percent of study participants were categorized as overweight with a BMI greater than the 95%ile. As BMI increased, the number of associated risk factors increased. For example, among all children, elevated insulin levels, defined as above the 95th age-, race-, and sex-adjusted percentile, increased from 1% to 27% as BMI increased from 25 to > 97%ile with the largest increase observed between the increase from 95-97 to > 97%ile (10% vs. 27% among 5-10 year olds, 10% vs. 25% among 11-17 year olds). The sensitivity of being overweight and having a cardiovascular risk factor varied from 23% for elevated DBP to 62% for elevated insulin levels. The PPV of being overweight also varied from 9% for elevated DBP to 24% for elevated triglycerides (TG > 130mg/dL). The largest calculated odds ratios (ORs) were seen with elevated insulin levels as overweight youth were 12.6 times more likely to have elevated insulin than youth of normal weight. Being overweight was considered effective in screening for cardiovascular risk with 61% of overweight 5- to 10 year-olds having at least 1 elevated risk factor and a 58% PPV of being overweight and having cardiovascular risk factors among 11- to 17-year-olds. Significant differences between race/ethnicity were seen between DBP and insulin levels with whites having elevated ORs in both when compared to blacks. As indicated by X^2 values above 20.5, elevated LDLC, SBP, and DBP values differed significantly by age group ($p < 0.001$). Additional analyses indicated that triceps skinfold thickness did not add additional information when BMI was known.

Freedman DS, Dietz WH, Srinivasan SR, Berenson GS. The Relation of Overweight to Cardiovascular Risk Factors Among Children and Adolescents: The Bogalusa Heart Study. Pediatrics. 1999 Jun 1;103(6):1175–82.

Kocher Criteria differentiates pediatric septic arthritis and transient synovitis of the hip

1. Children with septic arthritis of the hip could be accurately differentiated from transient synovitis of the hip on the basis of the presence or absence of four major clinical predictors: fever, lack of weight-bearing status, erythrocyte sedimentation rate (ESR) > 40 mm/hr, and leukocytosis greater than 12 000 cells/cm^3.

2. Several other variables increased the odds of septic arthritis, including radiographic evidence of joint effusion, fever with chills, female gender, and recent antibiotic use.

Original Date of Publication: December 1999

Study Rundown: When evaluating a child with acute hip pain, only a few diagnoses can be made primarily by radiographic appearance, including Legg-Calve-Perthes disease, slipped capital femoral epiphysis, and fracture. Differentiating between septic arthritis and transient synovitis of the hip remains a diagnostic dilemma. The appropriate management of septic arthritis requires timely initiation of intravenous antibiotics and surgical drainage of the infected joint, thus making rapid and accurate diagnosis vital in avoiding both the sequelae of a failure to treat and of the morbidity associated with treatment of those without a septic joint.

In the reviewed article, Kocher et al. set out to simplify the diagnostic process in differentiating between a septic hip and transient synovitis by developing and validating a set of clinical criteria by which an individual's risk for septic arthritis may be stratified. In a retrospective review of all cases of an acutely irritable hip in children between 1979 and 1996 at a major pediatric tertiary-care hospital, several variables were found to significantly differ between those with true septic arthritis and those with transient synovitis of the hip. The four variables that were most predictive of true septic arthritis were a history of fever, an inability to bear weight on the affected hip, an ESR greater than 40 mm/hr, and a leukocytosis of greater than 12 000 cells/cm^3. Patients with all four criteria were 99.6% likely to have septic arthritis, while those with zero of four criteria had septic arthritis effectively ruled out with less than 0.2% probability of an infected joint. Patients with true septic arthritis were also significantly more likely to be female, present with chills, have recent antibiotic use, and demonstrate radiographic evidence of a joint effusion at the affected site, although these features were not included in the final clinical decision algorithm due to reduced specificity. Following publication, Caird et al. prospectively evaluated these criteria in a separate pediatric population, finding that the algorithm remained effective, but inclusion of a C-reactive protein > 2.0 mg/dL was additionally predictive of septic arthritis as a fifth criterion and was independently more valuable than an ESR. However, with further prospective use of the Kocher criteria in alternative pediatric populations, such as that published in Luhmann et al. and rebutted by Kocher et al. in 2004, the clinical prediction rules demonstrated reduced but still reasonable diagnostic performance, possibly due to suboptimal modeling of the selected variables within a new population. This algorithm was the first and remains a lasting and effective evidence-based guideline for the clinical differentiation of septic arthritis from transient synovitis of the hip across multiple pediatric populations.

In-Depth [retrospective cohort]: A total of 282 children presenting with acute irritability of the hip between 1979 and 1996 at a major Northeastern pediatric hospital were included in this retrospective review. Patients were excluded if they presented with complicating factors, including immunocompromised status, renal failure, neonatal sepsis, postoperative hip infection, juvenile rheumatoid arthritis, subsequent development of Legg-Calve-Perthes disease or associated proximal femoral osteomyelitis. Patients were stratified into one of three categories of disease: True septic arthritis (38 patients), proven by positive bacterial growth from synovial fluid aspirate with associated fluid white blood cell (WBC) count > 50 000 cells/cm^3; presumed septic arthritis (44 patients) on the basis of a synovial fluid aspirate with > 50 000 WBCs/cm^3 but no bacterial growth on culture; or transient synovitis of the hip (86 patients), with < 50 000 WBCs/cm^3 on synovial aspiration, no bacterial growth on culture, and spontaneous resolution of symptoms without antibiotics or surgery. Multiple clinical variables were tracked to determine which differed most significantly between groups by univariate analysis and multiple logistic regression analysis.

Overall, children with true septic arthritis were significantly more likely to be female, and present with a history positive for fever > 38.5 degrees Celsius, chills, recent antibiotic use, radiographic evidence of a joint effusion, non-weight bearing status on the affected side, elevated ESR, reduced hematocrit, and leukocytosis (p < 0.05 for all). On further analysis, the four variables that were most predictive of septic arthritis formed the final Kocher Criteria and included fever > 38.5C, non-weight bearing status, ESR > 40 mm/hr, and leukocytosis > 12 000 WBC/cm^3. Meeting zero of the four criteria effectively ruled out septic arthritis (probability < 0.2%), while meeting all four criteria effectively ruled it in (probability of 99.6%).

With three of four criteria met, probability of disease was 93.1%, which reduced to 40.0% for two criteria and 3% for one criteria.

Kocher MS, Zurakowski D, Kasser JR. Differentiating between septic arthritis and transient synovitis of the hip in children: An evidence-based clinical prediction algorithm. The Journal of Bone and Joint Surgery. 1999 Dec 1;81-A(12):1662–70.

Additional Review:

Kocher MS, Mandiga R, Murphy JM, Goldmann D, Harper M, Sundel R, et al. A clinical practice guideline for treatment of septic arthritis in children: Efficacy in improving process of care and effect on outcome of septic arthritis of the hip. The Journal of Bone and Joint Surgery. 2003 June 1;85-A(6):994–99.

Table 1. Kocher Criteria.

Luhmann SJ, Jones A, Schootman M, Gordon JE, Schoenecker PL, Luhmann JD. Differentiation between septic arthritis and transient synovitis of the hip in children with clinical prediction algorithms. The Journal of Bone and Joint Surgery. 2004 May 1;86-A(5):956–62.

Kocher Criteria

1. Non weight-bearing
2. Temp > 38.5 C/101.3 F
3. ESR > 40 mm/hr
4. WBC > 12 000 cells/mm^2

Antibiotic Group B Streptococcus prophylaxis linked with reduced neonatal infection

1. During the 1990-1998 study period, which included the 1996 initiation of national Group B Streptococcus (GBS) guidelines, a significant, 65% decrease in early-onset neonatal disease was observed.

2. During the study's final year, an estimated 3900 early-onset neonatal GBS cases, along with 200 early- and late-onset neonatal deaths, were estimated to have been prevented by the recommended antibiotic prophylaxis.

Original Date of Publication: January 2000

Study Rundown: With the identification of GBS as a maternally-transmitted pathogen leading to significant neonatal morbidity and mortality, the United States instituted a national advocacy group and guideline recommendations to prevent and manage perinatal GBS infection during the 1990s. This study was the first to assess trends in GBS disease following the issuance of 1996 American Academy of Pediatrics (AAP)-, American College of Obstetricians and Gynecologists-, and Centers for Disease Control (CDC)-approved guidelines instructing practitioners on intrapartum antibiotic prophylaxis. Based on a high transmission risk or positive 35-37 week screening, women received intrapartum antibiotics. Researchers found a significant, 65% reduction in GBS early-onset neonatal disease, defined as disease manifesting before 7 days of life, but no difference in neonatal disease diagnosed at 7-89 days of life. When these findings were projected upon 1998 national data, it was estimated that about 3900 early-onset cases and 200 deaths due to neonatal GBS infection had been prevented. A significant, 21% reduction in GBS disease among pregnant women and girls was also seen.

This study was limited in its generalizability due to lack of racial diversity, particularly in its low numbers of Hispanic participants and in the likely higher alertness of practitioners in the study to GBS positivity. However, this large, multi-state study did allow for assessment of the guidelines among many laboratory-confirmed GBS cases. With this research indicating the effectiveness of preventative strategies in decreasing early-onset neonatal GBS infection, continued efforts to promote prevention, appropriate antibiotic intervention, and to determine why these strategies fail was and still are necessary. Antibiotic resistance, lack of education, and decreased compliance continue to be problematic today. The 1996 guidelines were later updated by the CDC in 2010 and an AAP policy statement followed in 2011.

In-Depth [cross-sectional study]: During 1993 to 1998, GBS cases in Maryland, California, Georgia, Tennessee, Connecticut, Minnesota, Oregon, and New York were reported through a laboratory-based surveillance protocol. Additional data from California, Georgia, and Tennessee for 1990-1993 were included to provide a greater temporal context for GBS rates prior to guideline initiation. GBS cases were reported if individuals tested positive for GBS in normally sterile body fluid. GBS isolated from either placenta, amniotic fluid, or urine was not included. GBS disease was classified by time of onset as follows: early-onset neonatal disease (< 7 days old), late-onset (7-89 days old), childhood disease (90 days to 14 years of age), or adult disease (> 15 years old). Disease in pregnancy was considered separately. National estimates of GBS incidence were calculated based on known population sizes.

During the 5-year study period, 7867 GBS cases were reported (84% from blood, 4% from cerebrospinal fluid, 4% from joint fluid, and the remainder from other sites). Early-onset disease remained constant throughout 1990-1993 and then declined by a significant 65% during 1993-1998 (1.7 per 1000 births in 1993 vs. 0.6 per 1000 in 1998, $X^2 = 121.0$, $p < 0.001$). African Americans had higher early-onset disease rates, but also underwent a steeper reduction during the study period than whites, with a 75% reduction in the difference between the 2 groups by 1998. No significant change in late-onset disease incidence took place in 1990-1998. Among pregnant women and girls, a significant, 21% reduction in GBS incidence was seen over the study course (0.29 per 1000 births in 1993 vs. 0.23 per 1000 births in 1998, $X^2 = 4.86$, $p < 0.03$). After projecting 1998 incidence from the selected states onto national data, it was estimated 3900 neonatal early-onset GBS cases and 200 early- and late-onset neonatal deaths were prevented through antibiotic usage.

Schrag SJ, Zywicki S, Farley MM, Reingold AL, Harrison LH, Lefkowitz LB, et al. Group B Streptococcal Disease in the Era of Intrapartum Antibiotic Prophylaxis. New England Journal of Medicine. 2000 Jan 6;342(1):15–20.

Parental input in oncology-related palliation and pain relief for children

1. When interviews with parents whose children died from cancer were compared to patient hospital records, researchers found that many children experienced substantial suffering toward the end of life with poorly managed symptoms.

2. There was significant discordance between parent and physician reports of patient discomfort, with parents being significantly more likely to report patient symptoms than physicians.

Original Date of Publication: February 2000

Study Rundown: While researchers previously investigated the quality of end-of-life care among adult oncology patients, no study explored palliative care for children. This study was the first to delve into the state of pediatric end-of-life care through interviews with parents whose children died from cancer and retrospective chart analysis of patient care. Results demonstrated that many children received aggressive care at the end of their lives, with nearly half dying in the hospital and many dying in the intensive care unit. In addition, 89% of children experienced substantial suffering in their last month of life, most of which went unresolved despite treatment attempts.

Through this retrospective analysis, it was found that parents were significantly more likely to report their child's fatigue, poor appetite, constipation, and diarrhea when compared to physicians. Parents were also significantly more likely to report their child to be in pain if they believed the child's oncologist to be less involved in direct end-of-life care. These findings suggested that care providers may not be optimally treating these patients due a lack of recognized patient discomfort. Also, results showed that earlier discussions of hospice care were significantly associated with parental descriptions of children as calm in the last month of life.

This study was limited by use of parental report and chart review. However, its findings had many implications for patient care. By encouraging early, direct discussions between physicians and patient families regarding symptoms, discomfort, and goals of care, researchers recognized that patient quality of life might improve as a patient progressed toward the end of life. Today, palliative care is better defined as care of the whole patient, involving an interdisciplinary team that is introduced to patients and their families at the time of a serious diagnosis

In-Depth [retrospective analysis]: A total of 103 parents (91% white, 86% female) of children who had died of cancer during 1990-1997 were interviewed by researchers based out of a large, tertiary children's hospital. The interview information was then combined with data obtained from chart reviews. In interviews, parents were asked to assess many aspects of his or her child's end-of-life care including, but not limited to, physical symptoms and suffering during the last month of life, treatment of these symptoms, and the perception of physician involvement at the end of life. Chart review was then completed to collect demographic data along with treatments administered, cancer care course, symptoms in the last month of life, cause and place of death, medical interventions close to the time of death, and discussions regarding end-of-life planning such as hospice and do not resuscitate orders (DNR).

Interviewed parents had children who died of leukemia or lymphoma (n = 50, 49%), brain tumors (n = 23, 22%), or other solid tumors (n = 30, 29%). Eighty-one children died from progressive disease, 21 died from treatment-related complications, with 1 child's records unavailable for review. On chart review, physicians discussed hospice care with 66% of children with progressive disease. Sixty-six percent of children had DNR orders in their charts. Nearly half, 49%, of patients died in the hospital and, of those, 45% died in the intensive care unit. From parental interview, nearly 100% of patients had at least 1 symptom toward the end of life with fatigue, pain, dyspnea, and poor appetite being the most common. Eighty-nine percent of children had "a great deal" of suffering as a result of 1 or more symptoms. Pain and dyspnea were the most commonly treated symptoms (76% and 65%, respectively), but few patients experienced relief from treatment (27% and 16%, respectively). During the last month of life, 21% of children were described by parents as being afraid. With regard to end-of-life discussions, the length of time between hospice care discussions and death were significantly longer for children whose parents found them to be calm during most of the last month of life ($p = 0.01$). Based upon parental report, lack of oncologist involvement in end-of-life care was associated with significantly more pain in the last month of a child's life (OR 2.6, 95%CI 1.0-6.7). In comparing parental interview to chart review, parents reported fatigue ($p < 0.001$), poor appetite ($p < 0.001$), constipation ($p < 0.001$) and diarrhea ($p < 0.05$) in their children significantly more often than physicians.

Wolfe J, Grier HE, Klar N, Levin SB, Ellenbogen JM, Salem-Schatz S, et al. Symptoms and Suffering at the End of Life in Children with Cancer. New England Journal of Medicine. 2000 Feb 3;342(5):326–33

Laboratory values and treatment associated with DKA-related cerebral edema in children

1. Among children admitted diabetic ketoacidosis (DKA) management, elevated serum urea nitrogen concentrations and low partial pressures of carbon dioxide were associated with a significantly increased risk of developing cerebral edema.

2. Lack of pronounced serum sodium rise and the use of bicarbonate for treatment were also associated with significantly increased cerebral edema risk.

Original Date of Publication: January 2001

Study Rundown: Among children presenting in DKA, about 1% will experience cerebral edema. At the time of this study, mortality occurred in 40-90% of these individuals, accounting for 50-60% of type 1 diabetes mellitus (T1DM)-related childhood deaths. However, before this study's publication, there was limited information regarding cerebral edema risk factors among children with T1DM. Researchers found that elevated serum urea nitrogen concentrations and low partial pressures of carbon dioxide were associated with significantly increased risk of children hospitalized for DKA developing cerebral edema. In addition, lack of pronounced increases in serum sodium with treatment and use of bicarbonate were also associated with significantly increased risk of cerebral edema development.

This study was limited by an inability to detect the possible influence of other confounders as well as to detect the potential role of variables that did not produce noticeable changes in clinical data. This was the first large, controlled study to investigate the role of cerebral edema-associated risk factors among children treated for DKA. It was proposed that each of these factors likely resulted in the development of cerebral edema due to potential contributions to cerebral ischemia. While this study helped lay the foundation for our understanding of cerebral edema risk, no exact pathophysiologic mechanism has been confirmed. Other risk factors found not to be statistically significant in this study have proven influential in subsequent studies. These include young age and DKA as the first presenting symptom of DM.

In-Depth [case-control study]: Through a review of records at 10 pediatric hospitals, all children with DM-related cerebral edema treated between1982-1997 were included in analyses. The record of any child who had died during admission in this time period was also included in analysis. Records of included patients had evidence of confirmed DKA (serum glucose > 300 mg/dL, venous pH < 7.25 or serum bicarbonate < 15 mmol/L, and urine ketones), altered mental status, and a radiologic or pathologic diagnosis of cerebral edema or clinical improvement following cerebral edema treatment. For each child with cerebral edema, 6 control patients were included for comparison: 3 patients selected randomly among the other patients with DKA and 3 patients matched by age among the other patients with DKA. Demographics, treatments, laboratory values, and calculated laboratory results were included for analysis. One-way analysis of variance was completed to analyze continuous variables and X^2 tests were used to analyze categorical variables.

Of the 6977 DKA-related admissions to the 10 centers, 61 (0.9%) had cerebral edema. After controlling for covariates, comparison of children with cerebral edema to the random control group revealed a 1.7 times increased cerebral edema risk per increase in urea nitrogen of 9 mg/dL from presentation. A 3.4 times increased risk of cerebral edema per 7.8 mmHg decrease in carbon dioxide partial pressure from presentation was also appreciated (RR 1.7, p < 0.003; RR 3.4, p < 0.001, respectively). Multivariate analysis, showed a significantly increased risk of cerebral edema with high urea nitrogen (RR 1.8 per 9 mg/dL increase, p < 0.01), low arterial carbon dioxide (RR 2.7 per decrease of 7.8 mmHg, p < 0.01), slow increases in serum sodium concentration during therapy (RR 0.6 per increase of 5.8 mmol/L/hr, p < 0.0.5), and bicarbonate treatment (RR 4.2, p < 0.01).

Glaser N, Barnett P, McCaslin I, Nelson D, Trainor J, Louie J, et al. Risk Factors for Cerebral Edema in Children with Diabetic Ketoacidosis. New England Journal of Medicine. 2001 Jan 25;344(4):264–9.

Earlier diagnosis and improved cystic fibrosis nutritional status with newborn screening

1. Among infants randomized to undergo either newborn screen with cystic fibrosis (CF) testing or undergo normal pediatric surveillance, those who underwent the screen were diagnosed with CF significantly earlier.

2. Infants diagnosed based on surveillance were significantly more likely to be severely malnourished compared to those diagnosed by newborn screen.

Original Date of Publication: January 2001

Study Rundown: CF is an autosomal recessive disease responsible for multi-system organ involvement most commonly secondary to impaired chloride channel transport. At the time of this study's publication, many patients were diagnosed through sweat testing following recognition of signs/symptoms linked to the disease. In 1996, the average age of diagnosis was 5 years and this delay in diagnosis was associated with worse nutritional status and lung disease. This clinical trial investigated the potential benefits of neonatal screening on nutritional outcomes. Infants were diagnosed using testing for elevated immunoreactive trypsinogen (IRT), which was later modified to include both IRT and DNA testing. A total incidence rate of 1:3938 was seen in the cohort, and those who underwent newborn screening were diagnosed significantly earlier than those diagnosed by surveillance. In addition, those who were diagnosed on newborn screening were at significantly lower risk of being severely malnourished when compared to those diagnosed by surveillance.

While strengthened by a randomized design, the study was limited secondary to the change of diagnostic technique partway through the study. Regardless, the study aided in establishing the value of early diagnosis and early intervention in the care of children with CF. Since the introduction of newborn screening, every state in the United States has adopted use of either IRT or combined IRT-DNA testing. Today, nearly 60% of cases of CF are diagnosed by newborn screen, increased from under 10% in 2001, with the average age of diagnosis under 2 years.

In-Depth [randomized controlled trial]: From April 1985 to 1998, 2 CF centers along with a newborn screening program in Wisconsin began a randomized clinical trial examining the effects of early screening for CF on nutritional and pulmonary outcomes. Children were randomized to either undergo newborn screening or traditional pediatric follow-up (i.e., monitoring for signs or symptoms of CF during acute and health maintenance visits). Initial newborn screening included the use of IRT analysis, with testing later modified in June 1991 to add DNA testing for ΔF508, the most common CF-related genetic mutation. All children were screened and then randomized such that the control group's lab results were blinded. These results were eventually unblinded. Positive testing on either the IRT or DNA testing in the screening group resulted in pediatrician-parental contact with the recommendation for a follow-up sweat test when the child was 4 to 6 weeks of age. Children with sweat chloride tests of ≥ 60 mEq/L were diagnosed with CF, those with 40-60 mEq/L were considered to have an indeterminate diagnosis, and those with sweat tests ≤ 40 mEq/L were not diagnosed with CF. Patients presenting with meconium ileus were also assigned to the "other CF group." Children diagnosed with CF (both through newborn screening and at a later age) were given the option to enroll for study inclusion. They then underwent standardized nutritional and pulmonary assessments along with therapeutic disease management starting at the time of diagnosis. Surveillance of patient outcomes was performed through healthcare provider-completed surveys and review of birth and death certificates.

A total of 650 341 babies born during the study period were randomized to either undergo newborn CF screening or be in the control group. Overall, 325 121 infants were included in the screening group and 325 120 were included in the control group. Among those in the screening group, 220 862 underwent IRT and 104 308 underwent both IRT and DNA testing. A total of 157 patients were identified as having CF. Additional diagnoses on autopsy and from sweat chloride testing in the 40-60 mEq/L range, resulted in a total incidence of CF in this cohort was 1:3938. Children who underwent initial newborn screen (n = 56) were diagnosed significantly earlier than those in the control group (n = 107; 13 ± 37 weeks in screening group vs. 107 ± 117 in control group, $p < 0.001$). At the time of diagnosis, those screened had significantly higher length ($p < 0.001$), weight ($p < 0.05$), and head circumference ($p < 0.01$) than those in the control group. Throughout the study, significantly greater odds of being severely malnourished, as determined by having a weight and height below the 10th percentile, was observed in the control group when compared to the screening group (odds ratio for weight = 4.12, 95%CI 1.64-10.38; odds ratio for height = 4.62, 95%CI 1.70-12.61). Odds of being below the 10th percentile for height disappeared by 9 years of age for those who were screened early.

Farrell PM, Kosorok MR, Rock MJ, Laxova A, Zeng L, Lai H-C, et al. Early Diagnosis of Cystic Fibrosis Through Neonatal Screening Prevents Severe Malnutrition and Improves Long-Term Growth. Pediatrics. 2001 Jan 1;107(1):1–13.

MMR vaccine not associated with autism

1. Among children born in Denmark during a 7-year study period, no increase in risk of developing autism was seen in those who were vaccinated against measles, mumps, and rubella (MMR) relative to unvaccinated children.

Original Date of Publication: November 2002

Study Rundown: There is considerable controversy surrounding the possible connection between the MMR vaccine and the development of autism in children. While previous studies did not find any associations, this was the first study on this topic to have adequate statistical power and appropriate design. In this retrospective cohort study, 537 303 files from children born in Denmark were analyzed to determine the relative risk of autism with MMR vaccination. No increased risk of autism diagnosis was seen among those receiving the vaccine nor was any association between the timing of vaccination and autism risk observed. This study provided strong evidence from a large cohort sample that an association between MMR vaccination and autism risk does not exist. Historically, the authors noted that the increase in autism incidence occurred much later than the release of the MMR vaccine - a temporal rift that makes a cause and effect relationship unlikely.

In-Depth [retrospective cohort]: Records from national registries of all children born between 1991 and 1998 in Denmark were studied and MMR vaccination status at 15 months of age, the typical age of first dose completion, was recorded. The primary outcome investigated was autism diagnosis. In total, 537 303 children, 440 655 vaccinated and 96 649 unvaccinated, were included in the study. Among those, 5811 children were diagnosed with autism or an autism-related disorder. A subgroup of diagnosed cases were validated with 93% meeting the Diagnostic and Statistic Manual of Mental Disorders-IV's criteria for autistic disorders. A log-linear Poisson regression model was used to assess the RR associated with the vaccine. When adjusted for potential confounding factors such as demographics and family socioeconomic status, no increase in relative risk of autism or related disorders was seen among those who received the vaccination (aRR 0.92, 95%CI 0.68-1.24 for autism and aRR = 0.83, 95%CI 0.65-1.07 for other autism-spectrum disorders). No associations were found between autism development and age at vaccination, time since vaccination, or year of vaccination.

Madsen KM, Hviid A, Vestergaard M, Schendel D, Wohlfahrt J, Thorsen P, et al. A Population-Based Study of Measles, Mumps, and Rubella Vaccination and Autism. New England Journal of Medicine. 2002 Nov 7;347(19):1477–82.

Clinical prediction rule stratifies pediatric bacterial meningitis risk

1. A Bacterial Meningitis Score (BMS) of 0 accurately identified all children with aseptic meningitis in the study's validation group.

2. The negative predictive value of a BMS score of 0 was 100% with a specificity of 73% in predicting bacterial meningitis. A BMS score of ≥ 2 was found to have a sensitivity and positive predictive value of 87% in predicting bacterial meningitis.

Original Date of Publication: October 2002

Study Rundown: Bacterial meningitis is associated with significant morbidity and mortality. At the time of this study, many children found to have CSF pleocytosis were admitted for intravenous antibiotic therapy and blood culture monitoring while distinguishing bacterial from aseptic meningitis. As individuals diagnosed with viral meningitis may be managed as outpatients, this study sought to create and validate a clinical prediction rule to aid in identifying patients at low risk for bacterial meningitis. This was the first study to create such a scoring system in the post-Haemophilus Influenzae Type b vaccination era. Researchers were able to create a scoring system that accurately stratified patients at low and high risk for bacterial meningitis diagnosis. This study was limited in both its design and potential referral bias as evidenced by the high percentage of patient participants with bacterial meningitis (18%). Through use of this prediction rule, clinicians may be able to better identify patients who could be cared for outside of the hospital setting. Of note, this scoring system was further validated in a follow-up analysis published in JAMA in 2007.

In-Depth [retrospective cohort]: A total of 696 patients from 29 days to 19 years old diagnosed with bacterial, viral, fungal, or tuberculous meningitis as identified by hospital diagnostic codes were recruited from 8 years of hospital records at a large, pediatric hospital. Patients were randomized into either a derivation or validation set. Patients were considered to have bacterial meningitis if their CSF sample grew bacteria or if they had CSF pleocytosis with a positive blood culture or positive CSF latex agglutination test. Patient charts were reviewed and analyzed for information regarding CSF characteristics, seizure occurrence, complete blood count data, CSF and blood culture results, and latex agglutination testing. One hundred and twenty-five (18%) of the patients identified were diagnosed with bacterial meningitis and 571 (82%) with aseptic meningitis.

Positive gram stain, CSF protein $\geq$ 80 mg/dL, seizure upon or prior to presentation, peripheral ANC $\geq$ 10,000 cells/mm^3, and CSF ANC $\geq$ 10,000 cells/mm^3 were identified as predictors of bacterial meningitis, with positive gram stain as the most significant predictor. A BMS ranging from 0 to 6 was created with presence of each predictor receiving 1 point except for a positive gram stain, which received 2 points. When applied to the validation set participants, a score of 0 accurately identified all children with aseptic meningitis and did not misclassify any cases of bacterial meningitis. The negative predictive value of a BMS score of 0 was 100% for bacterial meningitis with a specificity of 73%. A BMS score of $\geq$ 2 was found to have a sensitivity and positive predictive value of 87% in predicting bacterial meningitis.

Nigrovic LE, Kuppermann N, Malley R. Development and Validation of a Multivariable Predictive Model to Distinguish Bacterial From Aseptic Meningitis in Children in the Post-Haemophilus influenzae Era. Pediatrics. 2002 Oct 1;110(4):712–9.

Nigrovic LE, Kuppermann N, Macias CG, et al. Clinical prediction rule for identifying children with cerebrospinal fluid pleocytosis at very low risk of bacterial meningitis. JAMA. 2007 Jan 3;297(1):52–60.

RSV positivity associated with less serious bacterial infection risk in infants

1. Respiratory syncytial virus (RSV)-positive infants were significantly less likely to have a serious bacterial infection (SBI) relative to those who tested negative.

2. Infants ≤ 28 days old were significantly more likely to have an SBI than older infants.

Original Date of Publication: June 2004

Study Rundown: SBIs, such as meningitis and bacteremia, are sources of significant morbidity and mortality in febrile infants under 2 months of age. While many studies had investigated the risk factors for SBIs, at the time of this study no groups had investigated the potential interaction of viral infection in febrile infants with a simultaneous SBI. This study investigated the risk of SBI in febrile infants diagnosed with RSV infections. RSV was associated with a lower risk of concurrent SBI; however, many RSV-positive infants had simultaneous urinary tract infections (UTIs) and younger infants (≤28 days old) were found to have statistically similar SBI rates regardless of RSV positivity. Potential clinical implications of this study include limiting testing for infants > 1 month of age with RSV to urinalysis only, while continuing a full workup for younger infants regardless of their viral status.

In-Depth [cross-sectional study]: Data from 1248 patients, ≤ 60 days of age and with rectal temperatures ≥ 38°C, were gathered from 8 pediatric emergency departments over a period of 3 years. Patients underwent a history and physical examination, rapid RSV testing by nasopharyngeal aspirate, and further workup, treatment, and imaging at the discretion of their physician. Data was analyzed taking patients' RSV status into account while also considering the presence of SBI defined as bacterial meningitis, bacteremia, UTI, or bacterial enteritis. Over 11% of all study participants were found to have SBI with 0.7% having bacterial meningitis, 2% having bacteremia, 9.1% having UTI, and 1.9% having bacterial enteritis. Infants who tested positive for RSV were significantly less likely to have an SBI than those who tested negative (7% vs. 12.5%, RR 0.6, p < .05). Further analysis indicated that RSV-positive patients were at significantly lower risk for SBI. The highest concurrent bacterial infection was UTI, with 5.4% of RSV-positive infants having UTIs. In subanalyses, 82 RSV-positive infants ≤ 28 days old had SBIs; 6.1% of these infants had UTIs and 3.7% had bacteremia. There was no RSV-dependent significant difference between SBI rates in infants ≤ 28 days old. A total of 187 RSV-positive infants 29-60 days old were found to have an SBI rate of 5.5%, all of which were UTIs. Infants ≤ 28 days old were significantly more likely to have an SBI than older infants (10.1% vs. 5.5%).

Levine DA, Platt SL, Dayan PS, Macias CG, Zorc JJ, Krief W, et al. Risk of Serious Bacterial Infection in Young Febrile Infants With Respiratory Syncytial Virus Infections. Pediatrics. 2004 Jun 1;113(6):1728–34.

Computerized order system linked with increased pediatric mortality

1. The use of a computerized physician order entry (CPOE) program in a large, tertiary pediatric hospital was associated with over 3 times the risk of mortality when compared to patients admitted to the same center prior to CPOE implementation.

2. CPOE implementation resulted in increased physician time placing medication orders as opposed to providing patient care. It also increased delays in medication administration.

Original Date of Publication: December 2005

Study Rundown: CPOE systems were initially implemented to aid in reducing the tens of thousands of medical errors contributing to patient deaths across the United States. In 2002, the implementation of a CPOE in a large, tertiary pediatric hospital resulted in a significant reduction of adverse drug events (ADEs). This study was one of the first to evaluate long-term outcomes following CPOE implementation by examining mortality rates among children admitted to the same facility from the 2002 study. Retrospective analysis comparing patients transferred to the hospital before and after CPOE administration revealed a significant increase in mortality risk associated with care post-CPOE. Researchers attributed this result to changes in patient care following the implementation, including increased physician time spent entering orders and new challenges in acquiring medications as drugs were located in the hospital pharmacy as opposed to at the bedside.

This study was limited by its conduction in a single medical center, its short evaluation of time post-CPOE (which might have largely been an adjustment period to the new system), and potential lack of generalizability. However, these findings highlighted how promising technologic advances could pose serious underlying consequences and that decreases in ADEs are not necessarily an indication of improved clinical outcomes. This study argued that technologic advances require careful, thorough evaluation in order to ensure that unexpected consequences do not negatively influence patient care. Current CPOE implementation involves active incorporation of the findings from this study to ensure effective prevention of potential complications.

In-Depth [retrospective analysis]: From October 1, 2001 to March 31, 2003, 1942 patients (55% male, median age = 9 months) were recruited upon arrival to a tertiary care center via interfacility transport. Overall, 1394 patients were admitted before CPOE implementation and 548 after. The clinical condition for admissions, patient demographics, clinical characteristics, and mortality for each patient were recorded. Between group differences were calculated using Mann-Whitney rank sum and X^2 or Fisher's tests. Odds ratios were calculated as well. Patients were transferred for the following conditions: airway- (42.6%), infectious disease- (34.9%), and central nervous system- (19.4%) related. A total of 75 children died during the study.

Mortality increased significantly following CPOE implementation (2.80% before vs. 6.57% after, $p < 0.001$). Odds of mortality were increased significantly if a patient experienced shock (OR 6.24, 95%CI 2.94-13.26), was treated following CPOE introduction (OR 3.71, 95%CI 2.13-6.46), or severe coma (OR 3.43, 95%CI 1.88-6.25). Additional adjustment for covariation maintained significance between CPOE and mortality (OR 3.28, 95%CI 1.94 - 5.55). Researchers reported differences in clinical care following CPOE initiation. As the new system did not allow for orders to be entered prior to patient arrival, physicians spent longer times entering requests into the system as opposed to the shorter times required for handwritten orders. In addition, nurses were no longer at the bedside readily administering medications as CPOE implementation required all medications to be located within the pharmacy.

Han YY, Carcillo JA, Venkataraman ST, Clark RSB, Watson RS, Nguyen TC, et al. Unexpected Increased Mortality After Implementation of a Commercially Sold Computerized Physician Order Entry System. Pediatrics. 2005 Dec 1;116(6):1506–12.

Antibiotic prophylaxis and UTI prevention in children

1. Among children with low grade vesicoureteral reflex (VUR) recruited following febrile urinary tract infection (UTI) and randomized to receive either antibiotic prophylaxis or no medication, no significant difference in UTI recurrence was noted between groups.

2. Male children experienced a significant reduction in subsequent UTIs if treated with prophylactic antibiotics.

Original Date of Publication: February 2008

Study Rundown: In the years leading up to this study, physicians often prescribed antibiotic prophylaxis to children at perceived increased risk for repeat UTIs, particularly those with VUR). As multiple UTIs have been linked to renal scarring and nephropathy, preventing recurrence is highly important. However, since previous studies indicated that antibiotics might be ineffective at preventing UTIs, this study took a prospective, randomized approach to investigate the effectiveness of prophylactic antibiotics in pediatric patients with mild VUR. This randomized, multi-center prospective study found no significant difference in repeat UTI among children with mild VUR who did or did not receive prophylactic antibiotics. A significant increase in the risk for a second UTI was seen in those with grade III mild VUR and significant reduction in repeat UTI with treatment was observed in males. This study was limited in its lack of a blinded approach, lack of placebo for the control group, along with the use of potentially contaminated urine specimens from urine bags and uncircumcised males. It also lacked assessment for antibiotic compliance.

This study raised questions regarding the necessity to prescribe prophylaxis for all young children following first febrile UTI and the need to obtain voiding cystourethrograms (VCUGs) for all children in order to determine VUR presence. As unnecessary treatment is linked to potential adverse drug effects coupled with organism resistance, careful consideration should be taken in prescribing antimicrobial medication. In the time since this study's publication, many research projects have investigated UTI risk in children. The most recent American Academy of Pediatrics (AAP) practice guidelines for UTI management in young children recommend renal and bladder ultrasound prior to VCUG and VCUG only if abnormal findings are found on ultrasound. Use of prophylactic antibiotics following initial UTI is not recommended, but potential further investigation of prophylaxis value among males with higher grade VUR is proposed.

In-Depth [randomized controlled trial]: From June 2001 to December 2004, 225 patients (31% male) 1 month to 3 years of age with low grade VUR diagnosed on VCUG following febrile UTI were recruited from 17 French pediatric facilities. VUR was graded by severity into grade I, grade II, or grade III VUR and grouped by laterality (unilateral or bilateral). Participants were randomized to receive either trimethoprim (2 mg/kg)/sulfamethoxazole (10 mg/kg), also known today as Bactrim (n = 103, 46%), or no medication (n = 122, 54%). Follow-up renal ultrasound (US) was performed 9 and, 18 months after study initiation, both US and VCUG were completed. UTI was a study endpoint with children who experienced a UTI, defined as $> 10^5$ bacteria per mL of urine, excluded from the study and the UTI noted.

Following study initiation, 50 children, 18 in the treatment group (17%) and 32 in the control group (26%), experienced a second UTI. There was no significant difference between the 2 groups in terms of UTI rates (p = 0.15). There was also no significant difference between groups regarding the diagnosis of febrile UTI (13 or 13% in treatment group vs. 19 or 16% of the control group, p = 0.52). The majority of UTI recurrence occurred in females (78%). Males who received prophylactic treatments had a significantly lower rate of UTIs than those who went untreated (39, 57% in untreated vs. 30, 43% in treated, p < 0.05). This effect was not seen among females. No significant differences were seen between groups when analyzed by VUR grading or by VUR laterality. Multiple regression analysis indicated that grade III VUR was a significant risk factor for repeat UTI (p < 0.01).

Roussey-Kesler G, Gadjos V, Idres N, Horen B, Ichay L, Leclair MD, et al. Antibiotic Prophylaxis for the Prevention of Recurrent Urinary Tract Infection in Children With Low Grade Vesicoureteral Reflux: Results From a Prospective Randomized Study. The Journal of Urology. 2008 Feb 1;179(2):674–9.

PECARN Prediction rules for children at a low risk of clinically-important traumatic brain injury

1. The absence of 6 established predictors was found to have a near 100% negative predictive value (NPV) for clinically-important traumatic brain injury (ciTBI) when applied to head trauma patients under 18 years of age.

2. An algorithm was proposed, applying these predictors, in order to prevent physicians from using unnecessary computed tomography (CT) in pediatric patients at low risk for ciTBI.

Original Date of Publication: September 2009

Study Rundown: TBI continues to be one of the leading causes of morbidity and mortality among the pediatric population. At the time of this study, CT was the standard imaging technique for identifying TBI patients requiring intervention after head trauma. However, given the increase in malignancy risk associated with CT scans, investigators of this trial sought to identify patients at a low risk for ciTBI to potentially reduce CT imaging. Through the use of a large study cohort from various emergency departments, researchers analyzed the NPVs and sensitivities associated with a proposed "prediction rule", defined as having none of the identified ciTBI predictors versus having any cTBI predictors. The NPV and sensitivity of this prediction rule was then analyzed. Researchers found a NPV of > 98% and sensitivity > 94% in the prediction of ciTBI and TBI-negative CT scans in participants of all ages. Despite the fact that researchers did not CT scan all participants and sensitivities were not found to be 100%, this large, adequately powered study found similar results among both derivation and validation participant groups. With their findings, researchers were able to construct algorithms guiding physicians on appropriate CT scans use in head-injured patients. Altered mental status (AMS) and signs of skull fracture were established as branching points for patients at highest risk for ciTBI.

In-Depth [prospective cohort]: Data was analyzed from 42 412 patients under 18 years of age (mean 7.1 years ±5.5) who had experienced blunt head trauma within 24 hours from presentation and had Glasgow Coma Scale scores of 14-15. Patients were divided into derivation (n = 33 785) and validation groups (n = 8627) by recruitment date. ciTBI was defined as TBI-related death, need for neurosurgical intervention, intubation for more than one day following injury, or hospital admission for 2 or more nights. Research coordinators reviewed patient records during hospital admissions and completed telephone surveys of patient guardians for follow-up of patients discharged within 90 days of their ED visit. Predictors were chosen based upon established selection criteria and analyses were run to account for baseline development-related radiation risk with children under 2 years of age analyzed separately from those above 2 years of age.

Predictors for children under 2 years of age included: AMS, scalp hematoma, loss of consciousness (LOC), significant mechanism of injury (MOI), potential skull fracture, and changes in behavior. Predictors for those older than 2 years old included: AMS, LOC, vomiting, significant MOI, signs of basilar skull fracture, and headache. The number of predictors and risk of ciTBI in the derivation and validation groups were then compared. A total of 14 696 (35.5%) of participants underwent CT scan. Of these patients, 780 (5.2%) were found to have TBI on imaging and 376 (0.9%) with ciTBI (15.9% required surgical intervention, 0.02% required intubation for more than one day, 0% died from their injury). Among children under 2 years of age in the validation group, the prediction rule had an NPV of 100% and sensitivity of 100% for ciTBI. Among children over 2 years of age, this prediction rule had an NPV of 99.95% and sensitivity of 96.8% for ciTBI. In addition, among children under 2 years of age, the prediction rule had an NPV of 100% and sensitivity of 100% for patients having CT scan without evidence of TBI. Among children older than 2 years of age, the prediction rule had an NPV of 98.4% and sensitivity of 94% for patients having CT scans without evidence of TBI.

Kuppermann N, Holmes JF, Dayan PS, Hoyle JD, Atabaki SM, Holubkov R, et al. Identification of children at very low risk of clinically-important brain injuries after head trauma: a prospective cohort study. Lancet. 2009 Oct 3;374(9696):1160–70.

XIII. Surgery

"Nothing in life is to be feared, it is only to be understood. Now is the time to understand more, so that we may fear less."

- Marie Curie

The Lee index: Risk of perioperative cardiac events

1. The Lee index is a prospectively validated model that predicts the risk of a cardiac event in patients undergoing noncardiac surgery.

2. The 6 independent predictors are as follows: 1) high-risk surgery, 2) history of ischemic heart disease, 3) history of congestive heart failure, 4) history of cerebrovascular disease, 5) preoperative treatment with insulin, 6) preoperative serum creatinine > 2.0 mg/dL (>177 μmol/L).

Original Date of Publication: September 1999

Study Rundown: Patients undergoing noncardiac surgery are at risk of major cardiovascular complications. With the number of patients undergoing major noncardiac surgery consistently increasing, the incidence of surgery-associated cardiovascular complications has steadily risen. Numerous efforts have been made to identify potential interventions to reduce the likelihood of these complications, with several studies exploring the potential perioperative use of beta-blockers, calcium channel blockers, statins, aspirin, and cardiac revascularization. Several different groups have also attempted to develop tools to stratify patients with regards to their risk of perioperative cardiovascular complications. These include the Kumar, Detsky, and Goldman indices, as well as the American College of Cardiology/American Heart Association algorithm. The Revised Cardiac Risk Index, commonly referred to as the Lee index, was developed by modifying and simplifying the Goldman index. Initially published in 1999, the Lee index is considered the best validated tool for estimating perioperative cardiovascular risk. It uses six equally-weighted criteria to predict the likelihood of a cardiovascular event, and is widely used because of its simplicity.

In-Depth [prospective cohort]: Of the 4315 patients that took part in the study, 2893 were used in the development of the Lee index. The other 1422 patients took part in the prospective validation cohort. The major cardiovascular complications assessed were myocardial infarction, pulmonary edema, ventricular fibrillation/primary cardiac arrest, or complete heart block. Through logistic regression analyses, six predictors of perioperative major cardiovascular complications were identified: 1) high-risk surgery, 2) ischemic heart disease, 3) history of congestive heart failure, 4) history of cerebrovascular disease, 5) insulin therapy for diabetes, and 6) perioperative serum creatinine > 2.0 mg/dL (>177 μmol/L). The presence of any of these predictors contributes 1 point to the Lee index score. Higher Lee index scores were associated with higher rates of perioperative cardiac events.

Criteria	Points
High-risk surgery (e.g., emergency surgery, major thoracic procedures, cardiac procedures, aortic/major vascular procedures, procedures > 4 hours)	1
Ischemic heart disease	1
History of congestive heart failure	1
History of cerebrovascular disease	1
Insulin therapy for diabetes	1
Perioperative serum creatinine > 2.0 mg/dL (>177 μmol/L)	1

Table I. The Lee index.

Lee index score	Derivation cohort	Validation cohort
0	5/1071 (0.5%)	2/488 (0.4%)
1	14/1106 (1.3%)	5/567 (0.9%)
2	18/506 (3.6%)	17/258 (6.6%)
≥3	19/210 (9.1%)	12/109 (11.0%)

Table II. Cardiac event rates based on the Lee index score.

Lee TH, Marcantonio ER, Mangione CM, Thomas EJ, Polanczyk CA, Cook EF, et al. Derivation and Prospective Validation of a Simple Index for Prediction of Cardiac Risk of Major Noncardiac Surgery. Circulation. 1999 Sep 7;100(10):1043–9.

The NETT: Lung-volume-reduction surgery in emphysema

1. Lung-volume-reduction surgery significantly improved exercise capacity, but not overall survival, in patients with emphysema when compared with medical therapy.

2. Post hoc subgroup analyses showed that in patients with upper lobe emphysema and low baseline exercise capacity, lung-volume-reduction surgery significantly decreased mortality compared to medical therapy.

Original Date of Publication: May 2003

Study Rundown: While lung-volume-reduction surgery had been proposed as a treatment option for patients with severe emphysema, there was little evidence examining its effects. The National Emphysema Treatment Trial (NETT) was the first study to assess the morbidity, mortality, and therapeutic benefits of lung-volume-reduction surgery for emphysema patients. The findings of the trial showed that lung reduction significantly improved patients' exercise capacity compared to medical therapy, but did not significantly change overall survival. Post hoc subgroup analyses demonstrated that surgery significantly reduced mortality in patients with upper lobe emphysema and low exercise capacity and significantly increased mortality in patients with non-upper lobe emphysema and high exercise capacity when compared with medical treatment. A major criticism of this trial centers on the survival differences demonstrated in specific subgroups based on post hoc analyses, as opposed to predefined analyses. In summary, results of this study suggest that lung-volume-reduction surgery can significantly improve exercise capacity in patients with emphysema. While subgroup analyses did demonstrate survival benefits in patients with upper-lobe emphysema and low exercise capacity at baseline, these findings should be interpreted with caution given that they were performed post hoc.

In-Depth [randomized controlled trial]: This was a randomized, controlled trial that involved enrollment of 1218 patients from 17 clinics from across the United States. The list of inclusion and exclusion criteria is lengthy - generally, patients were eligible if they had clinical and radiological evidence of emphysema, were non-smokers for at least 4 months, completed all pre-rehabilitation assessments, and were considered fit for surgery. Each patient's distribution of emphysema (i.e., predominantly upper-lobe vs. predominantly non-upper-lobe) was determined by high-resolution CT. The primary outcome measures were overall mortality and maximal exercise capacity as measured by cycle ergometry. The secondary outcome measures included pulmonary function, distance walked within 6 minutes, and quality of life, as determined by self-administered questionnaires. Prior to randomization, patients underwent 6-10 weeks of supervised pulmonary rehabilitation. Patients were then randomly assigned to receive lung-volume-reduction surgery (i.e., bilateral stapled wedge resection via median sternotomy or video-assisted thoracic surgery) or medical therapy, and then re-evaluated after 6, 12, and 24 months of follow-up. Improved exercise capacity was defined as a 10 W increase in workload during cycle ergometry.

At 90 days, the mortality rate in the surgery group was significantly higher than the medical therapy group (7.9% vs. 1.3%, $p < 0.001$). There was no significant difference in mortality rates when comparing patients who underwent median sternotomy and video-assisted thoracic surgery (8.6% vs. 6.1%, respectively, $p = 0.33$). Total mortality rates were not significantly different between the two groups at a mean follow-up of 29.2 months (RR 1.01, $p = 0.90$). Patients receiving surgery had significantly improved exercise capacity as measured by cycle ergometry at 6 (28% vs. 4%, $p < 0.001$), 12 (22% vs. 5%, $p < 0.001$), and 24 months (15% vs. 3%, $p < 0.001$) than the medical-therapy group. Post hoc subgroup analyses revealed that surgery patients with upper-lobe disease and low-exercise capacity had a lower mortality rate (RR 0.47, $p = 0.005$) and experienced significantly improved exercise capacity (30% vs. 0%, $p = 0.005$) when compared with similar patients receiving medical therapy only. In patients with non-upper-lobe disease and high baseline exercise capacity, mortality was significantly higher in the surgical group (RR 2.06, $p = 0.02$).

Fishman A, Martinez F, Naunheim K, Piantadosi S, Wise R, Ries A, et al. A randomized trial comparing lung-volume-reduction surgery with medical therapy for severe emphysema. New England Journal of Medicine. 2003 May 22;348(21):2059–73.

The CARP trial: Preoperative revascularization prior to elective vascular surgery

1. In patients with stable coronary artery disease undergoing elective vascular surgery, preoperative revascularization did not significantly reduce short- or long-term mortality.

2. Patients undergoing revascularization experienced significant time delays prior to surgery.

Original Date of Publication: December 2004

Study Rundown: The Coronary Artery Revascularization Prophylaxis (CARP) trial demonstrated that in patients with stable coronary artery disease undergoing elective vascular surgery, pre-operative coronary revascularization did not provide any benefit in terms of reducing the risk of myocardial infarction or mortality (i.e., short- or long-term). Patients undergoing revascularization, however, waited significantly longer before having surgery compared to individuals who did not undergo revascularization (54 vs. 18 days). The findings of this study supported practice guidelines at the time, which recommended that coronary revascularization be reserved for patients with symptomatic coronary artery disease. Given the efficacy of perioperative beta-blockers and statins, medical management may be suitable alternatives to revascularization in patients with asymptomatic coronary artery disease.

In-Depth [randomized controlled trial]: Patients undergoing elective vascular surgery have a high prevalence of coronary artery disease and have high-risk of perioperative cardiac complications. The CARP trial, originally published in 2004 in NEJM, sought to explore the long-term effects of pre-operative coronary revascularization in patients undergoing elective vascular surgery, as retrospective studies until that point had mixed findings. Of the 5859 patients screened, 510 patients were eligible and underwent randomization. Patients were eligible if they were scheduled for elective vascular surgery (i.e., abdominal aortic aneurysm, severe occlusive arterial disease in the legs) and had stenosis of at least 70% in one or more major coronary artery that was suitable for revascularization (i.e., percutaneous intervention - PCI, coronary artery bypass graft - CABG). The primary endpoint was long-term mortality, as determined by follow-up. Of the 258 patients who were randomized to the revascularization group, 59% underwent

PCI, while 41% underwent CABG. The median time from randomization to surgery was 54 days in the revascularization group and 18 days in the non-revascularization group (p < 0.001). There were no significant differences between the groups in terms of the incidence of myocardial infarction or death in the 30 days following surgery. There were no significant differences between the two groups in terms of long-term mortality.

McFalls EO, Ward HB, Moritz TE, Goldman S, Krupski WC, Littooy F, et al. Coronary-Artery Revascularization before Elective Major Vascular Surgery. New England Journal of Medicine. 2004 Dec 30;351(27):2795–804.

The POISE trial: Perioperative use of beta-blockers

1. **The POISE trial was a randomized controlled trial exploring the effect of perioperative beta-blockade on cardiac death, nonfatal myocardial infarctions, and nonfatal cardiac arrest.**

2. **Perioperative oral extended-release metoprolol was found to reduce the risk of nonfatal myocardial infarction, while increasing the risk of stroke and mortality when compared to placebo.**

Original Date of Publication: May 2008

Study Rundown: With recent advances in non-cardiac surgery allowing for better treatment of diseases and improvements in quality of life, there have been substantial increases in the number of patients undergoing surgeries. These surgeries, however, are associated with increased risk of cardiac events. Numerous therapies have been investigated as prophylaxis against cardiac events in the perioperative state. The PeriOperative ISchemic Evaluation (POISE) trial was a randomized controlled trial published in 2008 exploring the effect of perioperative metoprolol in patients undergoing non-cardiac surgery. Perioperatively, beta-blockers are thought to protect against myocardial ischemia, while potentially increasing the risk of hypotension and bradycardia. In summary, the POISE trial demonstrated that perioperative beta-blockade significantly reduced the risk of perioperative myocardial infarctions compared to placebo. Patients treated with beta-blockers, however, also experienced significantly higher rates of stroke and death. Thus, patients must be carefully counseled regarding the risks and benefits of initiating perioperative beta-blockers for cardiac protection.

In-Depth [randomized controlled trial]: The final analysis involved 8351 patients from 190 hospitals in 23 countries randomized to either perioperative treatment with extended-release metoprolol or placebo. Patients were eligible for the trial if they were ≥45 years of age, were undergoing non-cardiac surgery, had expected hospitalization ≥24 hours, and had elevated risk of perioperative cardiac events (e.g., history of coronary artery disease, stroke, hospitalization for congestive heart failure, undergoing major vascular surgery). Exclusion criteria included heart rate < 50 beats per minute, second/third-degree heart block, asthma, treatment with a beta-blocker, and prior adverse reaction to beta-blocker. The primary outcome was a composite of cardiovascular death, non-fatal myocardial infarction, and non-fatal cardiac arrest at 30 days. Beta-blockers were found to significantly reduce the incidence of the primary endpoint compared to placebo (HR 0.84; 95%CI 0.70-0.99), due to a significant reduction in myocardial infarctions (HR 0.73; 95%CI 0.60-0.89). Compared to placebo, perioperative beta-blockade was also found to significantly increase the risk of stroke (HR 2.17; 95%CI 1.26-3.74), clinically significant hypotension (HR 1.55; 95%CI 1.38-1.74), and clinically significant bradycardia (HR 2.74; 95%CI 2.19-3.43). Furthermore, the metoprolol group had a significantly higher risk of mortality (HR 1.33; 95%CI 1.03-1.74).

POISE Study Group, Devereaux PJ, Yang H, Yusuf S, Guyatt G, Leslie K, et al. Effects of extended-release metoprolol succinate in patients undergoing non-cardiac surgery (POISE trial): a randomised controlled trial. Lancet. 2008 May 31;371(9627):1839–47.

The POISE 2 trial: Aspirin increases risk of major bleeding after noncardiac surgery

1. After noncardiac surgeries, patients treated with aspirin had significantly increased risk of major bleeding compared to those taking placebo.

2. There was no significant difference in death or nonfatal myocardial infarction between the aspirin and placebo groups.

Original Publication Date: April 2014

Study Rundown: After a noncardiac surgery, myocardial infarction is one of the most common major complications that patients can experience. It is suspected that surgery leads to greater platelet activation and higher risk of coronary thrombus, resulting in perioperative infarctions. A meta-analysis of data from randomized trials has shown that the use of aspirin in nonsurgical patients prevented cardiovascular events. Moreover, high-dose aspirin has not been shown to be superior to low-dose, but has been linked to higher risk of gastrointestinal adverse effects. Prior to this study, practice regarding the use of perioperative aspirin was inconsistent.

The Perioperative Ischemic Evaluation 2 (POISE-2) trial sought to determine whether low-dose aspirin would alter the risk of death or nonfatal myocardial infarction in patients who underwent noncardiac surgery. The results from this study show that there were no significant differences between the aspirin group and the placebo group in the composite endpoint of death or nonfatal myocardial infarction at 30 days. Treatment with aspirin, however, significantly increased the risk of major bleeding as compared with placebo, with the most common sites of bleeding being the surgical site and the gastrointestinal tract.

In-Depth [randomized controlled trial]: This trial utilized a 2×2 factorial design. A total of 10 010 patients from 23 countries were randomized to receive either aspirin or placebo, and clonidine or placebo. This study reported on the comparison between aspirin and placebo. Any patient undergoing noncardiac surgery, 45 years of age or older, expected to require at least overnight admission to hospital, and cardiovascular risk factors (e.g., coronary artery disease, peripheral vascular disease, stroke, undergoing major vascular surgery) was eligible for the study. Exclusion criteria included taking aspirin within 72 hours of surgery, hypersensitivity or known allergy to aspirin or clonidine, systolic blood pressure < 105 mm Hg, heart rate < 55 beats per minute without a pacemaker, and active peptic ulcer disease or gastrointestinal bleeding in the past 6 weeks. The primary outcome was a composite of death or nonfatal myocardial infarction in the 30 days after randomization.

The primary outcome occurred in 7.0% of the aspirin group and 7.1% in the placebo group (HR 0.99; 95%CI 0.86-1.15; p = 0.92). Major bleeding was significantly more common in patients taking aspirin (4.6% vs. 3.8%; HR 1.23; 95%CI 1.01-1.49; p = 0.04). Patients taking aspirin were found to have significantly higher risk of bleeding until post-operative day 6, at which point the bleeding risk was not significantly different between the 2 groups. Bleeding most commonly occurred at the surgical site (78.3%) and in the gastrointestinal tract (9.3%).

Devereaux PJ, Mrkobrada M, Sessler DI, Leslie K, Alonso-Coelle P, Kurz A, et al. Aspirin in patients undergoing noncardiac surgery. The New England Journal of Medicine. 2014;370(16):1494-1503.

The INVEST trial: Limited added utility of vertebroplasty versus sham surgery

1. Vertebroplasty does not reduce pain or pain-related disability in patients with osteoporotic compression vertebral body fractures when compared to sham surgery after 1 month.

Original Date of Publication: August 2009

Study Rundown: Osteoporotic fractures of vertebral bodies are often associated with pain and have historically been treated medically, including a combination physical therapy and pain management. These fractures are often a source of pain and disability for patients, and those who fail medical management may require hospitalization or extended care. Percutaneous vertebroplasty, which involves injecting medical cement (polymethylmethacrylate, or PMMA) into the fractured vertebral body, has typically been the next line of therapy in patients who have failed medical management. However, the efficacy of vertebroplasty in relieving pain in osteoporotic fractures has been limited to small case series and nonrandomized controlled studies. Prior to 2009, the best evidence of its efficacy was an open randomized trial involving 34 patients. Despite limited evidence, public institutions have recommended reimbursement for these procedures, which has led to increases in vertebroplasty volume.

The Investigational Vertebroplasty Safety and Efficacy Trial (INVEST) compared the efficacy of PMMA in patients with painful osteoporotic fractures against a sham procedure. The results of this trial showed no significant difference between groups in either the modified Roland-Morris Disability Questionnaire (RDQ) or in their pain scores after intervention, measured both at 24 hours and 1 month after intervention. These results suggest that there is no added beneficial effect in pain reduction or disability in patients undergoing vertebroplasty for osteoporotic compression fractures. A similar randomized controlled study published concurrently also examined vertebroplasty versus sham surgery, and found no beneficial effect of vertebroplasty at 1 week and up to 6 months after intervention. A Cochrane review confirmed these results in 2015, and concluded that that there was not enough evidence to support vertebroplasty for the treatment of osteoporotic vertebral fractures.

In-Depth [randomized controlled trial]: This prospective trial was conducted at 11 centers across the United States, United Kingdom, and Australia. These sites were chosen because they had established vertebroplasty practices, and a total of 1813 patients were screened for enrollment. Inclusion criteria included patients over the age of 50 that had one to three vertebral body compression fractures (between T4-L5 vertebral bodies) less than one year old who had failed medical therapy. Key exclusion criteria included evidence/suspicion of neoplasm in the target vertebral body, significant retropulsion of bony fragments, underlying hip fracture, active infection, and incorrigible bleeding diathesis. The main outcome measures were the modified RDQ and patients' rating of average back pain intensity during the preceding 24 hours on a 10-point scale. The minimal amount of change to be clinically significant was 30% in both pain intensity and RDQ. Patients were measured at various points up to one year after intervention, including 3, 14, and 90 days. The vertebroplasty interventionalists had performed a mean of 250 procedures (range of 50-800). All patients who were included in the study underwent fluoroscopically guided infiltration of skin and subcutaneous tissue with lidocaine and infiltration of the pedicle periosteum of the target vertebrae with bupivacaine. Patients were then randomized to either full vertebroplasty or the sham intervention (control procedure). Patients undergoing vertebroplasty had PMMA infused until it reached the posterior aspect of the vertebral body or it entered a paravertebral space. Patients were allowed to cross over to the other procedure 1 month or later after the intervention.

A total of 131 patients with similar baseline characteristics were enrolled between June 2004 and August 2008, with 68 patients who underwent vertebroplasty and 63 who underwent the control sham procedure. There was no significant difference between both groups with regards to either of the primary outcomes at one month. The mean RDQ score ($\pm$ SD) in the vertebroplasty group was 12.0 ± 6.3 versus 13.0 ± 6.4 in the control group (adjusted treatment effect: 0.7; 95%CI -1.3-2.8; $p = 0.49$). The mean pain-intensity rating was 3.9 ± 2.9 in the vertebroplasty group and 4.6 ± 3.0 in the control group (adjusted treatment effect: 3.9 ± 2.9, CI: -0.3-1.7; $p = 0.19$). Both groups had similar improvement in back related disability 3 days after intervention, which was maintained at 1 month. At 3 months, 9 patients in the vertebroplasty group and 32 patients in the control group had crossed over and underwent the alternative procedure ($p < 0.001$).

Kallmes DF, Comstock BA, Heagerty PJ, Turner JA, Wilson DJ, Diamond TH, et al. A Randomized Trial of Vertebroplasty for Osteoporotic Spinal Fractures. New England Journal of Medicine. 2009 Aug 6;361(6):569–79.

Additional Review:

Buchbinder R, Osborne RH, Ebeling PR, Wark JD, Mitchell P, Wriedt C, et al. A Randomized Trial of Vertebroplasty for Painful Osteoporotic Vertebral Fractures. New England Journal of Medicine. 2009 Aug 6;361(6):557–68.

The PANTER trial: Open necrosectomy vs. step-up approach for necrotizing pancreatitis

1. A minimally invasive step-up approach was associated with significantly reduced rates of major complications as compared to open necrosectomy in patients with necrotizing pancreatitis.

Original Date of Publication: April 2010

Study Rundown: Necrotizing pancreatitis with infected necrotic tissue is associated with high rates of both complication and death. Though first-line treatment is open necrosectomy, this study compared this with a minimally invasive step-up approach, consisting of percutaneous drainage, endoscopic drainage, and/or minimally invasive retroperotineal necrosectomy. The incidence of multiple organ failure was significantly lower in patients who underwent the step-up approach compared with those who had open necrosectomy. Though the rate of death did not differ significantly between the two groups, patients who were assigned to the step-up approach faced significantly lower rates of both incisional hernias and new-onset diabetes. One limitation of the study was that it was not powered to detect significant differences in death between the 2 groups.

In-Depth [randomized controlled trial]: Originally published in NEJM in 2010, this multicenter, randomized, controlled study involved 88 patients with acute pancreatitis and pancreatic necrosis. They were randomized to receive treatment with either open necrosectomy or a step-up approach, which included percutaneous or endoscopic drainage, and minimally invasive retroperitoneal necrosectomy. The primary end point was a composite of complications (i.e., new-onset multiple-organ failure, multiple systemic complications, bleeding, perforation of a visceral organ) and death. Patients managed using the step-up approach experienced a significantly lower rate of the composite primary endpoint compared to those treated with open necrosectomy (RR 0.57; 95%CI 0.38-0.87). This was largely driven by a significant reduction in new-onset organ failure (12% vs. 40%, $p = 0.002$), as there was no significant difference between the two groups in mortality. After 6 months of follow-up, patients who underwent open necrosectomy had a higher rate of incisional hernias (RR 0.29; 95%CI 0.09-0.95), new-onset diabetes (RR 0.43; 95%CI 0.20-0.94) and use of pancreatic enzymes (RR 0.21; 95%CI 0.07-0.67) when compared to those treated with the step-up approach. The study suggests that when treating necrotizing pancreatitis patients, a minimally invasive step-up approach reduces the rate of major complications and long-term complications when compared to open necrosectomy.

van Santvoort HC, Besselink MG, Bakker OJ, Hofker HS, Boermeester MA, Dejong CH, et al. A Step-up Approach or Open Necrosectomy for Necrotizing Pancreatitis. New England Journal of Medicine. 2010 Apr 22;362(16):1491–502.

The EVAR I trial: Endovascular vs. open abdominal aortic aneurysm repair

1. The EVAR I trial compared the safety and efficacy of endovascular and open abdominal aortic aneurysm repair.

2. There were no significant differences in all-cause mortality between the 2 groups.

3. The endovascular group experienced significantly higher rates of graft-related complications and reinterventions.

Original Date of Publication: May 2010

The Endovascular Aneurysm Repair (EVAR) trials were randomized controlled trials conducted to explore the safety and efficacy of repairing abdominal aortic aneurysms using endovascular methods. Two trials were conducted simultaneously and published in the same issue of The New England Journal of Medicine.

Study Rundown: Endovascular aortic aneurysm repair was first introduced in the late 1980s as an alternative for people considered unfit for open surgery. Several randomized controlled trials have demonstrated benefits of endovascular repair with regards to 30-day mortality, and it has become increasingly used to manage patients with abdominal aortic aneurysm. There was, however, a paucity of data with regards to the long-term follow-up of endovascular repairs. The EVAR I trial was a landmark study that compared mortality and graft-related complication/reintervention rates in patients who had undergone endovascular and open aortic aneurysm repairs. There were no significant differences between the 2 groups in terms of all-cause mortality. While early aneurysm-related mortality (i.e., 0-6 months after repair) was significantly lower in the endovascular repair group, this trend reversed in the longer run. More than 4 years after the repair, the endovascular repair group had significantly higher aneurysm-related mortality than the open group. Moreover, there were significantly higher rates of graft-related complications and reinterventions in the endovascular repair group.

In-Depth [randomized controlled trial]: Patients were eligible for the trial if they were at least 60 years of age, had an abdominal aortic aneurysm with a diameter of at least 5.5 cm on computed tomography, and were anatomically and clinically suitable for either endovascular or open repair. Eligible participants were then randomized to receive either endovascular or open aneurysm repair. The primary outcome was all-cause mortality, while other outcomes were aneurysm-related mortality, graft-related complications, and graft-related reinterventions. A total of 1252 patients were recruited for the trial from 37 hospitals across the UK. Approximately 90.7% of the study participants were male. There were no significant differences between the two groups in all-cause mortality at any timepoint. With regards to aneurysm-related mortality, there were significantly fewer deaths in the endovascular repair group until 6 months after the repair (adjusted HR 0.47; 95%CI 0.23-0.93), though this difference was not observed 6 months to 4 years after the repair. More than 4 years after the repair, there were significantly more aneurysm-related deaths in the endovascular groups compared to the open repair group (adjusted HR 4.85; 95%CI 1.04-22.72). There were significantly higher rates of graft-related complications and reinterventions in the endovascular repair group compared to the open group.

The United Kingdom EVAR Trial Investigators. Endovascular versus open repair of abdominal aortic aneurysm. Maedica (Buchar). 2010 Apr;5(2):148.

The EVAR II trial: Endovascular approach when unfit for open aortic aneurysm repair

1. The EVAR II trial compared endovascular abdominal aortic aneurysm repair with no intervention in patients unsuitable for the open procedure.

2. There were significantly fewer aneurysm-related deaths in the endovascular group, compared to no intervention.

3. The rates of complication and reintervention were similar to the rates observed in EVAR I.

Original Date of Publication: May 2010

Study Rundown: Endovascular aortic aneurysm repair was first introduced in the late 1980s as an alternative for people considered unfit for open surgery. The purpose of the EVAR II trial was to assess the benefits and risks associated with endovascular aortic aneurysm repair in patients who were unfit for the open procedure. There were no significant differences between the two groups in terms of all-cause mortality, though aneurysm-related mortality was significantly lower in the endovascular repair group. This benefit was largely attributed to the significant reductions observed in the 6 month to 4-year period following the repair procedure. Notably, the graft-related complication and reintervention rates were comparable to those observed in the EVAR I trial.

In-Depth [randomized controlled trial]: The EVAR II trial, originally published in 2010 in NEJM, focused on patients who were physically unsuitable for open abdominal aneurysm repair. The trial was supported by the National Institute for Health Research of the United Kingdom (UK). Patients were eligible for the trial if they were at least 60 years of age and had an abdominal aortic aneurysm with a diameter of at least 5.5 cm on computed tomography. Moreover, eligible patients were unsuitable for open repair, but candidates for endovascular repair. Eligible participants were then randomized to receive either endovascular aneurysm repair or no intervention. Again, the primary outcome was all-cause mortality, while other outcomes were aneurysm-related mortality, graft-related complications, and graft-related reinterventions. A total of 404 patients were recruited from 33 different hospitals across the UK. Approximately 86% of the participants were male. With regards to all-cause mortality, there were no significant differences between the two groups at any timepoint following the repair. Notably, there were significantly fewer aneurysm-related deaths in the endovascular group compared to the no intervention group (adjusted HR 0.53; 95%CI 0.32-0.89). This difference was driven by significant reductions in mortality in the 6 month to 4-year period following repair (adjusted HR 0.34; 95%CI 0.16-0.72). In total, 158 graft-related complications and 66 graft-related interventions were observed during the trial, and these rates were comparable to the rates observed in the EVAR I trial.

United Kingdom EVAR Trial Investigators, Greenhalgh RM, Brown LC, Powell JT, Thompson SG, Epstein D. Endovascular repair of aortic aneurysm in patients physically ineligible for open repair. New England Journal of Medicine. 2010 May 20;362(20):1872–80.

The CREST: Stenting versus endarterectomy for carotid stenosis

1. The rate of stroke, myocardial infarction or death did not differ significantly between patients treated with carotid artery stenting (CAS) compared to carotid endarterectomy (CEA).

2. The periprocedural rate of stroke was higher with stenting, while the rate of myocardial infarction was higher with endarterectomy.

Original Date of Publication: July 2010

Study Rundown: Carotid artery stenosis occurs as a result of atherosclerosis and leads to increasing risk of embolus and stroke. CEA and CAS are 2 procedures used to treat carotid artery stenosis but the evidence regarding their comparative efficacies is indecisive. The Carotid Revascularization Endarterectomy versus Stenting Trial (CREST) is one of the largest randomized controlled trials comparing these 2 treatment modalities. Prior to publication of these results, several trials had found higher rates of stroke and death associated with CAS, leading to a trend towards endarterectomy. The CREST trial found no significant difference in a composite outcome of stroke, myocardial infarction, and death between the 2 treatment groups and achieved lower rates of complications in both groups than those observed in previous trials. This supported both procedures as safe and effective treatment options; however, these results have been attributed to the highly trained interventionists involved in the study, which limits the external validity of the results. An interesting finding of the trial was that the rate of periprocedural stroke was higher in the stenting group, while the rate of myocardial infarction was higher in the endarterectomy group. This has led to debate regarding the relative harmful effects of suffering a stroke compared to myocardial infarction with some agreement that stroke results in more debilitating long-term consequences. In summary, the results of the CREST trial did not identify a definitive superior treatment for carotid artery stenosis. Treatment decisions should be individualized to patients' characteristics and needs.

In-Depth [randomized controlled trial]: This trial enrolled 2522 patients from 117 centers in the United States and Canada with symptomatic or asymptomatic carotid stenosis and randomized participants to receive CAS or CEA. Patients were considered eligible if they were symptomatic with ≥50% stenosis on angiography, ≥70% stenosis on ultrasonography, or ≥70% stenosis on computed tomographic/magnetic resonance angiography (CTA/MRA) but 50-69% stenosis on ultrasonography. Partway through the study, eligibility criteria were expanded to include asymptomatic patients with ≥60% stenosis on angiography, ≥70% stenosis on ultrasonography, or ≥80% stenosis on CTA/MRA but 50-69% stenosis on ultrasonography. Exclusion criteria included severe prior stroke, chronic atrial fibrillation, or paroxysmal atrial fibrillation. The primary outcome was a composite of stroke, myocardial infarction, and death during the periprocedural period, or ipsilateral stroke within four years of randomization.

There was no significant difference in the 4-year rates of the primary endpoint between CAS and CEA for the sample as a whole (HR 1.11; 95%CI 0.81-1.51), nor among symptomatic or asymptomatic patients separately (p = 0.84). The rate of the primary endpoint during the periprocedural period did not differ between treatment groups; however, when components were analysed separately, the rate of stroke was higher with CAS (4.1% vs. 2.3%, p = 0.01) while the rate of myocardial infarction was higher with CEA (1.1% vs. 2.3%, p = 0.03). Treatment effect was not modified by symptomatic status or sex; however, an interaction was detected between age and treatment efficacy, with CAS more effective in younger patients and CEA more effective in older patients.

Brott TG, Hobson RW, Howard G, Roubin GS, Clark WM, Brooks W, et al. Stenting versus Endarterectomy for Treatment of Carotid-Artery Stenosis. New England Journal of Medicine. 2010 Jul 1;363(1):11–23.

The PIVOT: Radical prostatectomy versus observation

1. Prostatectomy did not significantly reduce all-cause mortality or prostate cancer mortality when compared to observation.

2. These findings supported conservative management for men with localized prostate cancer, especially for those with prostate-specific antigen (PSA) values less than 10 ng/mL and low-risk disease.

Original Date of Publication: July 2012

Study Rundown: The incidence of prostate cancer in men is relatively high, but high long-term survival rates have been observed with conservative management. The treatment of localized prostate cancer is controversial, as few trials have compared surgical intervention to observation in the time since PSA testing has become a common screening tool. The Prostate Cancer Intervention versus Observation Trial (PIVOT) found no significant difference in all-cause or prostate-cancer mortality following radical prostatectomy compared to observation. These findings suggest that observation is a safe strategy in managing localized prostate cancer and avoids the unnecessary risks of intervention. The results also showed that PSA levels and tumor risk may be useful in identifying patients who will benefit from radical prostatectomy. Strengths of the study include the representative sample and measurement of all-cause mortality as the primary outcome, which avoids biased assessments of cause-of-death. Of note, the study may have been underpowered as the investigators intended to enroll 2000 participants, but reduced the sample size to 731. In addition, a substantial number of patients did not adhere to the assigned treatment in both groups, which could influence the observed treatment effect.

In-Depth [randomized controlled trial]: The trial included 731 men and followed participants for a median of 10 years. Patients were recruited from 44 Department of Veteran Affairs sites and 8 National Cancer Institute sites. In order to be eligible for the trial, patients had to be fit for radical prostatectomy, have histologically confirmed, clinically localized prostate cancer of any grade diagnosed within the previous 12 months, have PSA < 50 ng/mL, be ≤75 years of age, a negative bone scan, and life expectancy of at least 10 years from randomization. The primary outcome was all-cause mortality and a secondary outcome was prostate-cancer mortality, defined as death due to prostate cancer or prostate cancer treatment. The rate of all-cause mortality was not significantly different between the two groups (HR 0.88; 95%CI 0.71-1.08). There was also no significant difference between groups in prostate cancer mortality (HR 0.63; 95%CI 0.36-1.09). A significant interaction was found between study group and baseline PSA value. In men with a PSA value greater than 10 ng/mL, a significant reduction in all-cause mortality was observed with surgery (p = 0.04), though surgery did not reduce all-cause mortality in men with a PSA less than or equal to 10 ng/mL.

Wilt TJ, Brawer MK, Jones KM, Barry MJ, Aronson WJ, Fox S, et al. Radical Prostatectomy versus Observation for Localized Prostate Cancer. New England Journal of Medicine. 2012 Jul 19;367(3):203–13.

XIV. COVID-19

"What is necessary 'for the very existence of science,' and what the characteristics of nature are, are not to be determined by pompous preconditions, they are determined always by the material with which we work, by nature herself."

- Richard Feynman

COVID-19 pneumonia patients in Wuhan, China

1. This case series of patients with novel coronavirus–infected pneumonia (NCIP) found that 32% were admitted to the intensive care unit (ICU) and 15% died.

2. A significant proportion of patients (29%) developed acute respiratory distress syndrome.

Original Date of Publication: January 2020

Study Rundown: In this prospective case series, clinical features of NCIP patients in Wuhan, China were investigated during the beginning of the pandemic. The majority of patients were men without underlying chronic disease who had been exposed at the Huanan seafood market. The most common symptoms on initial presentation were fever, cough, myalgia, and fatigue. After admission, over half of patients developed lymphopenia and dyspnea. The present study was limited in that it evaluated a limited cohort of hospitalized patients. Thus, the findings cannot be extrapolated to the general population of COVID-19 patients. Additionally, only lower respiratory tract specimens were obtained to confirm diagnosis without information on viral load. In summary, COVID-19 infection may result in NCIP, severe respiratory distress, and subsequent ICU admission.

In-Depth [prospective case series]: This prospective case series evaluated the clinical presentation and course of NCIP inpatients (n = 41). Almost three quarters of participants were male (73%) with a median age of 49. Only 32% of patients had underlying chronic disease, the most common being diabetes (20%). The most common presenting complaints were fever (98%) and cough (76%). Dyspnea occurred in 55% of patients at a median time of 8 days after initial symptoms. Acute respiratory distress syndrome occurred in 29% of patients with 15% of patients being admitted to the ICU and a 15% mortality rate. During initial evaluation, significantly increased prothrombin time ($p = 0.012$) and D-dimer levels ($p = 0.0042$) were seen in patients who were admitted to the ICU. Most patients were treated with antiviral therapy (93%), and all patients initially received empirical antibiotic treatment. Additionally, 22% of patients received systemic corticosteroids.

Huang C, Wang Y, Li X, Ren L, Zhao J, Hu Y, Zhang L, Fan G, Xu J, Gu X, Cheng Z. Clinical features of patients infected with 2019 novel coronavirus in Wuhan, China. The lancet. 2020 Feb 15;395(10223):497-506.

COVID-19 epidemiologic characteristics in Wuhan, China

1. **This prospective cohort study found that novel coronavirus-infected pneumonia (NCIP) is transmitted via human-to-human contact.**

2. **The incubation period of NCIP was estimated to be 5.2 days.**

Original Date of Publication: January 2020

Study Rundown: In this prospective study, epidemiological data was collected on laboratory-confirmed cases of NCIP in Wuhan, China. Data was collected during the NCIP outbreak, with over half of the cases linked to the Huanan Seafood Wholesale Market. Epidemiological linking data demonstrated that human-to-human transmission occurred, the majority of which were in adults over the age of 60, although, these patients may be more likely to experience severe illness due to underlying health conditions and therefore overrepresented in the collected data. Additionally, detection of cases was limited by poor access to reliable testing resources as well as possibility of patients with asymptomatic infection. In summary, this study demonstrated that NCIP is likely transmitted between humans and that older patients may be at higher risk for severe infection.

In-Depth [prospective study]: This present prospective study evaluated patients in Wuhan, China with pneumonia of unknown etiology later confirmed as NCIP (n = 425). Approximately half of patients were male (56%) with a median age of 59 years and no cases in children below the age of 15. Based on data from 10 exposures, mean incubation period was approximately 5.2 days. NCIP case doubling time was estimated at 7.4 days (95%CI 4.2-14) with an $R0$¬ of 2.2 (95%CI 1.4-3.9). For patients with illness onset before January 1st, 2020 (n = 45), mean duration from onset to first medical visit was 5.8 days (95%CI 4.3-7.5). Comparatively, patients with illness onset between January 1st and January 11th (n = 207) was 4.6 days (95%CI 4.1-5.1).

Li Q, Guan X, Wu P, Wang X, Zhou L, Tong Y, Ren R, Leung KS, Lau EH, Wong JY, Xing X. Early transmission dynamics in Wuhan, China, of novel coronavirus–infected pneumonia. New England journal of medicine. 2020 Jan 29.

Characteristics of COVID-19 pneumonia patients

1. This case series found that the majority of patients with novel coronavirus–infected pneumonia (NCIP), the majority of patients were infected through hospital transmission (41.3%).

2. The majority of patients were admitted to isolation wards (73.9%) and the remainder to intensive care units (26.1%).

Original Date of Publication: February 2020

Study Rundown: This retrospective case series analyzed the characteristics of NCIP patients hospitalized in Wuhan, China. The most common presenting symptoms were fever, fatigue, and dry cough. Approximately one-fourth of patients had to be admitted to the intensive care unit, predominantly for respiratory distress syndrome. Hospital transmission was the primary method of contracting NCIP. Notably, viral load was not measured but may contribute to disease severity. Additionally, categorization of hospital-related transmission was based on contacts and proximity to infected individuals. It may have been overestimated, particularly in healthcare workers who were all presumed to have contracted NCIP in-hospital. In summary, the case series suggests that NCIP patients in Wuhan were most likely to become infected in-hospital and were primarily admitted to the intensive care unit for respiratory distress syndrome.

In-Depth [retrospective case series]: This case series involved retrospective analysis of NCIP progression in hospitalized patients (n = 138). The median age of participants was 56, and approximately half were men (54.3%). The majority of patients remained in isolation wards (73.9%) although some were moved to the intensive care unit due to decompensation (26.1%). Patients who were admitted to the intensive care unit were significantly older (median age 66 years versus 51 years; p < 0.001). Almost half of patients had underlying comorbidities (46.4%) including hypertension (31.2%), cardiovascular disease (14.5%), and diabetes (10.1%). Patients most commonly presented with fever (98.6%), fatigue (69.6%), and an unproductive cough (59.4%). In terms of treatment, antiviral therapy was preferred (89.9%) followed by moxifloxacin antibacterial therapy (64.4%).

Wang D, Hu B, Hu C, Zhu F, Liu X, Zhang J, et al. Clinical Characteristics of 138 Hospitalized Patients With 2019 Novel Coronavirus–Infected Pneumonia in Wuhan, China. JAMA. 2020 Mar 17;323(11):1061–9.

Novel coronavirus identified from patients with pneumonia in Wuhan, China

1. According to an investigation by a rapid response team, the Wuhan outbreak was most likely caused by a novel betacoronavirus.

2. This study reinforces the utility of next-generation sequencing and bioinformatics, especially in the identification of poorly-characterized pathogens.

Original Date of Publication: February 2020

Study Rundown: Coronaviruses, RNA-containing particles enveloped with protruding glycoproteins, are widely distributed in mammal and avian populations. In December of 2019, several cases of pneumonia with unknown cause were identified in Wuhan, the capital of Hebei province in China. An investigation launched by the Chinese CDC detected a novel strain of coronavirus (2019-nCov) that was traced back to a wet animal seafood market. Lower respiratory tract samples were collected from patients who presented with pneumonia of unknown cause as well as control patients with pneumonia of known cause. Following extraction of nucleic acids from these samples, viral RNA was isolated and sequenced, yielding an 87% match with a previously published bat SARS-like coronavirus genome. Virion particles were found to be generally spherical with ~10 nm spikes via transmission electron microscopy and cytopathic effects were observed in airway epithelial cells 4 days after inoculation. While this study did not fulfil Koch's postulates, evidence of seroconversion and pathogenicity have helped etiologically implicate 2019-nCov in the disease outbreak. Further research was needed to determine the coronavirus's modes of transmission and develop effective strategies to control its spread.

In-Depth [randomized control trial]: In this study designed to identify the cause of viral pneumonia in clusters of patients in Wuhan, China, various molecular techniques, high-throughput sequencing, and transmission electron microscopy were utilized to detect, isolate, and visualize a novel sarbecovirus. After collecting lower respiratory tract samples, including bronchoalveolar-lavage fluid, nucleic acids were extracted and tested for foreign material using polymerase chain reaction (PCR) and a real-time reverse transcription PCR (RT-PCR) assay. Supernatant from bronchoalveolar-lavage fluid samples was inoculated on special-pathogen-free human epithelial cell cultures and monitored daily with light microscopy and RT-PCR.

Cells that showed cytopathic effects were negative-stained and subjected to transmission electron microscopy; virion particles were found to be generally spherical with some pleomorphism and had an average diameter of 60 to 140 nm with prominent spikes characteristic of the coronaviridae family. Reads generated from Illumina and nanopore sequencing were assembled into contig maps, and genome gaps were filled using rapid amplification of cDNA ends. From these, three complete genome sequences were crafted, revealing a 86.9% nucleotide sequence identity to a known bat SARS-like Cov genome. Additional evidence supporting the discovery of a novel coronavirus include identification of a specific antigen through immunohistochemical analysis and confirmation of pathogenicity through monkey experiments.

Zhu N, Zhang D, Wang W, Li X, Yang B, Song J, et al. A Novel Coronavirus from Patients with Pneumonia in China, 2019. New England Journal of Medicine. 2020 Feb 20;382(8):727–33.

Sequencing of COVID-19: Comparison to SARS and bat coronavirus

1. This cross-sectional study found that coronavirus 2019 (COVID-19) shared 79.6% genome sequence identity with severe acute respiratory syndrome-related coronavirus (SARS-CoV).

2. Additionally, COVID-19 shares 96% whole genome sequence with bat coronavirus.

Original Date of Publication: February 2020

Study Rundown: In this cross-sectional study, full-length genome sequences were obtained from the early COVID-19 outbreak in Wuhan, China. The sequence was compared to SARS-CoV BJ01 and was identified to belong to the species SARS-related coronaviruses (SARSr-CoV). Additionally, COVID-19 uses the same cell entry receptor as SARC-CoV. Full-length sequencing was also performed on a bat coronavirus (BatCoV RaTG13) which was found through phylogenetic analysis to be the closest identified relative to COVID-19. Although, the generalizability of the study results is severely limited by small sample size and lack of robust epidemiological data confirming infection etiology. In summary, this study demonstrated that COVID-19 is a SARSr-CoV which whole-genome similarity to BatCoV RaTG13.

In-Depth [cross-sectional study]: The present cross-sectional study compared the whole-genome sequence of COVID-19 extracted from patients admitted to Wuhan Jin Yin-Tan Hospital (n = 5) to the whole genomes of SARS-CoV BJ01 and BatCoV RaTG13. Patients were originally presented with virus-induced pneumonia of unknown origin. Targeted PCR was used to obtain a COVID-19 genome which had 79.6% similarity to SARSr-CoV. The COVID-19 genome evaluated had six major open-reading frames and several accessory genes common to coronaviruses. Additionally, a virus infectivity study was conducted which determined that COVID-19 uses the same cell entry receptor-angiotensin converting enzyme II as SARS-CoV. Interestingly, overall sequence identity of COVID-19 had 96.2% similarity to BatCoV RaTG13.

Zhou P, Yang XL, Wang XG, Hu B, Zhang L, Zhang W, Si HR, Zhu Y, Li B, Huang CL, Chen HD. A pneumonia outbreak associated with a new coronavirus of probable bat origin. nature. 2020 Mar;579(7798):270-3.

COVID-19 patient characteristics across Mainland China

1. This cohort study of patients with novel coronavirus 2019 (COVID-19) found that a primary composite endpoint of intensive care unit (ICU) admission, mechanical ventilation, or mortality occurred in 6.1% of patients.

2. The majority of patients developed fever (88.7%) and cough (67.8%) throughout their hospitalization.

Original Date of Publication: April 2020

Study Rundown: In this cohort study, admission data was analyzed from patients with COVID-19 admitted to hospitals across mainland China. Approximately half of patients were female and 15 to 49 years old. The most common symptoms of COVID-19 were fever and cough. Nausea, vomiting, and diarrhea occurred in less than a tenth of patients. Patients with severe COVID-19 were more likely to be older and have another underlying illness. Additionally, those with severe COVID-19 were at increased risk of the primary composite endpoint of ICU admission, mechanical ventilation, or mortality. The major limitation of this study is the variation in available data for patients across different hospitals. Overall, COVID-19 patients seem to predominantly present as having fever and/or cough, with ICU admission, mechanical ventilation, and mortality more likely in those with severe disease.

In-Depth [cohort study]: This cohort study compared clinical presentations and outcomes of COVID-19 patients admitted to 552 hospitals across 30 provinces, autonomous regions, and municipalities in mainland China (n = 1099). Approximately half of patients were male (58.1%) with a median age of 47 years. The primary composite endpoint occurred in a total of 6.1% of patients, with 5.0% admitted to the ICU, 1.4% mortality, and 2.3% mechanically ventilated. During their hospital admission, 88.7% of patients experienced fever as compared to 67.8% reporting a cough. Over half of patients had ground glass opacity on chest computed tomography (56.4%) and most experienced lymphocytopenia (83.2%). Treatment principally consisted of intravenous antibiotic therapy (58.0%), oxygen therapy (41.3%), and antiviral therapy (35.8%) with a mean hospitalization of 12 days.

Guan WJ, Ni ZY, Hu Y, Liang WH, Ou CQ, He JX, Liu L, Shan H, Lei CL, Hui DS, Du B. Clinical characteristics of coronavirus disease 2019 in China. New England journal of medicine. 2020 Apr 30;382(18):1708-20.

5-day versus 10-day course of remdesivir in patients with severe COVID-19

1. Compared to patients who received remdesivir for 10 days, those in the 5-day group experienced no significant difference in either clinical outcomes or time to clinical improvement.

2. Although adverse events were slightly more frequent in the 10-day group, this effect may have been related to differences in baseline clinical status rather than treatment duration.

Original Date of Publication: May 2020

Study Rundown: Remdesivir is an adenosine analog prodrug whose metabolite directly inhibits RNA-dependent RNA polymerase and causes delayed chain termination. The medication has shown activity against SARS-CoV-2 *in vitro* as well as in primate models, and data from recent compassionate use studies and randomized controlled trials show that it may accelerate recovery from COVID-19. A 10-day course of treatment has been the standard in previous studies, but with millions of cases worldwide and the production of remdesivir proceeding at a crawl, shortening the treatment duration could reduce the length of hospital stays and increase the number of patients who can be treated with a limited drug supply. This study found that there was no significant difference in the likelihood of clinical improvement between the 5-day and 10-day groups. In fact, the 5-day group had numerically fewer deaths and a greater number of patients who had been discharged by day 14. The two groups had similar adverse event rates, but the 10-day group had over 10% more serious adverse events. This study had a high attrition rate because many patients were discharged prior to completing the full course of therapy, and the lack of a placebo arm precluded any analysis of the efficacy of remdesivir. Nonetheless, these results suggest that 10 days may not be the shortest effective duration of remdesivir therapy for COVID-19.

In-Depth [randomized control trial]: In this open-label phase 3 trial, 397 patients with PCR-confirmed SARS-CoV-2 infection not requiring ventilation were randomly assigned in a 1:1 ratio to receive either a 5-day or 10-day course of intravenous remdesivir. Demographic characteristics were similar between groups, but patients in the 10-day group had significantly worse baseline clinical status compared to those in the 5-day group (p = 0.02). All patients received a loading dose of 200 mg on day 1 and 100 mg per day thereafter. Efficacy was assessed using a 7-point ordinal scale with a score of 7 corresponding to discharge from the hospital and a score of 1 indicating death. At day 14, 65% of patients in the 5-day group had a clinical improvement of at least 2 points versus only 54% of those in the 10-day group. After adjusting for baseline clinical status, the distributions of final clinical status were similar between groups (p = 0.14). Additionally, no significant differences were detected in recovery, time to clinical improvement, or time to recovery. 70-75% of both groups experienced at least 1 adverse event of any severity, but 35% of patients in the 10-day group had serious adverse events, as compared with 21% in the 5-day group (p < 0.05). Acute kidney injury was observed in 15 patients in the 10-day group versus only 4 in the 5-day group. Some other common adverse events were nausea, constipation, and insomnia; the most common serious adverse event was respiratory failure.

Goldman JD, Lye DCB, Hui DS, Marks KM, Bruno R, Montejano R, et al. Remdesivir for 5 or 10 Days in Patients with Severe COVID-19. New England Journal of Medicine. 2020 Nov 5;383(19):1827–37.

The ACTT-1: Remdesivir for the treatment of COVID-19

1. This study determined that amongst adults hospitalized with COVID-19 wih evidence of lower respiratory tract infection, remdesivir was superior to placebo in shortening time to recovery.

2. Serious adverse events were reported as generally similar between the remdesivir and placebo group (24.6% of patients randomized to receive remdesivir, compared to 31.6% in patients receiving placebo).

Original Date of Publication: October 2020

Study Rundown: Since SARS-CoV-2 was first identified in December 2019, several therapeutic agents have been evaluated as treatment modalities; however, none have yet been shown to be efficacious. Remdesivir is an antiviral agent that has shown ability to inhibit SARS-CoV-2 in vitro but has not yet been studied in hospitalized patients with COVID-19. The objective of this randomized controlled trial was to evaluate the clinical efficacy and safety profile of remdesivir in hospitalized patients with COVID-19 and evidence of lower respiratory infection compared to placebo. Final results demonstrated remdesivir was superior to placebo in shortening time to recovery amongst patients hospitalized with COVID-19. Limitations of this study include a short follow-up period for patients with more severe disease (higher ordinal score); therefore, median recovery time in this population could not be estimated. Nonetheless, this study was significant in suggesting remdesivir as the first efficacious drug for COVID-19.

In-Depth [randomized controlled trial]: A total of 1062 patients hospitalized with COVID-19 and evidence of lower respiratory infection underwent 1:1 randomization in The Adaptive COVID-19 Treatment Trial (ACTT-1) across 60 trial sites. Patients were either randomized to receive remdesivir (n = 541) (intravenous 200 mg loading dose day 1, followed by 100 mg daily for up to 9 days) or normal saline placebo (n = 521) for up to 10 days. Results demonstrated that patients in the remdesivir group had shortened time to recovery compared to placebo (median = 10 days compared to 15 days; RR 1.29; 95%CI 1.12-1.49; $p < 0.001$). Patients who received remdesivir were also more likely to have clinical improvement at day 15 compared to placebo (OR 1.5; 95%CI 1.2-1.9, after adjustment for actual disease severity). Serious adverse events occurred in 24.6% (n = 131) of patients randomized to receive remdesivir, compared to 31.6% (n =

163) in patients receiving placebo. The incidence of adverse events was reported to be generally similar between the two treatment groups. Altogether, the results of this study support the use of remdesivir in patients hospitalized with COVID-19, suggesting decreased length of stay in this patient population. However, considering the high mortality despite remdesivir treatment, it is likely a single antiviral treatment is insufficient in the treatment of COVID-19.

Beigel JH, Tomashek KM, Dodd LE, Mehta AK, Zingman BS, Kalil AC, et al. Remdesivir for the Treatment of COVID-19 — Final Report. New England Journal of Medicine. 2020 May 22

BNT162b2 mRNA vaccine for COVID-19 prevention

1. This clinical trial determined the efficacy of the BNT162b2 mRNA vaccine at preventing coronavirus disease 2019 (COVID-19) infection (95%) based on comparison to a placebo control group.

2. Rates of serious adverse events did not differ significantly between the BNT162b2 vaccine and control groups.

Original Date of Publication: December 2020

Study Rundown: This clinical efficacy trial compared COVID-19 infection rates of patients receiving the BNT162b2 mRNA vaccine and of those receiving a placebo control. Participants in the treatment group had significantly reduced COVID-19 infection rates when compared to those receiving placebo controls. Vaccine efficacy did not vary based on demographic subgroup analysis. Overall adverse events were higher in the BNT162b2 group, but serious adverse event rates did not differ significantly between groups. The present study has limited generalizability to certain higher risk populations, including children as well as pregnant individuals and immunocompromised individuals, as they were not studied. These groups are commonly excluded from initial safety and efficacy trials to minimize confounding risk factors. In summary, this study demonstrates that the BNT162b2 mRNA vaccine provided a high-degree of COVID-19 protection with limited risk of serious adverse events.

In-Depth [randomized control trial]: This efficacy and safety trial randomized COVID-19 naïve participants to receive two doses of either the BNT162b2 mRNA vaccine (n = 21,720) or a placebo control (n = 21,728). Injections were given intramuscularly 21 days apart in both groups to adults aged 16 years or older. BNT162b2 mRNA vaccine efficacy was measured using rates of COVID-19 infection at least one week following second dose and was found to be 95% (95%CI 90.3-97.6). With only one dose, vaccine efficacy was 52% (95%CI 29.5-68.4). The safety profile of the BNT162b2 vaccine was measured at two-month follow-up. A higher rate of adverse events was reported in the intervention group (27%) as compared to the control group (12%). Serious adverse events did not differ significantly between groups, although safety monitoring will continue for two years after baseline.

Polack FP, Thomas SJ, Kitchin N, Absalon J, Gurtman A, Lockhart S, et al. Safety and Efficacy of the BNT162b2 mRNA COVID-19 Vaccine. N Engl J Med. 2020 Dec 31;383(27):2603–15.

The EMPACTA trial: Tocilizumab reduced COVID-19 disease-related adverse health outcomes

1. Tocilizumab reduced the need for mechanical ventilation and lowered death outcomes in patients infected with severe acute respiratory syndrome coronavirus 2 (SARS-CoV-2).

2. Treatment with tocilizumab did not improve survival among patients.

Original Date of Publication: December 2020

Study Rundown: Cases pertaining to the coronavirus disease 2019 (COVID-19) have led to severe clinical manifestations requiring mechanical ventilation. However, fatal outcomes have still resulted despite currently treatments and supportive care. This trial investigated the safety and efficacy of tocilizumab, an anti-interleukin-6 receptor monoclonal antibody, in patients hospitalized with COVID-19 pneumonia. These hospitalized patients were randomly assigned into one of two groups after informed consent was obtained. Patients were followed for two months and outcomes such as the need for mechanical ventilation or death were assessed on day 28. The trial results displayed both theefficacy and safety of tocilizumab treatment in managing patients with COVID-19 pneumonia. However, both groups revealed similar death outcomes. The study was strengthened by its focus on the inclusion of ethnic and racial minority patients. Conversely, the study was limited by the short follow-up period. Nonetheless, the study results are important as they showed tocilizumab reduces adverse health outcomes related to COVID-19.

In-Depth [randomized control trial]: This phase 3, double-blind trial enrolled 389 participants across multiple countries including Brazil, Kenya, Mexico, Peru, South Africa, and the United States. This study enrolled patients over the age of 18 with confirmed COVID-19 pneumonia who were hospitalized. Patients were excluded if they required additional breathing assistance such as continuous positive airway pressure, mechanical ventilation, or bilevel positive airway pressure. Patients were randomized in a 2:1 ratio to the standard of care including one or two doses of either tocilizumab or a placebo, respectively. On day 28, the primary endpoint of mechanical ventilation or death was evaluated for all participants. The results were further investigated using analysis and stratification, where the median follow-up time was 60 days.

By day 28, an overall of 12% (95%CI 8.5-16.9%) of the patients in the tocilizumab group had either received some form of mechanical ventilation or had died, whereas a total of 19.3% (95% CI 13.3-27.4%) of the placebo group had experienced these outcomes. The hazard ratio for mechanical ventilation or death between both groups was 0.56 (95%CI 0.33-0.97 p = 0.04). Furthermore, 15.2% of the patients reported serious adverse events in the study drug group compared to 19.7% were reported in the placebo. Consequently, more deaths were reported in the placebo group (29 patients) compared to the tocilizumab group (15 patients), although all-cause mortality at 28 days did not differ significantly between the two groups (weight difference 2.0; 95%CI −5.2 to 7.8). Overall, these findings demonstrate that tocilizumab is both safe and effective in treating patients with COVID-19 pneumonia.

Salama C, Han J, Yau L, Reiss WG, Kramer B, Neidhart JD, et al. Tocilizumab in Patients Hospitalized with COVID-19 Pneumonia. N Engl J Med. 2021 Jan 7;384(1):20–30.

The COVE Trial: mRNA-1273 vaccine for preventing COVID-19

1. In this phase 3 trial, the mRNA-1273 vaccine was found to be efficacious in preventing symptomatic infection from coronavirus disease 2019 (COVID-19) in comparison to a placebo control.

2. All serious cases of COVID-19 occurred in the placebo group and no major safety concerns were identified for the mRNA-1273 vaccine.

Original Date of Publication: February 2021

Study Rundown: The Coronavirus Efficacy (COVE) trial evaluated the efficacy of the mRNA-1273 at preventing symptomatic COVID-19 infection as compared to a placebo injection. The placebo group had significantly higher rates of COVID-19 infection at 14-day follow-up, which was consistent in subgroup analysis of participants with a previous COVID-19 infection and those aged 65 years or older. No cases of severe COVID-19 infection were seen in the intervention group and the incidence of serious adverse events did not differ significantly between groups. The primary limitation of the COVE trial was the short follow-up time for measuring efficacy and adverse events. Although, a two-year follow-up duration is planned for enrolled patients. The COVE trial was the first to demonstrate that the mRNA-1273 vaccine washighly efficacious at preventing COVID-19 infection with a low-risk safety profile for serious adverse events.

In-Depth [randomized control trial]: The participants of the COVE trial received two doses of either the mRNA-1273 vaccine (n = 15 210) or a placebo control injection (n = 15 210) with 28 days between doses and a 14-day follow-up time. The mRNA-1273 vaccine had 95.2% efficacy (95%CI 91.2-97.4) at preventing symptomatic COVID-19 infection as compared to placebo control. Notably, the mRNA-1273 vaccine was found to be 100% efficacious at preventing severe COVID-19 infection. Injection-site adverse events were higher in the mRNA-1273 group after both the first (84.2% versus 19.8%) and second injections (88.6% versus 18.8%). Similarly, systemic adverse reactions were also increased in the intervention group following the first (54.9% versus 42.2%) and second doses (79.4% versus 36.5%). Serious adverse event rates did not differ significantly between the mRNA-1273 and placebo injection groups.

This efficacy and safety trial randomized COVID-19 naïve participants to receive two doses of either the BNT162b2 mRNA vaccine (n = 21,720) or a placebo control (n = 21,728). Injections were given intramuscularly 21 days apart in both groups to adults aged 16 years or older. BNT162b2 mRNA vaccine efficacy was measured using rates of COVID-19 infection at least one week following second dose (95%; 95%CI 90.3-97.6). With only one dose, vaccine efficacy was 52% (95%CI 29.5-68.4). The safety profile of the BNT162b2 vaccine was measured at two-month follow-up. A higher rate of adverse events was reported in the intervention group (27%) as compared to the control group (12%). Serious adverse events did not differ significantly between groups, although safety monitoring will continue for two years after baseline.

Baden LR, El Sahly HM, Essink B, Kotloff K, Frey S, Novak R, et al. Efficacy and Safety of the mRNA-1273 SARS-CoV-2 Vaccine. New England Journal of Medicine. 2021 Feb 4;384(5):403–16.

The RECOVERY trial: Dexamethasone decreased mortality in hospitalized COVID-19 patients

1. Patients hospitalized with COVID-19 and treated with dexamethasone experienced lower 28-day mortality compared to those treated with usual care.

2. Patients treated with dexamethasone had a shorter hospitalizations compared to those in the usual care group.

Original Date of Publication: February 2021

Study Rundown: Although the majority of coronavirus disease 2019 (COVID-19) cases are asymptomatic or have minor symptoms, many patients need hospital care and can progress to respiratory failure and require ventilatory support. Furthermore, no therapeutic agent had been shown to reduce mortality in patients with more severe COVID-19 infections. This study assessed the use of dexamethasone in patients hospitalized with COVID-19. The study found that patients treated with dexamethasone experienced significantly lower mortality at 28 days when compared to patients in the usual care group. No benefit was found amongst patients who did not require supplemental oxygen therapy. Patients treated with dexamethasone were also noted to have shorter hospitalizations and a greater probability of being discharged within 28 days. The study was limited by the lack of long-term follow-up in patients treated with dexamethasone. Nonetheless, this was the first study to find a therapy that effectively prevented disease progression and lowere mortality in patients with severe COVID-19 infection.

In-Depth [randomized control trial]: This controlled, open-label trial enrolled 6425 patients. Eligible patients included those with confirmed SARS-CoV-2 infection, hospitalized for severe symptoms, and on ventilation or oxygen support. Patients were excluded if dexamethasone was not available at the hospital. Randomization occurred in a 2:1 ratio to receive either usual care alone or usual care plus dexamethasone (oral or IV 6 mg daily), respectively. The primary endpoint was all-cause mortality within 28 days after randomization. Overall, mortality at 28 days was significantly lower in the dexamethasone group (22.9%) compared to patients in the control group (25.7%) (rate ratio 0.83; 95%CI 0.75-0.93; $p < 0.001$). Subgroup analysis showed there was no benefit in treating patients who did not receive respiratory support in the form of supplemental oxygen with dexamethasone (17.8%) compared to usual care alone (14.0%) (rate ratio 1.19; 95%CI 0.92-1.55). Furthermore, patients treated with dexamethasone had a shorter duration in hospital stay compared to the control group (median 12 vs 13 days). Finally, patients treated with dexamethasone had a greater probability of discharge after 28 days when compared to usual care alone (rate ratio 1.10; 95%CI 1.03-1.17). Overall, dexamethasone was shown to decrease all-cause mortality, shorten the duration of hospitalization, and improve the probability of discharge in hospitalized patients with COVID-19.

The RECOVERY Collaborative Group. Dexamethasone in Hospitalized Patients with COVID-19. N Engl J Med. 2021 Feb 25;384(8):693–704.

Interleukin-6 receptor antagonist treatment improves outcomes in patients with COVID-19 infection

1. Treatment with tocilizumab and sarilumab increased the number of days without respiratory or cardiovascular organ support in patients with COVID-19 infection.

2. Interleukin-6 receptor antagonists improved in-hospital survival for patients diagnosed with COVID-19 and receiving organ support in the intensive care unit (ICU).

Original Date of Publication: April 2021

Study Rundown: Thus far, only glucocorticoids had been shown to improve survival in critically ill patients with coronavirus disease 2019 (COVID-19). Tocilizumab and sarilumab are monoclonal antibodies against receptors of interleukin-6 (IL-6), a key molecule in the acute-phase inflammatory response. This trial investigated the effectiveness of tocilizumab and sarilumab on organ support and survival in critically ill patients with COVID-19. Treatment with tocilizumab and sarilumab was found to improve the number of days critically ill patients in the ICU went without organ support. Furthermore, IL-6 receptor antagonist treatment improved 90-day survival in the same patient group compared to the control group. The study was not without limitations, such as the lack of reporting on long-term outcomes and small sample size in the sarilumab group. This study's results are significant, and its pragmatic, international design suggests results from this study may be generalized to use IL-6 receptor antagonist treatment in critically ill COVID-19 patients; however, caution must be taken as the standard of care may differ in other ICUs.

In-Depth [randomized control trial]: This randomized control trial randomized 895 patients at 113 sites across six countries. Critically ill patients admitted to the ICU on organ support and ≥18 years of age were included. Patients previously participated in another study within 90 days or a presumption of imminent death were excluded from the study. The patients were randomized to one of five interventions – tocilizumab, sarilumab, anakinra (IL-1 receptor antagonist), interferon beta-1a, and control. The primary outcome was number of respiratory and cardiovascular organ support-free days up to day 21. The median number of organ support-free days for treatment modalities were 10 days with tocilizumab treatment (interquartile range, -1 to 16); 11 days with sarilumab treatment (interquartile range, 0 to 16); and 0 days in the control group 0 (interquartile range, -1 to 15). The median adjusted odds ratios for organ support-free days were 1.64 for tocilizumab treatment (95%CI 1.25-2.14) and 1.76 for sarilumab treatment (95%CI 1.17-2.91). The in-hospital mortality for IL-6 receptor antagonist groups was 27% (108 of 395 patients) compared to 36% (142 of 397) patients in the control group. The median adjusted odds ratios for in-hospital survival were 1.64 in the tocilizumab treatment (95%CI 1.14-2.35) and 2.01 in the sarilumab treatment (95%CI 1.18-4.71). Therefore, IL-6 receptor antagonist therapy in critically ill ICU patients with COVID-19 was shown to improve outcomes, including survival.

The REMAP-CAP Investigators. Interleukin-6 Receptor Antagonists in Critically Ill Patients with COVID-19. N Engl J Med. 2021 Apr 22;384(16):1491–502.

Nationwide vaccination campaign with BNT162b2 (Pfizer–BioNTech) mRNA vaccine reports high immunogenicity across all age groups

1. There was a vaccine efficacy of 97.2% against symptomatic COVID-19 infection in individuals at least 7 days after their second vaccine dose.

2. Substantial and consistent declines in COVID-19 incidence were correlated with greater vaccine coverage.

Original Date of Publication: May 2021

Study Rundown: Beyond clinical trials, there is growing evidence of the practical value of vaccination in reducing the spread of COVID-19. Nationwide surveillance data of mass vaccination campaigns may contribute to our understanding of vaccine efficacy but has yet to be reported. This study uses national surveillance data to study the effects of the first 4 months of a nationwide vaccination campaign against SARS-CoV-2 in the Israeli population. The study found that after two doses of the BNT162b2 (Pfizer–BioNTech) mRNA vaccine, there were significant reductions in the incidence of asymptomatic COVID-19 infections, symptomatic COVID-19 infections, COVID-19 hospitalization and COVID-19-related deaths. Limitations include the lack of randomization and the observational nature of the study such that the observed outcomes cannot be casually linked to vaccination given the potential influence of confounding factors such as exposure. Moreover, the study setting has a unique population demographic and has experienced an equally unique vaccine roll out program. Nevertheless, this is one of the largest scale studies of the real-world vaccine efficacy and further supports the use of vaccinations in addressing COVID-19.

In-Depth [randomized control trial]: This study utilized national health records of individuals above the age of 16 in Israel from January 24 to April 3, 2021. Vaccine efficacy against COVID-19 infections, hospitalizations, and death was evaluated in fully vaccinated individuals, defined as being at least 7 days after their second dose of the Pfizer vaccine. The unvaccinated control group was defined as those in the national registry who had not received any vaccine doses and had not experienced a previous infection.

By the end of the study period, 4,714,932 of 6,538,911 (72%) individuals aged 16 years or older were fully vaccinated. Analysis was conducted by employing a negative binomial regression model with outcome adjustment age group, sex, and calendar week of vaccination. Vaccine effectiveness was determined to be approximately 95.3% (95%CI 94.9-95.7%) against infection, 97.0% (95%CI 96.7-97.2%) against symptomatic infection, 97.5% (95%CI 97.1-97.8%) against severe hospitalization, and 96.7% (95%CI 96.0-97.3%) against death. The incidence rate of SARS-CoV-2 infections was 91.5 per 100 000 person-days in unvaccinated individuals compared to 3.1 per 100 000 person-days in vaccinated individuals aged 16 years or older. Overall, increases in cumulative vaccine coverage corresponded to reductions in the 7-day daily moving average of incident SARS-CoV-2 infections across all age groups.

Haas EJ, Angulo FJ, McLaughlin JM, Anis E, Singer SR, Khan F, et al. Impact and effectiveness of mRNA BNT162b2 vaccine against SARS-CoV-2 infections and COVID-19 cases, hospitalisations, and deaths following a nationwide vaccination campaign in Israel: an observational study using national surveillance data. The Lancet. 2021 May 15;397(10287):1819–29.

Mixed vaccination with ChAdOx1-S followed by BNT162b2 induces a robust humoral immune response

1. Levels of antibodies against the trimeric spike protein and receptor-binding domain were 36- and 77-fold higher in the BNT162b2 group compared to control.

2. There were no vaccine-related serious adverse events.

Original Date of Publication: June 2021

Study Rundown: Current research on COVID-19 vaccination has revolved around a homologous dosing schedule (administering the same vaccine sequentially). With supplies becoming scarce globally, the need to interchange COVID-19 vaccines is growing. Until now, limited research has been conducted to assess the effect of a heterologous COVID-19 vaccine schedule in humans. This open-label randomized controlled trial aimed to assess the safety and efficacy of a second dose of BNT162b2 (Pfizer-BioNTech mRNA vaccine) in patients who received a first dose of ChAdOx1-S (AstraZeneca vaccine) approximately 8-12 weeks prior to study enrollment. The primary outcome for this study was immunogenicity to SARS-CoV-2 trimeric spike protein and receptor binding domain (RBD), measured by immunoassay at 14 days after second vaccination. Secondary outcomes included neutralizing antibody titers as measured by neutralization assay at two weeks. According to study results, IgG titers against the spike protein and RBD antibodies both increased from baseline to day 14 in the BNT162b2 booster group. There were no serious vaccine-related adverse events. This study was strengthened by a randomized trial that sampled a large group of individuals from multiple hospitals in Spain.

In-Depth [randomized control trial]: From April 24 to 30, 2021, 678 patients were assessed for eligibility across five university hospitals in Spain. Included patients were ≥18 years of age who previously received the ChAdOx1-S COVID-19 vaccine 8-12 weeks before screening. Altogether, 676 patients were enrolled and randomized, of which 673 completed the study to day 14 – 448 were assigned to BNT162b2, 441 were included in the immunogenicity analysis vs 448 in reactogenicity analysis, and 226 assigned to control with 222 included in immunogenicity analysis. Mean age among enrolled patients was 44 years (SD 9) and the majority (n = 382, 57%) were women.

Borobia AM, Carcas AJ, Pérez-Olmeda M, Castaño L, Bertran MJ, García-Pérez J, et al. Immunogenicity and reactogenicity of BNT162b2 booster in ChAdOx1-S-primed participants (CombiVacS): a multicentre, open-label, randomised, controlled, phase 2 trial. The Lancet. 2021 Jul;398(10295):121–30.

Inactivated whole-virion SARS-CoV-2 vaccine reduces rates of symptomatic COVID-19 infections

1. Incidence of PCR-confirmed symptomatic COVID-19 cases was lower in the vaccine group compared with the placebo group.

2. The majority of adverse events were mild and there was no vaccine-related mortality.

Original Date of Publication: July 2021

Study Rundown: Inactivated vaccines offer a variety of benefits against transmission of severe acute respiratory syndrome coronavirus 2 (SARS-CoV-2). One such inactivated whole-virion vaccine is CoronaVac, which is currently in phase 3 trials in Brazil, Indonesia, Chile, and Turkey. This phase III randomized controlled trial aimed to assess the safety and efficacy of CoronaVac in Turkey. The primary outcome for this study was the proportion of laboratory confirmed COVID-19 cases at least 14 days after administering the second dose, while key secondary outcomes included incidence of hospitalization, adverse events, and mortality. According to study results, the vaccine group reported significantly fewer cases of symptomatic COVID-19 compared with placebo; however, the frequency of adverse events was higher in the former. In addition, no individuals in the vaccine group required hospitalization for their infection. While this study was well done, a major limitation was that it did not explore the impact of vaccine interchangeability on the aforementioned clinical outcomes. Nevertheless, it provides valuable insight into the use of CoronaVac for safe and effective immunogenicity during the COVID-19 pandemic.

In-Depth [randomized control trial]: Between September 14, 2020, and January 5, 2021, 11 303 patients were assessed for eligibility across 24 centers in Turkey. Included patients were between 18-59 years of age with no previous history of COVID-19 and a negative SARS-CoV-2 PCR or antibody test. Those diagnosed with a bleeding disorder or on immunosuppressants were excluded. Altogether, 10 214 patients in the intention-to-treat group (65.1% in vaccine group vs. 34.9% in placebo group) and 10 029 patients in the per-protocol group (65.4% in vaccine group vs. 34.6% in placebo group) completed the trial. Median age among enrolled patients was 45 years (interquartile range [IQR] 37-51) and the majority (57.8%) were male.

Tanriover MD, Doğanay HL, Akova M, Güner HR, Azap A, Akhan S, et al. Efficacy and safety of an inactivated whole-virion SARS-CoV-2 vaccine (CoronaVac): interim results of a double-blind, randomised, placebo-controlled, phase 3 trial in Turkey. The Lancet. 2021 Jul 17;398(10296):213–22.

Heparin in noncritically ill COVID-19 patients

1. This study found that in patients hospitalized, but not critically ill, with coronavirus disease 2019 (COVID-19), heparin treatment was associated with significantly more organ support–free days as compared to normal thromboprophylaxis (98.6% posterior probability).

2. Probability of survival until hospital discharge was also increased in group receiving heparin (87.1% posterior probability).

Original Date of Publication: August 2021

Study Rundown: In this clinical trial, therapeutic use of heparin was compared to standard thromboprophylaxis in hospitalized but noncritically ill COVID-19 patients. The heparin group had a significant increase in organ support-free days as well as increased survival to hospital discharge. The benefit of heparin was greater in patients with an elevated D-dimer level. The main limitation of this study was that it was open-label. In summary, the present clinical trial demonstrated that in noncritically ill patients with COVID-19, heparin was superior to standard thromboprophylaxis in reducing in-hospital mortality and requirement for end-stage organ support.

In-Depth [randomized control trial]: The present study randomized hospitalized COVID-19 patients with moderate disease to receive either anticoagulation with heparin (n = 1190) or pharmacologic thromboprophylaxis as usual (n = 1054). The primary endpoint of organ support-free days was measured as a combination of in-hospital mortality and time without cardiovascular or respiratory organ support.

Treatment with therapeutic doses of heparin significantly increased the number of organ support-free days was when compared to controls receiving thromboprophylaxis (OR 1.27; 95%CI 1.03-1.58). Patients treated with therapeutic heparin also experienced significantly higher survival until hospital dischargewhen compared to thromboprophylaxis thromboprophylaxis (95%CI 0.5-7.2). Notably, the benefits of the therapeutic heparin was higher in patients with elevated D-dimer levels (97.3%) compared to those with a low D-dimer (92.9%). Rates of thrombotic events or in-hospital mortality were also lower in the heparin group (8.0%) than the control group (9.9%). Unsurprisingly, major bleeding was more common in the heparin group (1.9%) as compared to usual thromboprophylaxis (0.9%).

The ATTACC, ACTIV-4a, and REMAP-CAP Investigators. Therapeutic Anticoagulation with Heparin in Noncritically Ill Patients with COVID-19. N Engl J Med. 2021 Aug 26;385(9):790–802.

Third dose of BNT162b2 COVID-19 vaccine effective at decreasing risk of hospitalization

1. Compared to two doses of the BNT162b2 vaccine, a third booster dose was estimated to be 93% effective against admission to hospital due to COVID-19 infection.

2. A third dose was also associated less severe disease and lower COVID-19 related mortality.

Original Date of Publication: December 2021

Study Rundown: Despite a rigorous vaccination campaign in Israel, the country is still reporting vaccine "breakthrough" cases of COVID-19 infection. Israel, which has already rolled out many third doses of BNT162b2 mRNA vaccine, may be used as a pseudo-trial population to evaluate third dose vaccine effectiveness. This was the goal of this study, which compared individuals who had received a third dose at least 5 months after their second dose. Using demographically matched controls with only two doses, effectiveness of preventing hospitalization, severe disease and death was measured. This study found that a third dose of the BNT162b2 was highly effective at preventing hospitalization compared to two doses. Three doses were also more effective at preventing severe disease and death from COVID-19. Efficacy from a third dose was most pronounced in individuals over the age of 40. Limitations included lack of individual data for patients under 40. Nonetheless, this study provides key information which will help inform national vaccination strategies moving forward.

In-Depth [retrospective cohort]: This retrospective study utilized the highly vaccinated Israeli population to investigate the effectiveness of a third dose of the mRNA BNT162b2 (Pfizer) vaccine. The eligible population included individuals who had received two doses at least 5 months prior to their third dose. A matched control group included individuals matched to the treatment group by age, sex, place of residence, and risk factors for severe COVID-19 infection, but had only received two doses total. There were 728 321 matched pairs, of whom 51% were female and had a median age of 52 years. A total of 198 476 individuals were matched to themselves before and after third dose. Outcomes included risk of admission to hospital, severe disease, and death from COVID-19 infection. Outcomes were recorded 7 days after the third dosage was received and continued for a median follow-up of 13 days. Compared to two doses, a third dose conferred an effectiveness of 93% against hospital admission, 92% against severe disease and 81% against death from COVID-19. Effectiveness was found to be similar regardless of gender. The effectiveness of the third dose was to be greater in participants aged 40-69 years and >70 years, compared to those aged 16-39.

Barda N, Dagan N, Cohen C, Hernán MA, Lipsitch M, Kohane IS, et al. Effectiveness of a third dose of the BNT162b2 mRNA COVID-19 vaccine for preventing severe outcomes in Israel: an observational study. The Lancet. 2021 Dec 4;398(10316):2093–100.

INDEX

abscess, 293, 305, 306, 307, 443
acute coronary syndrome, 90, 117, 119, 127, 129, 130, 137, 138, 143, 157, 158, 167, 168, 226, 229, 240
Acute Ischemic Stroke, 216, 567, 568, 569, 570, 572, 579, 580
adrenal adenoma, 403, 413, 414, 415
adverse drug reactions, 391
Adverse events, 36, 38, 39, 186, 195, 498, 577
albumin, 238, 239, 288, 289, 480, 490, 527, 657
alpha-blocker, 103, 104, 518
alpha-fetal protein (AFP), 348
alpha-fetoprotein, 326, 327
alteplase, 566, 570, 571, 572
Alzheimer's disease, 548
American College of Radiology, 417, 444, 445, 455, 456
amiodarone, 101
amlodipine, 103, 104, 133, 134, 516
ANCA, 59, 60
angina, 58, 75, 104, 117, 127, 160, 227, 240
angiography, 119, 120, 240, 330, 431, 719
angiotensin converting enzyme inhibitor, 44, 45, 74, 76, 80, 82, 84, 85, 86, 88, 89, 97, 101, 103, 113, 114, 131, 132, 133, 222, 223, 516, 519
angiotensin-receptor blocker, 97, 111, 113, 127, 131, 132, 516
antibiotics, 246, 315, 318, 319, 480, 482, 483, 494, 498, 618, 619, 624, 640, 641, 656, 676, 677, 679, 695
Antiphospholipid Syndrome, 284

antiretroviral therapy, 488, 492, 496
aortic-valve replacement, 189
APACHE II, 218, 219, 228, 229
apixaban, 161, 162, 378
appendicitis, 387, 429, 430, 514
arrhythmia, 56, 70, 75, 139, 147, 206, 261, 262
arthritis, 58
aspergillosis, 232, 233
aspirin, 92, 119, 120, 125, 126, 129, 130, 139, 140, 143, 164, 226, 316, 320, 542, 544, 546, 550, 660, 661
atorvastatin, 90, 91, 117, 552
atrial fibrillation, 92, 93, 94, 105, 106, 139, 140, 141, 142, 147, 149, 150, 151, 154, 161, 165, 171, 173, 181, 182, 189, 190, 195, 196, 198, 275, 366, 368, 378, 538, 539, 542, 544, 546, 720
autism, 687
azathioprine, 59
back pain, 397, 398, 711
Balanced Crystalloids, 282, 283
barium enema, 436
benzodiazepine, 47
beta-agonist, 248
beta-blocker, 45, 80, 97, 101, 103, 105, 111, 125, 126, 127, 156, 210, 222, 319, 518, 700, 704, 706
Bezlotoxumab, 508, 509
biliary obstruction, 401
blood pressure, 40, 41, 44, 45, 88, 89, 103, 104, 126, 133, 134, 229, 261, 263, 298, 316, 484, 512, 513, 516, 526, 527, 555, 658, 659
BNT162b2 (Pfizer–BioNTech) mRNA vaccine, 748

Bosniak classification, 384, 385, 386
BRCA1, 424
BRCA2, 424
breast cancer, 333, 376, 377, 406, 416, 424, 425, 433, 434, 459
  ductal carcinoma in situ, 425, 460
  invasive ductal carcinoma, 460
Breast Imaging-Reporting and Data System (BI-RADS), 415, 416, 417, 418, 425
breast lumpectomy, 333, 334
bronchogenic carcinoma, 208
buproprion, 51, 53
buspirone, 51
C. difficile, 490, 494, 498, 508, 582
CA-125, 428, 449, 450
calcium channel blocker, 103, 105, 127, 133, 516, 518, 700
Canadian C-Spine Rule, 234, 235
Canadian CT Head Rule, 225
canagliflozin, 532
candesartan, 111, 112, 113
captopril, 76, 77
cardiac arrest, 70, 90, 91, 97, 105, 106, 126, 148, 230, 700, 706
cardioversion, 105
carotid endarterectomy, 56, 536, 546, 719
carotid stenosis, 536, 546, 719
carvedilol, 101, 102, 222
cervical cancer, 486
cervical-spine injury, 234
chemical shift imaging, 403
Child-Pugh score, 289, 318, 319, 327, 331, 332
chlorthalidone, 103, 104
cholangitis, 297, 298
choledocholithiasis, 297, 298, 401, 402
cholesterol, 49, 50, 55, 57, 78, 90, 117, 164, 552, 674
chronic obstructive pulmonary disease (COPD), 248, 254, 255
cirrhosis, 288, 301, 302, 312, 314, 315, 318, 319, 326, 327, 341, 342, 369, 412, 444, 480
cisatracurium besylate, 265, 266

Clopidogrel, 119, 120, 125, 126, 130, 139, 143, 144, 226, 320, 321, 546, 547, 579, 580
clostridium difficile, 490, 494, 495, 498
colloid solution, 238
colon cancer, 374, 375
colonoscopy, 375, 436, 437
colorectal cancer, 436
computed tomographic angiography (CTA), 431, 432, 719, 720
computed tomographic colonography, 436, 437
computed tomographic coronary angiography (CTCA), 137, 462, 463
computed tomographic venography (CTV), 431, 432
computed tomography, 138, 168, 208, 209, 225, 242, 243, 245, 258, 259, 269, 270, 327, 335, 336, 352, 353, 355, 362, 370, 371, 384, 385, 392, 404, 406, 407, 408, 413, 414, 415, 426, 427, 428, 430, 437, 438, 439, 444, 451, 452, 453, 454, 455, 456, 458, 462, 521, 557, 558, 559, 560, 561, 571, 562, 697, 698, 702, 715, 717
contrast, 390, 391, 393, 415, 424, 450
  gadolinium, 403, 404, 405, 440, 442, 528
  ionic contrast, 138, 391, 392, 401, 407
  nonionic contrast, 391, 392, 407
coronary artery bypass graft (CABG), 120, 135, 136, 157, 158, 159, 160, 518, 704, 705
coronary artery bypass grafting, 138
coronary artery disease, 44, 78, 79, 89, 103, 127, 135, 137, 138, 142, 167, 230, 320, 462, 464, 704, 706
coronary computed tomographic angiography (CTCA), 137, 138, 167, 168
coronary heart disease, 64, 65, 121, 595
corticosteroid, 248, 249, 250, 254, 310, 311, 343, 482, 483, 658

COVID-19, 723, 727, 736, 738, 742, 743, 744, 746, 748, 749, 754, 756, 757
C-reactive protein, 55, 56, 57, 439, 440, 657
Crohn's disease, 290, 310, 311, 439, 440, 441, 495
Crohn's Disease Activity Index, 290, 291, 439
Crohn's Disease Endoscopic Index of Severity (CDEIS), 440, 441, 442, 443
cryoballoon ablation, 198
crystalloid solution, 238
CTLA-4, 364
cyclophosphamide, 59, 60
cystic fibrosis, 685, 686
Dabigatran, 141, 142, 165, 173, 174, 278, 279, 366, 367
dalteparin, 337, 338
d-dimer, 345, 346
deep vein thrombosis, 329, 330, 337, 338, 345, 346, 347, 368, 369, 372, 378
depression, 51, 53, 126
Dexamethasone, 343, 344, 483, 744, 745
diabetes, 41, 44, 45, 58, 89, 92, 93, 103, 107, 112, 132, 134, 142, 210, 230, 252, 253, 343, 513, 516, 518, 524, 527, 555, 700, 701, 713
diabetic ketoacidosis, 683, 684
diabetic nephropathy, 480, 516, 518, 524, 525, 695
dialysis, 520, 521, 529
diffusion weighted magnetic resonance, 562, 563
digital subtraction angiography, 432
digoxin, 80, 85, 97, 105
dipyridamole, 550
disk herniation, 397
donepezil, 548
dopamine, 53, 261, 262
doppler imaging, 432, 546
Doppler ultrasound, 427, 428
doxazosin, 103, 104
ECASS, 559, 561, 566

ECG-gated CT, 138, 168
ectopic pregnancy, 394, 395, 396
efavirenz, 488
emphysema, 671, 702
emtricitabine, 488, 489
enalapril, 74, 75
encainide, 70
endocarditis, 187
endometrial cancer, 376, 377, 421
endometrial stripe, 421
endoscopic band ligation, 319
endoscopic retrograde cholangiopancreatography, 401, 402
endoscopy, 303, 308, 316, 317, 375, 439
endosonography, 305
endovaginal ultrasound, 421, 422
end-stage liver disease, 312
end-stage renal disease, 516, 518, 519, 528, 529
enoxaparin. *See* heparin
enterography, 439, 440
epilepsy, 654, 655
eplerenone, 107, 108, 155, 156
epoetin, 522, 523
erythrocyte sedimentation rate, 676, 677, 678
ESCAPE, 571, 572
esophageal varices, 288, 319
EXTEND-IA, 571, 572
ezetimibe, 55, 56
facet arthropathy, 397, 398
faecal calprotectin, 439, 440
famotidine, 303
febrile seizure, 654, 655
fecal transplantation, 498
fidaxomicin, 494
finasteride, 339, 340
fistulography, 305
flecainide, 70
Fleischner Society, 242, 243, 245, 269, 270, 471, 474, 475
fluticasone, 248, 249
Food and Drug Administration, 163
gadopentetic acid, 529

gastrointestinal bleeding, 142, 217, 300, 303, 308, 314, 316, 320, 480, 542, 709
Glasgow Coma Scale, 224, 225, 258, 259, 697
Glasgow Outcome Scale, 483, 542, 567
gradient echo imaging, 403, 404
ground-glass pulmonary nodules, 472
group B streptococcus, 679
Harvey-Bradshaw Index, 290, 291, 294, 439, 440
HbA1c, 44, 45, 252, 253, 524
heart block, 700, 706
heart failure, 56, 62, 64, 66, 68, 69, 72, 73, 74, 75, 76, 77, 78, 80, 82, 83, 84, 85, 86, 88, 89, 92, 93, 95, 96, 97, 99, 100, 101, 102, 103, 104, 107, 108, 109, 110, 111, 112, 113, 114, 115, 116, 123, 124, 125, 131, 132, 145, 146, 147, 148, 149, 150, 155, 156, 177, 178, 182, 191, 193, 197, 200, 201, 222, 226, 276, 319, 518, 522, 530, 531, 532, 700, 701, 706
hemorrhage, 44, 119, 120, 139, 141, 142, 161, 165, 166, 215, 217, 263, 303, 542, 544, 562
heparin, 181, 226, 329, 330, 337, 338, 372
hepatic encephalopathy, 288, 289, 318, 319, 480
hepatic hemangioma, 406
hepatitis, 299, 300, 326, 327, 348, 369, 588, 671
hepatitis B virus, 348
hepatitis C virus (HCV), 492
hepatocellular carcinoma, 319, 326, 327, 331, 332, 335, 336, 341, 342, 348, 349, 406, 407, 444, 445, 448
hereditary nonpolyposis colorectal cancer, 437
HIV, 488, 489, 493, 497, 500, 501, 506, 507, 604, 605
hormone replacement therapy, 421, 422
uman papillomavirus (HPV), 486, 487
hyaline membrane disease, 658
hydralazine, 66

hydrocortisone, 250
hypercholesterolemia, 55
hyperlipidemia, 41, 57
hypertension, 40, 41, 42, 43, 58, 64, 76, 88, 89, 92, 93, 103, 133, 139, 142, 151, 153, 177, 182, 221, 253, 275, 301, 319, 322, 343, 516, 518, 526, 527, 586, 589, 595, 635, 672
hypoglycemia, 45, 46, 253, 256, 257
hypotension, 112, 126, 143, 228, 261, 706, 707
hypothermia, 230, 231
iatrogenic injury, 36
Idarucizumab, 278, 279
ileocolonoscopy, 440
immune globulin, 344
immune thrombocytopenic purpura (ITP), 343
immune-related response criteria, 363
inflammatory bowel disease, 58, 310, 495
infliximab, 310, 311
insulin, 44, 45, 210, 256, 513, 524, 674, 675, 700
interferon beta, 540
intraabdominal infection, 504, 505
intraarterial therapy, 570, 571, 572
intracerebral hemorrhage, 572
intracranial arterial stenosis, 163, 164
intracranial hemorrhage, 567, 570
intracranial stenosis, 544
INVEST, 710
ipilimumab, 363
irbesartan, 516
isosorbide dinitrate, 66
Kawasaki disease, 660
Kocher Criteria, 676, 677, 678
lactate, 229, 267
lamivudine, 488, 489
Lee index, 701
leukemia, 451, 452, 682
Liraglutide, 183, 184
lisinopril, 86, 103, 104
Liver Imaging Reporting and Data System (LI-RADS), 444, 445, 448
liver transplant, 326

losartan, 518, 519
low-density lipoprotein, 55, 56, 57, 78, 79, 117, 552
lung cancer, 208, 209, 242, 243, 248, 352, 361, 362, 370, 371, 455, 456, 458, 473
Lung Imaging Reporting and Data System (Lung-RADS), 243, 244, 455, 456, 457, 473
lung-volume-reduction surgery, 702, 703
lupus, 58
lymphoma, 310, 682
magnesium sulfate, 206, 207, 620, 634, 635
magnetic resonance cholangiopancreatography, 401, 402
magnetic resonance enterography global score (MEGS), 440, 443
magnetic resonance imaging, 305, 355, 356, 397, 398, 424, 425, 426, 427, 428, 429, 430, 439, 444, 528, 540, 562
Magnetic Resonance Index of Activity (MaRIA), 439, 440, 442, 443
malignancy, 242, 269, 302, 326, 361, 384, 401, 402, 403, 413, 417, 418, 422, 427, 445, 451, 452, 458, 520
mammography, 415, 416, 417, 424, 425, 426, 433, 434, 459, 460, 461
mastectomy, 333, 334
measles, 687
mediastinoscopy, 208, 209
melanoma, 364
meningitis, 479, 482, 483, 689, 691
metformin, 44, 45
metoprolol, 82, 125, 126, 210, 706
metronidazole, 490, 494, 498
microscopic polyangiitis, 59
middle cerebral artery, 559, 560
Milan Criteria, 326
MMR vaccine, 687
MODS, 228, 229
MR CLEAN, 570, 571
mRNA-1273 vaccine, 742
multiple sclerosis, 540

mumps, 687
myocardial infarction, 42, 43, 45, 57, 58, 62, 63, 64, 66, 69, 70, 73, 75, 76, 77, 78, 79, 88, 89, 90, 91, 99, 103, 107, 112, 113, 115, 116, 117, 119, 120, 121, 122, 125, 126, 127, 129, 130, 131, 132, 133, 134, 135, 138, 140, 143, 144, 145, 150, 155, 156, 157, 158, 160, 168, 169, 170, 171, 172, 179, 180, 210, 211, 222, 223, 226, 227, 240, 253, 261, 320, 321, 432, 518, 522, 524, 525, 539, 550, 553, 595, 700, 704, 705, 706, 707, 708, 709, 719, 720
  non ST elevation myocardial infarction, 143, 160, 226, 240
  ST elevation myocardial infarction, 119, 120
National Emergency X-Radiography Utilization Study (NEXUS) Low-Risk Criteria, 234
National Institute of Health Stroke Scale, 567
neisseria meningitidis, 482
nephrogenic fibrosing dermopathy, 528, 529
nephrogenic systemic fibrosis, 528, 529
nephrolithiasis, 514
NINDS, 559, 566
Nintedanib, 273, 274
nitinol stent, 163
NLST, 244, 370, 455, 456, 473
norepinephrine, 53, 261, 262
novel coronavirus–infected pneumonia, 727
obesity, 64, 253, 322, 592, 632, 670
obstructive sleep apnea, 672
occult cancers, 381, 470
octreotide, 318, 319
olanzapine, 49
omeprazole, 303, 308, 316, 317, 320
Organ Procurement and Transplantation Network (OPTN), 335, 336
orthopedic infections, 581
osteoporosis, 710, 711, 712

Ottawa ankle rules, 212, 213, 214
Ovarian cancer, 350, 351, 427, 428, 449, 450
oxazepam, 47
pancreatitis, 271, 295, 296, 713
PCSK9 inhibitor, 185
penicillin, 478, 479
peptic ulcer, 139, 303, 308, 317
percutaneous coronary intervention, 135, 157, 169, 171, 172, 240, 518
percutaneous transluminal angioplasty and stenting, 163, 164
perianal fistula, 305
perphenazine, 50
PLCO, 371, 449, 450
pneumonia, 271, 272, 479, 484
polymethylmethacrylate, 710, 711
portal hypertension, 318
portal vein thrombosis, 302, 331, 406
pravastatin, 78, 79, 117
Prednisolone, 299
prednisone, 60, 310, 343
preexposure prophylaxis, 500, 506
pregnancy, 319, 394, 395, 429, 430, 434
primary biliary cirrhosis, 312
propranolol, 62, 63, 319
prostate cancer, 339, 340, 359, 360, 721
prostate-specific antigen (PSA), 339, 359, 360, 374, 721, 722
proton-pump inhibitor, 316
pseudopolyp, 440
puberty, 666
pulmonary embolism, 329, 330, 337, 338, 345, 369, 372, 373, 376, 378, 389, 431, 432, 584, 586, 588, 590, 592, 594, 596, 598, 600, 602, 604, 606, 608, 612, 614, 616, 618, 620, 622, 624, 626, 628, 630, 632, 634
Pulmonary Fibrosis, 273, 274
pulmonary nodules, 242, 243, 269, 270, 465, 471
pyelography, 514
quetiapine, 49
radiograph, 242, 371
radiotherapy, 353, 361
ramipril, 88, 131

RECIST criteria, 354, 355, 356, 357, 363, 364, 365
Remdesivir, 736, 737
renal cell carcinoma, 406, 520
renal cysts, 384
renal insufficiency, 41, 59, 75, 86, 512, 513, 522
respiratory distress syndrome (RDS), 220, 265, 271, 272
respiratory syncytial virus (RSV), 691, 692
REVASCAT, 572
risperidone, 49
rituximab, 59
Rivaroxaban, 165, 166, 196, 197, 280, 284, 285, 368, 372
ROMICAT 1, 137, 167
ROMICAT 2, 167
rosuvastatin, 57, 58
Rosuvastatin, 57, 58
rubella, 687
saline, 238, 239, 659
salmeterol, 248, 249
SAPS II, 228, 229
schizophrenia, 49, 50
Schmorl's node, 397, 398
seizure, 567, 654, 655, 689
semaglutide, 322
sepsis, 228, 250, 261, 271, 296, 298, 478, 479, 677
septic arthritis, 676, 677, 678
septic shock, 246, 247, 250, 275, 276
shock, 70, 101, 102, 120, 125, 126, 143, 158, 217, 238, 250, 261, 303, 316, 480, 694
sickle cell disease, 478
sigmoidoscopy, 359, 374, 375
simvastatin, 55, 56
skull fracture, 225, 259
spironolactone, 84, 85, 101, 107
splenic injury, 204, 205
spontaneous bacterial peritonitis, 480, 658, 659
St. James's University Hospital classification system, 306

statin, 55, 57, 78, 90, 117, 552, 553, 700, 704
streptococcus pneumoniae, 478, 479, 482
stroke, 45, 58, 88, 89, 92, 93, 103, 104, 105, 106, 112, 113, 117, 125, 126, 130, 131, 132, 133, 135, 139, 141, 142, 143, 147, 148, 151, 157, 158, 160, 161, 162, 163, 165, 168, 215, 216, 226, 227, 253, 320, 321, 368, 378, 522, 524, 525, 536, 542, 544, 546, 550, 552, 554, 556, 559, 560, 561, 562, 563, 566, 570, 571, 706, 719, 720
subarachnoid hemorrhage, 557, 558, 564
sudden infant death syndrome (SIDS), 662
SWIFT PRIME, 572
tamoxifen, 376, 377
tenofovir, 488, 489
testosterone, 339
thiazide diuretics, 103
Thrombectomy, 572, 573, 577, 578
thromboembolism, 141, 161, 337, 338, 366, 368, 369, 372, 378
TIMI risk score, 138
tiotropium, 254, 255
tissue plasminogen activator, 215, 216, 559, 560, 566, 570, 572, 573
tomosynthesis, 459
torsade de pointes, 105, 106, 206, 207
toxic megacolon, 495
tranexamic acid, 263
transfusion, 143, 151, 204, 218, 219, 227, 229, 263, 303, 304, 308, 317
transient ischemic attack (TIA), 92, 93, 129, 142, 320, 536, 544, 546, 550, 552, 554
transient synovitis, 676, 677, 678
transjugular intrahepatic portosystemic shunt (TIPS), 312, 318, 319
transvaginal ultrasonography, 394, 395, 449, 450
traumatic brain injury, 258, 259, 697

troponin, 137, 167, 240
tumor necrosis factor -α, 310
type 2 diabetes mellitus, 44, 183, 252, 516, 524
ultrasound, 327, 341, 342, 348, 355, 359, 374, 384, 387, 388, 389, 394, 399, 421, 423, 427, 429, 430, 432, 439, 449, 454, 480, 527, 546, 610, 611, 695, 696, 711
United Network for Organ Sharing (UNOS), 335, 336
urinary tract infection (UTI), 691, 695, 696
valsartan, 97
vancomycin, 490, 494, 495, 498
vena caval filter, 329, 330, 345
venography, 389, 390
venous thromboembolism, 173, 174, 285, 337, 366, 369, 373, 378, 380, 381, 469, 470, 622, 623
ventilation-perfusion scan, 431
ventricular dysfunction, 70, 76, 88, 99, 107
ventricular fibrillation, 125, 126, 230, 700
Vericiguat, 193, 194
vertebroplasty, 710, 711
vesicoureteral reflex, 695, 696
vitamin E, 548
voiding cystourethrogram (VCUG), 695
warfarin, 92, 139, 141, 142, 161, 162, 165, 173, 174, 182, 329, 337, 338, 366, 367, 368, 372, 378, 538, 539, 542, 544
Warfarin, 141, 142, 161, 162, 165, 166, 173, 181, 284, 367, 538, 542, 543, 544, 545
Wegner's granulomatosis, 59
Wells Criteria, 213, 347
World Health Organization, 354, 363, 364
zidovudine, 488, 489
ziprasidone, 50

BIBLIOGRAPHY

This bibliography includes any references, such as original trials and follow-up trials, in this text.
References are in ascending order by publication date.

1. Avery M, Mead J. Surface properties in relation to atelectasis and hyaline membrane disease. AMA Am J Dis Child. 1959 May 1;97(5_PART_I):517–23.

2. Douglas GJ, Simpson JS. The conservative management of splenic trauma. Journal of Pediatric Surgery. 1971 Oct 1;6(5):565–70.

3. Liggins GC, Howie RN. A controlled trial of antepartum glucocorticoid treatment for prevention of the respiratory distress syndrome in premature infants. Pediatrics. 1972 Oct;50(4):515–25.

4. Pugh RNH, Murray-Lyon IM, Dawson JL, Pietroni MC, Williams R. Transection of the oesophagus for bleeding oesophageal varices. Br J Surg. 1973 Aug 1;60(8):646–9.

5. Pizzo PA, Lovejoy FH, Smith DH. Prolonged Fever in Children: Review of 100 Cases. Pediatrics. 1975 Apr 1;55(4):468–73.

6. Parks AG, Gordon PH, Hardcastle JD. A classification of fistula-in-ano. Br J Surg. 1976 Jan;63(1):1–12.

7. Brenner WE, Edelman DA, Hendricks CH. A standard of fetal growth for the United States of America. Am J Obstet Gynecol. 1976 Nov 1;126(5):555–64.

8. Nelson KB, Ellenberg JH. Predictors of Epilepsy in Children Who Have Experienced Febrile Seizures. New England Journal of Medicine. 1976 Nov 4;295(19):1029–33.

9. Fujiwara T, Maeta H, Chida S, Morita T, Watabe Y, Abe T. Artificial surfactant therapy in hyaline-membrane disease. Lancet. 1980 Jan 12;1(8159):55–9.

10. Harvey RF, Bradshaw JM. A SIMPLE INDEX OF CROHN'S-DISEASE ACTIVITY. The Lancet. 1980 Mar 8;315(8167):514.

11. Weinstein L. Syndrome of hemolysis, elevated liver enzymes, and low platelet count: a severe consequence of hypertension in pregnancy. Am J Obstet Gynecol. 1982 Jan 15;142(2):159–67.

12. Merkatz IR, Nitowsky HM, Macri JN, Johnson WE. An association between low maternal serum alpha-fetoprotein and fetal chromosomal abnormalities. Am J Obstet Gynecol. 1984 Apr 1;148(7):886–94.

13. Kurman RJ, Kaminski PF, Norris HJ. The behavior of endometrial hyperplasia. A long-term study of "untreated" hyperplasia in 170 patients. Cancer. 1985 Jul 15;56(2):403–12.

14. Bosniak MA. The current radiological approach to renal cysts. Radiology. 1986 Jan 1;158(1):1–10.

15. Cohn JN, Archibald DG, Ziesche S, Franciosa JA, Harston WE, Tristani FE, et al. Effect of Vasodilator Therapy on Mortality in Chronic Congestive Heart Failure. New England Journal of Medicine. 1986 Jun 12;314(24):1547–52.

16. Gaston MH, Verter JI, Woods G, Pegelow C, Kelleher J, Presbury G, et al. Prophylaxis with Oral Penicillin in Children with Sickle Cell Anemia. New England Journal of Medicine. 1986 Jun 19;314(25):1593–9.

17. Newburger JW, Takahashi M, Burns JC, Beiser AS, Chung KJ, Duffy CE, et al. The Treatment of Kawasaki Syndrome with Intravenous Gamma Globulin. New England Journal of Medicine. 1986 Aug 7;315(6):341–7.

18. Freeny PC, Marks WM. Patterns of contrast enhancement of benign and malignant hepatic neoplasms during bolus dynamic and delayed CT. Radiology. 1986 Sep;160(3):613–8.

19. Puylaert JBCM, Rutgers PH, Lalisang RI, de Vries BC, van der Werf SDJ, Dörr JPJ, et al. A Prospective Study of Ultrasonography in the Diagnosis of Appendicitis. New England Journal of Medicine. 1987 Sep 10;317(11):666–9.

20. Tzivoni D, Banai S, Schuger C, Benhorin J, Keren A, Gottlieb S, et al. Treatment of torsade de pointes with magnesium sulfate. Circulation. 1988 Feb 1;77(2):392–7.

21. Lensing AWA, Prandoni P, Brandjes D, Huisman PM, Vigo M, Tomasella G, et al. Detection of Deep-Vein Thrombosis by Real-Time B-Mode Ultrasonography. New England Journal of Medicine. 1989 Feb 9;320(6):342–5.

22. Heiken JP, Weyman PJ, Lee JK, Balfe DM, Picus D, Brunt EM, et al. Detection of focal hepatic masses: prospective evaluation with CT, delayed CT, CT during arterial portography, and MR imaging. Radiology. 1989 Apr;171(1):47–51.

23. Balthazar EJ, Robinson DL, Megibow AJ, Ranson JH. Acute pancreatitis: value of CT in establishing prognosis. Radiology. 1990 Feb 1;174(2):331–6.

24. Katayama H, Yamaguchi K, Kozuka T, Takashima T, Seez P, Matsuura K. Adverse reactions to ionic and nonionic contrast media. A report from the Japanese Committee on the Safety of Contrast Media. Radiology. 1990 Jun 1;175(3):621–8.

25. Fleming PJ, Gilbert R, Azaz Y, Berry PJ, Rudd PT, Stewart A, et al. Interaction between bedding and sleeping position in the sudden infant death syndrome: a population based case-control study. BMJ. 1990 Jul 14;301(6743):85–9.

26. Matsui O, Kadoya M, Kameyama T, Yoshikawa J, Takashima T, Nakanuma Y, et al. Benign and malignant nodules in cirrhotic livers: distinction based on blood supply. Radiology. 1991 Feb;178(2):493–7.

27. Brennan TA, Leape LL, Laird NM, Hebert L, Localio AR, Lawthers AG, et al. Incidence of Adverse Events and Negligence in Hospitalized Patients. New England Journal of Medicine. 1991 Feb 7;324(6):370–6.

28. Leape LL, Brennan TA, Laird N, Lawthers AG, Localio AR, Barnes BA, et al. The Nature of Adverse Events in Hospitalized Patients. New England Journal of Medicine. 1991 Feb 7;324(6):377–84.

29. Echt DS, Liebson PR, Mitchell LB, Peters RW, Obias-Manno D, Barker AH, et al. Mortality and Morbidity in Patients Receiving Encainide, Flecainide, or Placebo. New England Journal of Medicine. 1991 Mar 21;324(12):781–8.

30. Cohn JN, Johnson G, Ziesche S, Cobb F, Francis G, Tristani F, et al. A Comparison of Enalapril with Hydralazine–Isosorbide Dinitrate in the Treatment of Chronic Congestive Heart Failure. New England Journal of Medicine. 1991 Aug 1;325(5):303–10.

31. The SOLVD Investigators. Effect of enalapril on survival in patients with reduced left ventricular ejection fractions and congestive heart failure. N Engl J Med. 1991 Aug 1;325(5):293–302.

32. North American Symptomatic Carotid Endarterectomy Trial Collaborators. Beneficial effect of carotid endarterectomy in symptomatic patients with high-grade carotid stenosis. N Engl J Med. 1991 Aug 15;325(7):445–53.

33. Stampfer MJ, Colditz GA, Willett WC, Manson JE, Rosner B, Speizer FE, et al. Postmenopausal estrogen therapy and cardiovascular disease. Ten-year follow-up from the nurses' health study. N Engl J Med. 1991 Sep 12;325(11):756–62.

34. McLoud TC, Bourgouin PM, Greenberg RW, Kosiuk JP, Templeton PA, Shepard JA, et al. Bronchogenic carcinoma: analysis of staging in the mediastinum with CT by correlative lymph node mapping and sampling. Radiology. 1992 Feb 1;182(2):319–23.

35. Ramond MJ, Poynard T, Rueff B, Mathurin P, Théodore C, Chaput JC, et al. A randomized trial of prednisolone in patients with severe alcoholic hepatitis. N Engl J Med. 1992 Feb 20;326(8):507–12.

36. Beck RW, Cleary PA, Anderson MM, Keltner JL, Shults WT, Kaufman DI, et al. A randomized, controlled trial of corticosteroids in the treatment of acute optic neuritis. The Optic Neuritis Study Group. N Engl J Med. 1992 Feb 27;326(9):581–8.

37. Lorincz AT, Reid R, Jenson AB, Greenberg MD, Lancaster W, Kurman RJ. Human papillomavirus infection of the cervix: relative risk associations of

15 common anogenital types. Obstet Gynecol. 1992 Mar;79(3):328–37.

38. Lai ECS, Mok FPT, Tan ESY, Lo C mau, Fan S tat, You K tjang, et al. Endoscopic Biliary Drainage for Severe Acute Cholangitis. New England Journal of Medicine. 1992 Jun 11;326(24):1582–6.

39. Pfeffer MA, Braunwald E, Moyé LA, Basta L, Brown EJ, Cuddy TE, et al. Effect of Captopril on Mortality and Morbidity in Patients with Left Ventricular Dysfunction after Myocardial Infarction. New England Journal of Medicine. 1992 Sep 3;327(10):669–77.

40. Mitchell DG, Crovello M, Matteucci T, Petersen RO, Miettinen MM. Benign adrenocortical masses: diagnosis with chemical shift MR imaging. Radiology. 1992 Nov;185(2):345–51.

41. Bellinger DC, Stiles KM, Needleman HL. Low-Level Lead Exposure, Intelligence and Academic Achievement: A Long-term Follow-up Study. Pediatrics. 1992 Dec 1;90(6):855–61.

42. Czeizel AE, Dudás I. Prevention of the First Occurrence of Neural-Tube Defects by Periconceptional Vitamin Supplementation. New England Journal of Medicine. 1992 Dec 24;327(26):1832–5.

43. Kinmond S, Aitchison TC, Holland BM, Jones JG, Turner TL, Wardrop CA. Umbilical cord clamping and preterm infants: a randomised trial. BMJ. 1993 Jan 16;306(6871):172–5.

44. Paty DW, Li DKB, Group the UMS, Group the IMSS. Interferon beta-1b is effective in relapsing-remitting multiple sclerosis II. MRI analysis results of a multicenter, randomized, double-blind, placebo-controlled trial. Neurology. 1993 Apr 1;43(4):662–662.

45. Sultan AH, Kamm MA, Hudson CN, Thomas JM, Bartram CI. Anal-sphincter disruption during vaginal delivery. N Engl J Med. 1993 Dec 23;329(26):1905–11.

46. Rossle M, Haag K, Ochs A, Sellinger M, Noldge G, Perarnau JM, et al. The Transjugular Intrahepatic Portosystemic Stent-Shunt Procedure for Variceal Bleeding. New England Journal of Medicine. 1994 Jan 20;330(3):165–71.

47. Klahr S, Levey AS, Beck GJ, Caggiula AW, Hunsicker L, Kusek JW, et al. The Effects of Dietary Protein Restriction and Blood-Pressure Control on the Progression of Chronic Renal Disease. New England Journal of Medicine. 1994 Mar 31;330(13):877–84.

48. Brown DL, Doubilet PM. Transvaginal sonography for diagnosing ectopic pregnancy: positivity criteria and performance characteristics. Journal of Ultrasound in Medicine. 1994 Apr 1;13(4):259–66.

49. Jensen MC, Brant-Zawadzki MN, Obuchowski N, Modic MT, Malkasian D, Ross JS. Magnetic Resonance Imaging of the Lumbar Spine in People without Back Pain. New England

Journal of Medicine. 1994 Jul 14;331(2):69–73.

50. Connor EM, Sperling RS, Gelber R, Kiselev P, Scott G, O'Sullivan MJ, et al. Reduction of maternal-infant transmission of human immunodeficiency virus type 1 with zidovudine treatment. Pediatric AIDS Clinical Trials Group Protocol 076 Study Group. N Engl J Med. 1994 Nov 3;331(18):1173–80.

51. van der Wee N, Rinkel GJ, Hasan D, van Gijn J. Detection of subarachnoid haemorrhage on early CT: is lumbar puncture still needed after a negative scan? J Neurol Neurosurg Psychiatry. 1995 Mar;58(3):357–9.

52. Malmberg K, Rydén L, Efendic S, Herlitz J, Nicol P, Waldenstrom A, et al. Randomized trial of insulin-glucose infusion followed by subcutaneous insulin treatment in diabetic patients with acute myocardial infarction (DIGAMI study): Effects on mortality at 1 year. J Am Coll Cardiol. 1995 Jul 1;26(1):57–65.

53. Stavros AT, Thickman D, Rapp CL, Dennis MA, Parker SH, Sisney GA. Solid breast nodules: use of sonography to distinguish between benign and malignant lesions. Radiology. 1995 Jul 1;196(1):123–34.

54. Stiell I, Wells G, Laupacis A, Brison R, Verbeek R, Vandemheen K, et al. Multicentre trial to introduce the Ottawa ankle rules for use of radiography in acute ankle injuries. Multicentre Ankle Rule Study Group. BMJ. 1995 Sep 2;311(7005):594–7.

55. Guibaud L, Bret PM, Reinhold C, Atri M, Barkun AN. Bile duct obstruction and choledocholithiasis: diagnosis with MR cholangiography. Radiology. 1995 Oct 1;197(1):109–15.

56. Livraghi T, Giorgio A, Marin G, Salmi A, de Sio I, Bolondi L, et al. Hepatocellular carcinoma and cirrhosis in 746 patients: long-term results of percutaneous ethanol injection. Radiology. 1995 Oct 1;197(1):101–8.

57. Korobkin M, Lombardi TJ, Aisen AM, Francis IR, Quint LE, Dunnick NR, et al. Characterization of adrenal masses with chemical shift and gadolinium-enhanced MR imaging. Radiology. 1995 Nov 1;197(2):411–8.

58. The National Institute of Neurological Disorders and Stroke rt-PA Stroke Study Group. Tissue Plasminogen Activator for Acute Ischemic Stroke. New England Journal of Medicine. 1995 Dec 14;333(24):1581–8.

59. Smith RC, Verga M, McCarthy S, Rosenfield AT. Diagnosis of acute flank pain: value of unenhanced helical CT. American Journal of Roentgenology. 1996 Jan 1;166(1):97–101.

60. Iams JD, Goldenberg RL, Meis PJ, Mercer BM, Moawad A, Das A, et al. The length of the cervix and the risk of spontaneous premature delivery. National Institute of Child Health and Human Development Maternal Fetal

Medicine Unit Network. N Engl J Med. 1996 Feb 29;334(9):567–72.

61. Rockall TA, Logan RF, Devlin HB, Northfield TC. Risk assessment after acute upper gastrointestinal haemorrhage. Gut. 1996 Mar 1;38(3):316–21.

62. Mazzaferro V, Regalia E, Doci R, Andreola S, Pulvirenti A, Bozzetti F, et al. Liver Transplantation for the Treatment of Small Hepatocellular Carcinomas in Patients with Cirrhosis. New England Journal of Medicine. 1996 Mar 14;334(11):693–700.

63. Baron RL, Oliver JH, Dodd GD, Nalesnik M, Holbert BL, Carr B. Hepatocellular carcinoma: evaluation with biphasic, contrast-enhanced, helical CT. Radiology. 1996 May 1;199(2):505–11.

64. Li H, Boiselle PM, Shepard JO, Trotman-Dickenson B, McLoud TC. Diagnostic accuracy and safety of CT-guided percutaneous needle aspiration biopsy of the lung: comparison of small and large pulmonary nodules. American Journal of Roentgenology. 1996 Jul 1;167(1):105–9.

65. Sacks FM, Pfeffer MA, Moye LA, Rouleau JL, Rutherford JD, Cole TG, et al. The Effect of Pravastatin on Coronary Events after Myocardial Infarction in Patients with Average Cholesterol Levels. New England Journal of Medicine. 1996 Oct 3;335(14):1001–9.

66. The Digitalis Investigation Group. The Effect of Digoxin on Mortality and Morbidity in Patients with Heart Failure. New England Journal of Medicine. 1997 Feb 20;336(8):525–33.

67. Herman-Giddens ME, Slora EJ, Wasserman RC, Bourdony CJ, Bhapkar MV, Koch GG, et al. Secondary Sexual Characteristics and Menses in Young Girls Seen in Office Practice: A Study from the Pediatric Research in Office Settings Network. Pediatrics. 1997 Apr 1;99(4):505–12.

68. Maisels MJ, Kring E. Transcutaneous Bilirubinometry Decreases the Need for Serum Bilirubin Measurements and Saves Money. Pediatrics. 1997 Apr 1;99(4):599–600.

69. Khuroo MS, Yattoo GN, Javid G, Khan BA, Shah AA, Gulzar GM, et al. A Comparison of Omeprazole and Placebo for Bleeding Peptic Ulcer. New England Journal of Medicine. 1997 Apr 10;336(15):1054–8.

70. Appel LJ, Moore TJ, Obarzanek E, Vollmer WM, Svetkey LP, Sacks FM, et al. A Clinical Trial of the Effects of Dietary Patterns on Blood Pressure. New England Journal of Medicine. 1997 Apr 17;336(16):1117–24.

71. von Kummer R, Allen KL, Holle R, Bozzao L, Bastianello S, Manelfe C, et al. Acute stroke: usefulness of early CT findings before thrombolytic therapy. Radiology. 1997 Nov 1;205(2):327–33.

72. Decousus H, Leizorovicz A, Parent F, Page Y, Tardy B, Girard P, et al. A Clinical Trial of Vena Caval Filters in the Prevention of Pulmonary Embolism in Patients with Proximal Deep-Vein Thrombosis. New England

Journal of Medicine. 1998 Feb 12;338(7):409–16.

73. Korobkin M, Brodeur FJ, Francis IR, Quint LE, Dunnick NR, Londy F. CT time-attenuation washout curves of adrenal adenomas and nonadenomas. American Journal of Roentgenology. 1998 Mar 1;170(3):747–52.

74. Felitti VJ, Anda RF, Nordenberg D, Williamson DF, Spitz AM, Edwards V, et al. Relationship of Childhood Abuse and Household Dysfunction to Many of the Leading Causes of Death in Adults. American Journal of Preventive Medicine. 1998 May 1;14(4):245–58.

75. Hansson L, Zanchetti A, Carruthers SG, Dahlöf B, Elmfeldt D, Julius S, et al. Effects of intensive blood-pressure lowering and low-dose aspirin in patients with hypertension: principal results of the Hypertension Optimal Treatment (HOT) randomised trial. HOT Study Group. Lancet. 1998 Jun 13;351(9118):1755–62.

76. Liberman L, Abramson AF, Squires FB, Glassman JR, Morris EA, Dershaw DD. The breast imaging reporting and data system: positive predictive value of mammographic features and final assessment categories. American Journal of Roentgenology. 1998 Jul 1;171(1):35–40.

77. Gozal D. Sleep-Disordered Breathing and School Performance in Children. Pediatrics. 1998 Sep 1;102(3):616–20.

78. UK Prospective Diabetes Study (UKPDS) Group. Effect of intensive blood-glucose control with metformin on complications in overweight patients with type 2 diabetes (UKPDS 34). Lancet. 1998 Sep 12;352(9131):854–65.

79. UK Prospective Diabetes Study (UKPDS) Group. Intensive blood-glucose control with sulphonylureas or insulin compared with conventional treatment and risk of complications in patients with type 2 diabetes (UKPDS 33). The Lancet. 1998 Sep 12;352(9131):837–53.

80. Smith-Bindman R, Kerlikowske K, Feldstein VA, Subak L, Scheidler J, Segal M, et al. Endovaginal Ultrasound to Exclude Endometrial Cancer and Other Endometrial Abnormalities. JAMA. 1998 Nov 4;280(17):1510–7.

81. Kupferminc MJ, Eldor A, Steinman N, Many A, Bar-Am A, Jaffa A, et al. Increased frequency of genetic thrombophilia in women with complications of pregnancy. N Engl J Med. 1999 Jan 7;340(1):9–13.

82. Hébert PC, Wells G, Blajchman MA, Marshall J, Martin C, Pagliarello G, et al. A Multicenter, Randomized, Controlled Clinical Trial of Transfusion Requirements in Critical Care. New England Journal of Medicine. 1999 Feb 11;340(6):409–17.

83. Freedman DS, Dietz WH, Srinivasan SR, Berenson GS. The Relation of Overweight to Cardiovascular Risk Factors Among Children and Adolescents: The Bogalusa Heart Study. Pediatrics. 1999 Jun 1;103(6):1175–82.

84. MERIT-HF Study Group. Effect of metoprolol CR/XL in chronic heart

failure: Metoprolol CR/XL Randomised Intervention Trial in-Congestive Heart Failure (MERIT-HF). The Lancet. 1999 Jun 12;353(9169):2001–7.

85. Sort P, Navasa M, Arroyo V, Aldeguer X, Planas R, Ruiz-del-Arbol L, et al. Effect of Intravenous Albumin on Renal Impairment and Mortality in Patients with Cirrhosis and Spontaneous Bacterial Peritonitis. New England Journal of Medicine. 1999 Aug 5;341(6):403–9.

86. Pitt B, Zannad F, Remme WJ, Cody R, Castaigne A, Perez A, et al. The Effect of Spironolactone on Morbidity and Mortality in Patients with Severe Heart Failure. New England Journal of Medicine. 1999 Sep 2;341(10):709–17.

87. Lee TH, Marcantonio ER, Mangione CM, Thomas EJ, Polanczyk CA, Cook EF, et al. Derivation and Prospective Validation of a Simple Index for Prediction of Cardiac Risk of Major Noncardiac Surgery. Circulation. 1999 Sep 7;100(10):1043–9.

88. Goodwin SC, McLucas B, Lee M, Chen G, Perrella R, Vedantham S, et al. Uterine Artery Embolization for the Treatment of Uterine Leiomyomata Midterm Results. Journal of Vascular and Interventional Radiology. 1999 Oct 1;10(9):1159–65.

89. Kocher MS, Zurakowski D, Kasser JR. Differentiating between septic arthritis and transient synovitis of the hip in children: an evidence-based clinical prediction algorithm. J Bone Joint Surg Am. 1999 Dec;81(12):1662–70.

90. Packer M, Poole-Wilson PA, Armstrong PW, Cleland JGF, Horowitz JD, Massie BM, et al. Comparative Effects of Low and High Doses of the Angiotensin-Converting Enzyme Inhibitor, Lisinopril, on Morbidity and Mortality in Chronic Heart Failure. Circulation. 1999 Dec 7;100(23):2312–8.

91. Mari G, Deter RL, Carpenter RL, Rahman F, Zimmerman R, Moise KJ, et al. Noninvasive Diagnosis by Doppler Ultrasonography of Fetal Anemia Due to Maternal Red-Cell Alloimmunization. New England Journal of Medicine. 2000 Jan 6;342(1):9–14.

92. Schrag SJ, Zywicki S, Farley MM, Reingold AL, Harrison LH, Lefkowitz LB, et al. Group B Streptococcal Disease in the Era of Intrapartum Antibiotic Prophylaxis. New England Journal of Medicine. 2000 Jan 6;342(1):15–20.

93. Yusuf S, Sleight P, Pogue J, Bosch J, Davies R, Dagenais G. Effects of an angiotensin-converting-enzyme inhibitor, ramipril, on cardiovascular events in high-risk patients. The Heart Outcomes Prevention Evaluation Study Investigators. N Engl J Med. 2000 Jan 20;342(3):145–53.

94. Therasse P, Arbuck SG, Eisenhauer EA, Wanders J, Kaplan RS, Rubinstein L, et al. New Guidelines to Evaluate the Response to Treatment in Solid Tumors. JNCI: Journal of the National

Cancer Institute. 2000 Feb 2;92(3):205–16.

95. Wolfe J, Grier HE, Klar N, Levin SB, Ellenbogen JM, Salem-Schatz S, et al. Symptoms and Suffering at the End of Life in Children with Cancer. New England Journal of Medicine. 2000 Feb 3;342(5):326–33.

96. Morris J, Spencer JA, Ambrose NS. MR Imaging Classification of Perianal Fistulas and Its Implications for Patient Management. RadioGraphics. 2000 May 1;20(3):623–35.

97. The Acute Respiratory Distress Syndrome Network. Ventilation with Lower Tidal Volumes as Compared with Traditional Tidal Volumes for Acute Lung Injury and the Acute Respiratory Distress Syndrome. New England Journal of Medicine. 2000 May 4;342(18):1301–8.

98. Hyams JS, Markowitz J, Wyllie R. Use of infliximab in the treatment of Crohn's disease in children and adolescents. The Journal of Pediatrics. 2000 Aug 1;137(2):192–6.

99. Lau JYW, Sung JJY, Lee KKC, Yung M yee, Wong SKH, Wu JCY, et al. Effect of Intravenous Omeprazole on Recurrent Bleeding after Endoscopic Treatment of Bleeding Peptic Ulcers. New England Journal of Medicine. 2000 Aug 3;343(5):310–6.

100. Hannah ME, Hannah WJ, Hewson SA, Hodnett ED, Saigal S, Willan AR. Planned caesarean section versus planned vaginal birth for breech presentation at term: a randomised multicentre trial. Term Breech Trial Collaborative Group. Lancet. 2000 Oct 21;356(9239):1375–83.

101. Nabholtz JM, Buzdar A, Pollak M, Harwin W, Burton G, Mangalik A, et al. Anastrozole is superior to tamoxifen as first-line therapy for advanced breast cancer in postmenopausal women: results of a North American multicenter randomized trial. Arimidex Study Group. J Clin Oncol. 2000 Nov 15;18(22):3758–67.

102. Peña CS, Boland GW, Hahn PF, Lee MJ, Mueller PR. Characterization of indeterminate (lipid-poor) adrenal masses: use of washout characteristics at contrast-enhanced CT. Radiology. 2000 Dec;217(3):798–802.

103. Farrell PM, Kosorok MR, Rock MJ, Laxova A, Zeng L, Lai HC, et al. Early Diagnosis of Cystic Fibrosis Through Neonatal Screening Prevents Severe Malnutrition and Improves Long-Term Growth. Pediatrics. 2001 Jan 1;107(1):1–13.

104. Glaser N, Barnett P, McCaslin I, Nelson D, Trainor J, Louie J, et al. Risk Factors for Cerebral Edema in Children with Diabetic Ketoacidosis. New England Journal of Medicine. 2001 Jan 25;344(4):264–9.

105. Kamath PS, Wiesner RH, Malinchoc M, Kremers W, Therneau TM, Kosberg CL, et al. A model to predict survival in patients with end-stage liver disease. Hepatology. 2001 Feb 1;33(2):464–70.

106. Gracia CR, Barnhart KT. Diagnosing ectopic pregnancy: decision analysis comparing six strategies.

Obstet Gynecol. 2001 Mar;97(3):464–70.

107. Kenyon SL, Taylor DJ, Tarnow-Mordi W, ORACLE Collaborative Group. Broad-spectrum antibiotics for preterm, prelabour rupture of fetal membranes: the ORACLE I randomised trial. ORACLE Collaborative Group. Lancet. 2001 Mar 31;357(9261):979–88.

108. Schwartz GG, Olsson AG, Ezekowitz MD, et al. Effects of atorvastatin on early recurrent ischemic events in acute coronary syndromes: The miracl study: a randomized controlled trial. JAMA. 2001 Apr 4;285(13):1711–8.

109. Dargie HJ. Effect of carvedilol on outcome after myocardial infarction in patients with left-ventricular dysfunction: the CAPRICORN randomised trial. Lancet. 2001 May 5;357(9266):1385–90.

110. Stiell IG, Wells GA, Vandemheen K, Clement C, Lesiuk H, Laupacis A, et al. The Canadian CT Head Rule for patients with minor head injury. Lancet. 2001 May 5;357(9266):1391–6.

111. Yee J, Akerkar GA, Hung RK, Steinauer-Gebauer AM, Wall SD, McQuaid KR. Colorectal neoplasia: performance characteristics of CT colonography for detection in 300 patients. Radiology. 2001 Jun;219(3):685–92.

112. Gage BF, Waterman AD, Shannon W, Boechler M, Rich MW, Radford MJ. Validation of clinical classification schemes for predicting stroke: Results from the national registry of atrial fibrillation. JAMA. 2001 Jun 13;285(22):2864–70.

113. Yusuf S, Zhao F, Mehta SR, Chrolavicius S, Tognoni G, Fox KK, et al. Effects of clopidogrel in addition to aspirin in patients with acute coronary syndromes without ST-segment elevation. N Engl J Med. 2001 Aug 16;345(7):494–502.

114. Brenner BM, Cooper ME, de Zeeuw D, Keane WF, Mitch WE, Parving HH, et al. Effects of Losartan on Renal and Cardiovascular Outcomes in Patients with Type 2 Diabetes and Nephropathy. New England Journal of Medicine. 2001 Sep 20;345(12):861–9.

115. Lewis EJ, Hunsicker LG, Clarke WR, Berl T, Pohl MA, Lewis JB, et al. Renoprotective Effect of the Angiotensin-Receptor Antagonist Irbesartan in Patients with Nephropathy Due to Type 2 Diabetes. New England Journal of Medicine. 2001 Sep 20;345(12):851–60.

116. Age-Related Eye Disease Study Research Group. A randomized, placebo-controlled, clinical trial of high-dose supplementation with vitamins C and E, beta carotene, and zinc for age-related macular degeneration and vision loss: AREDS report no. 8. Arch Ophthalmol. 2001 Oct;119(10):1417–36.

117. Rivers E, Nguyen B, Havstad S, Ressler J, Muzzin A, Knoblich B, et al. Early Goal-Directed Therapy in the Treatment of Severe Sepsis and Septic Shock. New England Journal of

Medicine. 2001 Nov 8;345(19):1368–77.

118. Mohr JP, Thompson JLP, Lazar RM, Levin B, Sacco RL, Furie KL, et al. A Comparison of Warfarin and Aspirin for the Prevention of Recurrent Ischemic Stroke. New England Journal of Medicine. 2001 Nov 15;345(20):1444–51.

119. Rose EA, Gelijns AC, Moskowitz AJ, Heitjan DF, Stevenson LW, Dembitsky W, et al. Long-term use of a left ventricular assist device for end-stage heart failure. N Engl J Med. 2001 Nov 15;345(20):1435–43.

120. Cohn JN, Tognoni G. A Randomized Trial of the Angiotensin-Receptor Blocker Valsartan in Chronic Heart Failure. New England Journal of Medicine. 2001 Dec 6;345(23):1667–75.

121. Herbrecht R, Greene RE, Ribaud P, Wingard JR, Chandrasekar PH, Pauw BD. Voriconazole versus Amphotericin B for Primary Therapy of Invasive Aspergillosis. The New England Journal of Medicine. 2002;8.

122. Hypothermia after Cardiac Arrest Study Group. Mild Therapeutic Hypothermia to Improve the Neurologic Outcome after Cardiac Arrest. New England Journal of Medicine. 2002 Feb 21;346(8):549–56.

123. Moss AJ, Zareba W, Hall WJ, Klein H, Wilber DJ, Cannom DS, et al. Prophylactic Implantation of a Defibrillator in Patients with Myocardial Infarction and Reduced Ejection Fraction. New England Journal of Medicine. 2002 Mar 21;346(12):877–83.

124. Henschke CI, Yankelevitz DF, Mirtcheva R, McGuinness G, McCauley D, Miettinen OS, et al. CT screening for lung cancer: frequency and significance of part-solid and nonsolid nodules. AJR Am J Roentgenol. 2002 May;178(5):1053–7.

125. Llovet JM, Real MI, Montaña X, Planas R, Coll S, Aponte J, et al. Arterial embolisation or chemoembolisation versus symptomatic treatment in patients with unresectable hepatocellular carcinoma: a randomised controlled trial. The Lancet. 2002 May 18;359(9319):1734–9.

126. Daeppen J, Gache P, Landry U, et al. Symptom-triggered vs fixed-schedule doses of benzodiazepine for alcohol withdrawal: A randomized treatment trial. Arch Intern Med. 2002 May 27;162(10):1117–21.

127. Kass MA, Heuer DK, Higginbotham EJ, Johnson CA, Keltner JL, Miller JP, et al. The Ocular Hypertension Treatment Study: a randomized trial determines that topical ocular hypotensive medication delays or prevents the onset of primary open-angle glaucoma. Arch Ophthalmol. 2002 Jun;120(6):701–13; discussion 829-830.

128. Altman D, Carroli G, Duley L, Farrell B, Moodley J, Neilson J, et al. Do women with pre-eclampsia, and their babies, benefit from magnesium sulphate? The Magpie Trial: a

randomised placebo-controlled trial. Lancet. 2002 Jun 1;359(9321):1877–90.

129. Gordon MO, Beiser JA, Brandt JD, Heuer DK, Higginbotham EJ, Johnson CA, et al. The Ocular Hypertension Treatment Study: Baseline Factors That Predict the Onset of Primary Open-Angle Glaucoma. Archives of Ophthalmology. 2002 Jun 1;120(6):714–20.

130. Rossouw JE, Anderson GL, Prentice RL, LaCroix AZ, Kooperberg C, Stefanick ML, et al. Risks and benefits of estrogen plus progestin in healthy postmenopausal women: principal results From the Women's Health Initiative randomized controlled trial. JAMA. 2002 Jul 17;288(3):321–33.

131. Fiebach JB, Schellinger PD, Jansen O, Meyer M, Wilde P, Bender J, et al. CT and Diffusion-Weighted MR Imaging in Randomized Order Diffusion-Weighted Imaging Results in Higher Accuracy and Lower Interrater Variability in the Diagnosis of Hyperacute Ischemic. Stroke. 2002 Sep 1;33(9):2206–10.

132. Heijl A, Leske MC, Bengtsson B, Hyman L, Bengtsson B, Hussein M, et al. Reduction of intraocular pressure and glaucoma progression: results from the Early Manifest Glaucoma Trial. Arch Ophthalmol. 2002 Oct;120(10):1268–79.

133. Nigrovic LE, Kuppermann N, Malley R. Development and Validation of a Multivariable Predictive Model to Distinguish Bacterial From Aseptic Meningitis in Children in the Post-Haemophilus influenzae Era. Pediatrics. 2002 Oct 1;110(4):712–9.

134. Fisher B, Anderson S, Bryant J, Margolese RG, Deutsch M, Fisher ER, et al. Twenty-Year Follow-up of a Randomized Trial Comparing Total Mastectomy, Lumpectomy, and Lumpectomy plus Irradiation for the Treatment of Invasive Breast Cancer. New England Journal of Medicine. 2002 Oct 17;347(16):1233–41.

135. Packer M, Fowler MB, Roecker EB, Coats AJS, Katus HA, Krum H, et al. Effect of Carvedilol on the Morbidity of Patients With Severe Chronic Heart Failure Results of the Carvedilol Prospective Randomized Cumulative Survival (COPERNICUS) Study. Circulation. 2002 Oct 22;106(17):2194–9.

136. Molyneux A. International Subarachnoid Aneurysm Trial (ISAT) of neurosurgical clipping versus endovascular coiling in 2143 patients with ruptured intracranial aneurysms: a randomised trial. The Lancet. 2002 Oct 26;360(9342):1267–74.

137. Madsen KM, Hviid A, Vestergaard M, Schendel D, Wohlfahrt J, Thorsen P, et al. A Population-Based Study of Measles, Mumps, and Rubella Vaccination and Autism. New England Journal of Medicine. 2002 Nov 7;347(19):1477–82.

138. de Gans J, van de Beek D. Dexamethasone in Adults with Bacterial Meningitis. New England Journal of Medicine. 2002 Nov 14;347(20):1549–56.

139. Wyse DG, Waldo AL, DiMarco JP, Domanski MJ, Rosenberg Y, Schron EB, et al. A comparison of rate control and rhythm control in patients with atrial fibrillation. N Engl J Med. 2002 Dec 5;347(23):1825–33.

140. The ALLHAT Officers and Coordinators for the ALLHAT Collaborative Research Group. Major outcomes in high-risk hypertensive patients randomized to angiotensin-converting enzyme inhibitor or calcium channel blocker vs diuretic: The antihypertensive and lipid-lowering treatment to prevent heart attack trial (allhat). JAMA. 2002 Dec 18;288(23):2981–97.

141. Gervais DA, McGovern FJ, Arellano RS, McDougal WS, Mueller PR. Renal Cell Carcinoma: Clinical Experience and Technical Success with Radio-frequency Ablation of 42 Tumors. Radiology. 2003 Feb 1;226(2):417–24.

142. Pitt B, Remme W, Zannad F, Neaton J, Martinez F, Roniker B, et al. Eplerenone, a Selective Aldosterone Blocker, in Patients with Left Ventricular Dysfunction after Myocardial Infarction. New England Journal of Medicine. 2003 Apr 3;348(14):1309–21.

143. Lim WS, Eerden MM van der, Laing R, Boersma WG, Karalus N, Town GI, et al. Defining community acquired pneumonia severity on presentation to hospital: an international derivation and validation study. Thorax. 2003 May 1;58(5):377–82.

144. Fishman A, Martinez F, Naunheim K, Piantadosi S, Wise R, Ries A, et al. A randomized trial comparing lung-volume-reduction surgery with medical therapy for severe emphysema. N Engl J Med. 2003 May 22;348(21):2059–73.

145. Kocher MS, Mandiga R, Murphy JM, Goldmann D, Harper M, Sundel R, et al. A clinical practice guideline for treatment of septic arthritis in children: efficacy in improving process of care and effect on outcome of septic arthritis of the hip. J Bone Joint Surg Am. 2003 Jun;85(6):994–9.

146. Meis PJ, Klebanoff M, Thom E, Dombrowski MP, Sibai B, Moawad AH, et al. Prevention of recurrent preterm delivery by 17 alpha-hydroxyprogesterone caproate. N Engl J Med. 2003 Jun 12;348(24):2379–85.

147. Lencioni RA, Allgaier HP, Cioni D, Olschewski M, Deibert P, Crocetti L, et al. Small Hepatocellular Carcinoma in Cirrhosis: Randomized Comparison of Radio-frequency Thermal Ablation versus Percutaneous Ethanol Injection. Radiology. 2003 Jul 1;228(1):235–40.

148. Lee AYY, Levine MN, Baker RI, Bowden C, Kakkar AK, Prins M, et al. Low-Molecular-Weight Heparin versus a Coumarin for the Prevention of Recurrent Venous Thromboembolism in Patients with Cancer. New England Journal of Medicine. 2003 Jul 10;349(2):146–53.

149. Thompson IM, Goodman PJ, Tangen CM, Lucia MS, Miller GJ, Ford LG, et al. The Influence of Finasteride

on the Development of Prostate Cancer. New England Journal of Medicine. 2003 Jul 17;349(3):215–24.

150. Cheng Y, Wong RSM, Soo YOY, Chui CH, Lau FY, Chan NPH, et al. Initial Treatment of Immune Thrombocytopenic Purpura with High-Dose Dexamethasone. New England Journal of Medicine. 2003 Aug 28;349(9):831–6.

151. Granger CB, McMurray JJV, Yusuf S, Held P, Michelson EL, Olofsson B, et al. Effects of candesartan in patients with chronic heart failure and reduced left-ventricular systolic function intolerant to angiotensin-converting-enzyme inhibitors: the CHARM-Alternative trial. Lancet. 2003 Sep 6;362(9386):772–6.

152. Yusuf S, Pfeffer MA, Swedberg K, Granger CB, Held P, McMurray JJV, et al. Effects of candesartan in patients with chronic heart failure and preserved left-ventricular ejection fraction: the CHARM-Preserved Trial. Lancet. 2003 Sep 6;362(9386):777–81.

153. Wells PS, Anderson DR, Rodger M, Forgie M, Kearon C, Dreyer J, et al. Evaluation of D-Dimer in the Diagnosis of Suspected Deep-Vein Thrombosis. New England Journal of Medicine. 2003 Sep 25;349(13):1227–35.

154. Pfeffer MA, McMurray JJV, Velazquez EJ, Rouleau JL, Køber L, Maggioni AP, et al. Valsartan, captopril, or both in myocardial infarction complicated by heart failure, left ventricular dysfunction, or both. N Engl J Med. 2003 Nov 13;349(20):1893–906.

155. Stiell IG, Clement CM, McKnight RD, Brison R, Schull MJ, Rowe BH, et al. The Canadian C-Spine Rule versus the NEXUS Low-Risk Criteria in Patients with Trauma. New England Journal of Medicine. 2003 Dec 25;349(26):2510–8.

156. Zhang BH, Yang BH, Tang ZY. Randomized controlled trial of screening for hepatocellular carcinoma. J Cancer Res Clin Oncol. 2004 Mar 20;130(7):417–22.

157. Cannon CP, Braunwald E, McCabe CH, Rader DJ, Rouleau JL, Belder R, et al. Intensive versus Moderate Lipid Lowering with Statins after Acute Coronary Syndromes. New England Journal of Medicine. 2004 Apr 8;350(15):1495–504.

158. Luhmann SJ, Jones A, Schootman M, Gordon JE, Schoenecker PL, Luhmann JD. Differentiation between septic arthritis and transient synovitis of the hip in children with clinical prediction algorithms. J Bone Joint Surg Am. 2004 May;86(5):956–62.

159. Finfer S, Bellomo R, Boyce N, French J, Myburgh J, Norton R, et al. A comparison of albumin and saline for fluid resuscitation in the intensive care unit. N Engl J Med. 2004 May 27;350(22):2247–56.

160. Levine DA, Platt SL, Dayan PS, Macias CG, Zorc JJ, Krief W, et al. Risk of Serious Bacterial Infection in Young Febrile Infants With Respiratory

Syncytial Virus Infections. Pediatrics. 2004 Jun 1;113(6):1728–34.

161. Kriege M, Brekelmans CTM, Boetes C, Besnard PE, Zonderland HM, Obdeijn IM, et al. Efficacy of MRI and Mammography for Breast-Cancer Screening in Women with a Familial or Genetic Predisposition. New England Journal of Medicine. 2004 Jul 29;351(5):427–37.

162. Landon MB, Hauth JC, Leveno KJ, Spong CY, Leindecker S, Varner MW, et al. Maternal and Perinatal Outcomes Associated with a Trial of Labor after Prior Cesarean Delivery. New England Journal of Medicine. 2004 Dec 16;351(25):2581–9.

163. McFalls EO, Ward HB, Moritz TE, Goldman S, Krupski WC, Littooy F, et al. Coronary-Artery Revascularization before Elective Major Vascular Surgery. New England Journal of Medicine. 2004 Dec 30;351(27):2795–804.

164. Bardy GH, Boineau R, Johnson G, Davidson-Ray LD, Ip JH. Amiodarone or an Implantable Cardioverter–Defibrillator for Congestive Heart Failure. The New England Journal of Medicine. 2005;13.

165. LaRosa JC, Waters DD, Fruchart JC, Greten H, Wenger NK. Intensive Lipid Lowering with Atorvastatin in Patients with Stable Coronary Disease. The New England Journal of Medicine. 2005;11.

166. Birchard KR, Brown MA, Hyslop WB, Firat Z, Semelka RC. MRI of acute abdominal and pelvic pain in pregnant patients. AJR Am J Roentgenol. 2005 Feb;184(2):452–8.

167. Gluckman PD, Wyatt JS, Azzopardi D, Ballard R, Edwards AD, Ferriero DM, et al. Selective head cooling with mild systemic hypothermia after neonatal encephalopathy: multicentre randomised trial. Lancet. 2005 Feb 19;365(9460):663–70.

168. Sabatine MS, Cannon CP, Gibson CM, López-Sendón JL, Montalescot G, Theroux P, et al. Addition of Clopidogrel to Aspirin and Fibrinolytic Therapy for Myocardial Infarction with ST-Segment Elevation. New England Journal of Medicine. 2005 Mar 24;352(12):1179–89.

169. Chimowitz MI, Lynn MJ, Howlett-Smith H, Stern BJ, Hertzberg VS, Frankel MR, et al. Comparison of Warfarin and Aspirin for Symptomatic Intracranial Arterial Stenosis. New England Journal of Medicine. 2005 Mar 31;352(13):1305–16.

170. Condous G, Okaro E, Khalid A, Lu C, Van Huffel S, Timmerman D, et al. The accuracy of transvaginal ultrasonography for the diagnosis of ectopic pregnancy prior to surgery. Hum Reprod. 2005 May;20(5):1404–9.

171. Villa LL, Costa RLR, Petta CA, Andrade RP, Ault KA, Giuliano AR, et al. Prophylactic quadrivalent human papillomavirus (types 6, 11, 16, and 18) L1 virus-like particle vaccine in young women: a randomised double-blind placebo-controlled multicentre phase II efficacy trial. Lancet Oncol. 2005 May;6(5):271–8.

172. Markus HS, Droste DW, Kaps M, Larrue V, Lees KR, Siebler M, et al. Dual Antiplatelet Therapy With Clopidogrel and Aspirin in Symptomatic Carotid Stenosis Evaluated Using Doppler Embolic Signal Detection The Clopidogrel and Aspirin for Reduction of Emboli in Symptomatic Carotid Stenosis (CARESS) Trial. Circulation. 2005 May 3;111(17):2233–40.

173. Petersen RC, Thomas RG, Grundman M, Bennett D, Doody R, Ferris S, et al. Vitamin E and Donepezil for the Treatment of Mild Cognitive Impairment. New England Journal of Medicine. 2005 Jun 9;352(23):2379–88.

174. Kinkel K, Lu Y, Mehdizade A, Pelte MF, Hricak H. Indeterminate Ovarian Mass at US: Incremental Value of Second Imaging Test for Characterization—Meta-Analysis and Bayesian Analysis. Radiology. 2005 Jul 1;236(1):85–94.

175. Israel GM, Bosniak MA. How I Do It: Evaluating Renal Masses. Radiology. 2005 Aug 1;236(2):441–50.

176. de Winter RJ, Windhausen F, Cornel JH, Dunselman PHJM, Janus CL, Bendermacher PEF, et al. Early Invasive versus Selectively Invasive Management for Acute Coronary Syndromes. New England Journal of Medicine. 2005 Sep 15;353(11):1095–104.

177. Lieberman JA, Stroup TS, McEvoy JP, Swartz MS, Rosenheck RA, Perkins DO, et al. Effectiveness of Antipsychotic Drugs in Patients with Chronic Schizophrenia. New England Journal of Medicine. 2005 Sep 22;353(12):1209–23.

178. MacMahon H, Austin JHM, Gamsu G, Herold CJ, Jett JR, Naidich DP, et al. Guidelines for Management of Small Pulmonary Nodules Detected on CT Scans: A Statement from the Fleischner Society. Radiology. 2005 Nov 1;237(2):395–400.

179. Chen ZM, Jiang LX, Chen YP, Xie JX, Pan HC, Peto R, et al. Addition of clopidogrel to aspirin in 45,852 patients with acute myocardial infarction: randomised placebo-controlled trial. Lancet. 2005 Nov 5;366(9497):1607–21.

180. Chen ZM, Pan HC, Chen YP, Peto R, Collins R, Jiang LX, et al. Early intravenous then oral metoprolol in 45,852 patients with acute myocardial infarction: randomised placebo-controlled trial. Lancet. 2005 Nov 5;366(9497):1622–32.

181. Han YY, Carcillo JA, Venkataraman ST, Clark RSB, Watson RS, Nguyen TC, et al. Unexpected Increased Mortality After Implementation of a Commercially Sold Computerized Physician Order Entry System. Pediatrics. 2005 Dec 1;116(6):1506–12.

182. Armstrong DK, Bundy B, Wenzel L, Huang HQ, Baergen R, Lele S, et al. Intraperitoneal Cisplatin and Paclitaxel in Ovarian Cancer. New England Journal of Medicine. 2006 Jan 5;354(1):34–43.

183. Gallant JE, DeJesus E, Arribas JR, Pozniak AL, Gazzard B, Campo RE, et al. Tenofovir DF, Emtricitabine, and Efavirenz vs. Zidovudine, Lamivudine, and Efavirenz for HIV. New England Journal of Medicine. 2006 Jan 19;354(3):251–60.

184. Pedrosa I, Levine D, Eyvazzadeh AD, Siewert B, Ngo L, Rofsky NM. MR imaging evaluation of acute appendicitis in pregnancy. Radiology. 2006 Mar;238(3):891–9.

185. Rush AJ, Trivedi MH, Wisniewski SR, Stewart JW, Nierenberg AA, Thase ME, et al. Bupropion-SR, Sertraline, or Venlafaxine-XR after Failure of SSRIs for Depression. New England Journal of Medicine. 2006 Mar 23;354(12):1231–42.

186. Trivedi MH, Fava M, Wisniewski SR, Thase ME, Quitkin F, Warden D, et al. Medication Augmentation after the Failure of SSRIs for Depression. New England Journal of Medicine. 2006 Mar 23;354(12):1243–52.

187. Best WR. Predicting the Crohn's disease activity index from the Harvey-Bradshaw Index. Inflamm Bowel Dis. 2006 Apr;12(4):304–10.

188. Grobner T. Gadolinium – a specific trigger for the development of nephrogenic fibrosing dermopathy and nephrogenic systemic fibrosis? Nephrol Dial Transplant. 2006 Apr 1;21(4):1104–8.

189. ESPRIT Study Group, Halkes PHA, van Gijn J, Kappelle LJ, Koudstaal PJ, Algra A. Aspirin plus dipyridamole versus aspirin alone after cerebral ischaemia of arterial origin (ESPRIT): randomised controlled trial. Lancet. 2006 May 20;367(9523):1665–73.

190. Caird MS, Flynn JM, Leung YL, Millman JE, D'Italia JG, Dormans JP. Factors distinguishing septic arthritis from transient synovitis of the hip in children. A prospective study. J Bone Joint Surg Am. 2006 Jun;88(6):1251–7.

191. Kumar A, Roberts D, Wood KE, Light B, Parrillo JE, Sharma S, et al. Duration of hypotension before initiation of effective antimicrobial therapy is the critical determinant of survival in human septic shock. Crit Care Med. 2006 Jun;34(6):1589–96.

192. Stein PD, Fowler SE, Goodman LR, Gottschalk A, Hales CA, Hull RD, et al. Multidetector Computed Tomography for Acute Pulmonary Embolism. New England Journal of Medicine. 2006 Jun 1;354(22):2317–27.

193. Amarenco P, Bogousslavsky J, Callahan A, Goldstein LB, Hennerici M, Rudolph AE, et al. High-dose atorvastatin after stroke or transient ischemic attack. N Engl J Med. 2006 Aug 10;355(6):549–59.

194. Fernández J, Ruiz del Arbol L, Gómez C, Durandez R, Serradilla R, Guarner C, et al. Norfloxacin vs ceftriaxone in the prophylaxis of infections in patients with advanced cirrhosis and hemorrhage. Gastroenterology. 2006 Oct;131(4):1049–56; quiz 1285.

195. Singh AK, Szczech L, Tang KL, Barnhart H, Sapp S, Wolfson M, et al.

Correction of Anemia with Epoetin Alfa in Chronic Kidney Disease. New England Journal of Medicine. 2006 Nov 16;355(20):2085–98.

196. Nigrovic LE, Kuppermann N, Macias CG, et al. Clinical prediction rule for identifying children with cerebrospinal fluid pleocytosis at very low risk of bacterial meningitis. JAMA. 2007 Jan 3;297(1):52–60.

197. Boyd NF, Guo H, Martin LJ, Sun L, Stone J, Fishell E, et al. Mammographic Density and the Risk and Detection of Breast Cancer. New England Journal of Medicine. 2007 Jan 18;356(3):227–36.

198. Johnston SC, Rothwell PM, Nguyen-Huynh MN, Giles MF, Elkins JS, Bernstein AL, et al. Validation and refinement of scores to predict very early stroke risk after transient ischaemic attack. Lancet. 2007 Jan 27;369(9558):283–92.

199. Calverley PMA, Anderson JA, Celli B, Ferguson GT, Jenkins C, Jones PW, et al. Salmeterol and Fluticasone Propionate and Survival in Chronic Obstructive Pulmonary Disease. New England Journal of Medicine. 2007 Feb 22;356(8):775–89.

200. Simon CJ, Dupuy DE, DiPetrillo TA, Safran HP, Grieco CA, Ng T, et al. Pulmonary radiofrequency ablation: long-term safety and efficacy in 153 patients. Radiology. 2007 Apr;243(1):268–75.

201. Boden WE, O'Rourke RA, Teo KK, Hartigan PM, Maron DJ, Kostuk WJ, et al. Optimal Medical Therapy with or without PCI for Stable Coronary Disease. New England Journal of Medicine. 2007 Apr 12;356(15):1503–16.

202. Lau JY, Leung WK, Wu JCY, Chan FKL, Wong VWS, Chiu PWY, et al. Omeprazole before Endoscopy in Patients with Gastrointestinal Bleeding. New England Journal of Medicine. 2007 Apr 19;356(16):1631–40.

203. Zar FA, Bakkanagari SR, Moorthi KMLST, Davis MB. A Comparison of Vancomycin and Metronidazole for the Treatment of Clostridium difficile–Associated Diarrhea, Stratified by Disease Severity. Clin Infect Dis. 2007 Aug 1;45(3):302–7.

204. Duffy JP, Vardanian A, Benjamin E, Watson M, Farmer DG, Ghobrial RM, et al. Liver Transplantation Criteria For Hepatocellular Carcinoma Should Be Expanded. Ann Surg. 2007 Sep;246(3):502–11.

205. Kim DH, Pickhardt PJ, Taylor AJ, Leung WK, Winter TC, Hinshaw JL, et al. CT Colonography versus Colonoscopy for the Detection of Advanced Neoplasia. New England Journal of Medicine. 2007 Oct 4;357(14):1403–12.

206. Wiviott SD, Braunwald E, McCabe CH, Montalescot G, Ruzyllo W, Gottlieb S, et al. Prasugrel versus Clopidogrel in Patients with Acute Coronary Syndromes. New England Journal of Medicine. 2007 Nov 15;357(20):2001–15.

207. Sprung CL, Annane D, Keh D, Moreno R, Singer M, Freivogel K, et al.

Hydrocortisone Therapy for Patients with Septic Shock. New England Journal of Medicine. 2008 Jan 10;358(2):111–24.

208. Roussey-Kesler G, Gadjos V, Idres N, Horen B, Ichay L, Leclair MD, et al. Antibiotic Prophylaxis for the Prevention of Recurrent Urinary Tract Infection in Children With Low Grade Vesicoureteral Reflux: Results From a Prospective Randomized Study. The Journal of Urology. 2008 Feb 1;179(2):674–9.

209. Kastelein JJP, Akdim F, Stroes ESG, Zwinderman AH, Bots ML, Stalenhoef AFH, et al. Simvastatin with or without Ezetimibe in Familial Hypercholesterolemia. New England Journal of Medicine. 2008 Apr 3;358(14):1431–43.

210. The ONTARGET Investigators. Telmisartan, Ramipril, or Both in Patients at High Risk for Vascular Events. New England Journal of Medicine. 2008 Apr 10;358(15):1547–59.

211. HAPO Study Cooperative Research Group, Metzger BE, Lowe LP, Dyer AR, Trimble ER, Chaovarindr U, et al. Hyperglycemia and adverse pregnancy outcomes. N Engl J Med. 2008 May 8;358(19):1991–2002.

212. POISE Study Group, Devereaux PJ, Yang H, Yusuf S, Guyatt G, Leslie K, et al. Effects of extended-release metoprolol succinate in patients undergoing non-cardiac surgery (POISE trial): a randomised controlled trial. Lancet. 2008 May 31;371(9627):1839–47.

213. Action to Control Cardiovascular Risk in Diabetes Study Group, Gerstein HC, Miller ME, Byington RP, Goff DC, Bigger JT, et al. Effects of intensive glucose lowering in type 2 diabetes. N Engl J Med. 2008 Jun 12;358(24):2545–59.

214. ADVANCE Collaborative Group, Patel A, MacMahon S, Chalmers J, Neal B, Billot L, et al. Intensive blood glucose control and vascular outcomes in patients with type 2 diabetes. N Engl J Med. 2008 Jun 12;358(24):2560–72.

215. Lencioni R, Crocetti L, Cioni R, Suh R, Glenn D, Regge D, et al. Response to radiofrequency ablation of pulmonary tumours: a prospective, intention-to-treat, multicentre clinical trial (the RAPTURE study). The Lancet Oncology. 2008 Jul 1;9(7):621–8.

216. Israel GM, Malguria N, McCarthy S, Copel J, Weinreb J. MRI vs. ultrasound for suspected appendicitis during pregnancy. J Magn Reson Imaging. 2008 Aug;28(2):428–33.

217. Rouse DJ, Hirtz DG, Thom E, Varner MW, Spong CY, Mercer BM, et al. A randomized, controlled trial of magnesium sulfate for the prevention of cerebral palsy. N Engl J Med. 2008 Aug 28;359(9):895–905.

218. Hacke W, Kaste M, Bluhmki E, Brozman M, Dávalos A, Guidetti D, et al. Thrombolysis with Alteplase 3 to 4.5 Hours after Acute Ischemic Stroke. New England Journal of Medicine. 2008 Sep 25;359(13):1317–29.

219. Tashkin DP, Celli B, Senn S, Burkhart D, Kesten S, Menjoge S, et al. A 4-Year Trial of Tiotropium in Chronic Obstructive Pulmonary Disease. New England Journal of Medicine. 2008 Oct 9;359(15):1543–54.

220. Ridker PM, Danielson E, Fonseca FAH, Genest J, Gotto AM, Kastelein JJP, et al. Rosuvastatin to Prevent Vascular Events in Men and Women with Elevated C-Reactive Protein. New England Journal of Medicine. 2008 Nov 20;359(21):2195–207.

221. Boland GWL, Blake MA, Hahn PF, Mayo-Smith WW. Incidental adrenal lesions: principles, techniques, and algorithms for imaging characterization. Radiology. 2008 Dec;249(3):756–75.

222. Jamerson K, Weber MA, Bakris GL, Dahlöf B, Pitt B, Shi V, et al. Benazepril plus Amlodipine or Hydrochlorothiazide for Hypertension in High-Risk Patients. New England Journal of Medicine. 2008 Dec 4;359(23):2417–28.

223. Buchbinder R, Mitchell P, Med M, Wriedt C, Murphy B. A Randomized Trial of Vertebroplasty for Painful Osteoporotic Vertebral Fractures. n engl j med. 2009;12.

224. Eisenhauer EA, Therasse P, Bogaerts J, Schwartz LH, Sargent D, Ford R, et al. New response evaluation criteria in solid tumours: Revised RECIST guideline (version 1.1). European Journal of Cancer. 2009 Jan 1;45(2):228–47.

225. Serruys PW, Morice MC, Kappetein AP, Colombo A, Holmes DR, Mack MJ, et al. Percutaneous Coronary Intervention versus Coronary-Artery Bypass Grafting for Severe Coronary Artery Disease. New England Journal of Medicine. 2009 Mar 5;360(10):961–72.

226. Andriole GL, Crawford ED, Grubb RL, Buys SS, Chia D, Church TR, et al. Mortality Results from a Randomized Prostate-Cancer Screening Trial. New England Journal of Medicine. 2009 Mar 26;360(13):1310–9.

227. NICE-SUGAR Study Investigators, Finfer S, Chittock DR, Su SYS, Blair D, Foster D, et al. Intensive versus conventional glucose control in critically ill patients. N Engl J Med. 2009 Mar 26;360(13):1283–97.

228. Kitahata MM, Gange SJ, Abraham AG, Merriman B, Saag MS, Justice AC, et al. Effect of Early versus Deferred Antiretroviral Therapy for HIV on Survival. New England Journal of Medicine. 2009 Apr 30;360(18):1815–26.

229. Davies DA, Pearl RH, Ein SH, Langer JC, Wales PW. Management of blunt splenic injury in children: evolution of the nonoperative approach. Journal of Pediatric Surgery. 2009 May 1;44(5):1005–8.

230. Hoffmann U, Bamberg F, Chae CU, Nichols JH, Rogers IS, Seneviratne SK, et al. Coronary Computed Tomography Angiography For Early Triage of Patients with Acute Chest Pain - The Rule Out Myocardial

Infarction Using Computer Assisted Tomography (ROMICAT) Trial. J Am Coll Cardiol. 2009 May 5;53(18):1642–50.

231. ACTIVE Investigators, Connolly SJ, Pogue J, Hart RG, Hohnloser SH, Pfeffer M, et al. Effect of clopidogrel added to aspirin in patients with atrial fibrillation. N Engl J Med. 2009 May 14;360(20):2066–78.

232. Baumann P, Nyman J, Hoyer M, Wennberg B, Gagliardi G, Lax I, et al. Outcome in a Prospective Phase II Trial of Medically Inoperable Stage I Non–Small-Cell Lung Cancer Patients Treated With Stereotactic Body Radiotherapy. JCO. 2009 Jul 10;27(20):3290–6.

233. Rimola J, Rodriguez S, García-Bosch O, Ordás I, Ayala E, Aceituno M, et al. Magnetic resonance for assessment of disease activity and severity in ileocolonic Crohn's disease. Gut. 2009 Aug 1;58(8):1113–20.

234. Kallmes DF, Comstock BA, Heagerty PJ, Turner JA, Wilson DJ, Diamond TH, et al. A Randomized Trial of Vertebroplasty for Osteoporotic Spinal Fractures. New England Journal of Medicine. 2009 Aug 6;361(6):569–79.

235. Wallentin L, Becker RC, Budaj A, Cannon CP, Emanuelsson H, Held C, et al. Ticagrelor versus Clopidogrel in Patients with Acute Coronary Syndromes. New England Journal of Medicine. 2009 Sep 10;361(11):1045–57.

236. Connolly SJ, Ezekowitz MD, Yusuf S, Eikelboom J, Oldgren J, Parekh A, et al. Dabigatran versus Warfarin in Patients with Atrial Fibrillation. New England Journal of Medicine. 2009 Sep 17;361(12):1139–51.

237. Moss AJ, Hall WJ, Cannom DS, Klein H, Brown MW, Daubert JP, et al. Cardiac-resynchronization therapy for the prevention of heart-failure events. N Engl J Med. 2009 Oct 1;361(14):1329–38.

238. Kuppermann N, Holmes JF, Dayan PS, Hoyle JD, Atabaki SM, Holubkov R, et al. Identification of children at very low risk of clinically-important brain injuries after head trauma: a prospective cohort study. Lancet. 2009 Oct 3;374(9696):1160–70.

239. Wolchok JD, Hoos A, O'Day S, Weber JS, Hamid O, Lebbé C, et al. Guidelines for the Evaluation of Immune Therapy Activity in Solid Tumors: Immune-Related Response Criteria. Clin Cancer Res. 2009 Dec 1;15(23):7412–20.

240. Schulman S, Kearon C, Kakkar AK, Mismetti P, Schellong S, Eriksson H, et al. Dabigatran versus Warfarin in the Treatment of Acute Venous Thromboembolism. New England Journal of Medicine. 2009 Dec 10;361(24):2342–52.

241. González AB de, Mahesh M, Kim KP, Bhargavan M, Lewis R, Mettler F, et al. Projected Cancer Risks From Computed Tomographic Scans Performed in the United States in 2007.

Arch Intern Med. 2009 Dec 14;169(22):2071–7.

242. De Backer D, Biston P, Devriendt J, Madl C, Chochrad D, Aldecoa C, et al. Comparison of Dopamine and Norepinephrine in the Treatment of Shock. New England Journal of Medicine. 2010 Mar 4;362(9):779–89.

243. Timmerman R, Paulus R, Galvin J, Michalski J, Straube W, Bradley J, et al. Stereotactic body radiation therapy for inoperable early stage lung cancer. JAMA. 2010 Mar 17;303(11):1070–6.

244. The United Kingdom EVAR Trial Investigators. Endovascular versus open repair of abdominal aortic aneurysm. Maedica (Buchar). 2010 Apr;5(2):148.

245. TOMA N. Endovascular versus open repair of abdominal aortic aneurysm. Maedica (Buchar). 2010 Apr;5(2):148.

246. Vermeire S, Schreiber S, Sandborn WJ, Dubois C, Rutgeerts P. Correlation between the Crohn's disease activity and Harvey-Bradshaw indices in assessing Crohn's disease severity. Clin Gastroenterol Hepatol. 2010 Apr;8(4):357–63.

247. Van Gelder IC, Groenveld HF, Crijns HJGM, Tuininga YS, Tijssen JGP, Alings AM, et al. Lenient versus Strict Rate Control in Patients with Atrial Fibrillation. New England Journal of Medicine. 2010 Apr 15;362(15):1363–73.

248. van Santvoort HC, Besselink MG, Bakker OJ, Hofker HS, Boermeester MA, Dejong CH, et al. A Step-up Approach or Open Necrosectomy for Necrotizing Pancreatitis. New England Journal of Medicine. 2010 Apr 22;362(16):1491–502.

249. Cortnum S, Sørensen P, Jørgensen J. Determining the sensitivity of computed tomography scanning in early detection of subarachnoid hemorrhage. Neurosurgery. 2010 May;66(5):900–2; discussion 903.

250. United Kingdom EVAR Trial Investigators, Greenhalgh RM, Brown LC, Powell JT, Thompson SG, Epstein D. Endovascular repair of aortic aneurysm in patients physically ineligible for open repair. N Engl J Med. 2010 May 20;362(20):1872–80.

251. Blake MA, Cronin CG, Boland GW. Adrenal imaging. AJR Am J Roentgenol. 2010 Jun;194(6):1450–60.

252. García-Pagán JC, Caca K, Bureau C, Laleman W, Appenrodt B, Luca A, et al. Early Use of TIPS in Patients with Cirrhosis and Variceal Bleeding. New England Journal of Medicine. 2010 Jun 24;362(25):2370–9.

253. Brott TG, Hobson RW, Howard G, Roubin GS, Clark WM, Brooks W, et al. Stenting versus Endarterectomy for Treatment of Carotid-Artery Stenosis. New England Journal of Medicine. 2010 Jul 1;363(1):11–23.

254. CRASH-2 trial collaborators, Shakur H, Roberts I, Bautista R, Caballero J, Coats T, et al. Effects of tranexamic acid on death, vascular occlusive events, and blood transfusion in trauma patients with significant

haemorrhage (CRASH-2): a randomised, placebo-controlled trial. Lancet. 2010 Jul 3;376(9734):23–32.

255. Stone JH, Merkel PA, Spiera R, Seo P, Langford CA, Hoffman GS, et al. Rituximab versus Cyclophosphamide for ANCA-Associated Vasculitis. New England Journal of Medicine. 2010 Jul 15;363(3):221–32.

256. Swedberg K, Komajda M, Böhm M, Borer JS, Ford I, Dubost-Brama A, et al. Ivabradine and outcomes in chronic heart failure (SHIFT): a randomised placebo-controlled study. Lancet. 2010 Sep 11;376(9744):875–85.

257. Jansen TC, van Bommel J, Schoonderbeek FJ, Sleeswijk Visser SJ, van der Klooster JM, Lima AP, et al. Early Lactate-Guided Therapy in Intensive Care Unit Patients. Am J Respir Crit Care Med. 2010 Sep 15;182(6):752–61.

258. Papazian L, Forel JM, Gacouin A, Penot-Ragon C, Perrin G, Loundou A, et al. Neuromuscular Blockers in Early Acute Respiratory Distress Syndrome. New England Journal of Medicine. 2010 Sep 16;363(12):1107–16.

259. Pisters R, Lane DA, Nieuwlaat R, de Vos CB, Crijns HJGM, Lip GYH. A novel user-friendly score (has-bled) to assess 1-year risk of major bleeding in patients with atrial fibrillation: The euro heart survey. Chest. 2010 Nov 1;138(5):1093–100.

260. Bhatt DL, Cryer BL, Contant CF, Cohen M, Lanas A, Schnitzer TJ, et al. Clopidogrel with or without Omeprazole in Coronary Artery Disease. New England Journal of Medicine. 2010 Nov 11;363(20):1909–17.

261. Symplicity HTN-2 Investigators, Esler MD, Krum H, Sobotka PA, Schlaich MP, Schmieder RE, et al. Renal sympathetic denervation in patients with treatment-resistant hypertension (The Symplicity HTN-2 Trial): a randomised controlled trial. Lancet. 2010 Dec 4;376(9756):1903–9.

262. EINSTEIN Investigators, Bauersachs R, Berkowitz SD, Brenner B, Buller HR, Decousus H, et al. Oral rivaroxaban for symptomatic venous thromboembolism. N Engl J Med. 2010 Dec 23;363(26):2499–510.

263. Grant RM, Lama JR, Anderson PL, McMahan V, Liu AY, Vargas L, et al. Preexposure chemoprophylaxis for HIV prevention in men who have sex with men. N Engl J Med. 2010 Dec 30;363(27):2587–99.

264. Zannad F, McMurray JJV, Krum H, van Veldhuisen DJ, Swedberg K, Shi H, et al. Eplerenone in Patients with Systolic Heart Failure and Mild Symptoms. New England Journal of Medicine. 2011 Jan 6;364(1):11–21.

265. Louie TJ, Miller MA, Mullane KM, Weiss K, Lentnek A, Golan Y, et al. Fidaxomicin versus Vancomycin for Clostridium difficile Infection. New England Journal of Medicine. 2011 Feb 3;364(5):422–31.

266. Felker GM, Lee KL, Bull DA, Redfield MM, Stevenson LW, Goldsmith SR, et al. Diuretic strategies

in patients with acute decompensated heart failure. N Engl J Med. 2011 Mar 3;364(9):797–805.

267. Jolly SS, Yusuf S, Cairns J, Niemelä K, Xavier D, Widimsky P, et al. Radial versus femoral access for coronary angiography and intervention in patients with acute coronary syndromes (RIVAL): a randomised, parallel group, multicentre trial. Lancet. 2011 Apr 23;377(9775):1409–20.

268. Park SJ, Kim YH, Park DW, Yun SC, Ahn JM, Song HG, et al. Randomized Trial of Stents versus Bypass Surgery for Left Main Coronary Artery Disease. New England Journal of Medicine. 2011 May 5;364(18):1718–27.

269. Buys SS, Partridge E, Black A, Johnson CC, Lamerato L, Isaacs C, et al. Effect of Screening on Ovarian Cancer Mortality: The Prostate, Lung, Colorectal and Ovarian (PLCO) Cancer Screening Randomized Controlled Trial. JAMA. 2011 Jun 8;305(22):2295–303.

270. Rimola J, Ordás I, Rodriguez S, García-Bosch O, Aceituno M, Llach J, et al. Magnetic resonance imaging for evaluation of Crohn's disease: validation of parameters of severity and quantitative index of activity. Inflamm Bowel Dis. 2011 Aug;17(8):1759–68.

271. National Lung Screening Trial Research Team, Aberle DR, Adams AM, Berg CD, Black WC, Clapp JD, et al. Reduced lung-cancer mortality with low-dose computed tomographic screening. N Engl J Med. 2011 Aug 4;365(5):395–409.

272. Cohen MS, Chen YQ, McCauley M, Gamble T, Hosseinipour MC, Kumarasamy N, et al. Prevention of HIV-1 Infection with Early Antiretroviral Therapy. New England Journal of Medicine. 2011 Aug 11;365(6):493–505.

273. Patel MR, Mahaffey KW, Garg J, Pan G, Singer DE, Hacke W, et al. Rivaroxaban versus Warfarin in Nonvalvular Atrial Fibrillation. New England Journal of Medicine. 2011 Sep 8;365(10):883–91.

274. Chimowitz MI, Lynn MJ, Derdeyn CP, Turan TN, Fiorella D, Lane BF, et al. Stenting versus aggressive medical therapy for intracranial arterial stenosis. N Engl J Med. 2011 Sep 15;365(11):993–1003.

275. Granger CB, Alexander JH, McMurray JJV, Lopes RD, Hylek EM, Hanna M, et al. Apixaban versus Warfarin in Patients with Atrial Fibrillation. New England Journal of Medicine. 2011 Sep 15;365(11):981–92.

276. Bosniak MA. The Bosniak renal cyst classification: 25 years later. Radiology. 2012 Mar;262(3):781–5.

277. EINSTEIN–PE Investigators, Büller HR, Prins MH, Lensin AWA, Decousus H, Jacobson BF, et al. Oral rivaroxaban for the treatment of symptomatic pulmonary embolism. N Engl J Med. 2012 Apr 5;366(14):1287–97.

278. Connolly ES, Rabinstein AA, Carhuapoma JR, Derdeyn CP, Dion J, Higashida RT, et al. Guidelines for the management of aneurysmal subarachnoid hemorrhage: a guideline for healthcare professionals from the American Heart Association/american Stroke Association. Stroke. 2012 Jun;43(6):1711–37.

279. Schoen RE, Pinsky PF, Weissfeld JL, Yokochi LA, Church T, Laiyemo AO, et al. Colorectal-Cancer Incidence and Mortality with Screening Flexible Sigmoidoscopy. New England Journal of Medicine. 2012 Jun 21;366(25):2345–57.

280. Wilt TJ, Brawer MK, Jones KM, Barry MJ, Aronson WJ, Fox S, et al. Radical Prostatectomy versus Observation for Localized Prostate Cancer. New England Journal of Medicine. 2012 Jul 19;367(3):203–13.

281. Hoffmann U, Truong QA, Schoenfeld DA, Chou ET, Woodard PK, Nagurney JT, et al. Coronary CT Angiography versus Standard Evaluation in Acute Chest Pain. New England Journal of Medicine. 2012 Jul 26;367(4):299–308.

282. Pearce MS, Salotti JA, Little MP, McHugh K, Lee C, Kim KP, et al. Radiation exposure from CT scans in childhood and subsequent risk of leukaemia and brain tumours: a retrospective cohort study. Lancet. 2012 Aug 4;380(9840):499–505.

283. Purysko AS, Remer EM, Coppa CP, Leão Filho HM, Thupili CR, Veniero JC. LI-RADS: a case-based review of the new categorization of liver findings in patients with end-stage liver disease. Radiographics. 2012 Dec;32(7):1977–95.

284. Farkouh ME, Domanski M, Sleeper LA, Siami FS, Dangas G, Mack M, et al. Strategies for multivessel revascularization in patients with diabetes. N Engl J Med. 2012 Dec 20;367(25):2375–84.

285. Naidich DP, Bankier AA, MacMahon H, Schaefer-Prokop CM, Pistolesi M, Goo JM, et al. Recommendations for the management of subsolid pulmonary nodules detected at CT: a statement from the Fleischner Society. Radiology. 2013 Jan;266(1):304–17.

286. van Nood E, Vrieze A, Nieuwdorp M, Fuentes S, Zoetendal EG, de Vos WM, et al. Duodenal Infusion of Donor Feces for Recurrent Clostridium difficile. New England Journal of Medicine. 2013 Jan 31;368(5):407–15.

287. Wald C, Russo MW, Heimbach JK, Hussain HK, Pomfret EA, Bruix J. New OPTN/UNOS Policy for Liver Transplant Allocation: Standardization of Liver Imaging, Diagnosis, Classification, and Reporting of Hepatocellular Carcinoma. Radiology. 2013 Feb 1;266(2):376–82.

288. Davies C, Pan H, Godwin J, Gray R, Arriagada R, Raina V, et al. Long-term effects of continuing adjuvant tamoxifen to 10 years versus stopping at 5 years after diagnosis of oestrogen receptor-positive breast cancer:

ATLAS, a randomised trial. Lancet. 2013 Mar 9;381(9869):805–16.

289. Dewilde WJM, Oirbans T, Verheugt FWA, Kelder JC, De Smet BJGL, Herrman JP, et al. Use of clopidogrel with or without aspirin in patients taking oral anticoagulant therapy and undergoing percutaneous coronary intervention: an open-label, randomised, controlled trial. Lancet. 2013 Mar 30;381(9872):1107–15.

290. Age-Related Eye Disease Study 2 Research Group. Lutein + zeaxanthin and omega-3 fatty acids for age-related macular degeneration: the Age-Related Eye Disease Study 2 (AREDS2) randomized clinical trial. JAMA. 2013 May 15;309(19):2005–15.

291. Mathews JD, Forsythe AV, Brady Z, Butler MW, Goergen SK, Byrnes GB, et al. Cancer risk in 680,000 people exposed to computed tomography scans in childhood or adolescence: data linkage study of 11 million Australians. BMJ. 2013 May 21;346:f2360.

292. Guérin C, Reignier J, Richard JC, Beuret P, Gacouin A, Boulain T, et al. Prone Positioning in Severe Acute Respiratory Distress Syndrome. New England Journal of Medicine. 2013 Jun 6;368(23):2159–68.

293. Miglioretti DL, Johnson E, Williams A, Greenlee RT, Weinmann S, Solberg LI, et al. The use of computed tomography in pediatrics and the associated radiation exposure and estimated cancer risk. JAMA Pediatr. 2013 Aug 1;167(8):700–7.

294. Agnelli G, Buller HR, Cohen A, Curto M, Gallus AS, Johnson M, et al. Oral Apixaban for the Treatment of Acute Venous Thromboembolism. New England Journal of Medicine. 2013 Aug 29;369(9):799–808.

295. Eikelboom JW, Connolly SJ, Brueckmann M, Granger CB, Kappetein AP, Mack MJ, et al. Dabigatran versus warfarin in patients with mechanical heart valves. N Engl J Med. 2013 Sep 26;369(13):1206–14.

296. M I, A B, R C, S F, S M, F B, et al. A randomized trial of colchicine for acute pericarditis. The New England journal of medicine [Internet]. 2013 Oct 17 [cited 2021 Aug 29];369(16). Available from: https://pubmed.ncbi.nlm.nih.gov/23992557/

297. Biro FM, Greenspan LC, Galvez MP, Pinney SM, Teitelbaum S, Windham GC, et al. Onset of Breast Development in a Longitudinal Cohort. Pediatrics. 2013 Nov 4;peds.2012-3773.

298. Makanyanga JC, Pendsé D, Dikaios N, Bloom S, McCartney S, Helbren E, et al. Evaluation of Crohn's disease activity: initial validation of a magnetic resonance enterography global score (MEGS) against faecal calprotectin. Eur Radiol. 2014 Feb;24(2):277–87.

299. Devereaux PJ, Mrkobrada M, Sessler DI, Leslie K, Alonso-Coello P, Kurz A, et al. Aspirin in Patients Undergoing Noncardiac Surgery. New England Journal of Medicine. 2014 Apr 17;370(16):1494–503.

300. Asfar P, Meziani F, Hamel JF, Grelon F, Megarbane B, Anguel N, et al. High versus Low Blood-Pressure Target in Patients with Septic Shock. New England Journal of Medicine. 2014 Apr 24;370(17):1583–93.

301. Zeuzem S, Dusheiko GM, Salupere R, Mangia A, Flisiak R, Hyland RH, et al. Sofosbuvir and Ribavirin in HCV Genotypes 2 and 3. New England Journal of Medicine. 2014 May 22;370(21):1993–2001.

302. Richeldi L, du Bois RM, Raghu G, Azuma A, Brown KK, Costabel U, et al. Efficacy and Safety of Nintedanib in Idiopathic Pulmonary Fibrosis. New England Journal of Medicine. 2014 May 29;370(22):2071–82.

303. Friedewald SM, Rafferty EA, Rose SL, Durand MA, Plecha DM, Greenberg JS, et al. Breast Cancer Screening Using Tomosynthesis in Combination With Digital Mammography. JAMA. 2014 Jun 25;311(24):2499–507.

304. McMurray JJV, Packer M, Desai AS, Gong J, Lefkowitz MP, Rizkala AR, et al. Angiotensin–Neprilysin Inhibition versus Enalapril in Heart Failure. New England Journal of Medicine. 2014 Sep 11;371(11):993–1004.

305. Holst LB, Haase N, Wetterslev J, Wernerman J, Guttormsen AB, Karlsson S, et al. Lower versus Higher Hemoglobin Threshold for Transfusion in Septic Shock. New England Journal of Medicine. 2014 Oct 9;371(15):1381–91.

306. Levine MS, Yee J. History, evolution, and current status of radiologic imaging tests for colorectal cancer screening. Radiology. 2014 Nov;273(2 Suppl):S160-180.

307. Mauri L, Kereiakes DJ, Yeh RW, Driscoll-Shempp P, Cutlip DE, Steg PG, et al. Twelve or 30 Months of Dual Antiplatelet Therapy after Drug-Eluting Stents. N Engl J Med. 2014 Dec 4;371(23):2155–66.

308. Berkhemer OA, Fransen PSS, Beumer D, van den Berg LA, Lingsma HF, Yoo AJ, et al. A Randomized Trial of Intraarterial Treatment for Acute Ischemic Stroke. New England Journal of Medicine. 2015 Jan 1;372(1):11–20.

309. Mitchell DG, Bruix J, Sherman M, Sirlin CB. LI-RADS (Liver Imaging Reporting and Data System): Summary, discussion, and consensus of the LI-RADS Management Working Group and future directions. Hepatology. 2015 Mar 1;61(3):1056–65.

310. Campbell BCV, Mitchell PJ, Kleinig TJ, Dewey HM, Churilov L, Yassi N, et al. Endovascular Therapy for Ischemic Stroke with Perfusion-Imaging Selection. New England Journal of Medicine. 2015 Mar 12;372(11):1009–18.

311. Goyal M, Demchuk AM, Menon BK, Eesa M, Rempel JL, Thornton J, et al. Randomized Assessment of Rapid Endovascular Treatment of Ischemic Stroke. New England Journal of Medicine. 2015 Mar 12;372(11):1019–30.

312. Douglas PS, Hoffmann U, Patel MR, Mark DB, Al-Khalidi HR, Cavanaugh B, et al. Outcomes of Anatomical versus Functional Testing for Coronary Artery Disease. New England Journal of Medicine. 2015 Apr 2;372(14):1291–300.

313. Pinsky PF, Gierada DS, Black W, Munden R, Nath H, Aberle D, et al. Performance of Lung-RADS in the National Lung Screening Trial: a retrospective assessment. Ann Intern Med. 2015 Apr 7;162(7):485–91.

314. Sawyer RG, Claridge JA, Nathens AB, Rotstein OD, Duane TM, Evans HL, et al. Trial of Short-Course Antimicrobial Therapy for Intraabdominal Infection. N Engl J Med. 2015 May 21;372(21):1996–2005.

315. Hamoen EHJ, de Rooij M, Witjes JA, Barentsz JO, Rovers MM. Use of the Prostate Imaging Reporting and Data System (PI-RADS) for Prostate Cancer Detection with Multiparametric Magnetic Resonance Imaging: A Diagnostic Meta-analysis. Eur Urol. 2015 Jun;67(6):1112–21.

316. Jovin TG, Chamorro A, Cobo E, de Miquel MA, Molina CA, Rovira A, et al. Thrombectomy within 8 Hours after Symptom Onset in Ischemic Stroke. New England Journal of Medicine. 2015 Jun 11;372(24):2296–306.

317. Saver JL, Goyal M, Bonafe A, Diener HC, Levy EI, Pereira VM, et al. Stent-Retriever Thrombectomy after Intravenous t-PA vs. t-PA Alone in Stroke. New England Journal of Medicine. 2015 Jun 11;372(24):2285–95.

318. Pollack CV, Reilly PA, Eikelboom J, Glund S, Verhamme P, Bernstein RA, et al. Idarucizumab for Dabigatran Reversal. New England Journal of Medicine. 2015 Aug 6;373(6):511–20.

319. Carrier M, Lazo-Langner A, Shivakumar S, Tagalakis V, Zarychanski R, Solymoss S, et al. Screening for Occult Cancer in Unprovoked Venous Thromboembolism. New England Journal of Medicine. 2015 Aug 20;373(8):697–704.

320. Douketis JD, Spyropoulos AC, Kaatz S, Becker RC, Caprini JA, Dunn AS, et al. Perioperative Bridging Anticoagulation in Patients with Atrial Fibrillation. N Engl J Med. 2015 Aug 27;373(9):823–33.

321. Molina JM, Capitant C, Spire B, Pialoux G, Cotte L, Charreau I, et al. On-Demand Preexposure Prophylaxis in Men at High Risk for HIV-1 Infection. New England Journal of Medicine. 2015 Dec 3;373(23):2237–46.

322. Siegal DM, Curnutte JT, Connolly SJ, Lu G, Conley PB, Wiens BL, et al. Andexanet Alfa for the Reversal of Factor Xa Inhibitor Activity. N Engl J Med. 2015 Dec 17;373(25):2413–24.

323. Marso SP, Daniels GH, Brown-Frandsen K, Kristensen P, Mann JFE, Nauck MA, et al. Liraglutide and Cardiovascular Outcomes in Type 2 Diabetes. New England Journal of Medicine. 2016 Jul 28;375(4):311–22.

324. Sweeting MJ, Patel R, Powell JT, Greenhalgh RM, EVAR Trial Investigators. Endovascular Repair of Abdominal Aortic Aneurysm in Patients Physically Ineligible for Open Repair: Very Long-term Follow-up in the EVAR-2 Randomized Controlled Trial. Ann Surg. 2017;266(5):713–9.

325. Wilcox MH, Gerding DN, Poxton IR, Kelly C, Nathan R, Birch T, et al. Bezlotoxumab for Prevention of Recurrent Clostridium difficile Infection. New England Journal of Medicine. 2017 Jan 26;376(4):305–17.

326. MacMahon H, Naidich DP, Goo JM, Lee KS, Leung ANC, Mayo JR, et al. Guidelines for Management of Incidental Pulmonary Nodules Detected on CT Images: From the Fleischner Society 2017. Radiology. 2017 Feb 23;284(1):228–43.

327. Sabatine MS, Giugliano RP, Keech AC, Honarpour N, Wiviott SD, Murphy SA, et al. Evolocumab and Clinical Outcomes in Patients with Cardiovascular Disease. New England Journal of Medicine. 2017 May 4;376(18):1713–22.

328. Nogueira RG, Jadhav AP, Haussen DC, Bonafe A, Budzik RF, Bhuva P, et al. Thrombectomy 6 to 24 Hours after Stroke with a Mismatch between Deficit and Infarct. N Engl J Med. 2018 04;378(1):11–21.

329. Albers GW, Marks MP, Kemp S, Christensen S, Tsai JP, Ortega-Gutierrez S, et al. Thrombectomy for Stroke at 6 to 16 Hours with Selection by Perfusion Imaging. N Engl J Med. 2018 22;378(8):708–18.

330. Campbell BCV, Mitchell PJ, Churilov L, Yassi N, Kleinig TJ, Dowling RJ, et al. Tenecteplase versus Alteplase before Thrombectomy for Ischemic Stroke. N Engl J Med. 2018 26;378(17):1573–82.

331. Self WH, Semler MW, Wanderer JP, Wang L, Byrne DW, Collins SP, et al. Balanced Crystalloids versus Saline in Noncritically Ill Adults. New England Journal of Medicine. 2018 Mar 1;378(9):819–28.

332. Johnston SC, Easton JD, Farrant M, Barsan W, Conwit RA, Elm JJ, et al. Clopidogrel and Aspirin in Acute Ischemic Stroke and High-Risk TIA. New England Journal of Medicine. 2018 Jul 19;379(3):215–25.

333. Pengo V, Denas G, Zoppellaro G, Jose SP, Hoxha A, Ruffatti A, et al. Rivaroxaban vs warfarin in high-risk patients with antiphospholipid syndrome. Blood. 2018 Sep 27;132(13):1365–71.

334. Iversen K, Ihlemann N, Gill SU, Madsen T, Elming H, Jensen KT, et al. Partial Oral versus Intravenous Antibiotic Treatment of Endocarditis. New England Journal of Medicine. 2019 Jan 31;380(5):415–24.

335. Li HK, Rombach I, Zambellas R, Walker AS, McNally MA, Atkins BL, et al. Oral versus Intravenous Antibiotics for Bone and Joint Infection. New England Journal of Medicine. 2019 Jan 31;380(5):425–36.

336. Mack MJ, Leon MB, Thourani VH, Makkar R, Kodali SK, Russo M, et al. Transcatheter Aortic-Valve Replacement with a Balloon-Expandable Valve in Low-Risk Patients. New England Journal of Medicine. 2019 May 2;380(18):1695–705.

337. Perkovic V, Jardine MJ, Neal B, Bompoint S, Heerspink HJL, Charytan DM, et al. Canagliflozin and Renal Outcomes in Type 2 Diabetes and Nephropathy. New England Journal of Medicine. 2019 Jun 13;380(24):2295–306.

338. McMurray JJV, Solomon SD, Inzucchi SE, Køber L, Kosiborod MN, Martinez FA, et al. Dapagliflozin in Patients with Heart Failure and Reduced Ejection Fraction. New England Journal of Medicine. 2019 Nov 21;381(21):1995–2008.

339. Huang C, Wang Y, Li X, Ren L, Zhao J, Hu Y, et al. Clinical features of patients infected with 2019 novel coronavirus in Wuhan, China. The Lancet. 2020 Feb 15;395(10223):497–506.

340. Zhu N, Zhang D, Wang W, Li X, Yang B, Song J, et al. A Novel Coronavirus from Patients with Pneumonia in China, 2019. New England Journal of Medicine. 2020 Feb 20;382(8):727–33.

341. Zhou P, Yang XL, Wang XG, Hu B, Zhang L, Zhang W, et al. A pneumonia outbreak associated with a new coronavirus of probable bat origin. Nature. 2020 Mar;579(7798):270–3.

342. Wang D, Hu B, Hu C, Zhu F, Liu X, Zhang J, et al. Clinical Characteristics of 138 Hospitalized Patients With 2019 Novel Coronavirus–Infected Pneumonia in Wuhan, China. JAMA. 2020 Mar 17;323(11):1061–9.

343. Li Q, Guan X, Wu P, Wang X, Zhou L, Tong Y, et al. Early Transmission Dynamics in Wuhan, China, of Novel Coronavirus-Infected Pneumonia. N Engl J Med. 2020 Mar 26;382(13):1199–207.

344. Zhou F, Yu T, Du R, Fan G, Liu Y, Liu Z, et al. Clinical course and risk factors for mortality of adult inpatients with COVID-19 in Wuhan, China: a retrospective cohort study. The Lancet. 2020 Mar 28;395(10229):1054–62.

345. Guan W jie, Ni Z yi, Hu Y, Liang W hua, Ou C quan, He J xing, et al. Clinical Characteristics of Coronavirus Disease 2019 in China. N Engl J Med. 2020 Apr 30;382(18):1708–20.

346. Armstrong PW, Pieske B, Anstrom KJ, Ezekowitz J, Hernandez AF, Butler J, et al. Vericiguat in Patients with Heart Failure and Reduced Ejection Fraction. New England Journal of Medicine. 2020 May 14;382(20):1883–93.

347. Beigel JH, Tomashek KM, Dodd LE, Mehta AK, Zingman BS, Kalil AC, et al. Remdesivir for the Treatment of Covid-19 — Final Report. New England Journal of Medicine [Internet]. 2020 May 22 [cited 2021 Nov 18]; Available from:

https://www.nejm.org/doi/10.1056/NEJMoa2007764

348. Kirchhof P, Camm AJ, Goette A, Brandes A, Eckardt L, Elvan A, et al. Early Rhythm-Control Therapy in Patients with Atrial Fibrillation. New England Journal of Medicine. 2020 Oct 1;383(14):1305–16.

349. Goldman JD, Lye DCB, Hui DS, Marks KM, Bruno R, Montejano R, et al. Remdesivir for 5 or 10 Days in Patients with Severe Covid-19. New England Journal of Medicine. 2020 Nov 5;383(19):1827–37.

350. Guimarães HP, Lopes RD, Silva PGM de B e, Liporace IL, Sampaio RO, Tarasoutchi F, et al. Rivaroxaban in Patients with Atrial Fibrillation and a Bioprosthetic Mitral Valve. New England Journal of Medicine [Internet]. 2020 Nov 14 [cited 2021 Nov 20]; Available from: https://www.nejm.org/doi/10.1056/NEJMoa2029603

351. Polack FP, Thomas SJ, Kitchin N, Absalon J, Gurtman A, Lockhart S, et al. Safety and Efficacy of the BNT162b2 mRNA Covid-19 Vaccine. N Engl J Med. 2020 Dec 31;383(27):2603–15.

352. Salama C, Han J, Yau L, Reiss WG, Kramer B, Neidhart JD, et al. Tocilizumab in Patients Hospitalized with Covid-19 Pneumonia. N Engl J Med. 2021 Jan 7;384(1):20–30.

353. Andrade JG, Wells GA, Deyell MW, Bennett M, Essebag V, Champagne J, et al. Cryoablation or Drug Therapy for Initial Treatment of Atrial Fibrillation. New England Journal of Medicine. 2021 Jan 28;384(4):305–15.

354. Baden LR, El Sahly HM, Essink B, Kotloff K, Frey S, Novak R, et al. Efficacy and Safety of the mRNA-1273 SARS-CoV-2 Vaccine. New England Journal of Medicine. 2021 Feb 4;384(5):403–16.

355. Wilding JPH, Batterham RL, Calanna S, Davies M, Gaal LFV, Lingvay I, et al. Once-Weekly Semaglutide in Adults with Overweight or Obesity. New England Journal of Medicine. 2021 Feb 10;

356. The RECOVERY Collaborative Group. Dexamethasone in Hospitalized Patients with Covid-19. N Engl J Med. 2021 Feb 25;384(8):693–704.

357. The REMAP-CAP Investigators. Interleukin-6 Receptor Antagonists in Critically Ill Patients with Covid-19. N Engl J Med. 2021 Apr 22;384(16):1491–502.

358. Haas EJ, Angulo FJ, McLaughlin JM, Anis E, Singer SR, Khan F, et al. Impact and effectiveness of mRNA BNT162b2 vaccine against SARS-CoV-2 infections and COVID-19 cases, hospitalisations, and deaths following a nationwide vaccination campaign in Israel: an observational study using national surveillance data. The Lancet. 2021 May 15;397(10287):1819–29.

359. Borobia AM, Carcas AJ, Pérez-Olmeda M, Castaño L, Bertran MJ, García-Pérez J, et al. Immunogenicity and reactogenicity of BNT162b2 booster in ChAdOx1-S-primed

participants (CombiVacS): a multicentre, open-label, randomised, controlled, phase 2 trial. The Lancet. 2021 Jul;398(10295):121–30.

360. Tanriover MD, Doğanay HL, Akova M, Güner HR, Azap A, Akhan S, et al. Efficacy and safety of an inactivated whole-virion SARS-CoV-2 vaccine (CoronaVac): interim results of a double-blind, randomised, placebo-controlled, phase 3 trial in Turkey. The Lancet. 2021 Jul 17;398(10296):213–22.

361. The ATTACC, ACTIV-4a, and REMAP-CAP Investigators. Therapeutic Anticoagulation with Heparin in Noncritically Ill Patients with Covid-19. N Engl J Med. 2021 Aug 26;385(9):790–802.

362. Falsey AR, Sobieszczyk ME, Hirsch I, Sproule S, Robb ML, Corey L, et al. Phase 3 Safety and Efficacy of AZD1222 (ChAdOx1 nCoV-19) Covid-19 Vaccine. N Engl J Med. 2021 Sep 29;NEJMoa2105290.

363. Anker SD, Butler J, Filippatos G, Ferreira JP, Bocchi E, Böhm M, et al. Empagliflozin in Heart Failure with a Preserved Ejection Fraction. New England Journal of Medicine. 2021 Oct 14;385(16):1451–61.

364. Barda N, Dagan N, Cohen C, Hernán MA, Lipsitch M, Kohane IS, et al. Effectiveness of a third dose of the BNT162b2 mRNA COVID-19 vaccine for preventing severe outcomes in Israel: an observational study. The Lancet. 2021 Dec 4;398(10316):2093–100.

STATISTICS ABBREVIATIONS

CI: Confidence Interval
HR: Hazard Ratio
RR: Relative Risk
RRR: Relative Risk Reduction
ARI: Absolute Risk Increase
NNH: Number Needed to Harm
X^2: Chi-square

NOTES

Made in the USA
Las Vegas, NV
21 August 2024

94169405R00439